Eighth Edition

DIAGNOSIS AND EVALUATION IN SPEECH PATHOLOGY

William O. Haynes
Auburn University

Rebekah H. Pindzola
Auburn University

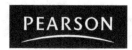

Boston Columbus Indianapolis New York San Francisco Upper Saddle River
Amsterdam Cape Town Dubai London Madrid Milan Munich Paris Montreal Toronto
Delhi Mexico City São Paulo Sydney Hong Kong Seoul Singapore Taipei Tokyo

Vice President and Editor in Chief: Jeffery W. Johnston
Executive Editor and Publisher: Stephen D. Dragin
Editorial Assistant: Jamie Bushell
Vice President, Director of Marketing: Margaret Waples
Marketing Manager: Weslie Sellinger
Senior Managing Editor: Pamela D. Bennett
Project Manager: Kerry Rubadue
Operations Supervisor: Central Publishing
Operations Specialist: Laura Messerly
Senior Art Director: Jayne Conte
Cover Designer: Bruce Kenselaar
Cover Art: Fotolia
Full-Service Project Management: Mohinder Singh/Aptara®, Inc.
Composition: Aptara®, Inc.
Printer/Binder: Courier/Westford
Cover Printer: Lehigh-Phoenix Color/Hagerstown
Text Font: Times

Credits and acknowledgments borrowed from other sources and reproduced, with permission, in this textbook appear on appropriate page within text.

Every effort has been made to provide accurate and current Internet information in this book. However, the Internet and information posted on it are constantly changing, so it is inevitable that some of the Internet addresses listed in this textbook will change.

Library of Congress Cataloging-in-Publication Data

Haynes, William O.
  Diagnosis and evaluation in speech pathology/William O. Haynes, Rebekah H. Pindzola.—8th ed.
    p.   cm.
  Includes bibliographical references and index.
  ISBN-13: 978-0-13-707132-6
  ISBN-10: 0-13-707132-9
  1. Speech disorders—Diagnosis.   2. Speech disorders—Case studies.   I. Pindzola, Rebekah H.
(Rebekah Hand) II. Title.
  [DNLM: 1. Speech Disorders—diagnosis. WL 340.2]
  RC423.H3826 2012
  616.85'5—dc22   2010054088

5 6 7 8 9 10 V092 16 15 14

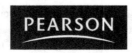

www.pearsonhighered.com

ISBN 10:   0-13-707132-9
ISBN 13: 978-0-13-707132-6

CONTENTS

PREFACE

With this eighth edition of *Diagnosis and Evaluation in Speech Pathology,* we invite a new group of students and practitioners to consider the complex and fascinating arena of assessment in communication disorders. For almost 40 years, this text has introduced diagnosis and evaluation as a *process* conducted in the context of an *interpersonal relationship* between clinicians and clients. This interesting and challenging process is a curious blend of science and art. On the science side, each case requires the clinician to think, solve problems, form hypotheses, gather data, and arrive at conclusions. Assessment, however, is much more than the simple administration of a few psychometrically adequate tests or scales, and this addresses the more artistic side of the process.

The diagnostician is much more than a neutral conduit through which test scores pass, and he or she must interact with clients to determine the real effects of communication impairment on their lives. The clinician must be able to interpret scores and measurements in the context of an individual client's problem. Thus, in this edition we again remind readers that most communication disorders have functional consequences for a person's life. The World Health Organization emphasizes the role of functional effects of disorders in its International Classification of Functioning, Disability, and Health (ICF). The American Speech-Language-Hearing Association addresses functional communication abilities in its Preferred Practice Patterns and in the National Outcomes Measurement System (NOMS). Another emphasis of the current edition is the ongoing nature of assessment. We must move beyond the notion of a single diagnostic session and think of assessment as including gathering baseline data, monitoring treatment progress, determining if generalization has occurred from training, and documenting functional gains in communication in a client's life.

Many readers of the prior editions have commented that they found the book to be both readable and clinically relevant. They have also made insightful suggestions, which we have endeavored to address in the present edition. Since the first edition appeared in 1973, the field of communication disorders has gone through many changes. With each successive revision of the text, we have attempted to reflect theoretical, clinical, and technological advances that have taken place in the field. The eighth edition is no different. The reader will notice we have attempted to maintain the strong points of the former edition while including new research and clinical tools.

NEW TO THIS EDITION

We have made every effort to bring this edition of the book completely up to date. A summary of these changes and additions includes:

- Completely updated content in every chapter
- Additional figures and tables to illustrate critical concepts
- Expansion of clinical interviewing to include discussion of ethnographic interviewing and curriculum-based assessment
- Expansion of sections dealing with early child language assessment and additional information on literacy assessment
- Expanded coverage of working memory and language processing in older children with language disorders

- Addition of resources to assess quality of life in adult clients
- Increased emphasis on measures to document treatment progress for all chapters dealing with disorders of communication
- Additional new information on adult and childhood apraxia of speech
- Major content and organizational changes to the chapter on fluency disorders

ACKNOWLEDGMENTS

The authors would like to express appreciation to our students, clients, colleagues, and teachers who helped to mould our thinking about the assessment process. We would also like to acknowledge Dr. Lon Emerick, who provided the initial impetus for this work. His basic philosophy, sensitivity, and enthusiasm still echo through the text. We also thank the reviewers of this book: Beverley Henke-Lofquist, SUNY Geneseo; Eva Hester, Towson University; and Julie Raplee, St. Joseph's College. Many of their helpful suggestions have been incorporated into this revision.

Finally, we should remember that the diagnostic session is our initial contact with clients; we never get a second chance to make a first impression. Every evaluation is unique, and each client deserves the best we can offer in terms of our ability, knowledge, judgment, and interpersonal sensitivity. We hope that this text can communicate both the method and the magic of this challenging task.

Introduction to Diagnosis and Evaluation
Philosophical Issues and General Guidelines

Speech-language pathology is a wonderfully diverse profession that requires a practitioner to possess a wide range of skills, knowledge, and personal characteristics. A speech-language pathologist (SLP) works as a case selector, case evaluator, diagnostician, interviewer, parent counselor, teacher, coordinator, record keeper, consultant, researcher, and student. Because the boundaries between these various duties are not clearly defined, and because the clinician must move continuously from one area to another, no one person can expect to be equally competent in all areas. The ultimate goal is to maximize one's strengths in all aspects to provide the best possible service to individuals with communicative disorders.

Diagnosis is one of the most comprehensive and difficult tasks of the speech-language pathologist. The diagnosis of a client requires a synthesis of the entire field: knowledge of norms and testing techniques, skills in observation, an ability to relate effectively and empathetically, and a great deal of creative intuition. Furthermore, because communication is a function of the entire person, the diagnostician must try to scrutinize all aspects of behavior. We must remember that we are not simply working with speech sounds, fluency, vocal quality, or linguistic rules but rather with changing people in a dynamic environment. The experienced diagnostician does not look at objective scores of articulatory skill, point scales of vocal quality, or standard scores as ends in themselves, but rather as aspects of an individual's communication ability—we diagnose communicators, not just communication. That revelation is a major factor in the transition from a technician to a professional clinician.

Because many of our diagnostic tools are imprecise, being largely in the experimental stages, and because communication disorders are by nature complex and perplexing, many of our diagnostic undertakings are incomplete and ambiguous. The lack of absolute and definitive answers to the various questions of diagnosis is often frustrating and demoralizing to the clinician. The ambiguous findings that sometimes culminate in a diagnostic evaluation must be dealt with in a fashion that perpetuates the evaluative undertaking rather than closes the door on further probing. Diagnosis is a continuous and open-ended venture that results in answers or partial answers that themselves are open to revision with added information.

DIAGNOSIS AND EVALUATION DEFINED

Some clinicians, at first glance, may consider the words *diagnosis* and *evaluation* to be synonymous. It is our intent in this text that diagnosis refer to the classical Greek definition of distinguishing a person's problem from the large field of potential disabilities. The term *diagnosis* in the original Greek means "to distinguish." The prefix *dia-* means "apart," and *-gnosis* translates as "to know." In order to distinguish a person's particular problem from the many possibilities available, we must know the client thoroughly and how he or she responds in many conditions, performing a variety of tasks. Evaluation refers to *the process* of arriving at a diagnosis. Thus, informal probes, trial therapy tasks, and gathering generalization data are part of evaluation. In the *American Heritage Dictionary* (1985), *diagnosis* is defined as "the act or process of identifying or determining the nature of a disease through examination." Our conception of diagnosis, then, includes a thorough understanding of the client's problem and not merely the application of a label. It is relatively simple to call a child "language impaired," but it is a more difficult matter really to understand how this child deals with linguistic symbols in a variety of tasks and situations. *This* is diagnosis in our view. We would also like to expand the notion of diagnosis to include distinguishing the nature of a person's problem at different points in time. Thus, diagnosis and evaluation are ongoing processes. We perform evaluation activities to arrive at an initial diagnosis, and we also examine the client repeatedly during the course of treatment. A client's diagnosis often changes over time. For example, a child may initially present with language delay and after a period of language treatment be characterized as primarily demonstrating a phonological disorder. A neurogenic patient may initially be diagnosed with aphasia, but may experience further neurological damage and be rediagnosed with aphasia and dysarthria. Another major thrust of this book is that diagnosis need not be confined to a 2-hour block of time in a university setting or a 30-minute period in a medical facility. The competent clinician will continue evaluation activities until the client's performance is understood to the extent necessary for effective treatment.

We perform evaluation tasks with two major goals in mind. First, we evaluate to arrive at a good understanding or diagnosis of a client's problem. Sometimes these evaluation activities will be confined to an assessment period, and at other times they will be performed well into the beginning of treatment. Often we must begin therapy with a client before arriving at a firm diagnosis. This approach is not optimal, but it is justified as long as we realize that (1) *any* treatment approach is experimental to a certain degree in the beginning, (2) most initial treatment goals will generally be "in the ballpark" in terms of appropriateness (e.g., we probably would not engage in voice therapy for a stuttering client), and (3) just because we have begun treatment, we have not abandoned our efforts in trying to define the parameters of the client's problem and arrive at a diagnosis. We can always "fine-tune" a treatment program based on an increased understanding of a client's problem and capabilities.

A second major reason to perform evaluation activities is to monitor the client's progress in treatment and describe changes in the communication disturbance. In this use of evaluation activities, we are not necessarily trying to diagnose the problem but to document treatment progress and determine possible changes in the course of treatment. In the chapters of the present text that deal with disorders, we will suggest evaluation tasks often used for these purposes that are not in the formal test category. Formal tests are designed more for categorizing clients as exhibiting certain disorders, whereas nonstandardized evaluation tasks are used to gain insight into specific client abilities and to gauge treatment progress. We will now discuss some of these purposes of diagnosis and evaluation in more detail.

BROADENING THE NOTION OF ASSESSMENT

Most people tend to think of diagnosis and treatment as two separate parts of the clinical process. We schedule clients for "assessment" and then if they evidence a problem, we arrange for them to receive "treatment." This distinction between assessment and treatment is somewhat arbitrary and nothing more than an administrative dichotomy made by school systems, medical settings, and insurance companies. In reality, we certainly do perform evaluations at the beginning of a clinical relationship with a client in order to determine the existence of and nature of a communication disorder, but the assessment does not stop there. Figure 1.1 shows a process in which diagnosis to determine the existence of a problem is only the first step in assessment. We diagnose the problem typically by using a combination of norm-referenced standardized tests coupled with nonstandardized communication tasks. Once the problem is confirmed, many additional evaluation tasks are performed to determine a client's baseline performance on very specific aspects of communication. These tasks are often performed after the initial diagnostic session and become part of measurements taken during the treatment phase of clinical work. One series of tasks is designed to determine treatment goals based on the client's initial performance in non-standardized tasks. A second type of evaluation concerns the person's functional level of communication at the beginning of treatment. This involves describing what a client can and cannot do with regard to communication for functional purposes in daily life. A third evaluative goal involves examining the client's environment (e.g., home, school, hospital setting) to determine communication levels in natural settings. When we understand the client's baseline performance levels for specific treatment goals, functional communication, and effectiveness in the natural environment, we must continue to evaluate in order to monitor treatment progress. Thus, even though treatment may have been going on for months, we continue to gather assessment data on the client's performance in the clinic, his or her changes in functional communication abilities, and the generalization of these abilities to other environments. These three levels of diagnosis and evaluation form a continuum ranging from diagnosis on one end, moving through establishing baseline performance data, and finally ending at measurement of treatment progress.

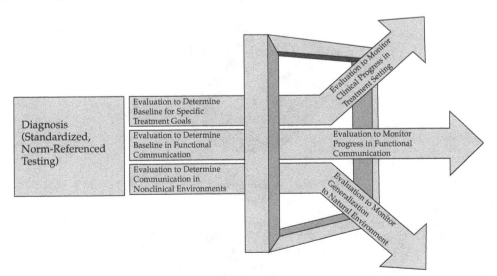

FIGURE 1.1   Diagnosis and evaluation involves determining the existence of a problem, taking baseline performance data, and monitoring treatment progress.

ILLUSTRATING THE IMPORTANCE OF MEASUREMENT IN CURRENT TRENDS

The assessment activities that take place after the initial diagnostic session have taken on increased importance in recent years with the emergence of three important influences in the field of communication disorders. These three influences have had and should continue to have far-reaching effects on our field in terms of research, theory, and clinical practice. The areas of which we speak are evidence-based practice (EBP), the response to intervention (RTI) initiative in public education, and research in dynamic assessment. You will soon see that the three areas are overlapping and in many ways are dealing with the same underlying construct of ongoing assessment or measurement of treatment progress. The three areas are illustrated in Figure 1.2.

We will briefly discuss each of these important influences in the following sections.

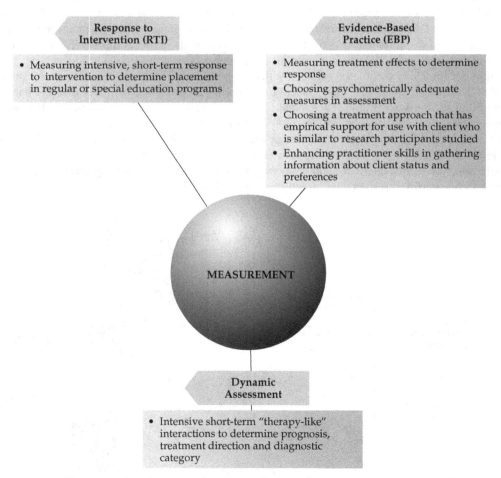

Response to Intervention (RTI)

- Measuring intensive, short-term response to intervention to determine placement in regular or special education programs

Evidence-Based Practice (EBP)

- Measuring treatment effects to determine response
- Choosing psychometrically adequate measures in assessment
- Choosing a treatment approach that has empirical support for use with client who is similar to research participants studied
- Enhancing practitioner skills in gathering information about client status and preferences

MEASUREMENT

Dynamic Assessment

- Intensive short-term "therapy-like" interactions to determine prognosis, treatment direction and diagnostic category

FIGURE 1.2   Three overlapping areas in current literature where measurement techniques are critical.

Evidence-Based Practice in Speech-Language Pathology

The Joint Coordinating Committee on Evidence-Based Practice of the ASHA produced a recent position statement (American Speech-Language-Hearing Association, 2005). Among the recommended skills for speech-language pathologists were the following (p. 1):

- Evaluate prevention, screening, and diagnostic procedures, protocols and measures to identify maximally informative and cost-effective diagnostic and screening tools, using recognized appraisal criteria described in the evidence-based practice literature.
- Evaluate the efficacy, effectiveness, and efficiency of clinical protocols for prevention, treatment, and enhancement using criteria recognized in the evidence-based practice literature.

These skills suggest two major implications of evidence-based practice. First, in selecting diagnostic measurements, it is our responsibility to choose those that have the most scientific support and psychometric adequacy. The second implication involves the notion that assessment is ongoing, and it is only through such continued evaluation that we can monitor treatment progress on the goals we have selected as targets. In short, what is the "evidence" in evidence-based practice? In many ways it all boils down to measurement of one type or another.

Evidence-based practice was initially developed in the medical profession as a means of promoting ". . . the integration of best research evidence with clinical expertise and patient values" (Sackett, Straus, Richardson, Rosenberg, & Haynes, 2000, p. 1). Obviously, this implies a three-part model with research evidence, clinical expertise, and patient values at each point, presumably each contributing significant importance to making clinical decisions. Figure 1.3 depicts the relationships in this model to the assessment process. This model has been recently applied to many other professions including education, social work, psychology, and communication disorders.

It is important to discuss how the three parts of the model in Figure 1.3 apply to assessment in communication disorders. The part of the model that deals with research evidence is critical in selecting both norm-referenced assessment instruments and nonstandardized measurements of client behaviors. As we will discuss in Chapter 3, all standardized tests should have been carefully developed so that they have psychometric qualities that make them both valid and reliable. These tests should have been normed on populations that make them applicable to clients from a

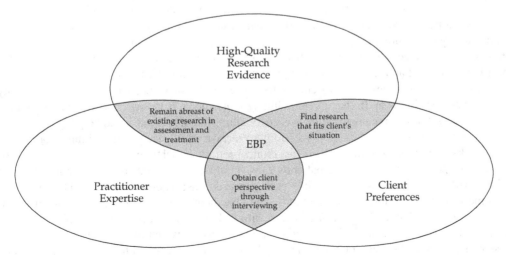

FIGURE 1.3   Three classical components of evidence-based practice.

variety of social and cultural groups. A clinician must be very careful to use standardized tests that meet exacting psychometric criteria and have been scientifically shown adequately to identify clients with communication disorders. When a clinician chooses a nonstandardized method of examining client communicative behavior, research evidence is even more critical. We should not simply design our own methods of gathering data on clients, but we should use nonstandardized methods that research has shown to be reliable and valid. For example, measurements such as mean length of utterance, type–token ratio, and maximum phonation time or percentage of disfluency are nonstandardized procedures that have well-documented definitions, procedures for sampling/calculation, and data on reliability/validity from many scientific investigations. It is almost always preferable to use a technique that has been implemented in research rather than develop an idiosyncratic approach with no empirical support.

Another way that knowledge of research evidence comes into play is in selecting a treatment procedure. There is no shortage of manuals and "programs" that tell the clinician how to do therapy. There are not, however, many scientific studies that actually document treatment effects on clients who underwent specific therapy procedures. The implication here is that clinicians should choose treatment methods that have scientific support in our research literature and not use untested techniques when others are available with evidence that shows effectiveness. Thus, research evidence is an extremely important component of the evidence-based practice model and applies to both assessment and treatment enterprises in communication disorders.

The second part of the EBP model includes clinical expertise of the practitioner. Clinical expertise is important for several reasons. First of all, one cannot be clinically competent unless he or she keeps up with the current research literature in the field. This is where the second part of the EBP model intersects with the first, research evidence. We assume that a competent clinician is familiar with latest developments in assessment and treatment. We also assume that if a practitioner uses new clinical methods that he or she will study and practice them so that they are used appropriately with the client. The practitioner is responsible for choosing appropriate assessment/treatment methods and knowing how to use them.

The third part of the EBP model involves the values and perspective of the patient with whom we are working. It is the responsibility of the practitioner to evaluate the client as a person, rather than merely a communication disorder. Every person has perceptions, values, and preferences that should be taken into account in a clinical relationship. For example, in the field of medicine, a person who has been diagnosed with cancer has many treatment options, ranging from surgery to chemotherapy and radiation. Each treatment has research data associated with it; these results can be communicated so that the patient and physician can make the decision that is best for the patient and family. Note that patients are not simply told which option to take; they have a choice. Sometimes they may choose to have a shorter survival chance, but a better quality of life. The decision is up to the patient. Although this choice is not as dramatic in communication disorders, there are many possible ways of dealing with most speech and language disorders. For example, it may be preferable for a family to receive an intense parent training program instead of having to make frequent visits to a clinical setting, which may be more of a strain on finances and scheduling. Again, the patient's view should always be taken into account. This part of the EBP model interacts with practitioner expertise because a good clinician will be able to assess the values and preferences of the family and take them into account when arriving at a clinical decision. In Chapter 2 we discuss interviewing, which is the mechanism by which we get to learn about patient concerns. There is also an interaction between the patient perspective and research evidence. As a clinician goes about choosing assessment and treatment techniques, he or she must determine if the technique has been used effectively on patients who fit the profile of the current client. That is, we should select treatment and assessment options that have been successful with clients similar to our patient.

It is easy to see from Figure 1.3 how research evidence, practitioner expertise, and patient preferences are not only important as individual entities but also in how they interact in carrying out the clinical transaction, both in assessment and in treatment.

The Response to Intervention (RTI) Model

Authorities in the field of education and learning disabilities have recently postulated a procedure for identifying and treating students with disorders using a model called response to intervention (RTI). The National Association of State Directors of Special Education (NASDSE, 2005) define RTI as "the practice of (1) providing high-quality instruction/intervention matched to student needs and (2) using learning rate over time and level of performance to (3) make important educational decisions." The legal groundwork for RTI was laid by PL 108-447: IDEA 2004, which states: "In determining whether a child has a specific learning disability, a local educational agency may use a process that determines if the child responds to scientific, research-based intervention." Similarly, No Child Left Behind (NCLB) advocates the use of scientifically based research, which is described as "research that involves the application of rigorous, systematic, and objective procedures to obtain reliable and valid knowledge relevant to education activities and programs." These two legal perspectives seem to be quite compatible. Moore-Brown and Montgomery (2006), Justice (2006), and Ukrainetz (2006) detailed how the SLP would fit into this type of approach to assessment and intervention for language, reading, and literacy disorders. We discuss RTI here only as an example of the important role that ongoing assessment will play in any program that involves continuous monitoring of client progress.

It is important to provide some perspective as to why RTI is a novel approach to evaluating students. Historically, students with learning disabilities, the majority of which are language/literacy based, were given special education services after being diagnosed with a particular learning problem. In most cases this was done by using outdated "discrepancy formulas," which showed a disconnect between a student's potential as measured through intelligence and aptitude testing and the student's performance on tests of specific abilities such as reading, writing, or oral language. Often, such evaluations were not completed until the end of second grade, and at this point, remediation is difficult and the social/psychological effects of failure may have already begun. The historical scenario described above has been called the "wait to fail" model. Currently, most authorities do not support the sole use of discrepancy models in diagnosis.

In an effort to be more proactive, educators have posited that variables other than just test scores could be used to determine the existence of a learning or language disorder. One such variable involves placing the student in a limited, intense period of treatment to determine if he or she can benefit from additional assistance. Proponents of RTI characterize the approach as having a number of "tiers" that provide progressively more specialized and intensive treatment. The number of tiers varies depending on the specific RTI model considered. Figure 1.4 generally illustrates a four-tier model of RTI. Movement through the tiers is dependent upon monitoring student response to treatment as revealed by continuous assessment and monitoring. Those students who benefit from the assistance could continue to be served in the general education classroom on a consultative basis by the SLP. The students who do not benefit from the intense treatment regimen could then be declared eligible for special education services by the speech-language pathologist. In this way, a student's actual learning response can be a significant consideration in the decision to enroll him or her for specialized services instead of just using arbitrary cutoffs and test scores. Enrollment

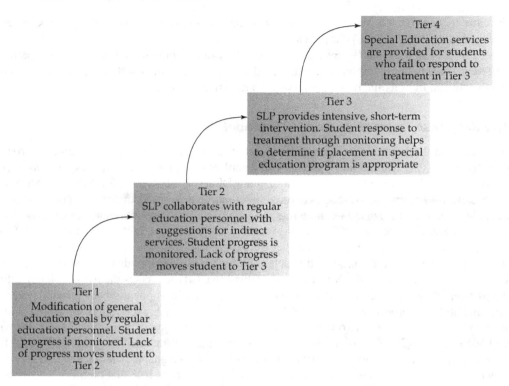

FIGURE 1.4 Illustrating the importance of monitoring in RTI: Ongoing assessment determines whether more intensive intervention is needed.

in specialized special education services often involves pulling the student out of the classroom, which could contribute to further academic problems caused by missing critical material. If a student can be adequately served in the general education setting in tiers 1–3 without having to be admitted to a special education program, such additional academic problems might be avoided.

RTI involves prevention and intervention goals in an outcomes-driven system. If RTI is going to be successful, it must include a team approach involving parents, educators, special educators, administrators, and related service providers (e.g., SLPs). The American Speech-Language-Hearing Association has developed guidelines regarding the role of the SLP in RTI (Ehren, Montgomery, Rudebusch, & Whitmire, 2007). Most of the early work with RTI was concerned with children who have learning disabilities, but currently it has been applied to all children receiving services in early childhood. According to Jackson, Pretti-Frontczak, Harjusola-Webb, Grisham-Brown, and Romani (2009, p. 425), "Common principles of RTI include (a) many tiers to insure maximum support for each child, (b) instruction implemented with high quality, (c) a core curriculum that encompasses a research base, (d) a data collection system consisting of both formative and summative sources of information, (e) interventions that have an evidence base, (f) procedures for identifying the selection and revision of instructional practices, and (g) measures to monitor the fidelity of implementation." It is clear from this statement that assessment and evaluation procedures are intimately related to almost every principle. Jackson et al. (2009) go on to point out that preferred methods of assessment should include naturalistic observation, family preferences, and functional outcomes. When monitoring treatment progress some allowance should be made not only for pre- and postintervention measures, but more frequent assessments on a daily or weekly basis to determine if the program needs modification. For some SLPs this may require an adjustment. For example, Jackson et al. (2009, p. 429) indicate: "Although SLPs have specific knowledge in the area of communication and language, the challenge is to shift their focus from the discipline's traditionally 'clinical,' norm-referenced assessment approaches to engagement in collaborative assessment practices that are authentic and focus on all areas of child development."

So, what does this have to do with assessment? It should be abundantly clear that evaluating a student's baseline abilities and then continuing to monitor his or her performance during an intensive, short-term treatment regimen involves copious measurements. In the RTI model, such assessment is very important because it can be used in the decision-making process to determine eligibility for special education services.

Dynamic Assessment

If diagnosis is to be of utmost benefit it must be goal oriented. Diagnosis is an empty exercise in test administration, data collection, and client evaluation if it fails to provide logical suggestions for treatment. Most clinicians would like to believe that for each client, there is a magic procedure that will work to improve communication. In almost every disorder area (fluency, voice, language, articulation), however, there is a multitude of procedures from which to select. Not only are there different types of treatment in terms of philosophy, entry level, and targets trained, but there are differences in the nature of the delivery system (e.g., highly structured, behavioral, client directed, cognitive, etc.). Thus, the SLP is faced with a number of avenues from which to choose in terms of making treatment recommendations.

The notion of using time in a diagnostic session to gain insight into performance on treatment tasks is known as *dynamic assessment* (Gutierrez-Clellen & Pena, 2001; Johns & Haynes, 2002; Lidz, 1991; Miller, Gillam, & Pena, 2001; Olswang et al., 1986; Pena, 1996; Wade & Haynes 1989). We feel that dynamic assessment is an important part of any diagnostic venture, because it is from these tasks that direction for treatment emerges. Table 1.1 illustrates salient differences between dynamic and static assessment. Static assessment is like a snapshot of a child's performance at a given moment in time. When we administer a standardized test, we are capturing a child's performance at a certain point, and we may characterize this behavior as a number or score. Static assessment, however, does not address how the child may be able to perform more effectively with assistance by the clinician or under altered circumstances. Dynamic assessment relies heavily on Vygotsky's (1978) notion of the "Zone of Proximal Development," which defines a range of performance that a child can produce with assistance from adults or peers. Standardized tests do not allow the clinician to assist a child or ask the client why he or she answered a question in a particular manner. In dynamic assessment we can determine a client's range of performance, given help by the clinician, and can find what types of circumstances result in improved performance. Wade and Haynes (1989) found that investing as little as 30 minutes of an evaluation in trial therapy demonstrated distinct performance differences in the types of cues responded to by children with language impairment.

Almost every communication disorder area has a variety of variables to experiment with during a diagnostic session. We are of the opinion that treatment should be viewed rather like a single-subject experimental design. No one really knows which type of treatment will be effective for a given client or which variables will have the most impact on performance. This is typically learned during the first stage of treatment as the clinician begins to fine-tune the management

TABLE 1.1	Comparison of Static and Dynamic Assessment
Static Assessment	**Dynamic Assessment**
Passive Participants	**Active Participants**
Child does task without help	Child participates with adult help; can ask questions and get feedback
Examiner Observes	**Examiner Participates**
Scores test; typically right/wrong responses	Give feedback; help child develop strategies
Results Identify Deficits	**Results Describe Modifiability**
Test results profile deficits, what child can/cannot do	Results profile how responsive the child is given help; describe strategies
Standardized Administration	**Administration Fluid, Responsive**
Given in standardized manner, no deviation from standard format	Nonstandardized administration; examiner responses contingent on child's behavior

Source: Adapted from Pena, E., Quinn, R., and Iglesias, A. (1992).

program. However, the diagnostic session can easily be used to gain some insight into client tendencies and preferences. Clients with aphasia may respond more favorably to certain combinations of cues in word retrieval. Clients with fluency disorders may become more fluent with one particular technique than with a second method. One client may express relief that the clinician is willing to talk about the psychological component of the stuttering problem during part of the diagnostic session, which may suggest that this covert dimension should at least be considered as a potential part of the treatment program. A child with a language impairment may respond better to a structured task as opposed to a child-directed one, or vice versa. A person with a voice disorder may be more able to alter vocal parameters by using feedback from certain instrumentation rather than not using this type of monitoring. A nonverbal child may show a marked tendency to learn a few gestures during a diagnostic session rather than to master vocal productions or words.

We could continue with examples of ways in which the clinician can use a portion of the diagnostic session to learn about the client's response to certain treatment variables. Although the diagnostician should never make treatment recommendations based only on hunches, the judicious use of evaluation tasks in the assessment can suggest a reasonable starting point for treatment in many cases. Of course, these recommendations should be treated as working hypotheses and should be stated as such in the diagnostic report. The initial selection of a treatment option is in most cases only an educated guess and is always subject to change based on client performance. This is why, we view evaluation as an ongoing process throughout the treatment experience.

THE IMPORTANCE OF FUNCTIONAL MEASUREMENTS: THE WORLD HEALTH ORGANIZATION, U.S. DEPARTMENT OF EDUCATION, AND ASHA

Over the years, the World Health Organization (WHO) has developed various conceptual frameworks to draw attention to the functional sequelae of an illness or disorder. Their International Classification of Functioning, Disability and Health, better known simply as ICF, provides a standard way of describing a person's health and health-related states (WHO, 2002). ICF is a multipurpose classification system that helps healthcare professionals describe a person's changes in two ways. The first concerns body function and structure: what the person can do in a standard environment. Such "levels of capacity" often are assessed through standardized testing. The second addresses what the person can actually do in his or her usual environment. These "levels of performance" often are assessed via nonstandardized probes and indexes of daily activity and participation. This ICF classification system is a radical change in healthcare diagnosis and evaluation—rather than emphasizing a person's disability, the focus is shifted to the level of health. Said another way, the focus is shifted from "cause" to "impact." We see this change echoed in recent clinical research literature. The speech-language pathologist, too, is no longer just diagnosing and evaluating a client's communication deficit. Rather, attention also is directed toward assessing a client's communicative functioning in his or her environment. What can the client do? What impact does the client's communication abilities have on their socialization? Their psychological state? Their education? Their vocation and avocations? Clearly, the modern SLP is concerned with the concepts of functioning and social disability as espoused in the International Classification of Functioning, Disability and Health (WHO, 2002). In each chapter of this text, we will present this ICF model as a reminder of our professional concerns with both functioning and disability in our realm of diagnosis and evaluation.

Beginning in 2008, the U.S. Department of Education required all states to submit accountability data regarding programs that serve young children with disabilities. Specifically, the types of data of interest concern functional outcomes as a result of treatment. Since most young children receiving services (e.g., 53%) require work on communication, the speech-language pathologist is clearly involved as part of the intervention team. The gathering of performance data on children with communication impairments goes well beyond the use of standardized tests. Hebbeler and Rooney (2009, p. 451) state, "Across professional organizations, the recommendations related to assessment contain similar themes, emphasizing the use of multiple sources of information, focusing on the child and family, and highlighting the use of assessment data for program planning and monitoring. . . . A balanced assessment, according to ASHA, includes gathering child-centered, contextualized, performance-based, descriptive and functional information from families, teachers and other service providers." The specific areas of interest involve social-emotional skills, acquiring and using knowledge/skills, and abilities to make their needs known to others. The form that these functional outcome assessments typically take is a 7-point rating scale—7 being age-appropriate skills and 1 being lack of foundational skills to accomplish the task. All of the seven levels carry operational definitions, and the values are assigned by the intervention team. Such scale values can be used to determine functional response to treatment and can also be used for required reporting to the Department of Education. Such rating systems are also prevalent in healthcare settings (FIM scores) and in the ASHA National Outcomes Measurement System (NOMS). Thus, there seems to be a convergence of the various professional organizations and governmental agencies on the value of initial and ongoing assessment, no matter what the age group or disability.

Since diagnosis and evaluation of communication disorders will require significant input from speech-language pathologists, it is important to review briefly the guidelines put forth by ASHA regarding assessment. First of all, ASHA develops what are called *preferred practice patterns* (PPPs) that generally define acceptable clinical approaches to assessment and treatment of communication disorders. These practice patterns are developed initially by an ASHA ad hoc committee and then circulated widely for peer review by practicing clinicians and experts in the field. Specifically, the preferred practice patterns "represent the consensus of the members of the professions after they considered available scientific evidence, existing ASHA and related policies, current practice patterns, expert opinions, and the collective judgment and experience of practitioners in the field. Requirements of federal and state governments and accrediting and regulatory agencies also have been considered" (American Speech-Language-Hearing Association, 2004, p. v). It is easy to see that such guidelines can have a far-reaching effect on knowledge and skills required in speech-language pathology training programs, and also on clinical practice in the field. The ASHA document on preferred practice patterns is driven in large part by "fundamental components and guiding principles," which are based on guidelines from the World Health Organization mentioned earlier. According to these fundamental guidelines, the evaluation must first of all be "comprehensive." This means that several important areas must be addressed:

1. *Body Structures and Functions.* Clearly, medically based problems are implicated in body structures (e.g., neurogenic disorders, cleft palate). Functions include "mental functions such as attention as well as components of communication such as articulatory proficiency, fluency and syntax" (p. vi). Thus, this first component would involve making a thorough diagnosis and defining the nature of a client's communication problem, similar to what professionals do in the assessment of any health-related condition. Obviously, we can accomplish the goal of a thorough diagnosis by administration of standardized and nonstandardized tests.

2. *Activities and Participation.* This component deals with the client's ability to participate in daily social, communicative, and self-help activities and perform tasks that may be relevant to educational and/or vocational enterprises. Essentially this means that part of an effective assessment must involve looking at how a communication disorder may affect a client's ability to perform in the real-life arenas of society, work, or education. Clearly, the use of tests is not the most efficient way of gaining information on the client's daily activities and communication skills in social, educational, or vocational environments. For this, there is no substitute for case history information, clinical interviewing, observing the client in the natural environment, and rating his or her functional abilities in communication and related activities.

3. *Contextual Factors.* These factors can include personal attributes of culture, education, social status, and environmental variables that may present obstacles or facilitate communication. Again, standardized testing may not be the most efficient vehicle for gaining information about cultural and environmental variables, but more nonstandardized approaches such as interviewing, patient rating scales, and observation in natural settings may provide the most relevant clinical data.

The ASHA preferred practice pattern document also provides other diagnostic and evaluation guidelines of a more general nature. Following are some selected principles that are especially pertinent to the present text.

1. *Measuring Outcomes.* According to the guideline, "Outcomes of services are monitored and measured in order to ensure the quality of services provided and to improve quality of those services" (p. vii). As we have stated previously, assessment is not confined to a "diagnostic session" but rather, it continues throughout the treatment phase as well.

2. *Going Beyond Static Assessment.* An emphasis of the present textbook is that diagnosis and evaluation is far more than simply administering a standardized test. While standardized tests can tell us if a problem exists, they rarely describe the nature of the

problem. The ASHA PPP document states: "Assessment may be static (i.e., using procedures designed to describe structures, functions, and environmental demands and supports in relevant domains at a given point in time) or dynamic (i.e., using hypothesis testing procedures to identify potential for change and elements of successful interventions and supports)" (p. vii). We will be covering both static and dynamic assessment in this text.

3. *Approaching Assessment Scientifically.* The ASHA PPP recommends that "services are consistent with the best available scientific and clinical evidence in conjunction with individual considerations" (p. vii). This notion is essentially what has become known as *evidence-based practice (EBP)* and is a current emphasis of ASHA and other disciplines that are following the lead of the medical profession in applying research to clinical practice. We will discuss selected aspects of EBP that apply to assessment later in the present text.

The American Speech-Language-Hearing Association has also been involved in examining functional outcomes of treatment for communication disorders. Since 1994 a variety of ASHA task force groups have been active in developing the National Outcomes Measurement System (NOMS), which includes functional communication measures (FCMs) for most speech, language, and swallowing disorders for the age range from children to adults. The FCMs are composed of 7-point rating scales that rate the patient from the least functional (level 1) to the most functional level (level 7). The ratings are based on clinical observations by the SLP and are not necessarily reliant on any formal assessment procedures. To date, FCMs have been developed in the following areas: alaryngeal communication, attention, augmentative-alternative communication, fluency, memory, motor speech, pragmatics, reading, problem solving, spoken language comprehension, spoken language expression, swallowing, voice, voice following tracheostomy, and writing. Currently, ASHA releases the FCMs only in the context of the National Outcomes Measurement System, and the scales are used mainly in this ongoing research. Eventually, the FCMs will be useful for widespread clinical use. It is important to note, however, that in most healthcare settings worldwide, professionals in speech-language pathology, physical therapy, occupational therapy and other disciplines have routinely used functional independence measurements (FIMs) to gauge client progress in the rehabilitation process. Typically such scores are on a 7-point scale, just like the FCMs described above; the scale runs from total assistance (level 1) to total independence (level 7). The scales are used for abilities such as ambulation, managing bowel/bladder functions, communication, grooming, bathing, dressing, memory, and social interaction. These FIM scores are used for many purposes ranging from discharge decisions to reimbursement guidelines. Anyone working in a medical setting will tell you that FIM scores are one of the most important determiners of the effectiveness/efficiency of rehabilitation programs and a favorite tool of healthcare administrators.

It can be seen from this discussion that functional outcome measurements are important components in initially assessing clients and in monitoring progress through treatment. We want clients not only to improve their abilities on standardized tests, but to be able to master functional abilities that will affect their lives. The term *activities of daily living* (ADL) refers to practical behaviors related to common activities such as eating, communicating, and ambulation, and these are often selected as targets for treatment and measured in terms of functional gains. Thus, assessment is not only about testing; it also includes educated clinical observations and functional estimates of a client's performance.

DIAGNOSIS TO DETERMINE THE REALITY OF THE PROBLEM

One function of diagnosis is to determine whether the presenting communication pattern does indeed constitute a handicap. Before this is possible, however, it is necessary to have a clear idea of what constitutes a communication disorder. Van Riper's classical definition of a speech disorder is widely quoted: "Speech is abnormal when it deviates so far from the speech of other people that it calls attention to itself, interferes with communication, or causes the speaker or his listeners to be distressed" (Van Riper & Emerick, 1984, p. 34). Figure 1.5 depicts three components that must be considered in determining a communication disorder.

1. *Speech Difference.* This refers to whether or not the speech signal calls attention to itself and when this might occur. We can quantify the physical characteristics of the speech signal through recording, measurement, and observation. Computer-assisted spectrographic analyses and pitch measurements are available to help the diagnostician obtain an objective measure of the acoustic nature of the individual's speech. In other words, we must scrutinize the physical characteristics of the speech signal and judge its quality. But these data are of limited value unless it can be determined what *difference* a particular speech parameter makes.

In most areas of communication disorders, the state of the art has not progressed to where we can simply take the quantified data, compare them with established numerical norms, and determine the correctness of the speech sample. Unfortunately, each diagnostician must develop a personal frame of reference. Vocal qualities are subject to individual impressions; and although a clinician may *know* that the voice is awry, evidence of the difference may often elude the sensors and algorithms of our high-tech instrumentation. On the other hand, physicians are able to scrutinize data from a laboratory test and make an immediate diagnosis regarding the normalcy of an individual's blood chemistry. This kind of reference information is not yet available to the SLP. The question of whether the presenting speech difference is different enough to be of concern thus becomes a matter of human judgment. This judgment involves filtering incoming data through the clinician's many synaptic junctions whose thresholds may have been worn thin by bias and experience. An inordinately critical or uncritical ear is a hazard with far-reaching implications.

What constitutes normal behavior? There are several definitions available, but we will discuss only two, representing the diverging philosophies with which each clinician must contend in establishing his or her own concept. The first theory we shall call the concept of *cultural norms.* The assumption is that there are behaviors that society considers aberrant in terms of group characteristics. According to this model, each bit of behavior can be judged against a real or theoretical standard, the nature of which is independent of the individual's personal idiosyncrasies.

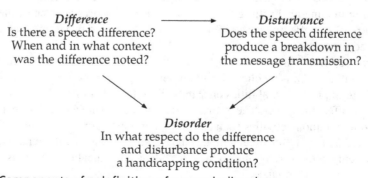

FIGURE 1.5   Components of a definition of a speech disorder.

Thus, even a 70-year-old person with a hearing threshold of 30 dB in the high frequencies may be thought of as exhibiting a significant hearing loss. The second theory we shall call the concept of *individual norms*. Advocates of this model assume that each individual has made a unique adjustment to life based on previous experiences, physical limitations, and the environment's reactions. Any judgment as to the normalcy of a bit of behavior must be contingent upon individual characteristics such as age, intelligence, and experience. Taken to the extreme, of course, the latter model would assert that each person is normal no matter what he or she does, since the behavior is the end product of all that plays upon the person, and to this extent the concept of individual norms loses meaning. But some case examples may help to clarify and give perspective.

The audiologist who examines the hearing of the 70-year-old individual referred to earlier and who obtains the typical presbycusic audiometric curve could make a case for the judgment that this person has "normal" hearing. According to individual norms, this is average or normal behavior for a person of 70; but according to cultural norms, the individual's hearing level is below the average for the total population. Follow-up procedures would be based, then, on the practical matter of getting a more efficient communication system for the individual and also on providing counseling so that the person will understand the nature of his or her hearing. Therefore, both cultural and personal norms play a part in diagnostic judgments and rehabilitative programs. A 10-year-old child with severe cognitive delays and an unstimulable distortion of the /r/ phoneme may not be judged to have seriously defective speech, whereas an 8-year-old presenting a similar speech pattern, but a different intellectual potential, may be recommended for treatment. Such judgments have implications for case selection, and the clinician must reconcile the variances between the physical differences in the sounds involved and the individual variables in conjunction with what is normal for the population as a whole. Each clinician must continually use both concepts of normalcy in diagnostic work.

There are all sorts of ways that a speech signal can call attention to itself and yet be perfectly appropriate. For example, an African American English (AAE) speaker may alter aspects of speech and language when style-shifting between members of one culture and another. Although Standard American English (SAE) speakers may notice the differences in AAE, these variations certainly would not be viewed as evidence of a communication disorder. Another example might be when speakers alter their rate, loudness, and vocal quality in order to tell a funny story or relate a particular experience in a dramatic way. Age is another variable. If the speaker is a child of 2 who exhibits many articulatory substitutions and omissions, does this difference constitute a problem? The answer can only lie in an examination of these errors against the context of normal 2-year-old communication. Thus, a difference is not enough to constitute a communication disorder if the context suggests normality. This points out the importance of the SLP's knowing the contextual effects on communication and the contributions of age and the wide variety of cultural, ethnic, and geographical dialects on the speech signal.

2. *The Intelligibility of the Message.* The second component of determining a communication disorder involves the perception of disturbance in the signal that is transmitted. Is the signal distorted or is its intelligibility affected? If the message transmission is adversely affected, there is a high probability of the existence of a problem. Many factors play a part in both the encoding and decoding processes, and the diagnostician must be capable of representing the standard for society when listening and making judgments.

We have, in the main, been content with clinical insight and intuitive estimates when we have judged the impact of speech differences upon intelligibility. The clinician is able to count the phoneme errors, quantify the number of repetitions or disfluencies per sentence, and establish various quotients of language ability, but it is still a challenge to assess the intelligibility of the transmitted message with any degree of reliability. In most cases the clinician resorts to scaling techniques to mark the impact of the disorder on intelligibility, and we have little way to know specific contributions of individual components of the speech signal or language used on overall signal distortion. Clearly, severe disfluency can interrupt a message, intermittent cessations of phonation and poor vocal qualities can distort transmission, inappropriate phoneme selection or production can lead to unintelligibility, and ambiguous vocabulary or sentence structure can lead to misinterpretations. Whatever the cause of the communication failure, we must document that it occurs. At present, however, we have no widely accepted system to use in this documentation for most areas of communication disorders.

3. *Handicapping Condition.* The final component in defining a disorder involves the determination of handicap in the life of the client. Emerick (1984) suggests:

> In the final analysis this third aspect justifies the existence of our profession. If the speech difference has no discernible impact on the child's behavior, and ultimately on his adjusting abilities and learning potential, there is little justification for concern on the part of the speech clinician. Although it is not feasible to compile a listing of all of the possible conditions under which a communication difference would become handicapping, it is generally agreed that communicative differences are considered handicapping when: (1) the transmission and/or perception of messages is faulty; (2) the person is placed at an economic disadvantage; (3) the person is placed at a learning disadvantage; (4) the person is placed at a social disadvantage; (5) there is a negative impact upon the emotional growth of the person; or (6) the problem causes physical damage or endangers the health of the person.

There are numerous examples of famous people who are highly successful and seemingly content with their lives despite manifesting a communication disorder. Some famous personalities have happy, fulfilling lives even though an SLP would have classified them as having a handicap. On the other hand, a minor deviation in a teacher or business executive may mean a significant handicap in terms of credibility and evaluation of job performance. Two people with hearing impairment can have identical audiograms and yet report significantly different effects that hearing loss has on their lives. If a person does not view his or her communication disorder as a handicap, it is difficult to justify clinical work or to motivate the client to improve communication skills.

DIAGNOSIS TO DETERMINE THE ETIOLOGY OF THE PROBLEM

Far too many clinicians view diagnosis simply as a labeling process; however, the actual labeling, or categorizing, is only a small part of the total assessment. Classification systems within our profession are poor at best, and high-level abstractions (e.g., stuttering) tend to emphasize the similarities within populations rather than the individual differences. The keen diagnostician looks upon classifications as communication conveniences to be viewed with suspicion. Of course, the convenience factor is important, and each clinician who makes a determination of the reality of the problem must be willing to label it. This must of necessity, however, follow an orderly description of the characteristics of the disorder so that it can be clear what route the diagnostician took in arriving at the final classification. A diagnosis that only describes the characteristics of the problem, without judging its type or class, is a dead end. Nelson (2010, p. 102) points to three major difficulties with categorization: "(1) lack of recognition of complexity of human differences, (2) unnecessary stigmatization, and (3) not enough benefits to overshadow the limitations." She goes on to say that categorization will not be abandoned in the real world since it is helpful in qualifying children for special services, funding, and admission to special programs run by state and federal governments.

The opposite path is also dangerous; the diagnostician who is willing to begin an evaluation by labeling the problem has reversed the orderly sequence of acquiring knowledge and often effectively closes his or her mind to factors that may later point away from the premature diagnosis. Nelson (2010) applies an old metaphor to the diagnostic process. If a clinician focuses only on the macrolevels of diagnosis such as applying a label to a client, he or she is likely to miss the trees for the forest. On the other hand, if the focus is only on microlevels, such as memory or auditory processing, the forest is often lost due to concentration on "trees." This is a wise notion to remember as we engage in diagnosis and evaluation. If we concentrate on macrolevels we do not become familiar with individual needs of the client, and if we focus on microlevels, we may not see how the client's abilities or impairments represent a broader syndrome.

The notion of "cause" has different meanings depending on its distance from the problem. As you look at a client in a diagnostic session, you search for reasons for the presenting behaviors. In fact, many of these reasons may be buried in the past and can only be revealed by painstaking effort. In many cases, cause and effect may be layered in complex patterns. Not only must we search through the client's past experience in order to uncover events that may help us alter current behaviors, but we must also guard against looking for causes in only one dimension of behavior. A child's brain damage, once identified, is probably not the only etiological factor, because communication is a complicated human function. Social, learning, motivational, and many other factors enter into the total process. Paul (2001) illustrates the complexity of determining causation in an example of babies who were exposed to cocaine because their mothers used the drug during pregnancy:

> Cocaine was usually not the only risk to which they were exposed. Mothers who abused cocaine during pregnancy also tended to abuse other street drugs, as well as alcohol. Alcohol itself is known to be a serious teratogen and could cause many of the problems thought to be present in these babies, even without any other substance abuse. Further, mothers who abused cocaine and other drugs during pregnancy frequently continued to do so after the child was born. These mothers would not be very available to their infants for either basic care or for social interaction. . . . Finally, mothers who abuse cocaine and other drugs tend to live in poverty. Poverty itself affects both general and communicative development through the tendency for poor children to have been born small and prematurely and to have poor nutrition, inadequate medical care and incomplete or absent inoculation against disease. (p. 99)

Thus, determining the etiology of a problem is not always straightforward, and we must be cautious about attributing the cause of a disorder to a particular event or factor. Classically, etiology has been defined in terms of predisposing, precipitating, and perpetuating factors. Predisposing factors are generally thought to be important because of their potential link with a third agent. A classic example of predisposing factors is the apparent genetic predisposition to stutter. We know that stuttering tends to run in families; however, it could be that environmental factors cause it to surface. The wary diagnostician must watch for factors that occur with high regularity in association with certain communication disorders. Such data could ultimately be instrumental in uncovering some basic information regarding the nature of the disorder.

Precipitating factors are generally no longer operating and as such may or may not be identifiable. For example, a child with a language disorder may have begun to lag behind in linguistic development during a period of recurrent ear infections that occurred when language was being learned. If the otitis has long since disappeared and the language disorder remains, it is difficult for the diagnostician to observe or even pinpoint the true cause of the disability. Even if the child did have recurrent bouts with ear infections, it can never be truly substantiated that these infections actually precipitated or played a role in language delay. This is especially true since many children experience frequent ear infections and manage to develop language normally. In many cases the precipitating factors are clear, as in instances of stroke, vocal abuse, structural abnormalities, and certain congenital conditions.

The perpetuating factors are those variables currently at work on the individual. Almost without exception, habit strength is a prime perpetuating factor in many disorders because the client has made various compensations for the problem in terms of cognitive/linguistic strategies and motoric adjustments. Other factors are also crucial, however, and it is the diagnostician's task to uncover the environmental and physical factors that are reinforcing and thus perpetuating the disorder. A hearing loss may be a precipitating and a perpetuating factor in a child's language delay. This child needs a thorough audiological evaluation and a prescription for amplification if indicated, or else the problem will perpetuate. We must always work to identify and, if possible, remove or reduce any factors that maintain a communication disorder.

DIAGNOSIS TO PROVIDE CLINICAL FOCUS

Although it is important to know the causes of the disorder, it is substantially more important to gain some insight into the possible ways to improve the client's communication. It is at this point that diagnosis and clinical management overlap. This is also where the importance of knowing a host of evaluation techniques becomes significant in the diagnostic enterprise. There is a series of questions that the diagnostician must ask:

1. What do I know about this condition?
   What are the usual etiologies?
   What are the usual effective treatment procedures?
   What is the typical prognosis?
2. What do I know about this person?
   What is the impact of the condition on the person?
   What are the person's strengths and needs?
   How is this person like others I have worked with?
   How is this person different from others I have worked with?
3. What do I know about my own skills in treatment of this disorder and this type of person?
   How have I effectively approached similar problems?
   How have I effectively worked with similar people?
4. What do I know about the services of other professionals available for this person?
   What referrals need to be made?
   What consultations do I need to make?
5. What factors need to be removed, altered, or added to improve the prognosis?
   What inhibiting environmental factors exist?
   What organic factors need alteration?
   What can enhance the person's motivation?
   How can the family be involved in treatment?

Note how many of the above questions address components of evidence-based practice discussed earlier.

DIAGNOSIS: SCIENCE AND ART

Diagnosis demands a unique blend of science and art (Silverman, 1984). The scientific method is applicable to our work as diagnosticians, both in guiding our procedures and in focusing our attitude of operation. The scientific method directs the diagnostician to observe all of the available factors, to formulate testable hypotheses by using clearly stated and answerable questions, to test those hypotheses to determine their validity, and to reach conclusions based on the tested hypotheses. The method demands rigorous adherence to standardized procedures and has as its favorable characteristics objectivity, quantifiability, and structure. The scientific diagnostician tends to rely on tests, test data, and other procedures that lend themselves to quantification. As an attitude of operation, the scientific method implies that the diagnostician has not predetermined the test findings and that there is no bias in seeking the proof or disproof of hypotheses. The diagnostician sees hypotheses as something to be tested rather than something to be defended.

The self-fulfilling prophecy is a lethal but almost universal human characteristic; it must be counterbalanced by a scientific approach to testing. We are familiar with parents of children with language impairment who had traveled all over the country in search of a diagnostic explanation for the linguistic delay. Often these children are victims of the "fat folder syndrome," in which a case file has accrued over the years with reports from various authorities and clinics. Each report often reveals more about the examiner than the child as it cites facts in support of a theory of etiology congruent with the diagnostician's particular specialty. For example, in the same client, the audiologist finds auditory processing disorder, the autism specialist diagnoses an autism spectrum disorder, the psychologist discovers attention-deficit disorder, and the speech-language pathologist finds language impairment. Finding what you want to find is not always in the realm of the scientific method. Diagnosticians often use their pet test instruments, to use a famous saying, as the drunk uses the street lamp—more for support than illumination!

The strict adherence to fact that is demanded by the pure scientific method is often a bit confining. That, in part, may explain why we all practice the art of diagnosis at times. The artistic approach has several specific characteristics. The artist is less dependent on specific observations than on casual and nonstructured scrutiny for the formation of hypotheses. This type of clinician is perfectly willing to disregard formal test results or standard testing procedures in favor of what appears obvious on the basis of clinical experience and expertise. The hunch, or clinical intuition, plays a significant part in such evaluations. The diagnostician will contend that facts can be approached from several directions and that we are capable of assessing the same kinds of behaviors that are measured on formal tests by using nonstandardized evaluation tasks. Such contentions are disconcerting to the test-bound person who has come to expect that the only valid way to gain information is through standardized procedures. One of the emphases in the present textbook is that these informal, nonstandardized evaluation procedures are valuable indeed in defining a client's problem and the potential response to treatment. In many ways these procedures may be more valid than standardized tests, as we will discuss in Chapter 3.

It is obvious that, in the extreme, there are weaknesses in both approaches. The scientist may tend to become so dependent on objective methods of measurement that there is a failure to see the client through the maze of percentiles and standard scores. The whole is greater than the sum of its parts, and every diagnostician must guard against simply measuring the isolated characteristics without getting a full picture of the individual. Do not build altars to any testing device; every objective instrument was once only an idea in someone's mind. The art end of the science–art continuum is just as precarious as the scientific end. The possibility of a diagnostician's projecting more than a modest amount of personal bias into the evaluation is greater when a less scientific approach is used. Clinical intuitions are often simply clinical biases, and it is very easy to make new evidence fit old categories. The diagnostician must find the proper mixture of each philosophy in establishing assessment procedures.

DIAGNOSIS VERSUS ELIGIBILITY

As our legal system, medical settings, and public school systems have become more complicated, clinicians are faced with increasing pressure to conduct their clinical work within parameters that are set by administrators. The resulting procedures for case selection, testing, and determining eligibility for services many times fall short of the ideal professional criteria used to make these decisions.

A prominent special education attorney of our acquaintance has won cases in almost every state of the union. When asked why his record of litigation was so impressive, he replied: "I win cases because schools make important decisions about children based on *administrative* criteria instead of *professional* criteria." We need continually to ask ourselves if we are doing the best thing for the client as dictated by the current state of knowledge in our profession. While we cannot always do everything optimally for a client in certain work settings, we need to be very careful in our decisions to streamline services and not make arbitrary decisions for administrative purposes that undermine our profession.

The influence of administrative decision making on our profession has blurred the distinction between diagnosis, on the one hand, and determining eligibility, on the other. For example, it is not unusual for private practitioners and community clinics to provide services to children who have clear language/phonological disorders but who are ineligible for such services in the local school system. Similarly, it is not unusual for private practitioners and university clinics to provide services to medically involved patients whose insurance carriers will no longer pay for treatment. Ehren (1993) states:

> Eligibility often shapes caseloads in ways that seem inconsistent with the state of the art. . . . In lieu of making a diagnosis, we ascertain whether the student meets eligibility criteria. Evaluation, then, becomes an eligibility determination process, rather than a process to describe a student's communication status. . . . We need to develop identification procedures that promote clinical decision making. Speech-language pathologists need to return to their clinical roots and employ their diagnostic skills in identifying students with communication disorders. First, we need to make a diagnosis; next, recommend the need for service; then, discuss eligibility. Diagnosis should drive eligibility; eligibility should not dictate the diagnosis. Eligibility criteria should be viewed as the last hoop to jump through in identifying a student. (p. 20)

THE DIAGNOSTICIAN AS A FACTOR

Ultimately, the most important diagnostic tool is the diagnostician. The clients we assess have seldom read the test manual, and the rigid structure of the testing situation may not be compatible with fluid and nonstructured styles of behavior. Tests are abstractions of behavior, and as such they represent only a fraction of the client's total repertoire of responses to the environment. What better measure of an individual's behavior than that behavior itself? Thus, the diagnostician becomes an important aspect of the evaluating situation in selecting measurements, interacting, responding, and assembling information.

What skills are necessary to develop in order to become an effective diagnostician? How do you develop them? There are no easy answers to these questions. Experience in the diagnostic process is an absolute necessity, but experience in number of clients seen is not enough. A pompous clinician once bragged, "I've had over 20 years of experience." The unfortunate thing, however, is that this person had the first year of experience repeated 19 times, which is altogether a different matter. The diagnostician must be able to gain from new experiences, and this demands *flexibility.* The stereotyped and stagnant diagnostician learns little from increased exposure to people and new situations, but those diagnosticians who use their experience as a pattern to be compared against, rather than as a mold into which all new experiences must fit, will continue to grow and learn. The diagnostician must be flexible enough within the testing situation to shift from predetermined plans to new modes of evaluation as the client presents unpredicted behaviors. The examiner who steadfastly plods through a series of tests even though a client is presenting some interesting new behavior or exhibiting valid instances of communication ability in nontest contexts will miss an important opportunity to gain insight into the problem. It is not atypical for beginning clinicians to panic in the face of an unexpected performance and become intransigent in their application of a series of formal tests because there is a certain degree of comfort in known processes. Continued experience in diagnosis may provide the flexibility needed to move freely to other avenues of information.

Another characteristic of a good diagnostician is a *healthy skepticism* and ability to *critically evaluate* new clinical techniques. Practicing clinicians often eagerly accept new and novel techniques as they become available. As the profession moves into new, uncharted areas of concern, many new materials, tests, and techniques become available. New techniques must not be accepted or rejected carte blanche but rather must be scrutinized for their merit. We must learn to keep up with new developments by participating in an active continuing education program, both personal and professional. On the other hand, the beginning student must guard against the "recent article" syndrome to which we all fall prey upon occasion. Typically, the behavioral pattern goes something like this: You read an article that depicts a particular syndrome and explains the distinctive characteristics of a disorder; for a few weeks thereafter every child you see appears to fall into the pattern described in the publication. The way to overcome the "recent article" syndrome, of course, is to be aware that it exists and to have a thorough understanding of the nature of human perception. With regard to new tests and measurements, techniques grossly foreign to experience tend to threaten and bewilder the inflexible clinician because these are perceived as attacks on trusted and time-proven methods. On the other hand, some clinicians get into the "recent test" syndrome and use the most popular test of the day simply because it is new. It is possible that training programs that emphasize formal testing, fixed therapy programs, and a focus on materials are more likely to produce an inflexible, nonevaluative clinician than are those programs that emphasize theory, problem-solving ability, creativity, and descriptive assessment techniques.

A clinician must possess many important *interpersonal relationship attributes.* Empathy, congruency, and unconditional positive regard are necessary characteristics of the clinician, and they most certainly apply to the diagnostic process as well. In many studies of clinical competence, both supervisors in speech-language pathology and adult clients perceive the interpersonal relationship to be a major factor in contributing to successful treatment (Haynes & Oratio, 1978; Oratio, 1977). Generally these qualities must be nurtured by consistent effort and proper guidance in training programs through analysis by clinical supervisors and review of session videotapes by clinicians in training.

If the term *sensitivity* may be defined as a keenness of sense or a heightened awareness of incoming sensory data, then this term has meaning for the diagnostician. The clinician must be able to detect subtle physical, psychological, or interactional changes in a client's behavior, since these small changes may have significant meaning in the diagnostic process.

The development of an *evaluative attitude* is often a rather difficult task for the beginning clinician. We are, to a large extent, slaves to our experience; each clinician tends to bring a social attitude into the testing setting. Rather than look upon the client's performance as having meaning for the evaluative process, we consult our own responses and formulate our own points of view in the give-and-take of the conversation. The critical, questioning attitude must be developed so that the clinician looks upon the behaviors in terms of their meaning rather than in terms of the response expected. Social interaction lends itself to superficiality, whereas the flow of the diagnostic interaction must, by design, lend itself to uncovering the meaning of the incorporated behavior. Effective diagnosticians tend to question the surface validity of behaviors and search for motivations, explanations, and interpretations that are not readily apparent.

Closely allied with the concept of the evaluative attitude is the idea of *persistent curiosity.* The diagnostician must develop an inquisitiveness that will make him or her persistent in searching for explanations. Answers are seldom apparent at first, and continuous effort is imperative. Training institutions often foster weakness in this area when they assign clients to students and expect therapy to get under way in a "reasonable" period of time. Additionally, they are so bound to the rigid university timetables that treatment is often discontinuous. In an attempt to give each student a variety of clinical experiences, training institutions often tend to sever clinical undertakings with a client at each semester's end, knowing full well that the diagnostic or therapeutic process is not best served in this way. The student may not always understand that these have been decisions based on program convenience rather than client need and may develop the notion that diagnosis is a temporary therapy-initiating exercise to be completed in an hour or two. The curious and persistent clinician, however, continues to place the client in situations that will permit additional scrutiny. It would be ideal, albeit probably unworkable in training programs, for students to follow their clients over longer periods of time so that the students could see how diagnosis is an ongoing process and an integral part of treatment as the client changes.

Objectivity comes from practicing the art of controlled involvement. The diagnostician must cultivate objectivity because we are all subject to human errors. We must be warm, understanding, and accepting, on the one hand, and objective, evaluative, and detached, on the other. Without some degree of balance between the two extremes, the diagnostician may so severely distort the interaction with the client that little information of value is obtained. Objectivity demands more than simply guarding against undue emotional involvement. To grow as a diagnostician, the examiner must be objective about his or her skills, knowledge, and personal characteristics and must take an objective attitude toward the client.

Rapport may be defined as the establishment of a working relationship, based on mutual respect, trust, and confidence, that encourages optimum performance on the part of both client and clinician. Rapport is developed over a period of time and is not easily established in a single session or during a few minutes at the initiation of one diagnostic encounter. Rapport must not only be developed, it must be maintained, and this calls for continued effort. We have known for decades that, especially with children, performance on formal tests varies with clinician familiarity (Fuchs et al., 1985). Children tend to perform better if they have had an opportunity to become familiar with an examiner. While the reasons for this phenomenon are not totally clear, the concept of rapport is obviously involved.

It is important that our *focus* be on the client as much as possible instead of on our own performance and internal states. Diagnosticians are people too, and we often forget that they occasionally have "a bad day." They too can experience the influence of pervasive personal problems and physical frailties that sometimes make them feel as though they should have stayed at home in bed. The most knowledgeable and skillful diagnostician, however, may fail to achieve adequate results if he or she lacks the inquisitiveness necessary to encourage continuous effort and if there is no professional drive to serve each individual to the maximum potential. Each of us is subject to individual variations in daily behavior (physical problems, depression, stress, etc.) that can have a direct effect on performance; however, it is incumbent upon every professional to control those variations so as to provide each individual with the best service available.

THE CLIENT–CLINICIAN RELATIONSHIP

Although much standardization is possible through strict adherence to test routines, the lowest common denominator in diagnostic evaluations is the examiner. Test results are the product of the subject, examiner, test, and test circumstance, each of which has a certain influence. Examinations are clearly selected as a result of the experiences and biases of the examiner. Just as the answers we receive to questions are in part a function of the questions we ask and how we ask them, the diagnostic findings we obtain are in part a function of the tests we administer and the way they are administered. An impaired communication pattern may be partially due to a defective testing pattern or an incompetent tester.

The most crucial factor in conducting a successful diagnostic session is the client–clinician relationship. When one person works with another, there is always human impact; even when clients are treated by computers, they come to accord human attributes to the machines. No matter how well prepared and rehearsed an examiner may be, if his or her approach to people is poor, failure will ensue. All tests, all examinations, all so-called objective diagnostic procedures are mediated by person-to-person contact.

We can be seduced into grave errors by test norms, percentile scores, and standard examination procedures: A human being is a total functioning unit, and the various tests are multiple and fragmented. Even if the instruments we use are relatively precise (which they are not), and we are deluded into thinking that the client is functioning with the same degree of precision in the testing situation, human elements may disturb the validity of the tests no matter how refined the scoring procedures or how calibrated the machines.

Impersonal, test-oriented clinical examination sessions can also make assessment more difficult because there is no absolute division between diagnosis and therapy. The first contact with a client initiates treatment. During a diagnostic session the client is forming opinions and conceptions about the clinician and the total clinical situation. Not all clients will require the full impact of this interpersonal dimension. Indeed, some individuals simply want to find out what is wrong and then rectify the situation. The point is, however, that the clinician should be able to discern what the client needs and then adjust his or her style appropriately.

THE CLIENT AS A FACTOR: CHILDREN, ADOLESCENTS, AND ADULTS

Although all age levels present unique diagnostic problems, three groups in particular—young children, adolescents, and to a lesser extent, older or elderly clients—require special effort and expertise. Since the present chapter is generic in nature, we will mainly talk about the general business of relating to the different age groups seen in diagnostic evaluations. The more specific chapters that follow will provide additional suggestions for dealing with the different age groups in the context of evaluating particular disorders. A major reason for including this generic section is that many readers of the present text are students in training to become speech-language pathologists. It is often difficult for a young person to capture the ephemeral guidelines for relating to people of different ages. It is not as simple as just "being yourself" or talking one way to a child and another way to an adult. There are certain common errors students have made over the years that we can at least alert you to so that you may avoid them. These precepts, of course, are drawn from the experiences of the authors, and there are obviously many more guidelines that could be added.

1. *Young Children.* Preschool and kindergarten children are often difficult to test and examine. Unlike most older children and adults, they just do not see the payoff for all the questioning and prodding. Often a major problem is dealing with the child's fear of the clinical situation. This apprehension may stem from one or more of the following related factors: (1) inadequate preparation for the examination by parents, (2) uncertainty as to what will be done to or with the child by the clinician, (3) vivid memories of trauma during visits to dentists and physicians, (4) the contagious anxieties and uncertainties experienced by the parents, and (5) stress and conflicts engendered by past listener reactions to the communication impairment. Children confront the clinical examination in a variety of ways, but the two most trying responses are shyness and withdrawal and, at the other extreme, aggressiveness and hyperactivity.

In many cases with very young children, it is possible to have the parent participate in the interaction, and this avoids any separation anxiety on the part of the child. The parents are typically willing to cooperate, the child is happy, and the parents can often get the child to do many things that the clinician would take several sessions of rapport building to accomplish. Parents can even be used to administer some formal tests that just involve turning picture plates and reading the cues on the backs of the pictures, while the clinician scores the child's responses. We have to choose our battles very carefully, and fighting an obstreperous child in a diagnostic session mainly leads to unsatisfying results for all concerned. In dealing with the children in the birth-to-2 age range, *most* of the pertinent information will be gleaned from parents, both from interview data and by observation of parent–child interaction. Not many 1-year-olds do well with an unfamiliar clinician, and we need to focus on the parent–child dyad anyway, because treatment will doubtless involve the entire family.

There are obviously many other considerations that could be discussed; additional suggestions will be offered in the chapters concerning various disorders. For the present, here are several basic precepts on the management of preschool children in a clinical examination:

- Help the parents prepare the child for the diagnostic session. They can tell him or her what will transpire, and maybe even bring along some stimulus items favored by the child (toys, picture albums, books, etc.).
- Play, rather than small talk, is the natural medium of expression for children. This is especially important when dealing with youngsters who may have a communication impairment. While we have all known children in the 3-to-5 age range that are impressive conversationalists, most children referred for communication disorders are not on this end of the conversational continuum. Try to arrange the diagnostic tasks with this in mind.
- As a general rule, ask less and observe more. Children usually lack the insight and cooperation necessary to analyze their problem rationally and objectively. Naturalistic observations—assessing a child's behavior in natural environments—yields more useful information.
- Learn everything possible about normal children in order to provide a baseline for observations of youngsters presenting problems. This can be done by taking courses, studying

relevant norms, but most of all by extensive scrutiny and interaction with children in day-care and preschool facilities. You should have a good idea of the typical or modal behavior for children at various age levels.

- Limit the choices you offer a child. Don't ask if he or she would like to go with you, do this or that, unless the alternatives do not conflict with the examiner's goals. The child will invariably say "No!" Also, refrain from saying "Okay?" after your utterances ("I want you to name these pictures, okay?"). This question suggests that there is an option available.

- Be flexible in your use of tests and examinations. If you cannot employ the rigid standardized format for administration, use the test to obtain all the data you can. If the child refuses to name the test pictures or objects, you may be able to get a language sample from other items. Also, if there is no standard order for administration of tests and tasks, go with the items the child appears to be interested in at a particular time. For example, if a test has some objects associated with it and the child is attending to these items, start this examination even if you had initially planned it for later in the session.

- Absolute honesty and candor is important in working with children. Do not make promises unless you can keep them.

- The whole assessment does not have to be done in one session; marathon diagnostics tend to be counterproductive. Remember that all we can hope to obtain in one time frame is a sample of a child's behaviors. It is better to terminate (preferably on a pleasant, successful note) than to continue an unproductive session until the child is fatigued or upset.

- Watch your language complexity when talking to children. For obvious reasons, the examiner should avoid sarcasm, idiomatic expressions, ambiguous statements, and indirect requests.

2. *Adolescents.* Experienced clinicians frequently report that adolescents, the classical teenagers, especially in grades 7 through 11, are often difficult to examine and resistant to treatment. The main problem seems to be getting through to the person. There is no magic formula for this, but we would like to make some suggestions that we have found helpful in guiding our work with adolescent clients:

- Acquire an understanding of the myriad pressures and changes the teenager is experiencing: rapid physical growth, sexual maturity, conflicts between dependence and independence, the development of self-confidence and interpersonal skills necessary to make decisions, a search for identity and life work, intense group loyalty and identification, and many more. It is a turbulent, trying period of behavioral extravagance and excess. Small wonder that teenagers are often overloaded with personal concerns and do not always welcome an overture of clinical assistance. Empathy that flows from understanding is a powerful force in establishing a working relationship.

- There is an intense desire to be like others, not to stand out from the group in any way that would suggest frailty. Hence, the adolescent may find it extremely difficult to reveal a communication impairment, even if help is desired. Often teenagers are simply sent for evaluation or treatment by parents. In some instances, the teenager with a chronic problem may have been in treatment for a long time and is weary of the idea of more therapy. Many will tend to cover up true feelings with a sullen bravado or a dense "it-doesn't-bother-me" shell. Denial is a particular forte. "Coolness" and image are very important. You can neither beat this down nor simply dismiss it with a shrug. Nor is silence a particularly effective tool in dealing with adolescent resistance. We advocate a straight-forward approach: Acknowledge the forces that are bearing on the individual; point up objectively the paths that others have taken; provide information about the economic and social penalties that accrue to the person with a communication disorder. Basically, try to demonstrate by your demeanor and what you say that you care about the client; a growing person needs lots of nourishment, and personal involvement and commitment are key factors.

- Do not abandon your professional role for that of a teenager. Be yourself. As Will Rogers pointed out, if they don't like you the way you are, they are sure not going to like you the way you are trying to be.

- Approach adolescents with tolerance and good humor. Do not be shocked or annoyed by their overstatements and superlatives; do not overreact to expressions of hostility or tempests of other emotions. Sometimes adolescents, in order to uphold their protective armor, will resort to all sorts of strategies to confuse, defeat, or anger the clinician. The ability to laugh at yourself and to use humor in a gentle, needling manner is an asset. Remember, though, to always treat the adolescent with honesty and dignity—don't make fun of intense or idealistic views.

- Explain the diagnostic process as much as possible by explaining what we are about, the reasons for the various tests and examinations, and how we will use the information. We encourage the adolescent to challenge and question what we are doing. Finally, we usu-ally give the client an idea of the route we would follow when therapy commences, or we even do some trial treatment activities.

- If the client is highly critical of parents or school officials, we must keep the person's confidences and not act in a judgmental manner. We do not enter into the criticism or side with the client against others, nor do we try to defend the institution or retreat to moralisms.

- Discuss the results of the evaluation with the client before talking with the parents or school personnel. Be sure to let the client know exactly what you intend to tell parents and teachers and determine any feelings the client has about these suggestions.

These recommendations have been distilled from our clinical experience and are not pre-sented as magical touchstones for all diagnosticians or all clients; nor do these recommendations represent the full range of possibilities for successful interaction with teenage clients. We present them here to encourage other workers to develop clinical generalizations on the basis of their ex-perience.

3. *The Elderly Client.* Older clients may present some rather special problems for the di-agnostician, or they may need no particular special handling. Although the concept of "elderly" is relative, we refer here to persons in their sixties or older. A word of caution: Although there are certain generalizations that are useful for planning and conducting evaluations, elderly people are not any more "all alike" than are children or adolescents.

The clinician should be alert to fatigue, disorientation, failing eyesight, and hearing loss. With advanced age, the person may find it more difficult to focus attention on a task and gener-ally may have trouble remembering directions because of possible short-term memory decline. Many of these potential problems are exacerbated when the person has experienced a neurologi-cal insult, as in a good number of elderly clients. We need, therefore, to explain each step of our clinical procedures at greater length and repeat instructions when necessary to ensure under-standing. Our pace should be geared to the client's abilities—if necessary, to a slower level.

Organize the testing sequence carefully to reduce distractions, noise, or interference. Older people are often more cautious and have a greater need to be certain before they respond, so adapt the tasks with this in mind; following standard procedure may not be as important as providing an environment in which the person is able to perform at an optimal level.

Since many older clients tend to feel useless and discarded in our youth-oriented culture and resentful that their bodies are betraying them, we may find it important to spend some time listening to their memories of past achievements. Older clients should always be treated with respect and not referred to by their first names. The clinician should also guard against using a louder vocal intensity and increased pitch range as if talking to a child. It is grossly offensive to infantilize an adult client. Many of our elderly clients will come to us with neurologically based disorders, serious vocal pathologies, and other medically related problems. There will be a tendency among many to talk about medical issues, since their problems have originated from this area. It is important for the diagnostician to be patient with these clients and listen to their concerns, while still not allowing conversation about medical issues to interfere with the testing.

In most cases, clinicians will find older clients to be interesting, socially adept individuals to be treated with courtesy and respect. The number of people over age 60 composes a significant proportion of the population, and we cannot afford to perpetuate the stereotype that old people are expendable or that they should be relegated to demeaning idleness. As with children and adolescents, the diagnostician should know as much as possible about aging. Many references pertinent to communication disorders are readily available (Heilbrun, 1998; Kirkwood, 2000; Morrison, 1998; Shadden, 1988; Sheehy, 1996).

PUTTING THE DIAGNOSIS TO WORK

Perhaps the most demanding of all diagnostic ventures is the ultimate synthesis of findings into a coherent statement of the nature of the problem. The skilled clinician draws the findings together by using the data available, past experience, knowledge, and intuition to formulate a total picture of the condition. At this point, textbooks, research findings, and academic lectures fail to provide all of what is needed to succeed. Maturation of skills will only develop in an extensive practicum under the close supervision of a knowledgeable diagnostician. The essence of the synthesis process is a comparison of what is observed with what we expect to observe from our knowledge of the normal process. The incongruities between the observed and the normal provide the building blocks for completion of the picture. Figure 1.6 identifies a model of diagnosis as a synthesis of findings and shows a number of outcomes to which the synthesis might lead. This figure points out several important concepts.

First, the bedrock of the entire model is the clinician's knowledge and skill base. Without adequate training and experience, the administration of tests and tasks becomes meaningless.

A second important point in the model is the series of six boxes that are immediately above the clinician's knowledge and skill base. These boxes highlight the diversity of information that the diagnostician should ideally obtain in order to make a principled judgment about a client's disorder (case history, prior reports, observation, interview, informal testing, and formal testing). Interestingly, it is not unusual for prior reports and tests to be missing or unrequested, case history information to be returned by the client at the time of evaluation instead of prior to it, the case history forms to be incomplete or lost, and the interview cut to a 10-minute conversation because of time pressure. It is also not unusual for the clinician to spend the entire assessment time giving tests with little opportunity left for informal testing or observation of clients in relevant situations. While it is difficult to obtain information from all six boxes in the model, we must try

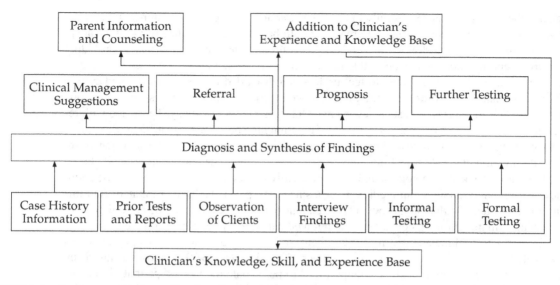

FIGURE 1.6 Components of an effective diagnosis/evaluation.

to get as close to the ideal as possible. In many settings, the evaluation will not take place unless the client has submitted all pertinent information and unless reports from other agencies have been received. It is certainly that way in many other professions (medicine, psychology, etc.). We must ask ourselves about the quality of the diagnostic evaluation that is done with incomplete information. What is the efficacy of performing an evaluation if we do not have access to critical information and are not willing to spend the time to carry on a decent interview and do informal testing and client observation? Again, remember that a crucial part of evidence-based practice is to understand the client's disorder and perspectives as fully as possible.

A third area in the center of the model is the synthesis of findings. This is where we begin to see overlaps in the data from case history, interview, reports, observations, and testing results. We should look for common threads among all of these information sources and tie them together in the synthesis and diagnosis. Often, this is where certain informational components begin to disagree with one another, which is also informative. For example, the parents indicate intense concern over their child's articulation in the case history and the interview. They also bring a host of prior reports that indicate the child has no clinically significant problem, and they look to you for guidance. If your own test results, informal task performance, and observations indicate that the child is performing within normal limits, the discrepancy between these components and the parents' perceptions is obvious. The prior reports also now gain significant importance in terms of counseling the parents and pointing out the disparity between their views and the perceptions of many professionals. Another example may point out the foibles associated with one or more of the sources of information. For instance, a child may not perform within normal limits on formal tests of language ability. Yet, that same child communicates well in informal tasks and observations of play interactions with caretakers and peers. The clinician must question the formal test results if the child's communication exceeds that which these measures suggest he or she is capable of.

A fourth series of five boxes in the model point out some important components of a diagnostic evaluation that are present after the synthesis of information. As we mentioned earlier, a good diagnostician will make suggestions for treatment in terms of which goals may be logically selected for initial intervention. The parents need to be counseled about the results of the evaluation, and any problems or feelings they express must be dealt with. Often we are so zealous in performing the evaluation and in scheduling time for doing everything we feel is necessary that we give the client or parents short shrift in explaining our results. In many cases, the results we report to parents or clients represent a significant affective burden. For example, even though parents usually know in their hearts that their child has a communication disorder, they often hold out the hope that their child really is typically developing and will grow out of a language or articulation difference. Telling parents that their child is indeed showing an impairment forces them to come to terms with this problem. Diagnosticians may experience parents or clients who cry at the culmination of the evaluation session when they are told something that confirms the idea of a disorder or commits them to an undetermined length of time spent in rehabilitation. Other emotions also emerge, such as anger and denial, which must sometimes be dealt with at the end of the diagnostic session. Emotions aside, it is enough of a challenge simply to communicate the complex evaluation results to parents of different educational levels and abilities. A skilled diagnostician has the ability to summarize assessment results and recommendations on the correct level of abstraction for different parents and spouses. Another aspect to deal with after synthesis is the possibility of referral. Many cases require a consultation by other professionals, such as audiologists, laryngologists, neurologists, special educators, psychologists, and others. Often the assessment raises more questions than it answers, and this is perfectly acceptable. We need to know the parameters of the patient's problem and many times this insight can only be gained from professionals who have expertise in areas with which we are not totally familiar.

Prognosis is another variable depicted in Figure 1.6. Prognosis may be defined as a prediction of the outcome of a proposed course of treatment for a given client: how effective treatment will be, how far we can expect the client to progress, and, perhaps, how long it will take. Inasmuch as diagnosis is a continuing process, prognosis should, like treatment planning, have both long-range and immediate facets. Immediate prognosis covers what the person can do now, what steps in therapy are possible, and what is the best route to take. Prognosis for specific communication disorders will be discussed in subsequent chapters; in this section we will present some generic purposes and a possible danger involved in predicting a client's response to treatment.

Patients and families want to know what they may expect in terms of progress. Some general factors that the clinician must consider when making predictions are as follows:

1. *Age.* The chronological age of the client is a gross predictor of treatment success. In general, the younger the client, the better the treatment outcome. This can be seen in childhood disorders where the earlier the intervention is begun, the more progress can be made prior to school entrance. The earlier we involve children in treatment, the more likely we are to prevent the formation of secondary problems (Shine, 1980; Starkweather, Gottwald, & Halfond, 1990) such as social, psychological, and educational penalties. In adult cases, it is well known that patients who develop neurogenic disorders at younger ages (40–60) are generally given better prognoses than patients who develop these problems at later ages (70–90) (Rosenbek, LaPointe, & Wertz, 1989). This, of course, is due to a variety of reasons that include psychological, motivational, and physical factors. Thus, age is a macrovariable that in and of itself is not a potent variable, but it subsumes many factors that do have an influence on prognosis.

2. *Length of Time Impairment Has Existed.* The length of time a client has had a disorder of communication may relate to prognosis. Obviously, if the impairment has a component of habitual activities (motor patterns, processing strategies, etc.), these are more difficult to alter in clients who have performed them for a lengthy period. In addition to the habit patterns developed over time, the client has also learned complex ancillary adjustment patterns to compensate for the communication impairment that may involve social, psychological, and motoric activities. These compensatory patterns eventually become part of the problem and often must be eliminated, as in the case of operant behaviors learned by people who stutter (head jerks, timing devices, etc.).

3. *Existence of Other Problems.* It is axiomatic that the more problems a client has, the more difficult it will be to deal with the disorder. A client with aphasia who is also hearing impaired will be more difficult than one with the language disorder alone. A child with a cleft palate and articulation problems will be more difficult than one with the articulation problem alone. A child who is language delayed and cognitively impaired is different from one who presents only a language disorder.

4. *Reactions of Significant Others.* A child with a communication disorder is going to make better progress in treatment if the parent takes an active role in the intervention. Many parents are interested in participating in treatment and will carry on home programs. On the other hand, if a child is brought to the clinic by a social worker and the parents do not appear interested in treatment, this child will probably take longer to succeed in remediation. If the spouse of a patient with aphasia is disinterested in facilitating communication, the client may make slower progress. The same can be said about the cooperation of teachers, aides, day-care providers, siblings, peers, and anyone else who comes in significant contact with the client and is in a position to help with treatment. Generally, the more assistance available from significant others, the better the prognosis.

5. *Client Motivation.* While we have no reliable way to measure motivation in a client, most diagnosticians can recognize it when they see it. If the client appears enthusiastic, interested, and anxious to begin treatment, it is clearly a plus. If the client is an adult, was he or she self-referred? This may be a positive indication as opposed to a person referred by an employer or teacher or dragged to the evaluation by a domineering spouse. There may also be some positive prognostic value in cases where the client has something to gain from successful treatment (better social life, higher-paying job, etc.). Motivation is always difficult to quantify, but few would totally disregard the importance of this admittedly blurry construct.

Accurate prognoses can help establish our credibility with other professions. The ability to predict with reasonable precision is perhaps the highest form of scientific achievement. Needless to say, however, these predictions should be based on something more than clinical intuition. Impressionistic conclusions, especially when made by experienced workers, can often be startlingly accurate, but they should always be labeled as impressionistic: A prognosis should be supported by a substantial amount of information. We never say that "the prognosis is favorable" without some documentation, both impressionistic and scientifically based. It is much better to say the following: "The prognosis is good because the child is stimulable for all error sounds, trial therapy has indicated good attention and a cooperative attitude, parents have committed to a home program, the client has stated he wants to change his speech, he has normal hearing, and language problems are not evident."

In what sense might a prognosis be dangerous? First, no one really knows the future. A client's prognostic variables might soon change with unforeseen circumstances (e.g., the uninterested parents become involved, the client develops motivation, the client makes a "breakthrough" in the ability to perform certain functions). This means that prognosis as a construct is dynamic, not static. A second danger is that the prognosis may well influence a client's performance and perceptions. If a clinician has certain expectations regarding the case's potential performance, this could be inadvertently communicated to the client or the family and could negatively affect the course of therapy. It could also influence the level of effort exhibited by the clinician. The old notion of a self-fulfilling prophecy is still alive and well. We must always be willing to alter prognostic judgments in light of new data; and perhaps more important, we must be willing to refrain from making prognostic statements in the first place if we do not know what we are talking about. It is better to say "I don't know how he will do in treatment; let's see what happens" than to jaundice the whole enterprise with a negative prognosis that has no real basis, or to disappoint all concerned with a positive prognosis that never is realized. This is *not* an exact science!

PRECEPTS REGARDING THE CLINICAL EXAMINATION

In this chapter we have presented some suggestions for general conduct of the diagnostic session. We dislike diagnostic formulas, and our purpose has not been to give out recipes, but rather to describe some way of approaching various problems without going too far astray. By way of summary, we now present a list of interrelated and overlapping precepts regarding the clinical examination.

- We examine persons, not communication problems. Our primary concern is with communicators, not just communication.
- The clinical examination is conducted interpersonally; the catalyst of a diagnostic session is the person-to-person relationship between clinician and client.
- There is an element of magic in every transaction between people. A diagnostic session can, in some instances, ameliorate a problem situation by engendering hope or be deeply disappointing to a client who hopes that a test or examination will resolve a difficulty.
- A most important requisite for conducting a clinical examination is a thorough understanding of normalcy.
- Diagnosis is the initial phase of treatment. The very first contact with a client—the manner in which he or she is treated during a clinical examination—is a crucial determining factor in response to therapy.
- Diagnosis is not necessarily confined to a single session.
- Treatment is often diagnostic; we often discover the nature of a client's problem in the initial stages of therapy.
- The clinical examination is performed to provide a working image of the individual; it is accomplished by interviewing, examining, evaluating, and testing.
- An important aspect in acquiring a working image of an individual is determining the person's self-perception and situation.
- An individual makes certain adjustments to a problem (attempts to solve the difficulty) that may include a protective cover of defenses. These may be a part of the problem, but must not be confused with the problem.
- Behavior is a function of the individual and the situation. We should be aware that our test results reflect not just the client's abilities but also performance in the diagnostic setting rather than the natural environment.
- Our diagnostic activities should include an assessment of a client's larger social context (home, family, peers, job, school, etc.).

- Tests are only tools to provide a systematic guide for our observations. They enable the clinician to scrutinize a client in a structured manner.
- Although for the examiner the testing situation may be very familiar and routine, for the client it is a novel experience.
- Examination and testing can be iatrogenic. It can suggest problems to the client that he or she had not previously considered.
- Simply because a testing device is made up of a series of precisely defined tasks, administered and scored in a rigidly structured manner, this does not mean that a client's responses are similarly precise.
- It is as important to observe *how* the client responds during a testing procedure as it is to obtain a score. Informal evaluation tasks are as important or more important than formal, standardized procedures.
- The needs of the client, not the work setting in which the clinician labors, should determine the scope of diagnostic activities. A good diagnostic is over when sufficient information about a client is gathered and should not be short circuited because of administrative red tape, arbitrary guidelines of a facility, or government regulations. A good clinician will find ways to obtain critical information even if the evaluation extends into the realm of treatment.

This chapter has served to generally introduce diagnosis and evaluation. The following chapters will focus more closely on important parameters of this interesting process with specific areas of communication disorders. We hope that students can see this is an exciting enterprise that combines instruments with interpersonal relationships, testing with talking, and measurement with personal magnetism. The assessment process is the portal through which real people with real problems come to us for help. We must offer them the best of scientific as well as human resources.

2

Interviewing

The clinician sets in motion the process of recovery at the very first contact with a client. This is accomplished through the vehicle of the spoken word—in short, by means of the initial interview. Because the intake interview ushers the client into treatment, it is the key link in the evaluation process. In order to assess and treat persons with communication disorders, it is essential that we know how to talk with them in a manner that reflects our expertise and inspires confidence and trust.

THE IMPORTANCE OF INTERVIEWING

Although clinical evaluation obviously involves more than proficiency at conducting interviews, it is central to the role of the diagnostician. By means of verbal exchange, we gather data about the individual, transmit information, and establish and sustain a working relationship. The interview is also the means by which treatment is carried out and, as such, serves both as a tool and as a relationship (Figure 2.1). For the clinical speech-language pathologist, interviewing, and professional communication in general, is an extremely important activity (Burrus & Haynes, 2009).

Although widely used, interviewing is often one of the least understood aspects of the worker's role. Prospective clinicians are expected to acquire an impressive array of knowledge, but often it is presumed that they know how to communicate effectively with clients. The mastery of interviewing is either taken for granted or expected to accrue somehow as an artifact of required course work and practicum experiences.

Some clinicians consider interviewing to be secondary; they use paper to replace personal interaction. An elaborate case history form containing a plethora of questions is mailed to the clients, and they are asked to fill it out and return it before the diagnostic appointment. The rationale for this procedure is that it saves the clinician time and reveals problem areas that can then be explored in the personal interview. Although the clinician certainly should get some idea of the problem before the diagnostic examination, there is no substitute for an in-depth interview. There are several reasons for disenchantment with an approach that only uses paper-and-pencil techniques. First, the questions on forms are often generic—they cover all possible respondents— and thus are ambiguous or not applicable to any particular clients; a parent may not understand the

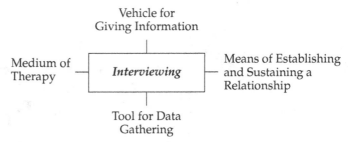

FIGURE 2.1   Interviewing is central in speech pathology.

relationship between the questions posed and the child's communication problems. Face-to-face interviews permit greater flexibility in formulating precise and germane inquiries. Second, the queries may be threatening or may engender guilt, and the clinician is not present to observe the respondent's reactions or to support and assist the respondent as he or she searches for an answer. Does the mailed questionnaire allow time for the respondent to plan a defense? Is it more likely that we end up with a view of what the respondent wants us to see? More complete information can be obtained in an interview, where primary questions may be followed up with pertinent secondary inquiries. Do not imply from the above that the present authors are opposed to obtaining information by having clients complete *well-designed* case history forms. Such data are critical for understanding the client's perspective. Our emphasis is that one should not rely *exclusively* on paperwork in assessment. In fact, see the section in Chapter 4 on "preassessment" as a valuable part of planning an evaluation.

THE NATURE OF INTERVIEWING

An interview is essentially a process, not an entity—a process of verbal and nonverbal intercourse between a trained professional worker and a client or parent who is seeking services. More specifically, an interview, in a clinical and diagnostic sense, is a *purposeful* exchange of meanings between two persons, a directed conversation that proceeds in an orderly fashion to obtain data, to convey certain information, and to provide counseling. The professional worker, by reason of his or her position and clinical expertise, is expected to (and usually does) provide the direction for the verbal exchange. Thus, an interview is not just an ordinary conversation in terms of a desultory exchange of opinions and ideas but rather a specialized pattern of verbal interaction directed toward a specific purpose and focused on specific content. The roles of interviewer and respondent are more highly specified in a professional interview than in a conversation. An interview differs from a social conversation in a number of other important respects. First, the time and location of an interview is specified formally. Second, the inquiries are generally unilateral—the clinician may ask about the parents' relationship with their child, for example, but it is not expected that the client will reciprocate with questions about the worker's children. Third, the clinician does not necessarily avoid unpleasant topics in the interest of social propriety.

In a good diagnostic interview, the clinician and client must become co-workers, multiplying their efforts by creating a mutual feeling of cooperation. It is futile to expect straightforward answers to simple questions. A good diagnostic interview always involves more than making queries and recording answers.

Interviewing is a unique kind of conversation. Perhaps for the first time, the respondent can talk freely without fear of criticism or admonishment. The *clinician* knows that an interview is a unique and distinct mode of verbal exchange. But does the *client* need to know? Probably not. Indeed, we typically advise students to refer to an interview as a "chat" or "a chance to share information" when they contact clients or parents to request an appointment time. An "interview" sounds rather ominous and frightening.

In summary, a diagnostic interview is a directed conversation, carried out for specific purposes such as fact finding, informing, or altering attitudes and opinions. The clinician's efforts are directed toward the creation of mutual respect and team effort in the understanding and solution of the communication problem.

COMMON INTERVIEWING CONSIDERATIONS

Several factors can prevent the establishment of effective communicative bonds between a speech clinician and those whom the clinician interviews. Although the list could obviously be expanded, we have picked several aspects that in our experience are the most common interviewing barriers.

Fears of the Clinician

There are two points in a student clinician's career when the anxiety rises to very high levels: the confrontation with his or her first therapy case and the first diagnostic interview. It is—and should be—an awesome responsibility to undertake the professional treatment of another human being. There is always an element of risk in offering help.

Perhaps the most common fear expressed by the beginning clinician is that clients will not accept the clinician in a professional role because of the clinician's youth. The clinician doubts that he or she can bridge the age gap, especially when the clinician deals with parents: "Who am I to be asking questions and giving suggestions to them when they are older and more experienced?" The clinician sighs, "Won't they look down on me if I don't have children?" Most of this is pure projection on the clinician's part (Haynes & Oratio, 1978). If the clinician indicates deep concern for the welfare of the client, then nearly every parent/client will respond in a positive manner, without scrutinizing the clinician for wrinkles, or gray hairs, or looking for photographs of children on the clinician's desk. The clinician, of course, should not communicate the uncertainty felt in the interview situation; otherwise, he or she will never establish competence or inspire confidence.

Another common fear among beginning clinicians—and one that is also largely projected—is that the client will become defensive or resentful during questioning. We have seen students omit a whole series of important questions when a client, especially a parent, responded curtly or showed mild annoyance. While it is not uncommon for parents to think of their child's communication disorder as an outward and visible sign of their own failure, in our experience few parents are resentful or defensive about the clinician's sincere efforts to determine the nature of the child's problem. The important point is, again, to make the clients and their families feel that they have done the best they could do, and now, with some assistance from the clinician, they can do better. The clinician should *always maintain a nonthreatened posture in the clinical transaction.*

Many beginning clinicians are leery of questions directed at them. "What do you do when the client starts asking *you* questions?" the beginning clinician frequently despairs. "Will I be able to explain to the client adequately what he or she needs to know? How will I know if I have communicated properly if the client just sits there and nods?" We shall return to this important topic of client questions in a later section of this chapter.

The Lack of Specific Purpose

Many beginning clinicians either have purposes that are too broad and general or interviewing goals that are too nebulous. It is important to write out carefully and rather explicitly the purposes for an interview before meeting with the client. We must know *why* we want the answers to the questions we ask. Specifying the purposes of an interview is also an effective way to reduce the interviewer's uncertainty and anxiety. Kadushin (1972) summarizes the importance of planning in this way: "To know is to be prepared; to be prepared is to experience reduced anxiety; to reduce anxiety is to increase the interviewer's freedom to be fully responsive to the interviewee" (p. 2). The clinician should keep in mind, however, that thorough planning does not mean the application of an inflexible routine.

AN APPROACH TO INTERVIEWING

We now present an interviewing approach, an eclectic product of our clinical experience together with an intensive study of relevant bibliographic materials. No doubt the reader will want to modify our approach in order to suit individual settings. It is desirable to do so, for only through critical self-evaluation and modification can any clinician acquire an interviewing procedure that is uniquely personal.

There are three basic goals in diagnostic interviews: to obtain information, to give information, and to provide counseling. For the purpose of discussion, each goal will be considered separately.

Goal One: Obtain Information

Although it may seem obvious, it is worth restating that as clinicians we must listen before we speak. There are essentially three reasons for this: (1) It gives clients an opportunity to talk out problems, to ventilate fears and feelings, thus enabling them to profit better from the direction and advice that the speech clinician will offer; (2) it gives the clinician an idea of the nature and scope of the information the client will need; and (3) it allows the clinician to formulate hypotheses concerning the individual's communication disorder.

SETTING THE TONE   The first important task of the clinician is to set the right tone for the interview, to get a structured conversation initiated and channeled in the proper direction. How does one go about that? We find that defining the roles is an effective procedure for setting the tone:

> Mrs. Taylor, I wanted to talk with you before we start our evaluation with Larry. I know you filled out the case history form we sent you and that provided a lot of important information. I did have a few questions about some of the things you said about Larry's early development and I also wanted to ask you about some of the speech and language he uses at home. It's hard for us to get an accurate picture of a person just by reading paperwork, so if we can talk a bit about Larry and get some examples of his communication from you it will help us to do a more effective evaluation.

It is helpful to think of the interview as a kind of role-playing situation. As the clinician, you define the roles for the client and indicate the rules and responsibilities that accrue to these roles. You tell who you are, what you intend to do, and what you expect of the client. In other words, you structure the situation by explaining the purposes of the interview—why the information is needed and what will be done with it. Initially, of course, the client accepts the respondent role because of the nature of the situation and the official sanction of the interviewer's position. Then it is up to you to demonstrate your empathy and clinical expertise in order to solicit further cooperation. Two problems sometimes arise here. First, some clients may be inhibited by such explicit role definitions; respondents from lower-middle or lower social classes may have had little experience in holding directed conversations. In this case, a clinician can prolong the small-talk phase, emphasize the nature of the interview as chatting, and gently ease into the more structured situation as the relationship develops. When two or more people get together, even for serious purposes, a certain amount of social and idle talk seems to foster positive attitudes toward continued interaction. There are a great many considerations related to cultural and socioeconomic variables as they relate to clinical interactions. These are covered in Chapter 12 of the present text. You may want to read this information while you are thinking about interviewing after completing this chapter.

The second, more difficult problem concerns the site of the interview. Although it is generally best to conduct interviews in a clinical setting, sometimes this is not possible, and you must seek the client or parents at home. This is rarely satisfactory, not only because of the distractions inherent in the situation (children, pets, and neighbors) but also because the interview frequently becomes a social visit.

It is vital that you convey sincere interest in the situation as the client sees it. Demonstrate to the client that you are genuinely trying to comprehend what the problem is and what it means to the client personally. Show interest by carefully attending to the respondent: Assume a relaxed, natural posture; maintain eye contact; and offer some verbal encouragements that reveal you are listening ("Yes," "I see," etc.).

Rapport, of course, is not a separate substance you can pour into a session; it is mutual respect and trust, a feeling of confidence on your part, and a large measure of understanding. Empathy, warmth, and acceptance are crucial aspects; strive for the ability to understand sensitively and accurately the interviewee's situation. Also try to be genuine, not contrived, with a professional demeanor. In addition to the words spoken, a number of forces shape the interview. Some things are conveyed by the setting and by the dress, manners, and expressions of the participants. In professional interviewing, the goal is to provide an atmosphere that fosters communication between client and clinician.

ASKING THE QUESTIONS   Preferably, you should use an interview guide or outline rather than read prepared questions. Word questions in keeping with your understanding of the individual's situation and thus conduct an interview that is much more spontaneous and meaningful. In most cases, formal questionnaires operate as another type of barrier or crutch for the insecure interviewer.

The specific content of the queries addressed to a respondent depend on, among other things, the age of the client, the nature of the problem, and the purposes of the interview. Most clinicians find that the younger the client being evaluated, the more important the parent interview. Because we intend to focus on style of interviewing in this chapter, we will not include lists of questions that pertain to particular disorders of communication. Many examples from specific areas are provided in later chapters. There are, however, seven general topics or areas of inquiry that are useful in any diagnostic session.

1. *What is the respondent's perception of the problem?*   We seek here a global description of the communication disorder. In a parent interview, for example, we frequently open the session with an open-ended question: "Tell me why you brought Jamie to the clinic" or "What concerns do you have about Jamie?"

2. *When and under what conditions did the communication disorder arise?* The purpose of this question is to determine the history of the development and of the onset of the problem. An example of where this etiology would be especially important might be the development of a voice disorder (e.g., rapid versus gradual onset, occurrence of vocally abusive behaviors, changes in medication).

3. *In what ways has the communication disorder changed since its onset?* When interviewing the parents of a child who is exhibiting early signs of stuttering, for example, we are interested in how the speech disfluency has changed since it was first noticed.

4. *What are the consequences (the handicapping conditions) of the problem?* In what manner—socially, educationally, occupationally—does the communication disorder affect the person's life? In what ways has he or she adapted to the disorder?

5. *How has the client and family attempted to cope with the problem?* What lay remedies have been tried by the client and family? How has the client responded to them?

6. *What impact has the client's communication disorder had on the rest of the family?* When a child has a handicapping condition, it creates fertile ground for familial conflict (see Featherstone, 1980). In order to obtain a description of the child's ongoing behavior and how he or she fits into the family regimen, ask the parents to describe a "typical" day, from the time the youngster gets up until he or she goes to bed.

7. *What are the client's (or parents') expectations regarding the diagnostic session?* The client often comes to a professional with an "agenda." The client may want the problem finally diagnosed after months of wondering about it. The parents may want a recommendation for treatment because they already know that their child has a communication problem. Sometimes parents have been agonizing over some hypothesis that has been advanced by a relative ("He's tongue-tied" or "We're afraid he is behind in his development") and their biggest concern is that the clinician address this issue. Whatever the client's expectations, do your best to determine what those expectations are and to provide some sort of resolution if possible.

A good diagnostic interview is characterized by a shifting of styles: objective questions that ask for specifics, subjective queries that deal with feelings and attitudes, and finally the indeterminate questions, like "Tell me more," that keep the respondent going.

Classically, the interviewer should start with the least anxiety-provoking queries, mostly objective questions that have high specificity, and then proceed to more subjective questions as the relationship develops. Quite often, however, we find it useful to employ a "funnel" sequence of inquiry during the course of a diagnostic interview—starting with broad, open-ended questions and then progressing to more specific or closed questions. Here is an example of a funnel sequence from a parent interview:

- How does Jimmy function in the family setting?
- How does he get along with his brothers and sisters?
- How does his older sister "help" him communicate?
- Can you describe an instance in which she talked for him?

The "inverted funnel" approach, proceeding from specific to general, is also useful. It is best to avoid the checklist or long series of "tunnel" questions that call for information on one level of specificity, all of which are asked in a similar style (e.g., "Did your child have earaches, fevers, head injury?").

THE PRESENTING STORY   Most persons who anticipate visiting a helping professional will have mentally rehearsed what they intend to say. Often you will have to contend with events that occurred prior to the session—the family car's failing to start, a burned breakfast, absence of a convenient parking place. A few words to reveal your understanding of the distracting antecedents will generally assist the respondent in shifting to the topic of the interview. In some cases, the client may even have a pseudoconversation with you while driving to the appointment. Think of the last time you visited your physician with a medical problem. While driving to the doctor's office, a person often rehearses how to describe his or her symptoms. We must allow this story to be unraveled, or the respondent will be left with a sense of frustration and lack of closure. A question such as "What seems to be the problem?" will permit the flow of conversation to begin. Remember that the client's description is how the *client* perceives the problem—it is the client's unique way of looking at the situation. The client's description may be grossly inaccurate, but you should hear it out; nothing turns a respondent off more quickly than for the interviewer to suggest by word or action that the respondent's views are silly or misguided. Sometimes the presenting story will become a motif that recurs again and again during the course of the interview.

This is generally a crucial point in an interview. The interviewee may cautiously extend a portion of himself or herself verbally, carefully scan the interviewer's response, and then decide whether or not to tell the whole story. Sometimes a respondent may even set up a straw man to see how the interviewer deals with it.

This is not the proper time to debate an issue with the client. The story can be accepted initially on the level of feeling, and later in the interview—when rapport is stronger—an issue can be discussed more fully. We feel very strongly that these initial stories, these primitive theories, should be respected as the best possible answer that clients have been able to come up with. It does not mean that you agree with a client's conclusions; it just means that you accept a client's judgment with understanding so you can form a basis for further communication.

Actually, the presenting information can be a very rich source of clinical hypotheses to be explored during the course of the interview. How do the client and parent present themselves—as long-suffering, anxious, diffident? How do they associate ideas or items of information sequentially? What priorities do they assign to issues they raise? Do they seem to be realistic in their expectations regarding the diagnostic session and treatment?

NONVERBAL MESSAGES   Respondents do not communicate by words alone, and the discerning clinician attends to body as well as oral language during an interview. As a matter of fact, some observers suggest that a large portion of the total message—particularly messages involving strong feelings—is carried by nonverbal cues. However, resist the urge to interpret a client's every twitch; each instance of nonverbal behavior should be related to the *content* of the oral message and to the *context* in which it occurs.

> If a parent leaves her coat on during an interview it may mean she feels vulnerable and the garment provides a bit of protective armor. It may also mean that she has a spot on her dress, or that all the hangers in the waiting room were taken again by forgetful students, or that the room is chilly. However, if she shifts her chair away from the clinician, sits with her arms and legs tightly crossed, avoids eye contact, and responds to questions with one-word answers, then it may be possible that she is defensive and guarded in the clinical setting.

The issue here is to avoid making one item of nonverbal behavior the sole basis for interpretation; be on the lookout for patterns. The most important thing to look for may be lack of congruence between the respondent's verbal and nonverbal messages; in cases where the two conflict, body language is generally a more accurate indicator of how a person feels about an issue.

THINGS TO AVOID IN THE INTERVIEW   Beginning interviewers commit several common errors. The list that follows is not meant to be exhaustive, but it does cover the most glaring mistakes.

1. *Avoid questions that may be answered by a simple "Yes" or "No."* Open-ended questions produce longer responses and more detailed information.

2. *Avoid phrasing questions in such a way that they inhibit freedom of response.* Do not say, "You don't have any difficulty with ringing in your ears, do you?" or "You don't tell Billy to stop and start over again, do you?" Such leading questions are not effective interviewing. The beginning interviewer tends to be anxious about asking open-ended questions. The interviewer is afraid that silence will result and that this will damage his relationship with the client. So the interviewer will ask an open-ended question and then close it: for example, "How do you feel about David's stuttering? Does it bother you?" Leave it open! Although open-end questions consume more time and may produce some rambling and irrelevant responses, there are many advantages to recommend their use.

Try also to avoid abrupt shifts in your line of questioning. For example, if you are exploring the client's feelings or attitudes on a particular issue (subjective questions), don't suddenly ask a question on a different topic. Inexperienced interviewers tend to jump around. If you are interested in learning about a child's play, ask all your play questions together. Do not skip around from play to language to book reading to medical history, and so on.

3. *Avoid talking too much.* This is perhaps the most common mistake of the beginning interviewer, who feels that every pause must be filled with verbiage. It is much better to rephrase what the respondent has said or make some comment like "I see," "Tell me more," or "Anything else?" Sometimes a smile and an understanding nod are effective when it seems that the client has more to say but needs some silent time to conjure it up. If there is a positive attitude—a good rapport—and if the client feels comfortable in the situation, then these encouragements increase the length of the response. If the topic or situation is neutral, these comments tend to expand the message.

4. *Avoid concentrating on physical symptoms and etiological factors to the exclusion of the client's feelings and attitudes.* There is a little bit of physician in all of us; we yearn to play the role of omniscient healer. The interviewer should remember to distinguish between items of information that are simply interesting and background information that is really important.

5. *Avoid providing information too soon.* There will be plenty of time to clear up misconceptions later in the interview. The surest way to cut off the flow of information is to stop a parent, for instance, after he says, "I just tell Michael to stop, take a deep breath, and start all over again," and counsel him on the proper responses to nonfluency.

6. *Avoid qualifying and hemming and hawing when asking questions.* Ask them in a straightforward fashion and maintain eye contact. Rather than asking, "Did you find that, well, you know, when you were, uh, shall we say . . . with child, did you experience any untoward conditions?" say, "Did anything unusual happen during your pregnancy?" Instead of inquiring, "Did you discover, hmm, I mean, well, after your father, uh, passed away, did your stuttering problem increase?" say, "What impact did your father's death have on your speech?"

7. *Avoid negativistic or moralistic responses, verbal or nonverbal, to the client's statements.* Avoid even the response "Good" since it implies a value judgment. The flow of information will stop rapidly and the relationship will be impaired severely if the individual senses that we find him or his behavior distasteful. We do not have to subscribe to a person's values or code of behavior for us to show compassion for and understanding of his or her situation. Use inquiries that begin with "Why . . .?" very sparingly because beginning a question with the word *why* is often perceived as a challenge or threat; this way of questioning is too reminiscent of disciplinary sessions ("Why were you late for class?" "Why can't you behave properly?"). In a clinical setting we must not let our values obscure our perception of the client's frame of reference. An interview is not the place to push the clinician's personal points of view. We had a student clinician who once talked about her political views during a diagnostic interview. This can immediately alienate certain clients. Another student wore a button that said, "Jesus is the answer," which certainly would not have been the case for her Jewish or Muslim clients.

8. *When the client causes the interview to wander, avoid abrupt transitions to bring it back to the point.* Most of those whom you will interview have had little experience in directed, orderly conversation. They tend to follow chance associations and wander far afield. The experienced interviewer has the ability to make smooth transitions. How does one go about getting the interview back on track? The best way is by building a bridge to the respondent's previous statements: for example, "That's interesting, Mrs. Davis, maybe we can come back to that in a little while. Now earlier you were mentioning that your child's loss of hearing occurred suddenly. . . ." The goal here is to use respondent antecedents—things that the person has said earlier in the interview.

9. *Avoid allowing the interview to produce only superficial answers.* We need ways to get deeper, more significant responses from our clients. There are several interviewing devices, termed *probes,* that the clinician will find helpful.

Crosshatch, or *interlocking,* questions are useful when we need to elicit more detail about a topic that has been glossed over. Often there are discrepancies that must be resolved. Essentially, the way to go about this is to ask the same thing in different ways and at different points during the interview. For instance, the father of a young child who stuttered responded in a superficial manner to our query about his relationship with the child. He assured us that he had a "loving relationship" with his son and then complained at length about his working conditions. Later in the interview when we asked him to describe the sorts of things he did with the child, he was unable to mention a single one. We don't mean to imply that the clinician should attempt to catch the client lying and then demand an explanation. The clinician must examine discrepancies, however, in order to enhance understanding of the problem, since such discrepancies could have a significant effect on the mode of treatment.

Pauses can be very helpful. When there is a lull in the interview, it may mean simply that the client has exhausted his or her store of information, that a memory barrier has prevented further recall, or that he or she senses lack of understanding by the clinician. It can also mean, however, that a sensitive area has been touched upon. Do not feel that pauses harm the interview. Much significant information can be forthcoming if we keep quiet and indicate with a smile or a nod that we expect more.

The *summary probe* is one of the best ways to keep the interview moving smoothly. The clinician summarizes periodically what the client has said, ending perhaps with a request for clarification or further information. Incidentally, this procedure also demonstrates to the interviewee that the interviewer is indeed trying to understand the former's problem. We generally use "min-isummary probes"—echo questions—all the way through an interview:

RESPONDENT: After my husband's stroke, my whole world collapsed.

INTERVIEWER: You were overwhelmed by the sudden change in your life.

RESPONDENT: Yes, one day he was happily planning our trip to Sanibel Island . . . and then, in just a moment, he was paralyzed and couldn't talk. Now all our plans are up in the air . . . the new car, the checking account, he took care of all that.

The *stumbling probe* is a variation of the summary probe; we have found it helpful, especially with the reticent respondent. The interviewer rephrases a portion of the respondent's communication and then, attempting to interpret or comment upon it, the interviewer pretends to halt or stumble. For example, when interviewing the mother of a child allegedly beginning to stutter, the clinician might say: "Now, you were saying that Bruce first started to repeat and hesitate after he caught his finger in the car door. Under these conditions, it would be natural for you to . . . uh . . ." The respondent's need for closure may precipitate significant information and, perhaps more important, significant insights.

Finally, there is the *assuming probe.* If the client has avoided an important area, leaving much unsaid regarding the speech or hearing problem and what it means to him or her, then it is up to the interviewer to bring this out. One adolescent boy, who had been vehemently denying that his stuttering bothered him, unburdened himself when we said, "It bothers you so much that you don't want anybody to know, do you?"

10. *Avoid letting the client reveal too much in one interview.* Sometimes a beginning interviewer makes the mistake of trying to get everything in one sitting. The client, sensing perhaps that this is the first person who really understands him or her, may want to provide more personal details than are necessary. Later, however, the individual will feel embarrassed and foolish, perhaps even exposed and guilty at revealing so much to a comparative stranger.

11. *Avoid trusting to memory.* Record the information as the interview progresses. Tell the client that you will take some notes during the interview so that you can plan the treatment program more effectively and make recommendations for other services. Such note taking, or even recording devices, are rarely questioned. Indeed, we have found that clients expect you to write down some of the information they are giving you; they doubt that you would be able to remember all of their answers. You obviously would lose your relationship, however, if you scribbled furiously while the client was revealing some sensitive information. It is axiomatic that the respondent's confidence will be respected, but we have mixed feelings about mentioning this explicitly to the client. The clinician's manner should suggest that all information received is to be held strictly confidential.

Prepare a report of the interview as soon as possible. Commit your observations to paper while the encounter with the respondent is still fresh in your mind (see Chapter 13 for information on writing reports).

Goal Two: Give Information

No one likes uncertainty. Ironically, all too frequently the information, if not supplied by the professional worker, will come distorted from other sources. We can do an admirable job on our evaluation, but if we drop the ball on communicating the results to our client, we have not been successful. When not correctly informed, parents become misinformed, and this misinformation leads to confusion, misunderstanding, and further compounding on the problem. It is our responsibility, therefore, to provide accurate, unemotional, objective information of the status of the individual's problem. This forwarding of information is generally accomplished during the postdiagnostic conference.

Summarize the findings of the clinical examination in simple, nontechnical language, using common terms compatible with the client's background. We prefer to commence, if possible, with results that show a client's area of normal functioning, to review findings that indicate what is good before describing deficiencies. Relate comments to normative values whenever possible. Clarify and help the respondent to ask questions by using examples and simple analogies. If you are in doubt concerning the client's understanding of the diagnostic material (clients will rarely ask if they don't understand), talk more slowly, employ longer descriptions, and use many examples and more redundant language. Providing information to clients who are bilingual or from a culture different from that of the clinician can be a challenge and is discussed in more detail in Chapter 12.

THE QUESTIONS CLIENTS ASK   An interview is much more than a clinician's posing questions and recording the client's answers. It is an important forum for *exchange*—a reflexive, dynamic experience of sharing between the diagnostician and the informant. Indeed, we find that a client—especially a parent of a young child being evaluated—frequently is eager to probe the clinician's expertise. But often the questions the clinician asks may have a hidden meaning or purpose. The clinician must evaluate the informant's inquiries and determine, What is the person *really* asking? Is there an unstated concern behind the questions? Luterman (1979) divides the questions clients ask into three categories: *content, opinion,* and *affect.* We will describe and illustrate these three types of inquiries with excerpts from an initial interview with the mother of a 3-year-old child brought to the clinic because she was concerned that her child was beginning to stutter.

1. *Questions Dealing with Information or Content.*   In this instance, the client seeks an informative or factual response from the clinician. The inquiry usually takes the form, "I want to know about something, and I hope you have the right information."

MRS. BELL:	The type of choppy speech [disfluency] Jesse has—is it common among children his age?
CLINICIAN:	It sure is. Most children between the ages of two-and-a-half and five do a lot of repeating and hesitating.

2. *Questions with Predetermined Opinions.*   Here the client has an opinion regarding a particular subject and wants to determine if the clinician agrees with it. The clinician must be careful not to merely demolish the client's opinion until the clinician understands *why* and *how strongly* the client holds it.

MRS. BELL:	Um, on TV a couple of times, I've seen a demonstration of the airflow technique for stuttering. What do you think of it?
CLINICIAN:	Those demonstrations are very dramatic, aren't they? What's your impression of the technique as it applies to Jesse?

3. *Questions That Are a "Faint Knocking on the Door."*   In this case, the client is not asking for information or to determine the clinician's opinion, but rather for emotional support and reassurance. The question conceals a feeling that the client either is unaware of or is reluctant to reveal.

> MRS. BELL: Do you think my divorce and remarriage had anything to do with Jesse's speech problem?
>
> CLINICIAN: It's pretty common for parents to feel guilty about something they might have done to cause their child to begin stuttering.

You may have already detected a flaw in the triad: On the surface, each question posed by Mrs. Bell could be classified in any of the three categories. How does a clinician know *what* the client means? The clinician doesn't know in every case, but he or she tries to determine the purpose of a question by scrutinizing *how* a client asks it—by vocal inflection and body language—and by examining the context in which the inquiry appears. Interestingly, as long as the clinician is *trying to understand,* a client will not be alienated by an inaccurate interpretation.

In our experience, beginning clinicians, probably because the bulk of their training focuses on information, do a good job of responding to content questions. However, many clinicians in training find it difficult to respond appropriately to a client's expression of emotion.

Avoid superficial statements of reassurance. The client's anxiety and uncertainty will be better relieved once he or she begins to understand his or her particular speech problem; the best antidote to fear and uncertainty is knowledge. Do not use terms or suggest consequences that will precipitate more stress for the client. Do not communicate any negative expectations regarding the outcome of therapy to the client. It is possible that such statements could influence the client's performance in treatment.

Following are six basic principles, addressed to the beginning clinician, for imparting information to clients that we have found useful:

1. Emotional confusion may, and often does, inhibit the client's ability to understand cognitively what you are trying to say. Just because you have once reviewed the steps of therapy is no reason to expect that their importance will be grasped.
2. Refrain from being didactic; do not lecture your clients. Focus on sharing options rather than giving advice.
3. Use simple language with many examples and illustrations. If you must err, err in the direction of being too simple rather than too complex. And repeat, repeat, repeat the important points—rephrasing each time.
4. Try to provide something that the client—especially a parent—can do. Action reduces the feelings of futility and anxiety. The activity should be direct and simple and should require some kind of reporting to the clinician.
5. Say what needs to be said pleasantly—but frankly. Do not avoid saying something that must be said on the assumption that the client cannot take it or that you will be rejected. People often display an amazing reserve of courage in difficult situations.
6. Remember, however, that the one who finally communicates what the client may have been dreading to hear is often hated and maligned. If you are the first to say the feared words, you may become the focus for all the hostile, negative feelings thus aroused. As a professional worker, you will have to be strong enough to be the lightning rod for these emotions.

Clients and parents expect to receive help from the clinician but often will resist change. No matter how maladaptive a client's behavior may seem from an objective point of view, it represents the client's best solution. In fact, the client will often resist attempts to alter his or her equilibrium, precarious as it may appear to others. Change is stressful; diagnosis and treatment imply change; therefore, assessment and therapy are stressful.

We must listen for two aspects of our clients' utterances: a *cognitive* aspect (the content) and an *affective* aspect (the feelings). In order for genuine understanding to take place, both aspects must be included in the interviewer's response to the client's statement. If you are successful in crystallizing both aspects of your response, you provide an *interchangeable base* that allows the interview to move forward to levels of helping that involve direct action. Here are some examples taken from diagnostic interviews:

CLIENT: (in response to a query regarding his marital status): No, I'm single. . . . Who would want to marry someone who stutters like me?

CLINICIAN: You feel rejected because of your speech problem, is that right?

PARENT: We tried to be good parents, we really did . . . but somehow we messed up in helping Peter learn to talk.

CLINICIAN: You feel a sense of failure, perhaps even guilt, that your child has a speech problem.

CLIENT: I stutter so badly that life is worthless. . . . I can't get a job. . . . The business of living just doesn't seem to meet expenses.

CLINICIAN: You feel thwarted and frustrated by your speech problem. Sometimes you wonder if you can go on.

Note the clinician's responses carefully. The clinician does not simply repeat the client's comment but attempts to restate it in clarified form. Observe that the interviewer used the second-person singular "you" in referring to the client's affect. Feelings are commonly stated first, since they are more important than content. We sometimes add a tag question ("Is that right?") to check on the client's intake of our responses.

Goal Three: Provide Release and Support

The clinician does not, of course, wait until the end of the interview to provide release for the frustrations and fears of the client. Most of the parts of the interview already discussed will serve this purpose. By helping the client talk out his or her problems, the clinician is providing an excellent escape for pent-up feelings. We maintain that our purpose is not just to remove discomfort but also to promote a state of comfort and well-being.

More than advice is needed during interviews for the purpose of helping a client take some specific action or move in a particular direction. The client needs help in sorting out confusing choices. To support a respondent's real strengths, we need to make it clear that we understand what the situation means to him or her and that we uncritically sympathize with his or her feelings and attitudes. We can restore the client's self-esteem and ability to function more appropriately if we convey our interest in him or her as a person and our solid acceptance of the client's importance.

There is an unfortunate tradition of "sweetness and light" in client counseling. A person has a problem. The person is sad and depressed, and we try to cheer that person up. Sometimes this degenerates into a debate, with the interviewer attempting to persuade the person not to feel miserable. A person who feels depressed, anxious, and fearful does not want to count his or her blessings. That person wants you to feel miserable, too, and to share and identify with him or her on the same level. Thus, you are given a basis for communication with the person. Start where he or she is, accept it as the proper place to start, and agree that it is a sad state of affairs that would make anyone sad and depressed. Then, using this bond of identification, which becomes a basis for communication, you can assist in solving the problem. The main ingredient is *empathy,* the capacity to identify with another's feelings and actions. The best way to demonstrate an attempt to understand a client's point of view is by listening creatively. In our judgment, of all the skills inherent in effective interviewing, the most important is the ability to listen carefully and empathically. This skill can be learned, although beginning clinicians find it difficult to employ remarks that facilitate a client's expression of feelings.

How does one handle emotional scenes? They are bound to arise at some point in your interviewing experience. Some clinicians excuse themselves from the room and allow the respondent to recover his or her dignity alone. Others try to change the subject to something less emotional. Both of these approaches may, with certain clients, give the impression that you are rejecting their feelings. It is more effective to indicate understanding of the feelings that are being expressed and accept them as natural human reactions: for example, "That's okay to let it come out, Mrs. Moody. You have been holding it back too long. Sometimes it helps to get it out in the open."

Not all clients seen by the speech clinician will need or even want extensive supportive interviewing. In some cases, the procedures discussed here would be grossly inappropriate. Visualize an interview as ranging along a continuum from affective concern, such as feelings and attitudes, to objective matters, such as goals and advice. Some respondents simply need objective information so that they can take over and modify their behavior. The clinician's role in some interviews may consist of simply listening to and supporting a client. A good relationship is a *necessary* but not a *sufficient* condition for good interviewing. Although it may sound trite, it is true that the secret of care *of* a client is caring *for* the client. The sense of being understood by a helping professional is a powerful stimulant to the client's growth.

USING INTERVIEWING SKILLS BEYOND THE DIAGNOSTIC EVALUATION

As we mentioned in Chapter 1, evaluation is not confined to a 2-hour block of time in a university or a 1-hour session in a school district. The speech-language pathologist constantly gathers data on clients as treatment progresses in order to determine if the remediation is successful or if goals should be adjusted. In many types of cases seen by the SLP the treatment plan is jointly formulated by the clinician, parents or family members, and other professionals. In such instances, the amount of information gathered in the diagnostic evaluation is not sufficient to generate a meaningful treatment plan that takes into account both the clinician's and the family's perspectives. Thus, more extensive interviewing is necessary to discover information on family strengths, concerns, and needs. More interviewing of related professionals is needed to determine how the client is performing in a variety of contexts. We will briefly illustrate this notion with two popular clinical techniques.

1. *Ethnographic Interviewing.* Especially in cases where the SLP is working with infants, toddlers, and preschool children, the law requires that families be an integral part of treatment planning and monitoring. In fact, the clinician, along with other professionals and the family, must generate an Individualized Family Service Plan (IFSP) that states specific information related to the treatment program (see Chapter 4 for more details). Most authorities in early child language recommend an approach known as ethnographic interviewing

(Nelson, 2010). In this type of interview, the focus is on the parent and the goal is to obtain the parent's perspective on the problems, goals, and approaches used in treatment. The clinician asks both specific and broad-based questions that are not meant to necessarily lead the parent, but just to guide the conversation. The goal is to let the parent set the direction of the interview toward what is important to him or her, and ideally the parent will do most of the talking with encouragement and structure from the clinician. This type of in-depth interview is used to effectively understand the family situation and its goals and aspirations for the child with a communication disorder. Parents are encouraged to tell the clinician what goals are most important to them and which ones they would like to see incorporated first into the remediation plan. If you consider the wealth and depth of possible information to gather in such a case it should be no surprise that ethnographic interviews take hours of conversation to complete effectively.

2. ***Curriculum-Based Assessment.*** In cases where a school-age student is being treated for a language disorder, there are many considerations to planning therapy that go beyond the diagnostic evaluation. Curriculum-based assessment is concerned with finding out the demands placed on a child by the educational environment in which he or she must use language and literacy skills (Nelson, 2010; Paul, 2007). In order to determine the types of communication, language, and literacy skills necessary to compete in the classroom environment, the SLP must interview teachers and examine curricular materials. This, again, requires conversation with other professionals to design treatment programs and monitor progress/generalization of the skills focused upon in therapy.

Hopefully, you can see that interviewing never stops from the beginning to the end of our clinical relationships. The same types of skills that we use in our initial intake interview are used again or modified as we gather and disseminate information through therapy and dismissal. The more practice and experience in talking with families and clients you can obtain, the better your clinical skills will become.

IMPROVING INTERVIEWING SKILLS

We hope the material in this chapter will be useful to students majoring in clinical speech pathology and to our colleagues working in various settings. However, no one ever became proficient in interviewing solely by reading about it. Nor, it seems, are interviewing skills enhanced by increasing knowledge about communication disorders. It took us many years of constant searching and experimenting to evolve the interviewing approach presented here. And, with the indulgence of our clients and many long-suffering parents, we continue to explore for better ways.

We have included a series of activities and projects for your own practice. Let them serve as the beginning steps in a continual learning effort toward improved interviewing. You will find that the time devoted to such training exercises is well spent. Now, consider these steps on how to improve your interviewing skills:

1. ***Read widely from a variety of sources.*** Find out what people are like by reading in sociology, psychology, anthropology, and philosophy. This is, of course, a lifetime project, which we feel is delightful since there is always a new frontier, an open horizon toward which we can set our sails.

2. ***Listen to all sorts of people.*** Listen to their dreams, their rationalizations, their insights—or lack of them—and their gripes. Get acquainted with the way people think and talk by following the example of others (Least Heat-Moon, 1982; Terkel, 1980, 1986, 1993, 2001).

3. *Form small heterogeneous groups of students majoring in speech pathology and audiology.* Conduct some sensitivity and values clarification training, particularly as it relates to your self-concept, your assets and liabilities, your responses to people, and your relationship with your own parents and other older adults (Kaplan & Dreyer, 1974). In order to provide assistance to others, we must know our own foibles and potential blind spots and have them under reasonable control.

4. *Role-play to prepare for interviewing.* Set up several typical interview situations in front of a class and play, for example, the roles of the reluctant parent, the spouse of a patient with aphasia, or a hostile father. Discuss the interaction and replay the situations with others assuming the roles. Write out interview purposes prior to the role-playing and determine, or have the class determine, how effectively the interviewer accomplished avowed purposes. Whenever the viewers feel that the interview went wrong or the responses were ineffective, see how many different ways the interview could have been handled. This builds up the beginning interviewer's repertoire of adaptive responses. You can do a surprising amount of intrapersonal role-playing in your spare time. While we are waiting for a class to begin or for a light to change, we frequently imagine ourselves in various interviewing situations and then explore alternate statements, probes, and so forth.

5. *Record your first few interviews, then analyze them carefully with your clinical supervisor or a colleague.* Finally, we suggest you evaluate your diagnostic interviews by using the Checklist of Interviewing Competencies (Figure 2.2). Obviously, no beginning clinician will remember, let alone exhibit, all the skills delineated in the checklist; practice only a few at a time, and provide constructive feedback for each other.

We would like to end this chapter with a challenge: Utilize the interviewing approach delineated above, find the errors, the things that just don't work for you, and then develop your own methods. We have given you the foundation blocks. Can you use them to make stepping-stones?

Interviewer: _____   Date: _____

Client/Respondent: _____

I. *Orienting the Respondent*
   A. Attends to comfort (coats, seating, and so on)
   B. Engages in appropriate "flow" talk
   C. Explains purposes, procedures
   D. Structures roles
II. *Engendering Communication*
   A. Attending behaviors (demonstration receptiveness)
      1. Relaxed, natural posture
      2. Appropriate eye contact
      3. Responses that follow the client's comments (restating, overlapping the client's message)
   B. Open invitation to share (open-ended questions)
   C. Nondistracting encouragement to continue talking
      1. Verbal ("Yes," "I see," and the like)
      2. Nonverbal (nodding, shifting posture toward client)
   D. Obtains an overview of the presenting problem

FIGURE 2.2 Checklist of interviewing competencies.

Note: This checklist is designed to help monitor the performance of beginning interviewers. It can be used as a self-rating device or a format for supervisory feedback.

III. *Use of Questions and Recording*
    A. Orderly, sequential questions
    B. Nondistracting note taking
IV. *Active Listening*
    A. Reflects feelings (empathic statements)
        1. Matches affect
        2. Matches content
    B. Periodic summarizing of affect and content message
V. *Monitoring Nonverbal Clues*
    A. The diagnostician's
    B. The respondent's
VI. *Skills in Presenting Information*
    A. Transmission of information
        1. Content
        2. Style and language
    B. Responds to questions appropriately
    C. Appropriate use of humor, "flow" talk
VII. *Closing the Interview*
    A. Summary, review of findings
    B. Recommendations
    C. Supportive comments
VIII. *Analysis of Information*
    A. Major themes in the client's presentation, association of ideas, inconsistencies and omissions
    B. Descriptive report

FIGURE 2.2   *(continued)*

Psychometric Considerations in Diagnosis and Evaluation

Let us interest you in purchasing a standardized test to use in assessing communication disorders. It has the following characteristics:

1. Test administrators have trouble agreeing on whether a response on the test is correct or not.
2. Clients seem to perform differently on the test each time they take it.
3. The test really does not focus on the aspects of communication that are relevant to treatment or diagnostic decision making.
4. The test manual is vague about how to administer the instrument and how to interpret the results.
5. The test does not really examine the true process that you are attempting to assess.
6. The test was normed on 200 normal, white children from Idaho.
7. The test does not adequately discriminate between clients with disorders and those who have none.

No one in their right mind would buy the instrument described above because it would provide little valid and reliable information to use in assessment. Do tests in communication disorders ever have this many shortcomings? Unfortunately, *many* formal tests in our field suffer from the problems listed above (Huang, Hopkins, & Nippold, 1997; McCauley & Swisher, 1984a, 1984b; McFadden, 1996; Muma, 1983, 1984, 1986, 2002; Muma, Lubinski, & Pierce, 1982; Plante & Vance, 1994; Spaulding, Plante, & Farinella, 2006)! The authors of these tests no doubt begin with the notion of designing a useful instrument; however, when conceptual and psychometric limitations manifest themselves, the test designer is typically reluctant to scrap the whole enterprise. Usually, the test is submitted, warts and all, to a publisher because, even though it suffers from inadequacies, it represents a significant amount of work in its development. It is therefore up to the consumer carefully to evaluate any instrument in terms of psychometric adequacy before purchasing it. We must become educated in evaluating any instruments that we buy, not only because purchasing an inadequate test is a waste of our money but, more important, a waste of our time. We have just mentioned the effects of buying and using inadequate tests on the clinician, but it also affects our clients, since they must spend money paying for the administration of these tests and also must invest their time to take the tests. In addition, a client can be misdiagnosed, mislabeled, and mistreated on the basis of testing with psychometrically poor instruments. One can readily see that psychometric adequacy of standardized tests is a significant issue and one that we must deal with in a textbook on diagnosis and evaluation.

It is important to note that it is not only standardized instruments that require some measure of psychometric adequacy. Although many clinicians associate psychometric principles only with standardized, norm-referenced tests, it is the feeling of the present authors that most of the informal or descriptive measures that we use in communication disorders are also susceptible to considerable error. Just because we are not using a standardized test does not relieve us of the responsibility of checking our validity and reliability. The same psychometric rigor applied to standardized examinations could easily be applied to our informal evaluation procedures (Hegde, 1987). Informal measures can clearly vary in the degree to which they are valid and reliable. Validity is the degree to which a procedure actually measures what it purports to measure. Validity can be compromised in both formal or informal procedures. For instance, we can ask a person with velopharyngeal incompetency to blow a pinwheel, and we can time how long it spins to get an indication of velopharyngeal closure. This measure may have good reliability in that two clinicians could time the pinwheel with a stopwatch and agree on how long the wheel spins. Perhaps the client could even be reliable in terms of blowing the wheel in a similar fashion over several trials and making the wheel spin a fairly consistent length of time each trial. The problem, however, is validity. We know that blowing a pinwheel may not relate at all to the ability to maintain velopharyngeal closure during speech production. Reliability is useless if the measure being taken is not valid.

There are many potential problems with reliability as well with the use of informal measures. For instance, many behaviors that we observe, count, or time are often not clearly defined, and this imprecision contributes to a lack of reliability. In order to have good agreement, two examiners would have to be looking for the same behavior and coding it in a similar manner. The difficult aspect of informal assessment is that many behaviors that we examine are transient (phonemes, disfluencies, facial grimaces, laryngeal tension, slight head jerks, etc.), while others may be ill defined and subjective (pitch changes, topic changes, cohesive adequacy, voice quality changes, stress alterations, intelligibility, severity, etc.). In research reports, it is incumbent on the investigator to provide evidence that measurements of behaviors studied are both valid and reliable. Clinicians must devote the same attention to these issues if they use informal measures so that these measures can be replicated over time as indications of treatment progress. Without validity and reliability, informal measures are nothing more than the "artsy," subjective judgments of one person that may tell us little about client performance.

COMMON TYPES OF TESTS

Most textbooks on psychometric issues focus on norm-referenced tests. Norm-referenced tests also are called standardized tests or formal tests, depending on the designer's preference. Just because a test is standardized, however, does not mean that it is norm referenced. Standardization may imply only that the *procedures* for test administration are standard, not that norms are provided with the instrument. In developing norm-referenced tests, the designers have created some tasks they feel are relevant (valid) and have administered the instrument to large groups of subjects who hopefully represent the population on whom the test is to be used. From these large-scale administrations, the designers are able to calculate normative data that reflect the performance of the large sample. When an individual is given the test, his or her score is compared to the performance of the normative sample and it is determined how this person performed relative to the large group. The purpose of norm-referenced tests is to determine if an individual obtains a score similar to the group average or, if not, how far away from average the score is. Generally, if the individual scored within 1.5 to 2 standard deviations above or below the mean, he or she is said to reflect performance within "normal limits." If the score was more than 2 standard deviations above or below the mean, the performance is said to be exceptional, since only about 5% of the normative population scored in a similar manner. Thus, norm-referenced tests have the major purpose of determining if there is a problem, or a significant enough difference from standard performance to warrant concern with regard to normalcy. We will have more to say in a later section regarding some qualifications that must be taken into account when considering this purpose of standardized tests.

The other type of test typically mentioned in psychometric texts is the criterion-referenced instrument. Criterion-referenced examinations also appear under other terminologies such as mastery testing, domain-referenced testing, objectives-referenced testing, and competency-based testing. These measurements are designed to distinguish specific levels of client performance in a clearly specified domain. The client's performance can be interpreted using raw scores because the goal is to determine performance in relation to a particular performance standard instead of determining how an individual scores in relation to a normative group. Functional outcomes are often criterion-referenced behaviors that describe what a person can do after treatment that he or she could not do prior to intervention. We mentioned functional outcomes in Chapter 1 when we discussed the initiatives of ASHA and the World Health Organization in developing measures that reflect patient progress in "real world" activities.

The criterion-referenced test serves a different purpose compared to a norm-referenced instrument. It is clearly more related to defining specific skills in assessment and treatment and emphasizes individual performance, while the norm-referenced tests focus on group similarity (Muma, 1973b). McCauley (1996) provides guidelines for the evaluation, selection, and development of informal criterion-referenced measures in communication disorders. Unfortunately, there are precious few criterion-referenced measures in our field. Current emphases on evidence-based practice and functional outcome measures will promote the development of more criterion-referenced tests in the near future. Most of our formal instruments are norm-referenced, so the focus of the rest of the chapter will be on these types of tests.

VALIDITY: THE FOUNDATION OF THE TEST OR MEASURE

As we mentioned, a test can be reliable but may lack validity. Validity basically refers to the extent to which a test measures what it sets out to measure. Validity is highly related to the purpose for which the test is used, and a particular test can be valid for one purpose and invalid for another (Plante, 1996). If we say we are going to measure a child's language comprehension, we hopefully select a test that can accomplish this goal. If the test is measuring something other than the child's language comprehension, then the test is invalid. So many of the behaviors we assess in communication disorders are extremely complex and involve multiple systems. Language, for example, has many areas (semantics, syntax, morphology, phonology, pragmatics), and it is influenced by other systems (cognitive, social, psychological, neurolinguistic, etc.). If we develop a test of "language ability" that can be administered and scored in 20 minutes, and this test has the child imitate, name pictures, and point to photographs, we have not really looked at language ability completely. We have taken a few tasks and we are willing to make judgments about a very complex linguistic system based on the child's ability to perform these operations, which are totally unnatural and unrelated to normal language use. This is tantamount to a cardiologist's making a clinical judgment about a significant heart condition only by feeling the patient's pulse. Such a judgment is just not valid, especially when we have the technology available to do a thorough evaluation of heart function by using EKG and other measures. The major point here is that without validity we are fooling ourselves as we look at complex behaviors. Even if we can demonstrate that the items on the test are reliable, it does not matter. We have only developed a reliable way of looking at "garbage." This point is made painfully clear by several authors who raise ethical concerns about the administration of tests that lack validity (Messick, 1980; Muma, 1984). If we use such tests, we not only waste time and money, but we can arrive at erroneous judgments about our clients, resulting in incorrect goal selection or, worse, placement in inappropriate programs.

Classically, discussions of validity focus on three types: construct, content, and criterion-related validity. Construct validity is "the degree to which a test measures the theoretical construct it is intended to measure" (Anastasi, 1976, p. 151). To obtain this type of validity "the test author must rely on indirect evidence and inference" (Salvia & Ysseldyke, 1981, p. 108). Thus, a test in any area of communication disorders must ideally reflect the underlying construct it is attempting to assess. A second type of validity is content validity. Typically, content validity is derived by "a careful examination of the content of a test. Such an examination is judgmental in nature and requires a clear definition of what the content should be. Content validity is established by examining three factors: the appropriateness of the types of items included, the completeness of the item sample, and the way in which the items assess the content" (Salvia & Ysseldyke, 1981, p. 102). Typically, expert judges are included to examine the content of the test in order to make the determination of content validity.

A final type of validity is criterion-related. There are two types of criterion-related validity. First, concurrent validity is a measure of how an individual's current score on one instrument can be used to make an estimate of his or her current score on some other criterion measure, typically another test in a related area. Predictive validity is a measure of how an individual's current score on one instrument can estimate scoring on a criterion measure taken at a later time. A critical variable, however, is the validity and reliability of the criterion measure selected for use in criterion-related validity. The instrument you design must be valid, and so must the criterion measure.

The three types of validity mentioned above would ideally be used in concert to determine the overall validity of a test instrument. There is, however, a tendency among some test designers to believe that only one or two types of validity are required to validate an instrument and that perhaps the three types of validity are equally powerful and thus interchangeable. This is *not* the case. The most potent type of validity is construct validity. Construct validity is viewed by most authorities as the *keystone* of test development (Messick, 1975, 1980; Muma, 1985). Muma (2002) provides an excellent summary of construct validity and reviews many contemporary language tests showing that most of these instruments are found lacking in construct validity. We agree that this is a serious problem with the standardized tests (especially in language and phonology) in our field. This once again shows that there is no substitute for a thorough analysis of real communication in assessment. We have separated this section on validity from the rest of the psychometric background in this chapter and discuss it first because it is probably the most important issue in psychometric adequacy. It does not matter how popular a test is, how easy it is to administer, or how much statistical hocus-pocus is found in the examiner's manual. If the test lacks validity, it is nothing more than a wasteful, empty exercise.

RELIABILITY

The notion of reliability is critical to formal as well as informal measures. If one were to develop a valid norm-referenced test or informal measure, it would be useless if the test developer could not demonstrate that different examiners could use it with similar facility and that clients performed consistently from one occasion to another. Several types of reliability are classically discussed.

1. *Interjudge Reliability.* This term refers to the agreement of two independent judges on the occurrence and type of responses performed by a client. Almost every clinician has had the experience of asking another SLP to take a look at a difficult case. We question our abilities to judge aberrant vocal qualities and pitches. We often want another opinion on a child's intelligibility or pragmatic abilities. Clients who stutter often present many complex avoidances and timing devices that we ask our peers to scrutinize, just to make sure we are on the right track. Sometimes, even in standardized tests, we ask the opinions of others to check some arbitrary scoring convention that we have used because the manual did not tell us what to do in enough detail. All of these factors have to do with interjudge reliability.

The types of responses that we ask children and adults to perform in diagnosis and evaluation tasks are many and varied. Some responses are relatively straightforward and easily agreed upon by two independent judges. For example, if we ask a client to point to one of four pictures in response to an auditory model (e.g., "Point to 'running'"), most judges would agree on the correctness of the client's response. Other types of responding may not be quite as clear to judges. For instance, judges may not be able to agree on the occurrence of a distorted /s/ or /r/ phoneme.

Judges may have difficulty determining whether a response was correct if the client initially makes the wrong response and then self-corrects it. Does the test provide guidelines for examiners in terms of accepting a self-corrected response as "correct"? In informal tasks, it is often difficult for judges to agree on certain behaviors, such as the amount of time spent in symbolic play. An adequate operational definition of symbolic play would be necessary, and criteria for when such play begins and ends would be required, if two judges are to agree on time sampling of behavior. Thus, we can see that the behaviors that judges must agree upon vary in terms of their observability, definition, and subjectivity. If judges cannot agree on what they are observing, then the test or procedure is unreliable. There are some obvious contributing factors that decrease interjudge reliability:

- ***Incomplete or Ambiguous Definitions.*** If a behavior is to be counted, timed, observed, or interpreted, there must be an adequate definition of the behavior so that independent judges can agree on behavioral occurrences. For example, if one goal of treatment is to reduce behavior problems in a client with language impairment, the measurement of this construct (behavior problem) must be guided by a specific definition. Do behavior problems include only tantrums, or do actions such as pushing the materials away, whining, repetitive vocalizations, and refusal to participate in tasks also constitute behavior problems? One can readily see that two examiners could experience major disagreement on this measure unless the definition was quite precise. The two judges need to know what to count or time and what behaviors to exclude from the concept of behavior problems. Sometimes the operational definition selected by an examiner may not be universally agreed upon, and this may affect the *validity* of the measure. Even if the definition is somewhat incomplete, however, reliability can be increased by limiting the behaviors under scrutiny so that everyone can agree when they occur. Regardless of whether the measure is a formal, standardized test or an informal evaluation measure, interjudge reliability is critical to psychometric adequacy of the test. Formal tests should include data on interjudge reliability. Test manuals should include detailed definitions of the behaviors to be scored and as many guidelines as possible about potential response modes that may be difficult for the examiner to interpret as a correct or incorrect response. Some tests (Porch, 1981) have multidimensional scoring systems in which the client's response is not merely judged for correctness but also for the way the response occurred and for levels of acceptability. If the scoring system is complex enough, the test developer may even recommend taking a training course in test administration. This training is routinely done for tests of intelligence that require many judgment calls about client responses and some consistency in these decisions.

- *Training.* For any procedure to be reliable, the judges need to receive similar training in the observation, coding, and interpretation of the data. Most researchers put reliability judges through training periods, sometimes lasting several hours, prior to actual computation of the reliability scores. It makes good sense that prior to using any procedure a clinician will have adequate exposure to the methods and some practice using them.

- *Practice.* Reliability is a function of practice. Both formal tests and informal evaluation measures require practice to efficiently administer and score. If one judge has much experience with a particular test or measurement and another judge has had none, lack of reliability can be expected. The more we perform procedures, the more systematic and consistent our decision making becomes.

- *Response Complexity.* Generally, the more complex the response, the greater the lack of reliability. If the system you are using to examine teacher–child interactions has a host of teacher and child variables, it will be more difficult to use than one with fewer aspects to examine. Another common example is the poor reliability associated with narrow phonetic transcription. The more molecular we become in what we do, the more difficult it is to obtain adequate reliability. In this age of writing generative phonologies from children's spontaneous samples, you can imagine how many specific disagreements could occur between two clinicians. First, there is error in just transcribing the sample, and there is the opportunity for many disagreements. Second, there is error in detecting the specific errors within the transcript. Third, there is further error in trying to arrive at a list of phonological processes or idiosyncratic rules that account for the child's sample. Finally, there is error in determining the frequency or percentage of occurrence of each rule derived from the sample. The result could be a catalog of chaos. The more guidelines these clinicians have in making decisions, the better the reliability; in addition, the less complex the decisions, the better the reliability. This is why, some authors have developed specific guidelines and definitions to use in phonological analyses (Ingram, 1981; Shriberg & Kwiatkowski, 1980).

- *Live Scoring Versus Tape Analysis.* Scoring behaviors "online" is always more difficult than being able to replay video- or audiotapes for second and third opportunities to examine a behavior. Probably, videotape scoring would tend to be more reliable simply because it is difficult to accurately observe behaviors in rapid sequence and to take the time to note their occurrence on an observation form (which further takes away from one's ability to observe).

There are several ways to compute reliability. One method involves statistical procedures known as reliability coefficients or correlation coefficients (Hegde, 1987; Salvia & Ysseldyke, 1981). Typically, formal tests compute such correlations on judges to determine if the scores they derive are in general agreement as far as moving up and down together is concerned. It is preferable for standardized tests to have interjudge reliability coefficients of .90 or above to show good agreement among examiners. For example, if Judge A scored a series of tests as 89, 62, 53, and

36 and if Judge B scored the same tests as 90, 60, 50, and 35, there would be general agreement and a possible correlation of .99. The closer a coefficient of reliability is to 1.0, the more reliable the scoring. Some reliability coefficients take into account variance in the examiner's judgments (e.g., intraclass correlation, Winer's Coefficient of Reliability). Other test developers have used a simple correlation coefficient (e.g., Pearson Product Moment), which is far less effective in evaluating reliability (Bartko, 1976). In the example above, the judges did not agree exactly on any of the test scores, but there was a general trend for the two judge's scores to go up and down together. There was also a tendency for the scores to be rather close (within 3 points of each other). This type of reliability may be acceptable for general responses, but if we want to gain insight into more specific behaviors, the correlation coefficient is too general a measure.

For instance, if we wanted to count specific articulatory errors, it would be important to agree on the type of error produced. It also would be important for the judges to be counting the *same* errors. The following scenario is possible. A child is asked to produce 10 words for two-judges who are going to count misarticulations. Both judges come up with five misarticulations. If the two judges made these kinds of responses over many subjects, they would appear to represent perfect agreement (1.0 in a correlation). Further analysis, however, reveals that Judge A found errors in the first five words and Judge B found errors in the last five words. In essence, they did not agree on *any* of the misarticulations, but came up with the same total number.

This example points out the importance of a different type of reliability measure called *point by point* or *percent exact agreement*. In this type of reliability, a formula such as the following is used:

$$\frac{\text{Agreements}}{\text{Agreements} + \text{Disagreements}} \times 100 =$$

Thus, one takes the total number of specific agreements and divides this number by the total number of agreements plus the disagreements and arrives at a percentage of exact agreement. In this way, we get a good idea of the behaviors that judges rate in exactly the same way. Any clinician can compute such a simple formula and determine interjudge reliability for almost any clinically relevant behavior in a diagnostic or treatment context. Often it is good to check our perceptions every once in a while to see if we are fooling ourselves with regard to the occurrence of client behaviors. This type of reliability is especially important in behaviors that lend themselves to error because of subjectivity. Unfortunately, this includes many of the relevant measures in communication disorders.

2. Test–Retest Reliability. Some behaviors are highly stable over time. We would hope that most of the responses we assess to gain insight into various processes underlying communication are of this variety. If we are attempting to examine language comprehension, we assume that client performance on one day will be similar to that on another day. Vocal differences found one week would hopefully be observed the next week. If it were not for these behavioral consistencies, we really would have difficulty justifying treatment. A person's voice is either disordered, or it is not. Clearly, there are behavioral fluctuations in some disorders (e.g., stuttering, voice problems that vary with fatigue, etc.), but in others one can expect a fairly consistent occurrence (e.g., articulation errors, language errors). Tests are supposed to be designed to probe a particular error in such a way as to show consistent problems with a client's communication. If a patient with aphasia showed drastically different performances from week to week, it would be impossible to formulate a treatment program, because the targets would always be changing. If a person's IQ was not relatively stable from week to week, it would be impossible to diagnose cognitive deficits. If a laboratory test for cancer varied from day to day in its diagnosis of tissue samples, it would be unusable. It is easy to see that test–retest reliability has much to do with the behavior being evaluated, and also with the test items chosen to reveal the skill you are testing. Reliability coefficients, as described above, also are used to examine test–retest reliability, and those coefficients close to 1.0 indicate stability in performance on a particular task. One could also use the point-by-point procedure to determine if the errors made on one day are similar to those made at a later time. It depends on how molecular the clinician wants to be in examining client performance.

3. *Split-Half Reliability.* Many formal test developers want to evaluate the internal consistency of the items on their instrument. In essence, they want to determine if both halves of the test tend to be reliable or agree in terms of scores obtained.

SOME QUANTITATIVE BACKGROUND FOR TEST INTERPRETATION

There are some basic concepts in measurement that are necessary in order to appreciate most standardized tests. Many traditional quantitative aspects will not be covered, since they rarely are found on tests we use (e.g., mode, median, semiquartile range, types of curves, kurtosis, and skewedness). Although we are omitting these, we are certainly not suggesting they are of diminished value. We simply want to discuss aspects that are useful for interpreting most tests in communication disorders. For more detailed accounts of these concepts, consult other sources that provide more in-depth coverage (Anastasi, 1997; Messick, 1980; Salvia & Ysseldyke, 1995, 2004).

CENTRAL TENDENCY, VARIATION, AND THE NORMAL CURVE

Whenever someone takes a test they earn one or more scores. Part of test interpretation involves placing the score(s) of an individual in the context of others who also have been administered the instrument.

The most frequently encountered measure of central tendency in formal tests is the mean or arithmetic average of the normative sample. This is computed simply by adding up all the scores of the standardization sample and dividing by the total number of scores. As a clinician, you will probably not have to compute many mean scores on clients you test. You will see means in formal tests that have been used to examine differing age groups on a particular skill, and you will use this information as a reference point to compare the score of a specific child or adult you have tested. For example, if we have tested a 4-year-old on a vocabulary test, we are interested in how his or her score compares to the normative sample of 4-year-olds who took the same test as part of the standardization procedure. While some tests report data on other measures of central tendency (e.g., mode, median), the most frequently reported scores are means, and they are perhaps the most meaningful to a clinician.

The other important score we must deal with in order to make sense of normative data is some measure of variability (variance) in the standardization sample. The *variance* is "a numerical index describing the dispersion of a set of scores around the mean of the distribution" (Salvia & Ysseldyke, 1981, p. 50). In computing the variance, the statistician first derives the amount by which each person's score deviates from the sample mean (e.g., if the score is 70 and the test mean is 60, the deviation is 10). After this is done for each subject in the sample, the deviation scores are all squared. Then, these squared scores are added up and divided by the total number of subjects minus one. This results in the variance. One can easily see that we are essentially obtaining a very gross measure of the average amount of variation from the mean (squared) by computing the variance. The variance is not particularly meaningful in test interpretation so its square root, the *standard deviation,* is used because it is a more interpretable measure of variation. Thus, if the variance is 25, the square root of this is 5, which is the standard deviation. This measurement is more interpretable since it is in the same units as the mean instead of squared values as in the variance. If the mean on a test is 50 points and the standard deviation is 5 points, one can actually use these numbers together to gain a picture of variability. If we used a mean of 50 points and the variance of 25, we are no longer talking about the same types of numbers (points), because the variance is the average number of points of deviation squared.

In most cases, whenever researchers gather data on a particular skill from a large sample of people, the scores tend to form what statisticians call a *normal curve.* This means that there will be a tendency for most of the scores to fall around an average value, while some scores will be scattered toward very high and very low values. If researchers weighed a random sample of two thousand adults between the ages of 20 and 40, they would probably find an average weight, with most people clustered around this value, and a much smaller number of people who were very fat and very thin who deviated markedly from this value. This is where means and standard deviations are helpful in describing the performance of a given population of subjects.

Figure 3.1 shows a normal bell-shaped curve that could theoretically depict the performance of a sample of people on any variable. For our purposes, let us say that the curve represents scores on a vocabulary test. Several things are important to note. First, the line in the center of the normal curve at the score of 45 represents the mean performance or the average score in the distribution. Notice that it is the tallest line in the curve because height represents the largest number of people (9) who earned this score. The lines on either side of the mean are shorter and represent smaller numbers of subjects (8) who earned these scores (e.g., 40 and 50). As the lines become shorter it indicates that fewer subjects earned the scores as they moved progressively higher and lower than the mean of 45. The two subjects scoring 10 and the two subjects scoring 80 are in the tails of the normal curve and are called "outliers."

Look again at Figure 3.1 that depicts vocabulary scores. Previously, we said that the mean was 45. If we said that the standard deviation was 10, this would mean that +1 standard deviation would be located at 55 and −1 standard deviation would be located at 35. Taking the example further, +2 standard deviations would be at the score of 65, and −2 standard deviations would be at

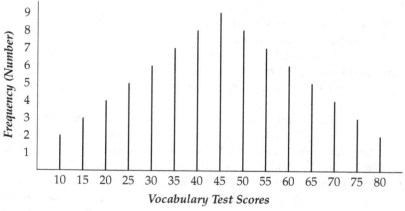

FIGURE 3.1   Example of normally distributed data.

25. Now look at Figure 3.2, which depicts the percentage of cases under portions of the normal curve and the standard deviations at the bottom. We can see that about 68% of cases in the sample would probably score within −1 and +1 standard deviations from the mean. This means that on the vocabulary test, about 68% of the subjects would earn scores somewhere between 35 and 55. If we considered the cases scoring between −2 and +2 standard deviations, about 96% of the subjects would earn scores in this area, somewhere between 25 and 65. Finally, if we looked at cases scoring between −3 and +3 standard deviations, around 99% of the cases would earn scores between 15 and 75.

Thus, the use of means and standard deviations helps researchers and test developers to determine scoring patterns that are characteristic of the majority of a particular population. It often has been stated in the assessment literature that scores falling at or below −1.5 to −2.0 standard deviations from the mean are thought to be abnormal enough to be clinically significant (Ludlow, 1983; McCauley & Swisher, 1984b). This, of course, indicates that the score in question was lower than some 95% of the population included in the standardization sample. Thus, it should be clear that we use the means and standard deviations of the normative sample as a context for comparing an individual client's score on a standardized test. If the client's score falls below a particular standard deviation level (e.g., −2.0), we may decide to make a judgment about lack of normality in performance. This is why, it is important to understand some basic facts about means and standard deviations. Although many authorities advocate the use of cutoff scores as mentioned above, others (Plante & Vance, 1995; Spaulding, Plante, & Farinella, 2006) dispute the use of such arbitrary guidelines and suggest that clinicians empirically derive specific cutoff scores for each test they use on local populations. This suggestion is based on research that shows variability in the ability of specific tests to discriminate normally developing children from those with disorders (Plante & Vance, 1995). If tests are going to be used to establish whether a child has a problem, they should have demonstrated discriminant validity. All distributions, however, are not normal. Some are skewed positively (many low scores) or negatively (many high scores); others have much variation (platykurtic) or very little variation (leptokurtic). It is significant that most standardization samples tend to be normally distributed, which is important for the statistical analyses that are applied to them. There are many special problems in dealing with abnormally distributed data that are beyond the scope of the present text. It is enough if we are clear about normally distributed data and about the ways of describing these distributions.

Types of Scores Found on Formal Tests

There are several kinds of scores that the diagnostician will encounter when dealing with standardized, norm-referenced tests. The first type of score we will mention is the *raw score*. The raw score is the actual number you arrive at when grading the client's test. Many times the raw score amounts to the number of correct responses that the client gave to the test items. So, if the test has 75 items on it and the client got 50 of them correct, the raw score might be 50. On some tests the raw score is not simply the number correct but is some other number (e.g., maybe each test item is worth 2 points). At any rate, you score the test and arrive at some number that the test manual typically refers to as the raw score.

Most standardized, norm-referenced examinations include a manual to be used by the diagnostician in scoring and interpreting the test results. These test manuals typically contain a series of tables that are designed to convert raw scores into more interpretable numbers. Raw scores by themselves are not readily meaningful. For instance, the raw score of 50 out of 75 does not tell us anything about how our client's score compares to the performance of the normative sample. Perhaps this is normal performance for the client's age group and perhaps it is not. Thus, we must convert the client's raw score into a more meaningful type of number to allow comparison with the normative sample. Another reason to convert the raw scores to some other type of derived score is that one cannot compare the results of two different tests by using raw scores. For instance, if a child obtains a raw score of 50 out of 75 on a vocabulary test and then earns a raw score of 125 out of 200 on a metalinguistics test, it would be difficult to compare these results. If, however, the raw scores were converted to some derived score, we could generally compare the performances on the two measures.

One type of converted score is called the *percentile rank*. Percentile ranks reflect the percentage of subjects or scores that fall at or below a particular raw score. For example, if a child scored in the 20th percentile, this means he or she scored as well or better than 20% of the children of the same age in the normative sample. Likewise, if a child was in the 90th percentile, the score was as good or better than 90% of the children taking the test. Another way to look at it is that only 10% of the normative population scored higher than a child who performed in the 90th percentile. If you look at Figure 3.2, you will see that percentile ranks are arranged under the normal curve. It can be seen that the 50th percentile rank basically represents the middle or median performance of the normative sample. A percentile rank of 10 is slightly more than –1 standard deviation below the mean. Remember from the prior discussion that some authorities view performance below –1.5 or –2.0 standard deviations to constitute clinical significance or abnormality. Some authorities suggest that consistent performance below the 10th percentile is cause for clinical concern (Lee, 1974), because this is between –1 and –2 standard deviations. One can see that conversion of the raw score into a percentile rank allows the clinician to put an individual client's performance into the context of the normative sample. It is meaningless to say that the client got a raw score of 90, but it is much more valuable to be able to say that a client scored in the 90th percentile.

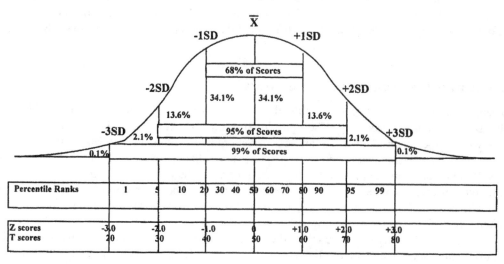

FIGURE 3.2 Relationship of various types of derived scores to the normal curve.

Another way to derive more interpretable data from a client's raw score is to convert it into a *standard score*. There are a number of types of standard scores that the diagnostician will encounter on formal tests; however, we will discuss only the two most common types: *z-scores* and *T-scores*. Standard scores transform the raw scores into sets of scores that have the same mean and standard deviation. A *z*-score has a mean of 0 and a standard deviation of 1. One can see from Figure 3.2 that the *z*-scores are exactly equivalent to the standard deviations in the normal curve. Thus, a *z*-score of –1.0 is in the same place on the curve as a standard deviation of –1.0. A raw score can be converted to a *z*-score by subtracting the raw score from the mean of the normative sample and dividing the resulting number by the standard deviation of the normative sample. Test manuals typically include tables for the conversion of raw scores into *z*-scores so that the clinician will not have to perform the mathematical operation mentioned above. It is easy to see that when a client's raw score is converted to a *z*-score, it is much more interpretable. For instance, it is meaningless to that say a client had a raw score of 59 on a test, because it does not relate to the normative sample. If, however, the client has a *z*-score of –2.0, we can look at Figure 3.2 and see that this is equivalent to performing at –2.0 standard deviations, which is a clinically significant abnormality according to the criteria mentioned earlier.

Another standard score is the *T*-score. This operates basically the same way as the *z*-score, except that the mean is 50 and the standard deviation is 10. Thus, the performance of a client with a *T*-score of 30 would be equivalent to –2.0 standard deviations.

A final type of standard score is the *stanine*. Tables for conversion of raw scores to stanines are not found as often in standardized tests. As stated by Salvia and Ysseldyke (1981),

> Stanines are standard score bands that divide a distribution into nine parts. The first stanine includes all scores that are 1.75 standard deviations or more below the mean, and the ninth stanine includes all scores 1.75 or more standard deviations above the mean. The second through eighth stanines are each .5 standard deviation in width and the fifth stanine ranging from .25 standard deviation below the mean to .25 standard deviation above the mean. (p. 73)

It can be seen from this discussion that standardized, norm-referenced tests provide the diagnostician with a variety of possible scores to use when interpreting a particular client's performance. Remember, however, that although standard scores are useful to the diagnostician, they are valid only if the score distribution in the normative sample is normal. Percentiles do not require a distribution to be normal and can be computed on any distribution shape; thus, they have fewer requirements than standard scores for accurate use and interpretation.

The Age and Grade Score Trap

Many formal tests include tables for converting raw scores into age-equivalent or grade-equivalent scores. Thus, a 9-year-old child who earns a raw score of 50 might be said to have an age-equivalent score of 7.5 (7 years, 5 months). A fourth grader might earn a grade-equivalent score of 2.2 (second grade, second month). It is easy to be seduced into using these types of scores because they appear to relate to development. On the surface, these age and grade equivalents seem to place the child in a developmental context with peers who took the test. It is tempting to say that the 9-year-old mentioned above is really at the 7-and-a-half-year-old level, or the fourth grader is performing at the second-grade level. All of these assumptions could be wrong. Most authorities who focus on psychometric interpretation indicate that age-equivalent and grade-equivalent scores are the *least* useful and *most dangerous* scores to be obtained from standardized tests because they lead to gross misinterpretations of a client's performance (Lawrence, 1992; McCauley & Swisher, 1984b; Salvia & Ysseldyke, 1981). Basically, age-equivalent scores indicate that the client's raw score approximated the average performance for a particular age group. In the example above, the 9-year-old earned a raw score that was the average of the children in the 7-year-old group of the normative sample. A similar relationship holds for grade-equivalent scores.

There are several commonly discussed difficulties with age- and grade-equivalent scores. McCauley and Swisher (1984b) discuss these problems:

> For most tests, as age increases, similar differences in age-equivalent scores are the result of smaller and smaller differences in raw scores. Therefore, an age-equivalent score that is 6 months behind an individual's chronological age may indicate a larger difference in actual test performance for younger test takers than for older ones. . . . The 1-year delay . . . reported for Paul, who is 4 years old, may have resulted from 12 missed items; whereas a 1-year delay for a 10-year-old child taking the test might be due to only one or two missed items. This causes the reliability of age-equivalent scores to be poorer for developmentally more advanced test takers. A second psychometric problem with age-equivalent scores is that they are not necessarily based directly on evidence collected for children of that chronological age. . . . Instead, a given age-equivalent score is often calculated indirectly either by interpolating between two ages for which data are available or by extrapolating from ages for which data are available to older or younger ages, for which data were not gathered. For example, Paul's raw score . . . probably fell between the average scores of the 3-year-olds and 4-year-olds in the normative sample, and he was assigned the age-equivalent of 3:2 by interpolation although no children of age 3:2 were sampled in the normative studies. (p. 340)

The psychometric problems above lead to a number of misinterpretations of age-equivalent scores. First, as Salvia and Ysseldyke (1981) indicate, it leads to "typological thinking." As they say, "The average 12-0 child does not exist. The child is a composite of all 12.0 children. Average 12-0 children represent a range of performances" (p. 68).

A second misinterpretation is that laymen and some professionals may believe that a 9-year-old child who earns an age-equivalent score of 7-0 is *performing like* a 7-year-old. This is probably not true. While the 9-year-old may have earned the score obtained by the average 7-year-old, the test items that were correct and missed may be totally different in the client and the normative sample of 7-year-olds. As McCauley and Swisher (1984b) state: "Similarly, a 60-year-old suffering from aphasia might receive an age-equivalent score of 10 years on the vocabulary test. It is unlikely, however, that such a client would make the same kind of errors as the 10-year-old or that he would exhibit similar communication skills" (p. 341).

A final danger in using age-equivalent scores is their use in attempting to define impairment in a client. Often, the assumption is made that a child exhibits a disorder if his or her age-equivalent score is lower than his or her chronological age (e.g., a 4-year-old earning an age-equivalent score of 3.0). It is important to understand that these age-equivalent scores do not take into account the variation in performance expected in a particular age group. If a child performs below the average score for his or her age group, it may be within the range of normal variation for that group and not an indicator of impairment at all (McCauley & Swisher, 1984b).

It is almost universally agreed that the least useful and most perilous types of scores are the age-equivalent or grade-equivalent scores mentioned above. They tend to distort a client's performance and lead to misinterpretations by laymen and professionals alike. Yet, many state departments of education mandate use of age-equivalent scores for purposes of determining eligibility for services (Lawrence, 1992). Most authorities advocate the use of percentile ranks and standard scores for test interpretation, because these do not suffer from the problems mentioned in relation to developmental scores. Perhaps the percentile rank is the easier of the scores to use in communicating with parents and spouses since most people can understand this concept readily. Clinicians who are consumers of formal, standardized, norm-referenced tests would be wise to refuse to purchase examinations that offer only age-equivalent scores and that omit standard scores and percentile ranks.

Standard Error of Measurement and Confidence Intervals

Two final concepts that we will deal with regarding standardized tests are the notions of *standard error of measurement* and *confidence intervals*. When used with the concepts previously discussed (mean, standard deviation, standard scores), these measurements give the diagnostician some very powerful quantitative tools to use in evaluating test performance.

Even though a standardized test may be developed very carefully, a client's responses to test items may not really reflect the underlying ability that the examination is attempting to tap. Statisticians realize that *any* measure is susceptible to error. Error is ubiquitous—it is in everything we measure, and especially in evaluating human performance. Thus, we know that no test is perfectly reliable (1.0) and that some distortion is present in any measurement device. Some statisticians use the terms *observed score* and *true score* to refer to the actual raw score that the test taker earns and to the "ideal" score that the person would have earned if there were no error in the measuring instrument. The true score, then, does not really exist; it is only hypothesized. We would ideally like the observed score to be highly similar to the true score, and this is the case in using tests that have high reliability. As the reliability of a test decreases, the disparity between true and observed scores increases.

A statistic called the standard error of measurement (SEM) has been developed to increase our precision in determining whether the observed score of a client is reasonably close to his or her possible true score. Although one could calculate the SEM and associated confidence intervals from one of several statistical formulas, most tests provide tables from which to arrive at this information. Basically, the calculation of SEM involves three things (McCauley & Swisher, 1984b): "(a) an estimate of the test's reliability, (b) the mean and standard deviation of scores obtained by the normative sample to which the test taker's score is to be compared, and (c) the test taker's observed score" (p. 339). We should be able to look up the SEM in a test manual and find a table that indicates the confidence intervals around the client's true score for at least a 95% level of confidence. Thus, if a subject had an observed score of 50 on a test and we calculated the true score and it was 53, there would be a pretty good correspondence between the observed and true scores. If we look up the 95% confidence interval in a table included in the test manual, we might find that the confidence interval is 5. Next, we subtract 5 from the subject's true score, arrive at 48, add 5 to the true score, and get 58. Thus, we have a range from 48 to 58, with the subject's true score in the middle. We can have confidence that the subject's true score would fall in this range 95 times out of 100 test administrations.

McCauley and Swisher (1984b) point out the importance of using confidence intervals, especially when attempting to determine cutoffs for abnormality. This problem becomes especially important in cases where psychometrists are attempting to determine if a child is cognitively impaired.

If an IQ below 70 is indicative of significant impairment, it would be important for the client's true score *and* confidence interval to be well below 70 to make a judgment. If the confidence interval overlaps the cutoff, it is possible that the true score could lie in the area above the cutoff even though the observed score is below it. Important decisions should not be dealt with lightly, and clients should be given the benefit of the doubt, especially where program placements are concerned.

SENSITIVITY AND SPECIFICITY: KEY CONCEPTS IN EVIDENCE-BASED PRACTICE

When a diagnostic test is developed, it is critical that the instrument be able to distinguish people who have the disorder from those who do not. In the process of test development, researchers have used the concepts of sensitivity and specificity to characterize the ability of an instrument to "fail" the people with disorders and to "pass" the people who do not have the disorder. In Chapter 1, we mentioned evidence-based practice and the importance of using scientifically sound assessment instruments. Specificity and sensitivity are critical concepts in evidence-based practice. Imagine that you have a group of 83 people. Of the 83 people, there are 21 who have a particular communication disorder and 62 who have normal communication. Ideally, a standardized test would fail all 21 of the people with disorders and pass all of the normal communicators. Most tests, however, are not ideal. Figure 3.3 illustrates four possible scenarios of administering this examination depicted in the four boxes.

Target Disorder

	Present	Absent	
Positive (failed the test)	True Positive (People with disorder failed the test) a Ex: 19	False Positive (People who were normal failed the test) b Ex: 12	a + b
Negative (passed the test)	False Negative (People with disorder passed the test) c Ex: 2	True Negative (People who were normal passed the test) d Ex: 50	c + d
	a + c	b + d	

(Test Result)

Sensitivity = a/(a + c), or the percentage of people with the disorder who failed the test

Specificity = d/(b + d), or the percentage of people who were normal who passed the test

Example Sensitivity: 19/(19 + 2) = 90%
Example Specificity: 50/(50 + 12) = 80%

FIGURE 3.3   Sensitivity and specificity values for standardized tests: The concept and an example.

One outcome of testing (box a: true positive) is that the instrument would accurately iden-tify people who have the disorder. That is, the people with the disorder would fail the test, or test positive for the impairment. Another outcome could be that people who are normal fail the test (box b: false positive). In this case, you have identified people who have no problem and you now must spend time doing further evaluation ultimately to determine that they should not be added to your caseload. A third scenario could be that some people who have the disorder actu-ally pass the test, or test negative for the impairment (box c: false negative). In this case, you would be missing people with the disorder, and they might not be eligible for services. A final outcome might be that people who do not have the disorder pass the test (box d: true negative). This, of course, is exactly what one would want to happen; normal speakers are actually identi-fied as such. Since no diagnostic test is without error, it is most often the case that all four scenar-ios occur simultaneously with test administration. Test developers and clinicians should be inter-ested in the rates of true positives, false positives, false negatives, and true negatives associated with any particular instrument. Thus, the terms *sensitivity* and *specificity* are used to characterize two of the most important scenarios: the percentage of true positive scores and the percentage of true negative scores.

The notions of sensitivity and specificity would be simple indeed if people with disorders and those with normal communication performed in such a way that there was a clear demarca-tion between their performances on a test instrument. Figure 3.4 (top example) illustrates the "ideal" situation in which people with disorders have a distribution of scores on a test that does not overlap at all with the normal speakers. Deriving a cutoff score to use in identifying people with a disorder from those who are normal would be quite easy. In the real world, however, the distributions tend to overlap to a considerable degree, and choosing a cutoff will result in the errors (false positives, false negatives) discussed above. The sensitivity and specificity are dependent on

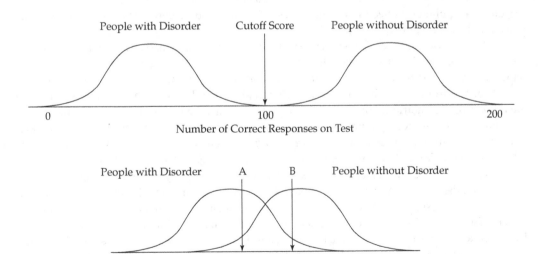

Cutoff "A" misses many people with disorders and passes most people without the disorder (poor sensitivity)

Cutoff "B" identifies most people with disorders, but fails many people with normal communication (poor specificity)

FIGURE 3.4 Illustration of "idealized" nonoverlapping distributions of normal and abnormal populations (top) and the "typical" overlapping distributions (bottom).

where the test developer sets the cutoff score. In the bottom example in Figure 3.4, we illustrate the consequences of choosing a cutoff in terms of committing false positive and false negative errors.

Figure 3.3 illustrates an example in which the sensitivity was 90% and the specificity was 80%. This example test is not as good at identifying normal speakers (80%), and one would expect that more people without disorders than acceptable would tend to "fail" the test. The test can, however, identify people with disorders fairly well at 90%. When test developers design diagnostic instruments, they should use a reference standard to identify initially people who have disorders. This reference standard should be independent of the test being developed, and the assumption is that it is a gold standard for identifying the particular disorder. Thus, sensitivity and specificity are always viewed in juxtaposition to the reference standard. Most authorities would expect sensitivity and specificity measures to be over 85% for a test to be of clinical use, and most test developers strive for figures in both sensitivity and specificity to be over 90%. When you are going to purchase a test, it is important to examine the test manual for data showing the sensitivity and specificity of the instrument.

CRITERIA FOR EVALUATING STANDARDIZED TESTS

We present this section for use by consumers of standardized tests. Every year clinicians in most work settings may be lucky enough to be given a budget for purchasing new materials. Among these new acquisitions are standardized tests. If you have had the occasion recently to peruse publisher's catalogs containing new tests, you have doubtless found that these instruments are quite expensive. It is rare to find a test for less than one hundred dollars, and many examinations may sell for between two and five hundred dollars. Even new packets of test response forms cost considerable money to replace each year for the examinations already owned by a facility. Thus, if your budget is five hundred dollars, it can be easily expended on a single test. For economic reasons alone, clinicians need to evaluate seriously any test they consider for purchase and not make the decision lightly.

The expense, however, is just one consideration in deciding whether to purchase a particular test. Another major issue is whether the test was developed using rigorous scientific standards. Does the test have good reliability and validity? Can it adequately discriminate clients with disorders from those who have normal communication? If you purchase a test that does not have good psychometric qualities, you have wasted your money. Even worse, you have done your clients a disservice by administering a useless instrument. Administering a test that lacks good psychometric qualities is at best a waste of your client's time and money, and at worst an ethical problem. We wish that we could tell you that all tests advertised by publishing companies are of high quality. Unfortunately, there is a wide variety to the psychometric adequacy of tests available on the market. While some companies pay careful attention to the science of test development, there are still many instruments advertised in catalogs that are not psychometrically adequate. Therefore, it is up to the consumers of test instruments to examine carefully the process by which a test was developed prior to purchasing it. In Chapter 1 we talked about the importance of evidence-based practice. A major tenet of evidence-based practice is that we should use measurements that have been developed using correct scientific methods. We need to be assured that a test instrument can, in fact, do what the publisher indicates in the test manual.

What are the most important psychometric considerations in evaluating standardized tests? The criteria have been reported by many authors (Andersson, 2005; Hutchinson, 1996; McCauley & Swisher, 1984a; Salvia & Ysseldyke, 2004), but basically flow from the *Standards for Educational and Psychological Tests* compiled by the American Psychological Association.

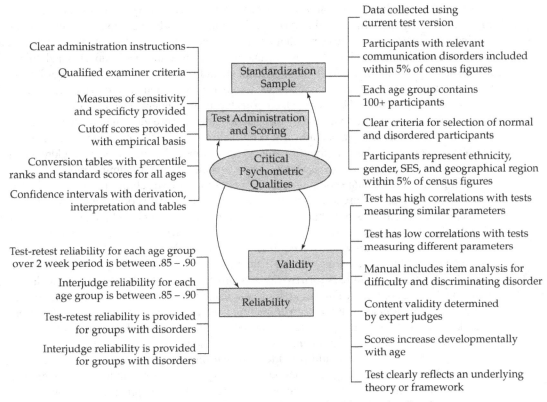

Clear administration instructions

Qualified examiner criteria

Measures of sensitivity and specificty provided

Cutoff scores provided with empirical basis

Conversion tables with percentile ranks and standard scores for all ages

Confidence intervals with derivation, interpretation and tables

Standardization Sample

Test Administration and Scoring

Critical Psychometric Qualities

Test-retest reliability for each age group over 2 week period is between .85 – .90

Interjudge reliability for each age group is between .85 – .90

Test-retest reliability is provided for groups with disorders

Interjudge reliability is provided for groups with disorders

Validity

Reliability

Data collected using current test version

Participants with relevant communication disorders included within 5% of census figures

Each age group contains 100+ participants

Clear criteria for selection of normal and disordered participants

Participants represent ethnicity, gender, SES, and geographical region within 5% of census figures

Test has high correlations with tests measuring similar parameters

Test has low correlations with tests measuring different parameters

Manual includes item analysis for difficulty and discriminating disorder

Content validity determined by expert judges

Scores increase developmentally with age

Test clearly reflects an underlying theory or framework

FIGURE 3.5 Selected critical psychometric qualities associated with standardized tests.
Source: Adapted from Andersson (2005); McCauley & Swisher (1984b); Salvia & Ysseldyke (2004).

Figure 3.5 shows selected psychometric qualities usually associated with standardized tests. We will briefly sketch those considerations here, but the reader should know that the actual standards go into much more detail.

Test Administration and Scoring

Some clinicians wonder why every test comes with a fairly extensive manual that goes into painful detail about (a) the rationale behind the test, (b) the psychometric development of the instrument, (c) the specific purposes for which the test is to be used and not used, (d) qualifications of the test administrator, and (e) detailed instructions for administering, scoring, and interpreting the test. It is the tendency of most students and beginning clinicians to skip over the part of the test having to do with the development of the instrument. Some students read just enough of the manual to be able to administer the test, and then revisit it when it comes time to score it.

Manuals are detailed for several reasons. First of all, the portion dealing with psychometric qualities of the test should be read in detail prior to purchasing the test in the first place. This is where you see the information on reliability, validity, sensitivity, specificity, the normative sample, and all sorts of other important information. There is no point in purchasing a test that is psychometrically inadequate. Usually, these tests have very brief manuals and leave consumers with many unanswered questions. The part of the manual that talks about its rationale and purposes lets the consumer know if the instrument is well grounded in current theory about the disorder. In some cases, examiners may require training or specific educational background in order to administer and interpret a test. In the field of psychology, for instance, one has to have highly specific training in order to administer and interpret tests of intelligence. Since the test has been standardized, it is important that it be administered to an individual client in exactly the same manner as it was given to the normative sample. If you administer the test to a client without regard to the instructions, then you cannot compare his or her score to the norms for the instrument. The more questions about administration that cannot be answered by the test manual, the more idiosyncratic decisions that must be made by the clinician. For example, if you ask a client to point to a particular picture and he says "Huh?" are you allowed to tell him the name a second time? The manual should address concerns such as this, or else the test will have a lot of error associated with its administration.

Similarly, the manual should include detailed scoring instructions, because we do not want individual clinicians making idiosyncratic judgments about what is or is not correct. It should all be spelled out as much as possible. One way that test manuals assist clinicians is that they provide detailed tables to be used in converting raw scores to percentile ranks and standard scores. Tables should also be provided for confidence intervals. You can easily see how much error would be injected into the testing process if each clinician had to put raw scores into a formula of some type and crunch numbers to arrive at standard scores. Probably you can ask a class of students to add up a column of numbers with a calculator and there will be many different answers provided. Even with tables, there is error in clinicians running their fingers down the wrong row or looking up conversion factors in tables for the wrong age group. The tables, however, help to reduce error to an acceptable level and are indispensable to a good test instrument.

A good test manual should provide information to aid clinicians with interpreting the scores. If there is a cutoff score that defines the existence of a problem, it should be explained in the test manual. Measures of sensitivity and specificity should be provided to show that the test can discriminate adequately between people with disorders and those who exhibit normal communication. In a prior section, we indicated that it is ideal for these two measures to be above 90%.

Reliability

Earlier in this chapter we discussed the importance of reliability in developing a standardized test. It is important that the test manual reports both test–retest and interjudge reliability scores for the normative sample. The test–retest reliability for each age group over a 2-week period should be between .85 and .90. The desired coefficients for interjudge reliability should also be near .90. Interestingly, some test developers report reliability across an entire age span of the normative population. That is, if the normative sample is for children between the ages of 5 and 10 years, they report a single reliability coefficient. Ideally, reliability coefficients should be reported for each age group and separately for groups with communication disorders. It is quite possible for reliability to change with age and with the presence/absence of disorder.

The Standardization Sample

If a client is going to be compared to norms on a standardized test, it is important to know about the makeup of the normative sample. It was not that many years ago that test developers normed standardized tests on groups of white, middle-class, Standard English speakers. The result, of course, was that people from different ethnic/cultural backgrounds who were dialect speakers "failed" the test, and our caseloads contained a disproportionate number of clients who did not exhibit real communication disorders. More recently, test developers have tried to take into account socioeconomic and ethnic considerations in selecting participants for the normative sample to which people will be compared. Generally, participants should represent ethnicity, gender, SES, and geographical region within 5% of national census figures. Thus, if African Americans represent 15% of the population, the normative sample should also have 15% from this cultural group. Another consideration in addition to culture is the size of the age groups represented in the normative sample. Historically, it was not unusual for individual age groups to be represented by fewer than 50 participants in the normative sample. We now know that the number of participants is an important factor in adding stability and strength to the normative data. A contemporary instrument should have age groups that contain a minimum of 100 participants. If the test is focusing on communication disorders, participants with relevant communication disorders should be included in the normative sample within 5% of the current census figures. Also, there should be clear criteria for selecting the participants who represent normal and disordered groups. This is the reference standard referred to in an earlier section.

Validity

In an earlier section we discussed the importance of validity and some common measures test developers use to confirm whether an instrument measures the parameters it is designed to assess. First, the examination manual should detail the underlying theory or framework that the test is based upon. Second, there should be some measure of content validity as determined by expert judges. Thus, if a test is purported to measure cognitive development in Piaget's sensorimotor period, judges should be able to examine the test items and link those to the pertinent theory of cognitive development. A third type of validity reports how well the instrument correlates with other known tests of the same construct. Therefore, a new instrument should have high correlations with tests measuring similar parameters, and low correlations with tests measuring different parameters. So, a test of receptive vocabulary should correlate highly with other receptive vocabulary tests, and less of a relationship might be found with tests of syntax or phonology. Test developers should also include an item analysis by which test items are evaluated statistically for difficulty level, changes in scores with age, and the ability of particular test items to discriminate between people with and without disorders.

It should be clear that selection of a standardized, norm-referenced test should not be just an arbitrary decision on the part of a diagnostician. Every month we are inundated with flyers and catalogs attempting to sell tests. The choice of whether to purchase one of these instruments is significant in terms of cost and, more important, in terms of serving our clients well. Try to examine these tests at conferences and conventions, read reviews in professional journals, and examine the *Buros Mental Measurements Yearbook* for critical reviews (ASHA, 1995; Compton, 1996; Impara & Plake, 1998). Many libraries have access to the *Buros Mental Measurements Yearbook* on the Internet. Although it is published only every few years, an online database includes reviews for upcoming issues, and the Internet resources may be more timely than bound volumes.

Test brochures and catalogs may not tell you enough to make an accurate judgment. If possible, order a test "on approval," and pay for it only if you are satisfied with its psychometric adequacy and what it will actually tell you about a client. Most reputable publishers allow a customer to return an instrument that he or she is not satisfied with.

COMMON ERRORS IN THE USE OF NORM-REFERENCED TESTS

With very few exceptions, norm-referenced tests are designed to help the clinician determine if a client is performing within normal limits on a particular behavior. We compare an individual's score to the normative data and decide if our client is impaired or not. Muma (1973b) has said that the purpose of formal tests is to solve the "problem/no problem" issue. Often, the clinician could do this just by observation alone, but many institutions (e.g., school systems) may require some formal test score to include in a client's record instead of relying solely on clinical judgment. IDEA requires a standardized test be used in assessment. At any rate, solving the problem/no problem issue is a rather narrow payoff for taking the time to administer and score a standardized test. As a result, some clinicians try to make more of the test results than they should. Formal tests are only designed to go so far; and if we make other judgments about our clients based on these data, we are violating the assumptions of the tests. The following are some of the common ways in which clinicians misuse standardized tests:

1. ***Measuring Treatment Progress with Norm-Referenced Tests.*** We mentioned earlier that the purpose of norm-referenced tests is to determine if a client is performing in a way that is similar to a large standardization sample. The tests were not designed for the purpose of measuring progress in treatment. If the clinician administers a formal test at the beginning of treatment and readministers the test (or even an alternate form of the test) after a period of treatment, the resulting scores can lead to gross misinterpretations. First of all, the formal test samples a broad range of behaviors and may sample the behavior trained in therapy only in a few trials. Thus, much of the time spent in test administration would be devoted to assessing behavior that is unrelated to therapy. It would be much more logical to examine the trained behavior in detail by using an informal format that focused more fully on the particular behavior of interest. Second, a child who scores abnormally low on an initial administration of an instrument will tend to score higher on a subsequent administration of the same test. This is a well-known phenomenon called *statistical regression,* which states that subjects earning extreme scores (either high or low) will tend to regress toward the mean of the sample population on subsequent administrations. Thus, a client may receive a higher score, not because of treatment effects but because of statistical regression. Third, clinicians may unconsciously "teach to the test" and prepare the client to do well on a second administration by practicing items in a format similar to the formal test. Fourth, all tests include elements of unreliability. It could very well be that an increase in an overall score on a formal test is simply the result of chance. We urge clinicians to never use standardized, norm-referenced tests as measures of progress. Criterion-referenced tests and informal probe tasks are the best way to gauge treatment progress.

2. ***Analyzing Individual Test Items for Treatment Target Selection.*** After administering a norm-referenced test, it is always tempting to examine the client's responses to particular test items and to try to determine some pattern of impairment. For example, on a receptive vocabulary test one might find that particular prepositions are in error. A natural tendency would be to include the understanding of prepositions in a treatment program based on the analysis of the formal test performance. There are several problems with this. To begin with, clients cannot be expected to take tests that are of an inordinate length. As a result, a formal test must be relatively brief in order to be practical. On the other hand, most formal tests are fairly broad based in that they cover a number of areas (e.g., syntax, morphology, vocabulary) or one area that has several facets to it (e.g., assessment of all relevant, bound morphemes). This characteristic creates a dilemma for the person who is developing a test instrument. In order to cover all of the areas of interest, or even all aspects of one area, the test developer must be very selective in deciding how many items to include and how many times a particular behavior will be sampled. In assessing bound morphemes, for instance, the test developer must determine how many times each morpheme of interest will be sampled and in what contexts. Often, a particular form will only be sampled two or three times in order to make the length of the test manageable. Herein lies the tradeoff: Making a test of reasonable length necessitates the use of small samples of each behavior of interest. Thus, it would be difficult to make a judgment about a particular grammatical morpheme (e.g., plurals) based on only two or three occurrences. This observation is especially true when client responses on formal tests can be due to a variety of reasons. As much as test developers would like to believe that an incorrect response indicates lack of ability on a particular item or that a correct response suggests mastery of an item, it is well known that test takers are human. Clients make lucky guesses, are distracted during test administration, do not fully understand instructions, experience a variety of internal states (fatigue, boredom, pain, need to use the bathroom, etc.) that could all affect test performance. Research has clearly indicated that use of individual standardized test items targeting specific structures for treatment planning is not advisable (McCauley & Swisher, 1984b; Merrell & Plante, 1997; Plante & Vance, 1994). Be wary of selecting treatment objectives from any norm-referenced test.

   3. *Forgetting That Formal Tests Almost Always Distort What They Are Designed to Examine.* Almost every construct one might desire to measure in communication disorders is highly complex. Whenever we deal with human behavior and try to translate a complex activity into a single score, there is a considerable amount of information lost in the process. Is it valid to say the child's vocabulary is a 74 because he or she earned this score on a test? Does this tell us how many words are in the lexicon, or are understood? Does it tell us how words are retrieved? Does it tell us if the child's internal definition of the word is equivalent to an adult's? Do we know how the word is used for communication? Do we know how the word will be used in sentences or written language? We could continue to ask questions about how deeply we have examined the child's vocabulary by obtaining a formal test score, but you probably have the idea by now that such a score is quite superficial. In designing a test, developers have competing goals that make it almost impossible to create the perfect instrument. Figure 3.6 illustrates this dilemma. As the test becomes more specific and controlled, it becomes more unnatural. As we move toward a naturalistic task, we lose control over stimuli, tasks, and responses. Standardized tests have a number of ways in which they tend to distort the constructs that we wish to examine.

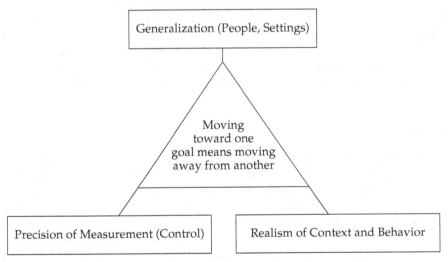

FIGURE 3.6 Competing goals of measurement: The test developer's dilemma.
Source: Adapted from Sabers (1996).

First, almost all tests that are standardized imply a circumscribed method of administration. The testing must be done in a particular setting, specific instructions must be given, and items must be administered in a particular order. In addition, the client's responses must be graded as pass or fail, based on the criteria set forth by the test developer (some tests do not classify client responses as pass/fail, but these are few in number). The vast majority of formal test scenarios involve a highly artificial, regimented way of assessing performance.

A second reason for distortion is that most of these tests designed to assess communication rarely examine *real* communicative efforts. The interactions are typically artificial. The client has no real communicative intent, communications are often about trivial topics (e.g., telling the examiner what is going on in a picture while both client and clinician look at it), and the topic of each task is constantly changing as the clinician flips the test plates. Thus, we must *always* remember that we have not examined real communication until we have analyzed the client's communicating in a natural situation.

A third source of distortion is the fragmentation of integrated systems often seen in formal testing. As Muma (1973b) points out, many systems interact with one another in communication and to single out a particular area to analyze is in many cases ludicrous. For instance, how can one separate semantics from cognition, syntax from semantics, syntax from morphology, phonology from syntax, motor speech skills from language, intonation from meaning, or structural language from pragmatics? Although this can be done on the formal test level, it certainly cannot be done on a construct validity level. We cannot evaluate a system or subsystem independently of the context in which it typically operates. If we do, we have not really evaluated the system of interest. Always be aware that when we use an artificial task as found on most formal tests, we are always a dimension or more away from looking at the reality of communication.

4. *Ignoring the Cultural Makeup of the Normative Sample.* With the progressive increase in the cultural diversity of the United States, it is important to consider the type of normative data gathered by test developers. A more in-depth discussion of this issue is presented in Chapter 12 on multicultural issues, but we wanted to mention it here as well because it is a common error in the use of standardized tests. Clearly, if we want to compare a child's score to norms, those norms should have been generated from a large sample of children that includes members of a variety of cultural groups. Many test developers use current census figures in selecting their normative samples so that the percentages of groups in the sample are roughly equivalent to representation in the general population. In some cases, clinicians are in areas that are heavily populated by certain cultural groups, and in these instances it may be advisable to develop local norms so that test performance might be compared to a relevant population.

CONCLUSION

Some students and clinicians feel frustrated when confronted with the type of information presented in this chapter. This is especially true if the clinician has emphasized formal tests in his or her approach to diagnosis and evaluation. Others also may feel a bit guilty if they have misused norm-referenced tests or have used instruments and techniques uncritically without ensuring the validity and reliability of those instruments or techniques. These practices, however, are probably the rule rather than the exception. Others might feel lost if all of their traditional tools are suddenly taken away from them, and they may ask, "What are we supposed to do without our tests?" There is no simple answer. One obvious response would be that we can still use tests for the purposes they are intended to serve, but we need to tighten up our criteria for test selection, use, and interpretation. The other response would be that we need to develop and use more informal methods for diagnosis and evaluation that will give us insight into the nature of a client's problem and the means for treating it. In many areas of communication disorders, we are beyond the basic question of the "problem/no problem" issue. We need ways to describe client performance and gain insight into individual differences, dynamism, ecological relevance, processes, and patterns of behavior (Bates, Bretherton, & Snyder, 1988; Bronfenbrenner, 1979; Chafe, 1970; Donaldson, 1978; Muma, 1978, 1981, 1983, 1984, 2002). The field of communication disorders is moving more toward descriptive and criterion-referenced measures rather than toward norm-referenced tests. This trend, however, does not absolve each of us from the ultimate responsibility of incorporating sound scientific principles into our measurements. An informal probe or task used to describe client behavior is just as susceptible as a norm-referenced test to psychometric and examiner error. Students, professors, and working clinicians should adhere to high standards of measurement and should refuse to use inadequate test instruments or descriptive procedures that cannot be effectively replicated.

4

Assessment of Children
with Limited Language

Our discussion of evaluation of child language disorders will be divided into two chapters. This chapter considers clients whose language does not exceed simple multiword combinations. Because most clients with limited language are children, we will refer to them as such in this chapter. Chapter 5 focuses on children who are using longer sentences and are typically school age or older.

THE PROCESS OF BECOMING A COMMUNICATOR: GETTING THE "BIG PICTURE"

MacDonald and Carroll (1992) have presented a useful conception of the developmental progression children must follow on their way to becoming effective communicators. The steps are deceptively simple, yet elegant. The following steps should be easy to remember, and they are important to consider in development, assessment, and treatment:

- *Play Partners (Implication: Cognitive Assessment).* Does the child play with objects appropriately? A child's play tells us about his or her conceptions of objects, events, and relationships in the world. A child who exhibits primitive play strategies with objects (e.g., mouthing, banging, sensorimotor exploration) is likely to have quite different cognitive abilities than a child who engages in functional object use and symbolic play. A child who does not know how to play with objects in productive ways is unlikely to learn to communicate about objects and events in an appropriate manner.
- *Turn-taking Partners (Implication: Social Assessment).* After children learn some appropriate play strategies with objects, they begin to involve adults in their play interactions. This social development is a critical prerequisite for communication. The development of reciprocity is important because communication involves social turn-taking between partners.
- *Communication Partners (Implication: Assessment of Communicative Intent and Gesture System).* The initial communications of children are gestural in nature. They point, pull, push, give, take, and reach while looking at adults and objects. These initial

nonverbal communications precede the use of words to regulate adult action and attention. Nonverbal communicative intents or functions such as declaratives and imperatives are included here. These communicative acts may or may not be accompanied by vocalizations.

- *Language Partners (Implication: Language Model Analysis and Language Structure Analysis).* After the "flow" of communication is established through the use of gestures, children begin to approximate word productions that are modeled by their caregivers.
- *Conversational Partners (Implication: Pragmatic Analysis).* When the use of language is firmly established, the child gradually learns the pragmatic rules for taking into account listener perspective, topic manipulation, and appreciation of social context in participating in dialogue.

One can easily see that the five areas mentioned above build upon one another, and in assessment we can locate a child on this continuum. Each step implies a different evaluation focus and different treatment implications.

FOCUSING ON THE CHILD'S LANGUAGE LEVEL: NONVERBAL, SINGLE-WORD, AND EARLY MULTIWORD COMMUNICATORS

In talking about children with language disorders, it is not uncommon for authorities to refer to children's presenting linguistic-development level (Carrow-Woolfolk & Lynch, 1982; McLean & Snyder-McLean, 1978; Paul, 2007). Often, training programs in speech-language pathology offer one course that deals with language disorders in infants/toddlers and another course that focuses on language disorders of school-age children and adolescents. It is not the chronological age per se that is important here, because a client with limited language can be from any age group (e.g., there are nonverbal teenagers and adults with cognitive impairments). Thus, it is unlikely that a single assessment procedure would be appropriate for *every* 4-year-old, because some of these children could be using advanced syntax while others could be using nonverbal communication. It is much more meaningful to discuss techniques that would be useful for a client who is communicating at the single or early multiword level regardless of his or her chronological age. For example, Tager-Flusberg et al. (2009) propose recommendations for defining spoken language benchmarks for children with autism. They recommend: ". . . moving away from using the term functional speech, replacing it with a developmental framework . . . they recommend multiple sources of information to define language phases, including natural language samples, parent report and standardized measures. They also provide guidelines and objective criteria for defining children's spoken language expression in three major phases that correspond to developmental levels between 12 and 48 months of age" (p. 643).

Interestingly, this is similar to the developmental phases recommended for assessment in the present text, which rely on developmental language levels (nonverbal, single word, early multiword, syntax). Assigning such developmental benchmarks can not only be used to track clinical progress in treatment but also be used by researchers to equate groups for empirical study rather than exclusively using standardized tests.

For purposes of assessment, it is useful to consider children with limited language in three general categories. First, there are children who are largely nonverbal. They use vocalizations and perhaps gestures, but their caretakers report no real use of language to control the child's environment. Obviously, in dealing with a nonverbal child, a "test of language ability" would be too advanced. Faced with the virtual elimination of an entire shelf of standardized language tests, the clinician must focus on more informal assessment procedures. The following areas are especially important to consider in evaluation of nonverbal communicators:

- General developmental level/adaptive behavior
- Biological prerequisites (audiometry, neurological, medical)
- Case history (preevaluation questionnaire, detailed interview)
- Caretaker–child interaction analysis
- Communicative intent inventory (types, frequency, level)
- Vocalization analysis (use of phonetically consistent forms, syllable shape, phonetic inventory)
- Gestural analysis
- Cognitive analysis (play analysis, screening tasks, formal scales)
- Lexical comprehension (parent reports, scales, tasks)

We will discuss each of the procedures mentioned above in more detail later in this chapter.

A second group of children consists of those who speak largely at the single-word level. The single-word stage has long been reported in the developmental literature (Nelson, 1973). According to some authorities, the child may accrue a lexicon of about 50 words before starting the use of word combinations for generative language. Clearly, the assessment of a "single-word child" is both similar to and different from dealing with a child who is nonverbal. In terms of similarities, we are still interested in general developmental levels, biological prerequisites, case history, caretaker–child interaction, communicative intent, the phonetic inventory, cognitive development, and understanding of semantic elements. At the single-word level, however, we can add the following assessment areas to the ones listed above:

- Length measures from spontaneous sample (e.g., mean length of utterance, or MLU)
- Form/function analysis of single-word productions (What functions do the child's single-word utterances serve?)
- Analysis of presyntactic devices (transitional elements related to development of multi-word utterances)
- Analysis of lexical production (grammatical types of words, number of words in lexicon)
- Phonological analysis and phonetic inventory

The measures listed above will be discussed more specifically in later sections.

A third type of child is one who is using early multiword combinations. For this type of child, it is clear that some basic cognitive capacity for using a symbol system exists because the child is, in fact, using one. In studying an early multiword child, it is more important to focus on the types of word combinations used and the functions for which the child uses the utterances. The phonetic inventory and phonological-process analysis also become important for this type of case, because a child's oral language can only be functional if it is intelligible to listeners. Thus, for the child who uses early multiword utterances, we must examine the language, but not necessarily in the same way as we would a language sample of a child who has a longer length of utterance. Thus, we would add the following to the prior measures:

- Analysis of semantic relations (types, frequency, productivity)
- Specific language development test
- Comprehension of simple commands
- Assessment of emerging literacy skills (e.g., joint book reading)

We have seen that there are at least three categories into which we can place children with limited language. The clinician's first step is to determine in which category the client is placed based on preponderant communication behaviors. The next step involves considering the high-probability diagnostic areas associated with the category. Finally, the clinician can use some of the specific procedures referred to later in this chapter, which will allow evaluation of the pertinent areas. Implied in the categories are different assessment targets, most of which cannot be evaluated by using formal test instruments (Wetherby & Prizant, 1992). McCathren, Warren, and Yoder (1996) identify four proven predictors of later language development in prelinguistic children: (1) use of babbling, (2) development of pragmatic functions, (3) vocabulary comprehension, and (4) the development of combinatorial/symbolic play skills. Unfortunately, most available formal assessment instruments do not measure these variables adequately. Notable exceptions are the *Communication and Symbolic Behavior Scales* (CSBS) (Wetherby & Prizant, 2002) and *Assessing Prelinguistic and Early Linguistic Behaviors in Developmentally Young Children* (ALB) (Olswang et al., 1987). Crais and Roberts (1991) provide a useful conceptual framework for the clinician in the form of decision trees to help generate assessment questions, select procedures, and link these procedures to intervention recommendations. Nelson (2010) provides a useful flowchart of clinical questions the diagnostician must ask while moving from initial evaluation to setting goals and finally to monitoring progress.

CONSIDERING ETIOLOGY

Although we have characterized children with language disorders by their general linguistic development level, some students may be tempted to describe those disorders by using etiology (e.g., autism spectrum disorder, cognitive impairment, or hearing impairment). We agree with those who suggest that classification of language disorder by etiology does not relate productively to assessment (Lahey, 1988; Nelson, 2010; Newhoff & Leonard, 1983; Paul, 2007). The various etiological groups themselves are highly heterogeneous, and thus to refer to a child who is "mentally retarded" really means little in terms of predicting what he or she might be like. In addition, the language disorders manifested by these various groups may not be significantly different. Therefore, the language samples gathered from children who are hearing impaired, cognitively impaired, learning disabled, autistic, and language delayed but with normal intelligence may be highly similar. Diagnostic grouping, then, does not necessarily provide the clinician with valid guidelines for assessing language skills. On the other hand, a focus on the language abilities of a child will help us to understand the strengths and limitations of communication and assist in development of treatment objectives.

WHY IS EARLY LANGUAGE ASSESSMENT SO DIFFICULT?

Language assessment in children is one of the most difficult and challenging tasks faced by the SLP, and many clinicians are insecure about their diagnostic ability in this area.

    1. *Heterogeneity of the Population.* One complicating factor for the diagnostician is that the population that exhibits a language disorder is extremely heterogeneous (Wolfus, Moscovitch, & Kinsbourne, 1980). In addition, children from a wide spectrum of etiological groups manifest language impairment, and the practitioner is faced with youngsters who are cognitively impaired, autistic, hearing impaired, learning disabled, or who exhibit a variety of other organically based conditions. This heterogeneity appears to make diagnosis quite difficult, especially for the clinician who knows only one approach to language assessment.

2. *Highly Varied Severity Levels.* A second variable that makes language diagnosis difficult is the difference in the degree of severity found in the language-impaired population. The children range from those who are nonverbal with a lack of social and cognitive bases for language, on the one hand, to youngsters who inconsistently misuse grammatical morphemes or exhibit subtle pragmatic problems on the other. Thus, for each evaluation the clinician must be prepared to assess the broad representation of linguistic and prelinguistic behaviors.

3. *Language Is a Complex Phenomenon.* A third variable that makes language assessment confusing is the complex nature of language itself. Most introductory courses discuss language as an area that is comprised of various domains. In fact, many textbooks are organized with reference to such language areas as semantics, syntax, morphology, phonology, and pragmatics. Any or all of these areas can be affected in a language disorder. Most theorists agree that these domains are not isolated from one another but have complex interactions that proceed from "top-down" and "bottom-up" in models of language processing. Complicating the problem further is the fact that authorities in the area of psycholinguistics are not in total agreement regarding exactly how these domains of language interact with each other in spontaneous communication.

4. *A Multitude of Assessment Instruments/Procedures.* Another variable that makes it difficult to know what to do in language evaluation is the proliferation of assessment devices and procedures available on the market. We are inundated with flyers and catalogs, many reputed to offer "the best language assessment device." How does one select a test? Is one test really enough? The fact that people have designed tests of language for children with oftentimes very inclusive titles suggests that it is possible to find out all one needs to know from a single test. Unfortunately, the disclaimers that some authors place in their test manuals regarding the shortcomings of the instruments are forgotten, and the perhaps overambitious title remains in the mind of clinicians and parents. Also, tests are based on different theoretical points of view or models. The differing theoretical underpinnings result in dramatically different types of tasks and areas of emphasis on tests. The plethora of tests, then, is a source of confusion to many clinicians.

5. *Language Is Profoundly Affected by Multiple Processes and Domains.* It is also difficult to know what to do in language assessment because language development and disorders encompass so much more than just linguistic ability. In the literature on language acquisition, for instance, one routinely reads about cognitive development, neurolinguistics, linguistic theory, adaptive behavior, play development, social development, self-help skills, phonology, motor ability, emergent literacy, caretaker–child interaction, and other areas that may not appear to be directly related to linguistic symbols but are critical to language development. Since language itself has many domains (semantics, syntax, phonology, morphology, pragmatics, etc.) and the related areas mentioned above are numerous, language assessment may take on quite different guises, depending on the focus of the evaluation. This complexity is clearly a source of confusion for clinicians and requires a very broad base of skill and knowledge.

The difficulties mentioned above probably contribute to many clinicians' uncertainties in the area of language assessment. Models, as we indicate in the following section, are sometimes helpful in reducing the difficulties in understanding an area and in assisting diagnosticians to develop workable clinical procedures.

MODELS TO CONSIDER IN LANGUAGE ASSESSMENT

If we were to travel around the country and eavesdrop as SLPs evaluate children, we would find a confusing conglomeration of activities performed under the aegis of linguistic assessment:

A clinician has a child repeat sentences.

A child plays silently while the clinician takes notes.

A child is trying to obtain a toy, and the clinician resists.

A clinician is asking a child to point to one of three pictures.

A clinician is instructing a child to act out a scene with dolls.

A child is trying to get a piece of candy by pulling a string tied to the candy, and the clinician is scribbling on a clipboard.

A clinician is watching a child and the parents play.

A clinician with a child is pushing a car back and forth and suddenly pushes a horse on wheels instead of the car back to the child.

A child is trying to complete open-ended sentences presented by the clinician.

A child is describing pictures for a clinician behind a cardboard barrier.

What does it all mean? Are all these clinicians really performing language assessments? How does a clinician know which thing to do with a particular child? One thing is clear: Language assessment requires the clinician to possess more varied skills and diversity of educational background than ever before.

The clinician in a language evaluation must have some framework upon which to gather and organize the data. For years, authorities have been "model building." Many people, however, tend to think that the models that are built in paneled dens across the country are exclusively the stuff of intellectualization and idle theorizing. There is a point, however, where some models begin to have clinical relevance. When a clinician has some sort of guiding principle to use in assessment and treatment, the model appears as a relevant clinical concept. You cannot operate effectively unless you have some organization of your database. Models, then, are "organizing principles" that help to make the clinician more operational. The way in which the clinician conceptualizes language and communication will largely dictate how language disorders are assessed and treated. For instance, a strict behavioral model of language and communication would not necessarily consider cognitive or social prerequisites. It may not deal with intent or other unobservable phenomena. If a clinician subscribes exclusively to this model, there may be no evaluation of the areas mentioned above. Models that emphasize modalities of input and output, such as Kirk and Kirk's (1971), do not particularly focus on linguistic aspects such as syntax, morphology, and pragmatics. Prerequisite areas (cognitive, social, biological) also are ignored. These are just two examples of how the model of language that is adopted by a clinician can constrain thinking and clinical behavior. Thus, all models are not equally useful to a clinician, and certain important aspects of the language process can be missed.

Kamhi (2004) discusses the notion of "meme" in accounting for the perpetuation of diagnostic labels. Most diagnostic labels such as "language disorder" and "phonological disorder" represent very complex phenomena, which are not easily understood. Both laypeople and professionals, however, like to use categories like "auditory processing disorder" and "sensory integration problem" to represent complex problems, because they are easy to remember and perpetuate.

Such memes may offer an oversimplification of the nature of a particular disorder and overlook the true complexity of the problem. In reality, such memes may be plausible on a superficial level, but may not generally be supported by theory or empirical data. While memes are attractive, they do not explain or account for complex disorders, and the diagnostician must be aware of existing "memeplexes."

There are some cautions. First, general semanticists have said for decades that the "map is not the territory." So it is with models. They are not the knowledge or behavior they represent. Clinicians should never forget that it is what they know that is important, far beyond any model. Models are perspectives and guides for organizing clinical information, nothing more. If the clinician is confronted with a real child who is performing at odds with a model's prediction, the validity of the child's behavior is not questionable, but the applicability of the model in this case is certainly a bit dubious. A second caution is that at the present time no one knows for certain all the details of exactly how language is developed, processed, or most efficiently assessed. Thus, any model is likely to be inaccurate or at least, incomplete. Clinicians, like theorists, must be open to change in their conceptualizations and evaluations of language and its evaluation.

THEORETICAL CONSIDERATIONS IN LANGUAGE ASSESSMENT

Following the lead of Muma (1973b, 1978, 1983), we would like to echo some basic diagnostic precepts that we feel should underpin language assessment. First, the best language assessment device, as Siegel (1975) stated, is a well-trained clinician who keeps up with current developments. There is no "best" language test, just as there is no ideal language treatment program.

Second, language is a multidimensional process that has many facets of structure and use. There are also the prerequisite areas discussed earlier to consider in evaluation (e.g., cognitive, social). The existence of the multidimensional process makes it unrealistic to separate structure and function or syntax from semantics or pragmatics. The most ecologically valid methods of analyzing the process are preferable. Whenever we fractionalize the communicative process, we are no longer really looking at it. If we are interested in a child's communication abilities, we should look at real communication, not some artificial task from which we have to infer communication abilities.

Third, Muma (1978) has reminded us that whatever we do in assessment must apply to treatment of the language disorder. If we administer tests and then do not consider these results in planning our treatment, the time spent in assessment is wasted. Our assessment and treatment procedures also should be based on similar assumptions about the communication process.

A fourth important concept also was articulated by Muma. He stated that the diagnostic paradigm seems to have two levels or issues associated with it. The most basic issue is the "problem/no problem" issue. Standardized tests help to solve the problem/no problem issue by comparing a child's test performance to that of other children. This type of testing emphasizes group similarity and minimizes individual variability. The "nature of the problem" issue, however, must be addressed through description of the individual child's communicative performance. This assessment is best accomplished through nonstandardized, descriptive techniques that are more ecologically valid. Fortunately, the problem/no problem issue is solved by many parents when they have referred their children for evaluation. These parents typically know that something is wrong when they compare the communication of their child with his or her peers. A standardized test can confirm this, but it rarely can be prescriptive in terms of specifying treatment targets (Millen & Prutting, 1979).

A fifth important notion has to do with sampling. All we ever do in a diagnostic evaluation is obtain a sample of communicative behavior. There are several important implications that stem from the sampling idea. First, the samples we obtain should be "representative" of the child's communicative performance. The notion of representativeness has been with us for a long while, and we must not forget that a sample we obtain may or may not represent a child's typical or "best" performance. Second, speech pathologists have subscribed for years to the idea that an evaluation can and must take place within a 1- or 2-hour block of time. This kind of thinking can result in frustrated clinicians when they do not obtain the data they need in the allotted time, or if the child is uncooperative. Evaluation is ongoing, and there should be no pressure to find out all there is to know in a limited time frame. The medical profession does not feel compelled to diagnose in a limited time with short, abbreviated procedures. Physicians order examinations that they feel are appropriate, and the diagnostic process takes place over as much time as is necessary. This is not to say that we should emulate the lengthy testing procedures of the medical profession; but on the other hand, we should not become like purveyors of fast food. Third, whenever possible, the clinician should attempt to obtain multiple samples. Many children behave differently in the clinical setting than they do at home or in the preschool.

A sixth basic premise of language assessment is that for every technique or test that the clinician uses, he or she must realize that certain assumptions are implied about child language. To use an instrument, you should "buy the assumptions" that underlie it. Whenever we receive the myriad flyers and announcements of new language assessment instruments, we should remember that each is based on assumptions. We should ask ourselves, "What do I have to believe about language to use this instrument?"

These suggestions should not be taken to mean that we are opposed to the use of standardized tests. We do, in fact, recommend the use of such instruments for the purpose they are most able to accomplish, namely, to determine if a child is performing similarly to other children of his or her age group. Standardized tests, however, cannot make a principled clinical judgment; clinicians make decisions. Assessment has aspects of both art and science (Allen, Bliss, & Timmons, 1981). We advocate the use of a combination of standard measures coupled with nonstandardized tasks and more naturalistic sampling of communicative behavior (Lund & Duchan, 1988; Nelson, 2010; Paul, 2007). We believe that exclusive reliance on either type of procedure will not provide as complete a picture of a child's performance as the use of both types. Additionally, school systems and other work settings typically require some form of standardized testing. Figure 4.1 illustrates the components, goals, and example procedures we recommend for the assessment of children with limited language. The areas of nonstandardized testing and evaluating relevant environment address pertinent aspects of the World Health Organization ICF model presented in Chapter 1.

ASSESSMENT THAT FOCUSES ON EARLY COMMUNICATION AND VARIABLES THAT PREDICT LANGUAGE GROWTH

Wetherby and Prizant (1992) called for a new approach in evaluating early communicative competence. They were in the process of developing the *Communication and Symbolic Behavior Scales* (CSBS) and wanted to capture relevant features of early communication use. Wetherby and Prizant listed several features that they viewed as critical to such early assessment: (1) assessing communicative functions, (2) analyzing preverbal communication, (3) evaluating social-affective signaling, (4) profiling social, communicative, and symbolic abilities, (5) using caregivers as informants and as active participants in the evaluation, and (6) assessing a child's

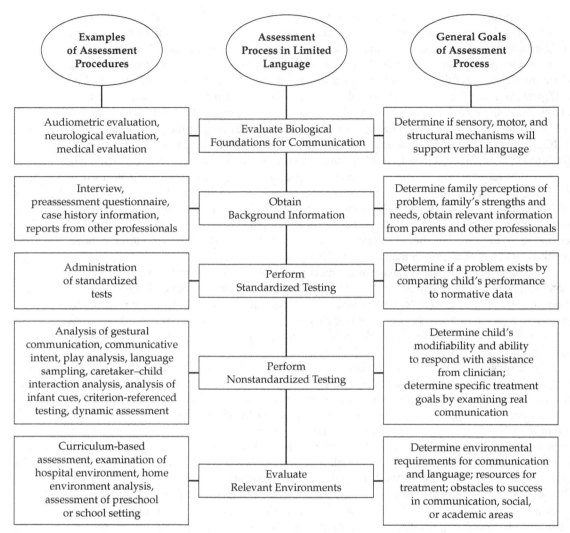

FIGURE 4.1   Critical assessment process in limited language.

communication directly in spontaneous child-initiated interactions. Interestingly, when these authors examined the 10 most frequently used standardized test instruments for the limited-language population, it was clear that most of these examinations did not address relevant features or only addressed them in a limited manner. In most cases, there were no standardized tests that focused on the most relevant variables, and we must rely on nonstandardized approaches to evaluate domains such as communicative intent, play, social behavior, affective states, gestural communication, and caregiver–child interaction.

In the time since Wetherby and Prizant suggested this new approach to assessment of limited language, several studies have shown that many of the variables listed above have predictive value in terms of communication development. For example, McCathren, Warren, and Yoder (1996) reviewed literature to determine which variables in prelinguistic children were effective predictors of language development. They found four major areas that were important. First, the amount of babbling vocalizations and use of consonants in those vocal productions was an important predictor (the more the better). Second, the use of pragmatic functions in behavioral regulation (protoimperative), joint attention (protodeclarative), and social interaction (e.g., showing off, taking turns, social reciprocity) was another good predictor of language development. A third area that was predictive of language development was vocabulary comprehension as measured on the *MacArthur-Bates Communicative Development Inventories* (CDI) (Fenson et al., 2006). Finally, the combinatorial and symbolic play skills of children were predictive of later language development. Yoder, Warren, and McCathren (1998) studied fifty-eight children with developmental delay and gathered a baseline sample of their communication. One year later they divided the children into two groups based on their expressive language. Prefunctional speakers were those children with fewer than five different nonimitative spoken words in a language sample. Functional speakers were those children with more than five different nonimitative words in a sample. Three variables predicted 83% of the children in terms of group membership (functional or prefunctional): (1) number of canonical vocal communication acts (CVCV combinations), (2) CDI discrepancy score (number of words said divided by number of words understood and said), and (3) rate of protodeclarative production. Similarly, Calandrella and Wilcox (2000) examined relations between children's prelinguistic communication and language ability one year later. They found that nonverbal communication acts involving intentional gestural communication and social interaction signals predicted receptive and expressive language outcomes one year later. Brady, Marquis, Fleming, and McLean (2004) conducted a longitudinal study of 18 children with developmental disabilities who were between 3 and 6 years old and followed for 2 years. The three most potent predictors of language outcome as revealed on the SICD-R were the initial level of gestural attainment, rate of communication, and parental response contingency. Many other studies of language prognosis in children described as "late talkers" have also found the variables mentioned above to be valuable in predicting language development. The CDI has recently been used to attempt predictions of language development for populations such as children with developmental delay and autism spectrum disorders (Luyster, Qiu, Lopez, & Lord, 2007). Prelinguistic skills are critical predictors of language development in many groups of children. For example, specific skills such as vocabulary size, verbal imitation ability, pretend play with objects, and use of gestures to initiate joint attention have been shown to be important predictors of vocabulary development in children with autism (Smith, Mirenda, & Zaidman-Zait, 2007).

The predictive variables for children with limited language have two important assessment implications. First, as indicated by Wetherby and Prizant (1992), the exclusive use of standardized tests with this population will miss most of the critical behaviors that are relevant to assessment and prognosis. McCathren, Warren, and Yoder (1996) examined the most popular prelinguistic assessment instruments and, similar to Wetherby and Prizant, found that those instruments ignored relevant areas or only examined them in a limited fashion. McCathren, Warren, and Yoder suggested that only two assessment procedures at that point in time addressed the four critical predictive areas of babbling, pragmatic functions, vocabulary comprehension, and combinatorial/symbolic play. One of the measures was the CSBS (Wetherby & Prizant, 1993) and the other measure was the ALB (Olswang, Stoel-Gammon, Coggins, & Carpenter, 1987).

A second implication of the research on predictive variables is that there is no substitute for communication sampling, play evaluation, caretaker involvement, gestural communication, and evaluation of communicative intent in limited-language cases. This sampling and evaluation can be done using a published procedure such as the CSBS or the ALB or any number of nonstandardized procedures that focus on specific areas of interest. We will mention some of these nonstandardized approaches in the following sections.

SPECIFIC ASSESSMENT AREAS: PROCEDURES, CONSIDERATIONS, AND DIRECTIONS FOR FURTHER STUDY

In the sections that follow, we discuss specific techniques for assessing important areas related to the communication of a child with limited language. We try to provide guidelines and references for the clinician to use in learning about these various aspects of language assessment. In cases where we cannot adequately summarize a procedure (which is most of the time), we refer you to a primary source with the hope that you will critically evaluate and perhaps learn techniques that will be clinically useful.

At the beginning of most sections, we provide a brief sketch of some important developmental trends reported in the existing research. It is imperative to appreciate that each assessment technique mentioned is basically grounded in the research on communication development. While it is beyond the scope of this chapter to present an adequate view of any aspect of language acquisition, we would be remiss if we did not touch upon some highlights of the process that are related to language assessment. Many fine textbooks are available that summarize research in language acquisition, and you should become familiar with this information before engaging in any language assessment.

Preassessment and Pertinent Historical Information

PREASSESSMENT In most clinical settings, prospective clients are required to complete a case history before being seen by the speech-language pathologist or other professionals. It is especially unnerving to meet a client for the first time without first receiving the completed case history information, because it is impossible to prepare for the evaluation. Especially in the area of language disorders, the client could be at levels ranging from totally nonverbal to a syntax level with only subtle language problems. Thus, it is crucial for SLPs in any work setting to avoid performing an evaluation without access to important historical information. Prior knowledge of historical information can allow the clinician to plan the evaluation to maximize the use of time and resources during the initial contact with the child and parents.

Gallagher (1983) suggested a preassessment procedure for use with language cases and outlined the advantages of such a process for the clinician in planning and conducting evaluations. Preassessment is more than the typical process of having the parents merely fill out a case history form. The notion of preassessment includes finding out some clinically useful data that could affect the way in which the initial evaluation is conducted. In our university setting, we use a preassessment form that contains components from a variety of research projects. Clients are asked to return the completed form before the evaluation appointment is scheduled. In some cases where the parents cannot read or have difficulty completing the form, an interview session is scheduled in which the parents are questioned about each item on the preassessment before we see the child. The important thing is that the clinician has a fairly good picture of the child's cognitive, social, play, and communicative behavior before the evaluation session. Typically, to provide additional information on noncommunicative behaviors that relate to cognitive, social, and language development, we also include a short adaptive-behavior scale that focuses on motor skills, self-help skills, and personal/social abilities. Gallagher (1983) gives a concrete example of the value of preassessment information:

> One child who was particularly sensitive to the communicative partner had an MLU value of 1.6 in the clinician–child sample and an MLU of 3.96 when she talked with her brother. One boy produced his most structurally complex utterances while he

was playing with water toys in a plastic pan filled with water, an activity his mother had indicated "he would talk most about." One boy's most structurally complex language performance was obtained when he played with a younger friend who was his neighbor. For one child, it was talking about pictures in a family album. (p. 14)

None of these language-facilitating situations would have been known to the clinician if the appropriate questions had not been asked on a preassessment instrument. The clinician can plan ahead and ask family members to bring specific stimulus items, toys, or interactants that would provide the best sample of a client's communication abilities.

THE PARENT INTERVIEW   Many questions will be raised by parent responses on the preassessment packet. The interview is a good place to clarify any missing information or inconsistencies in a parent's responses. The information obtained from caretakers of limited-language children is highly important. First of all, many of these children may not have the linguistic means or cognitive development to express themselves well, and the parent or guardian must be relied upon to provide pertinent background details and estimations of present skill levels. Second, recent research has suggested that expressive language disorders tend to run in families (Lahey & Edwards, 1995), and information regarding symptoms, treatments, and outcomes related to disorders in other family members is most easily obtained in the interview format that allows for examples and follow-up questions. Third, the Individuals with Disabilities Education Act (IDEA) of 2004 mandates that families are critical team members and requires professionals to work closely with them when assessing and treating children with communication disorders. We will discuss this more specifically later in the present chapter. Thus, parent involvement is not just a "nice touch" to incorporate into early intervention, it is the law. As mentioned in Chapter 1, evidence-based practice (EBP) requires a clinician to fully understand the client's perspective on the disorder prior to recommending treatment. The parent interview is an important information-gathering mechanism in this regard.

As mentioned in Chapter 2, we do not recommend that the diagnostician write specific questions prior to the evaluation. Appendix A contains an interview protocol for assessing the limited-language child. The protocol is divided into broad areas covering the prerequisites to language as well as the beginnings of linguistic development. Much of the specific information can be filled in from responses to the preassessment packet, and the interview can simply follow up areas of interest to the clinician. The interviewer should ask questions in the broad areas, obtaining information in each subarea. The exact wording of questions is not provided owing to the pragmatics of the interview situation. Parents represent differing levels of education, intelligence, socioeconomic status, and experience, and we have found it more feasible to tailor interview questions for each individual case. The protocol was designed only to "jog the mind" of the clinician, who, it is hoped, will ask questions in specific topic areas. When remarkable information is reported in any area, the interviewer should formulate appropriate follow-up questions to clearly illuminate the area of interest. The major interview areas represent biological, social, and cognitive prerequisites to language as well as linguistic level and were gleaned from a variety of child-language-acquisition and language-impairment sources. The interviewer should especially focus the interview on the most applicable portions of the protocol and not ask unnecessary questions. For instance, if a child is using a wide variety of multiword utterances and is communicating effectively in the environment, it would not be productive for the interviewer to spend inordinate time on cognitive and social attainments.

One of the most revealing questions about the child's home environment is the item that asks a parent to describe a typical day in the life of his or her child. It is often surprising how much important information can be uncovered in the answer to this question. For instance, a parent may report that the child spends many hours watching television, or playing alone outside, or engaging in self-stimulatory activities—activities that have been allowed to continue despite their lack of productivity. Often, a pattern emerges that shows that the child spends little time in meaningful social interactions. Another pattern that reveals much about a child's problem is lack of a schedule or rules in the household. One mother reported that her nonverbal 3-year-old child typically went to bed at 11:30 P.M. after a late-night talk show and liked to sleep until 9:30 A.M. The child also ate all his meals while walking around inside the house, refused to wear pajamas, threw frequent tantrums, and was prone to writing on the walls. This scenario suggests that the parents and child may be in some need of counseling regarding behavior management. Much of this information would not have been gleaned from the preassessment packet or a formal test, but the information would be quite important when it comes to making recommendations for treatment. If, for example, we wanted these parents to begin to withhold desired items from this child in order to create communicative opportunity, they would have extreme difficulty with this procedure, since there appear to be few existing rules in the home. Tantrums would inevitably increase, and the treatment plan would have a high probability of being aborted by the family.

Assessment of Social Prerequisites and Caretaker–Child Interaction

Language development takes place in a social context. From the moment of birth, a child interacts with his or her caretakers and is bombarded with visual, auditory, and tactile stimuli that occur in this relationship. The Individuals with Disabilities Education Act (IDEA) also mandates the involvement of the family in both assessment and treatment, and it is especially important in cases of nonverbal, single-word, and early-multiword-level children to observe them as they interact with their caretaker. There are two reasons for this.

First, we want to observe the child with someone with whom he or she is familiar and feels comfortable being around. It is often the case that the best sample of the child's communication is obtained in this portion of the evaluation. When unfamiliar clinicians attempt to establish rapport with a child in strange surroundings, it may be quite difficult to observe natural communication, especially in a limited time period. Occasionally, we have seen children who refused to interact with us in an evaluation. In these cases the caretaker–child interaction provides the only database available. In the early years of our field, we were frequently told that the initial step in an evaluation was to separate the child from the mother. Often, this resulted in a catastrophic reaction on the part of the child, and little information was gained from the evaluation (other than the fact that the child did not "separate well from the mother"). We must not lose sight of our goal, namely, to observe the child's communicative and prelinguistic skills through talking and play. If the caretaker can provide a more effective demonstration of certain skills than the clinician can, then we must take advantage of this opportunity and not feel that we have failed as clinicians. Rather, we have succeeded in getting the data we were after as the result of making a sound clinical judgment. Establishing a relationship with a child can always be accomplished in the initial treatment sessions where we are not under as severe time constraints. In communication samples gathered by either the clinician or the caretaker, the caretaker should always be asked whether the child's communicative behavior is representative of his or her typical interaction.

A second goal of the caretaker–child interaction is to observe the quality of the language model provided by the parent. Research has shown that caretakers alter many aspects of their communicative behavior. Suprasegmentally, they raise their vocal fundamental frequency, increase their pitch range, speak more slowly, and use double primary-stress patterns.

The caretaker is less disfluent when talking to an infant and pauses at major linguistic constituent boundaries. Linguistically, the mean length of utterance is reduced, and the vocabulary and syntactic complexity are simplified. Developing children, in addition to being exposed to a simpler language model, are given an introduction to the reciprocity of communicative interchange. Snow (1977) has shown that with neonates as young as three months of age, mothers engage in turntaking, reciprocal behavior. Early on, the child's "turn" is a biologically programmed nonverbal action, such as smiling, sneezing, or burping. The mother simply responds to this with some sort of language response and often takes the child's turn for him or her linguistically. As the child develops, the caretaker demands that the youngster's turn more closely resemble the adult correct model.

As important as the model itself are the circumstances under which it is delivered. The youngster benefits cognitively from interacting with the caretaker. Mothers and fathers typically show the child "how the world works" by demonstrating the functional use of objects and body parts, the attributes of objects, and many other conceptual aspects of the environment. Children have been observed to follow a caretaker's line of visual regard (to look at an object a parent is focused on) very early in development (McLean & Snyder-McLean, 1978). Adults also show the child how to play with a variety of objects and even stimulate symbolic play. We see then, that caretakers demonstrate language structure, language use, concepts, and the reciprocity of communication. Children are highly sensitive to their social environment, and they learn that language is a tool to be used for a variety of social and nonsocial purposes (Dore, 1975; Halliday, 1975). With young children, it is clear that their early exposure to language and their early use of it is highly social.

One important aspect of caretaker–child interaction involves book sharing. Parents share books with their children from infancy onward. This activity carries with it reciprocal roles and redundancy in language stimulation. The roles taken by parent and child change over time as the child develops language and cognitive abilities. Initially, the child just looks at the book with the caretaker and visually follows the caretaker's pointing responses. Later, the child takes on the role of "pointer" as language comprehension develops, and the caretaker asks questions about pictures in the book (e.g., "Where's the kitty?"). During this time the child is also becoming oriented to the nature of literacy activities such as page turning, book positioning, and the differences between text and pictures. When the child reaches the single-word period, the caretaker asks questions and the child names pictures in the book. Ultimately, when the child has connected speech, the caretaker asks more difficult questions about what events will happen next and how characters feel. Many authorities suggest sampling joint book reading as part of an evaluation to determine caretaker–child interaction strategies and get a sense of how both participate in literacy activities. Kaderavek and Sulzby (1998) developed a protocol for evaluating parent–child joint book reading behaviors and strategies, which would be a useful adjunct to assessment. Similarly, Rabidoux and Macdonald (2000) described caretaker–child interactive parameters during joint book sharing, including communicative styles, child roles/styles, and strategies for maintaining interactions. This taxonomy may be useful in assessing the climate of children's emergent literacy. One might assume that the nature of a child's language impairment itself would be the best predictor of emergent literacy. McGinty and Justice (2009), however, found that differences in language ability were not particularly good at explaining variability in print knowledge in children with language impairment. Instead, they found that quality of home literacy experience was the best predictor of print knowledge, especially in language-impaired children with attentional difficulties. This again underscores the importance of examining the literacy opportunities available in the family for children when we are examining emergent literacy.

Research has shown that teachers can also provide important information on preschoolers' emergent literacy skills, and it is wise to enlist their input to determine in which skills a child has strengths. Teachers, however, have not necessarily been effective in identifying or diagnosing children who are at risk for literacy difficulties (Cabell, Justice, Zucker, & Kilday, 2009).

The clinician needs to answer many questions about the caretaker–child interaction. Does the caretaker talk about the "here and now" (Holland, 1975) or about things removed in time and space? What kind of joint referencing takes place in the interaction? Does the caretaker talk about and participate in things that the child appears to be interested in? Does the caretaker direct the child's play to things that the former feels are significant and disregard the child's preferences? Is there a balance between when the parent joint references with the child and when the child joint references with the parent? Regarding the uses of language, does the parent force the child into limited or respondent modes of communicative function? It is not unusual to observe parents of early language-disordered children who ask incessant questions (e.g., "What's this?" "What color is this?") or who ask the child to constantly imitate (e.g., "Say 'ball'"). We are not intimating that the parent's interactive style is in any way causally related to the child's language disorder. In fact, a parent's way of talking to a child could be a result of the disorder rather than a cause. Whatever the relationship, the caretaker's model as it presently exists may not be conducive to language development and should be changed. The only way to determine the quality of this relationship is through the observation of caretaker–child interaction. Evaluating and working with caretaker–child interaction is especially important when dealing with infants and toddlers who are at "high risk" for language disorder. Providing the best-quality stimulation for these children will go a long way toward preventing, or at least reducing, the severity of potential language disorders. Table 4-1 provides an example of a checklist that the clinician could use in examining caretaker behaviors during interaction in the evaluation session. The clinician's impressions of the caretaker modifications could lead to treatment recommendations involving work with interaction patterns.

It is also important to examine specific aspects of the child's social behavior in the caretaker–child interaction. Socially, the child's eye contact and willingness to participate in reciprocal nonverbal activities should be observed. A child who does not tolerate or seek out the participation of another person may not have any need for a communication system. Perhaps this child might need to work on some prelinguistic social skills along with the development of language. Recall that MacDonald and Carroll (1992) said that a child must first become a play partner and a turntaking partner before a communication partnership develops. Language is, after all, a social tool, and a child who is not "social" has little need of a code to use around people with whom he does not even communicate nonverbally. Children with autism spectrum disorders require close examination of social skills because these may play a major role in determining diagnosis and monitoring treatment. Parents are a rich source of information on social behavior and so are teachers, because they spend many hours observing and interacting with the child. The input from these two groups, however, may not provide equivalent information. For instance, Murray, Ruble, Willis, and Molloy (2009) found that while there was general agreement between parents and teachers on overall social skill ratings, there was poor agreement on individual social behaviors. The implication is not that one group is more correct than another, but that there can be contextual differences in a child's behavior, and multiple informants provide a more complete picture of social skill than relying on a single source. Bopp, Mirenda, and Zumbo (2009) followed children with autism over a 2-year period and tried to predict vocabulary production and comprehension from an initial sample of behavior. Specifically, they found that high rates of inattentive behaviors such as not paying attention to the environment, distractiveness, failure to listen to instruction, and looking away from a joint task tended to predict less progress in vocabulary

TABLE 4.1	Caretaker–Child Interaction Attributes

Child: _____ Date: _____ Age: _____

Nature of interaction in terms of toys, room, and interactants:

General Parameters	**No**	**Yes**

1. Encourages communication by looking expectantly
2. Responds to communication by reinforcing it with action or utterance
3. Joint references with child
4. Alternates adult/child direction in joint referencing
5. Talks about present context (here and now)
6. Model is timed to coincide with joint referencing
7. Talks at child's eye level
8. Successful attempts at interpretation of child's utterances and communicative intents
9. Creates communicative opportunities by using sabotage or pause time
10. Does not anticipate child's needs ahead of time, thus reducing communicative attempts

Language Model Parameters
1. Reduces sentence length
2. Reduces sentence complexity
3. Repeats utterances frequently (redundancy)
4. Paraphrases utterances ("throw the ball; throw it")
5. Uses exaggerated intonation patterns
6. Places stress on important words
7. Uses concrete, high-frequency vocabulary
8. Does not talk too much and dominate conversation
9. Does not use excessive questions and commands
10. Uses slower speech rate

Use of Teaching Techniques
1. Self-talk
2. Parallel talk
3. Expansion
4. Expatiation (enlargement)
5. Buildup/breakdown sequences
6. Recast sentences

production and comprehension. Additionally, the more socially unresponsive the child was, such as not making eye contact, failing to respond to his or her name, and rarely smiling, also associated with less language progress. Again, this suggests that the SLP should examine not only linguistic skills, but ancillary behaviors that are associated with social abilities. Some past investigations have suggested that about 50% of the population of children with language impairment have been reported to manifest behavior problems.

In some of the early research, however, the diagnosis of children with language disorder may not have been confined to those with specific language impairment. For example, children with developmental delay or pervasive developmental disorder might have been included. Interestingly, Rescorla, Ross, and McClure (2007) found that children with language delay did, in fact, show more total behavior problems, and language scores were significantly correlated. However, when the researchers eliminated children with neurodevelopmental delay and pervasive developmental disorder, total behavior problems and language scores were no longer significantly related. With this exclusion, only the variable of social withdrawal remained correlated with language ability. Harrison and McLeod (2010) gathered data on almost five thousand Australian children to determine risk and protective factors related to language impairment. The variables considered spanned the child, family, parent, and community. They found that risk factors involved being male, having persistent hearing difficulties, and being more reactive in temperament. The major protective factors were having a sociable temperament and higher scores on maternal well-being. The implication of this study is that we must look beyond the child's test performance on language measures and into social/emotional and family contexts to understand prognostic factors.

ADAPTIVE BEHAVIOR SCALES Adaptive behavior scales typically rate a child's development of motor skills, social behavior, self-help skills, and language ability. Children are given tasks to perform, or the parents are asked to respond to items on the interview protocol. The advantage of such scales is that their use helps to broaden the perspective of the SLP beyond exclusively examining language ability. Although we will assess social cognitive development as it relates to language, much of a child's adaptive behavior depends on cognitive and social attainments. We can obtain a better overall picture of the child's level of functioning, and this information, when coupled with our other assessment data, can be valuable. In addition, many conditions (e.g., cognitive impairment) may show that a child is generally low functioning in most areas and that language is only part of the problem. Knowledge of adaptive behavior also will be important to the clinician in making referrals. Language-treatment activities also can be designed to incorporate motor, social, and self-help areas so that the child is learning a variety of needed skills as well as the language associated with them. Several adaptive behavior scales are available (Bricker, Squires, & Mounts, 1995; Furuno et al., 1994; Sparrow, Balla, & Cicchetti, 1984). In most work settings, including public schools and many medical settings, SLPs are part of a transdisciplinary or multidisciplinary team. Other professionals such as psychologists, psychometrists, occupational therapists, physical therapists, special-education teachers, and medical personnel can provide valuable interpretations of the noncommunication domains included on such behavior scales as self-help, motor skills, and social adjustment (Haynes, Moran, & Pindzola, 2011). The advantage of such a team approach is not only in interpreting assessment findings but also in programming goals for multiple domains across the treatment regimen.

Assessment of Play to Gain Insight into Cognitive Attainments Associated with Communication

As mentioned by MacDonald and Carroll (1992) in the "big picture" of language acquisition provided at the beginning of this chapter, typically developing children first become "play partners" and "turn-taking partners." This involves learning how to joint reference with the caregiver and manipulate objects together, both in exploration and in functional use of items. Play assessment helps us to determine if a child is capable of being a productive play partner and social participant with adults in his or her environment. Evaluation of cognitive attainments is simultaneously simple and elusive. First of all, it appears that relationships between cognitive and linguistic skills change significantly with development. Although a particular cognitive attainment may relate strongly to a communication skill at one age, this relationship may disappear as the child continues to develop. If anything, there is a general as opposed to a specific relation between cognition and language. Yet, when we see a prelinguistic child for an evaluation, we would like to get a sense of what he or she seems to understand about the objects, events, and actions in the world. Obviously, a nonverbal child cannot provide this information through language and speech. Many authorities have suggested that a child's play strategies reflect, to some degree, his or her concepts and understanding of the world. The main vocation of a child is play, and an examination of play routines can allow the clinician to make some general inferences about the child's worldview. It is unlikely that a child with primitive play routines that involve sensorimotor exploration, shaking, banging, and mouthing of objects has an understanding of objects and events that lends itself well to coding with a linguistic system. A child with no concept of functional object use (using an object appropriately, as in pushing a toy car) is unlikely to need language to code the name of this object (*car*) or the relationships this object enters into (e.g., *push, go, big*).

Conceptual holdings are thought to be important to linguistic acquisition for several reasons. First, language is a representational act. It represents reality or stands for objects and relationships in the world. Second, language is an abstract symbol system. In order to appreciate abstract symbols, we must be able to represent them mentally. Third, language is a tool that we use in social interactions. Tool use implies certain conceptual underpinnings such as the apprehension of relationships like means–end. Fourth, language use involves talking about objects, events, and relationships in the world. It is necessary that one knows and can remember the properties of these objects and relationships before talking about them coherently. As Nelson (1974) said, we use words as *tags* for the concepts that we have.

Perhaps the best known researcher in the area of children's cognitive development has been Jean Piaget. A most significant period in language development occurs between birth and 2 years (Beard, 1969; Ginsburg & Opper, 1969; Morehead & Morehead, 1974). By the age of 2, a child is typically beginning to use multiword utterances and has clearly demonstrated the symbolic capacity for dealing with language. Piaget calls the period between birth and age 2 the sensorimotor stage of cognitive development, because most learning takes place through active sensorimotor exploration of a child's environment. Piaget has divided his sensorimotor period of cognitive development into six substages. In typical development, a child attains at least stage 4 of the sensorimotor period to evidence gestural communication and stages 5 or 6 for expressive single- and early multiword constructions. In reviewing the cognitive development literature, however, there seem to be certain skills that are included on cognitive assessment scales and often referred to by authorities as potentially being language related.

Functional object use has been related to the development of communication (Steckol & Leonard, 1981). Using an object for its intended purpose (e.g., combing hair with a comb) requires the mental representation of both the object and its use. Also, when a child begins to talk about basic relations in the environment, utterances typically concern objects, their functions, and all the relationships an object enters into (Nelson, 1974).

Imitation and *deferred (delayed) imitation* also have been related to the development of language (Bates, 1979). Imitation requires mental representation of an act for a short time period, and deferred imitation requires holding onto an event for a longer duration. Both suggest at least an ability to represent reality for a length of time and to not depend on immediate stimulus support.

Finally, *symbolic play* (pretend behavior) is frequently regarded as evidence of a child's general symbolic capacity. One can think of symbolic play on a continuum from playing with exemplars of an object that are physically similar to the real object (e.g., a box representing a car), to playing with exemplars that are dissimilar to the real object (e.g., a comb for a car), and finally to playing with no object at all (*pantomime*). The use of one object to stand for another is similar to the way that words represent objects in the real world. A basic symbolic capacity must be present in order to use a symbolic play routine, and these routines should be noted in a child's behavior as a positive sign of increased symbolic capacity.

A primary reason to assess cognitive level is to determine a child's ability to represent reality and deal with symbols. As we mentioned in an earlier section, some of the specific behaviors that have been associated with language development are imitation, deferred imitation, means–end, functional use of objects, and symbolic play (pretend). These cognitive attainments will be the focus of discussion here because they are the behaviors included in cognitive test batteries and have been referred to most often as being possibly related to language development.

An important notion to keep in mind when assessing cognitive attainments is that we watch a child's behavior and *infer* his or her conceptual holdings. We should obtain as much information as possible about the child's typical play routines and object use. The preassessment questionnaire and parent interview are invaluable here. The child may exhibit evidence of more sophisticated play at home and not demonstrate it in the clinical setting. The failure of a child to perform a task that we set up to evaluate a particular cognitive attainment is not necessarily evidence of a lack of the concept. A child can fail a cognitive task due to inattention, disinterest, or some other reason that has nothing to do with his or her cognitive status.

With the above admonitions in mind, how does one perform a play assessment, and what type of child undergoes the evaluation? We have found it productive to take note of cognitive attainments in children who are nonverbal and those who are at the single-word level. Children who currently use productive early multiword utterances already are evidencing some representational ability and symbolic ability just by using language normally. It is not useful to routinely administer a lengthy and complex cognitive test battery initially. We recommend that the diagnostician move from general analyses to more specific ones.

The first level of analysis can be a lengthy behavioral observation of the child engaged in play. In our experience, children whose cognitive levels are lower will exhibit primitive play routines and perseverative use of objects. Westby (1980) outlines some useful stages and a scale to use in assessing the developmental relationship between cognitive development, language, and play. The clinician can set up a play situation and watch the child interact with objects and people. It is important to remember that the toys and objects provided give the child an opportunity to exhibit higher levels of play. For example, if only a car, ball, blocks, and a toy horse are provided, the child would be limited in his or her ability to demonstrate combinatorial symbolic play. On the other hand, if a doll, doll bed, spoon, bowl, baby bottle, and blanket were provided, the child would have the opportunity to show how he or she could pretend using these objects in combinations. The examiner should be looking for behavior that suggests functional use of objects, symbolic play, means–end, combinatorial play, sensorimotor exploration, imitation, and searching for hidden objects. On the Westby (1980) scale we should "triangulate" a child's chronological age, language stage, and play level to determine if there are discrepancies. For example, a 3-year-old child may exhibit a play level of 3 years of age, but a language level of 1 year of age. This suggests that the child's language level is lagging behind his or her cognitive development, and this is likely to be more of a language problem than a cognitive one. If, on the other hand, a 3-year-old child is at the 1-year level for both language and cognition, it is possible that both cognitive and linguistic goals should be targeted in treatment. Chappel and Johnson (1976) recommend looking at a child's play behavior and coding play on three levels, such as sensori-motor exploration, functional use of objects, and symbolic/combinatorial play.

The most important thing to determine is the child's *modal level* of play, which is the most frequently occurring type of interaction. It is optimal to videotape the play interaction for later specific analysis (Lund & Duchan, 1988). We recommend the following general steps as you analyze a videotape. First, divide the play session into play episodes that represent a particular theme. For instance, if the child is playing with a farm set, call the play episode "farm." Then, look at each interaction the child has with the objects and people in each play episode. If a child picks up a cow and puts it in his mouth, this should be documented as mouthing or sensorimotor exploration. If the child makes the cow walk and jump into the back of a truck, take note of this behavior as possibly symbolic play, because pretending is involved. If the child brushes a doll's hair and puts it to bed covered up with a blanket, this may be combinatorial symbolic play. A summary of behaviors in play episodes can easily result in a modal level of play in terms of sensorimotor exploration, functional object use, or symbolic play. In all cases, view the specific behaviors in terms of the context in which they occurred. For instance, pretending that a block is a car can qualify as symbolic play only if the clinician did not demonstrate this activity earlier in the session. At any rate, it is important to view children's nonverbal play behaviors contextually and, if possible, obtain some historical data on their play routines.

After observing play routines, consider whether a cognitive delay is suggested, based on the quality of play exhibited. Sometimes, there will clearly be no representational problem, based on the sophisticated levels of observed play routines. Other times, behavior will occur that strongly suggests a rather primitive representational ability. Many cases fall between these two ends of the cognitive continuum, and these children may require further testing to determine which level of cognitive development they have attained.

A final level of analysis is to administer a more detailed scale such as that developed by Uzigiris and Hunt (1975). Dunst (1980) has developed some helpful procedures for use with the Uzigiris and Hunt scales that make the clinical administration of the tasks more streamlined. Such lengthy measures should be administered to a child who is strongly suspected of exhibiting cognitive deficits.

The speech-language pathologist should be careful when assessing cognitive attainments related to language and not allow other professionals or parents to perceive this evaluation procedure as the testing of a child's *intelligence*. We should make no judgments about how "smart" a child is or necessarily even his or her potential for cognitive growth. Children whose play behavior and performance on cognitive scales indicate that they lack some cognitive basis for language should be referred to other professionals (e.g., psychologist, special educator) for a program that includes many domains of child development including cognitive, social, self-help, and motor abilities. SLPs examine cognitive attainments only because they appear to be related to the acquisition and use of abstract language systems. If we determine that a child does not possess the cognitive attainments for acquiring the abstract and arbitrary symbol system of language, we then can consider attempting to train cognitive goals (Kahn, 1984) or training a communication system that is less abstract, such as simple signs or augmentative communication devices that code concrete and frequently occurring activities. In fact, it is common to use augmentative devices to train children about specific cognitive attainments such as means–end, as children learn that pushing a button or level can activate a toy or communication device. Snyder-McLean, McLean, and Etter (1988) provide many useful suggestions in evaluating the cognitive status of older, severely involved clients.

Cognitive assessment is not just smoke and mirrors; this information has practical clinical applications. Recall the earlier section in this chapter on prediction and prognosis in early language development. Among the strongest predictors of language development in children was the level of play, symbolic play, and use of combinatorial play. This is also one of the potent predictors for discriminating whether a child is a "late talker" or is language impaired, along with other measures of language production, comprehension, communicative intent, phonology, and social behavior. Another practical aspect of looking at children's play is its relationship to social behavior. Some studies have shown that children with language impairment also exhibit social deficits. Children who play appropriately will be able to form social relationships with others, while those who are limited to sensorimotor exploration will have difficulty being accepted by their peers. Incorporating play/cognitive goals into language treatment is relatively easy and has a potentially large payoff for a child's social interactions.

The CSBS of Wetherby and Prizant (2002) is respected by many clinicians and researchers as a useful measure of early language development, because it focuses on many aspects of communication, including cognitive, social, affective, phonetic, and linguistic domains. The CSBS uses a relatively natural sampling procedure for communication and play and provides normative data on all areas examined. This is also a reasonable initial step in cognitive assessment. The CSBS has also been extended to include a shortened procedure that can be administered and scored in significantly less time than the entire CSBS battery (Wetherby & Prizant, 1998).

Assessment of Communicative Intent and Function

The third step toward becoming a communicator is to interact with caregivers as communication partners (McDonald & Carroll, 1992). It is important to realize that *communication* is not synonymous with speech and language. That is, children communicate gesturally long before they do so with words. A thorough analysis of a child's gestural communication is an important part of early language evaluation to determine if a child is in fact a communication partner. Preverbal communication is fairly easy to see in children. They communicate profusely by pushing adults, pulling adults, pointing at objects or events, reaching for objects, giving objects to adults, and showing objects to adults. They also use gaze shifts as very important components of their preverbal communication. Children will point at an object and alternate their gaze between the caregiver and the object. They will also engage in visual checking to see if a caregiver is watching their gestural communication while they are pointing or reaching. We cannot emphasize enough that the analysis of communicative intent is critical to assessment of early language cases. There is a strong rationale for this notion. First, function/intent precedes form/structure in communicative development. Children exhibit intentional communication before they produce words. Second, training forms/structures in the absence of functions is not efficacious. That is, it is not particularly useful to train a child to say words when he or she has no reason to use them. This type of case probably needs a focus on training social reciprocity, communicative intent, and gestural communication in addition to learning words. In therapy we would much rather see a child who is a little puller, pusher, and pointer than one who has no intentional gestural communication with others in the environment. Again, standardized tests typically do not examine communicative gestures, so the clinician must rely on nonstandardized communication sampling. Steigler (2007) showed that an in-depth analysis of interactions using conversation analysis and speech act analysis can provide important insight into variables such as conversational sequencing, diversity of speech acts, gazing, smiling, initiations, and communicative output of a child with autism. Such measurements are not often found on standardized tests and instead focus on actual social or clinical interactions. Shumway and Wetherby (2009) evaluated rate, communicative functions, and means of communication on the Communication and Symbolic Behavior Scales for 125 children between the ages of 18–24 months who were categorized as typically developing, children with autism spectrum disorders, and children who were developmentally delayed. They found that children with autism produced communicative acts at a significantly lower rate and used fewer acts to establish joint attention, which were the strongest predictors of language development at age 3. The children diagnosed with autism who did use joint attention acts tended to coordinate vocalizations, eye gaze, and gesture with these bids, so just because a child with autism coordinates means of communication does not rule out the diagnosis of autism spectrum disorder.

Crais, Douglas, and Campbell (2004) conducted a longitudinal study of 12 typically developing children between the ages of 6 and 24 months. The results show a detailed summary of gestural development in the broad categories of regulating behavior, gaining joint attention, and social interaction. Within each category, means and variability data are provided for individual gestures, which would be valuable in assessment of gestural communication. Similarly, Capone and McGregor (2004) outline the development of communicative gestures in early childhood in both typical children and those with language impairment. They discuss implications of examining gestural development for diagnosis, prognosis, and intervention. Determining a child's semantic representations is almost always a difficult task for the clinician. This is especially challenging when a child has a limited vocabulary. From studies of gesture and gesture/speech combinations in typically developing children, we have gained considerable insight into what a child knows about the world. For instance, if a child looks at a picture of a fish and makes a swimming motion with the hands, it tells us that he or she knows how a fish moves. Detailed analysis of a child's gestural system and how gestures are coupled with words and vocalizations are a rich source of data for early language assessment (Capone, 2007).

Some authorities have indicated that a frequent manifestation of early language disorder in children is their failure to use language (Fey, 1986; Lucas, 1980; Wetherby & Prutting, 1984). As mentioned previously, a prelinguistic or nonverbal child has no expressive language. This does not imply, however, that the child is not communicating. Any mother of a prelinguistic child will attest that her child communicates profusely about his or her desires, moods, and a variety of pleasing and noxious biological states. Bates (1976) studied the sensorimotor performatives of young children and determined that those children have primitive forms of imperatives or commands by which they use adults to obtain access to objects in their environment. The goal is to gain access to the object. One can initially see the child physically manipulating the adult, as in putting the adult's hand on a jar to open it. Later, the child may use pointing coupled with vocalizations to indicate to the adult what he or she wants done. Bates also noted primitive forms of the declarative in which the child uses an object to gain adult attention as the goal. There appears to be a progression that begins with the child's showing and giving objects to adults. Ultimately, the child exhibits the declarative by pointing toward objects with an alternating gaze between the adult and object. Bates (1979) reported a "gestural complex" that, in part, may be related to language development. Thus, communication is taking place quite vividly in the preverbal child.

There are also preverbal evidences of the "functions" of language alluded to by Halliday (1975) and Dore (1975). That is, children use the greeting function nonverbally by waving, they question by exhibiting a quizzical look, and they regulate adults physically before they use language for these purposes. In preverbal children, the primary evidence for their communication ability is found in gestures, facial expressions, and/or vocalizations. These phenomena can be observed by a clinician in a diagnostic session, or caretakers can be asked in an assessment interview about how the child makes his or her needs known at home and at school.

Communicative intents can be realized on a gestural, vocal, or verbal level. Dore et al. (1976) noted that a prelinguistic child is not simply uttering "jargon" vocalizations. At a certain point in development, Dore et al. noted the presence of phonetically consistent forms (PCFs) that he termed "transitional phenomena." Phonetically consistent forms are vocalizations that are stabilized around certain situations. They are not word approximations but are fairly stable phonetic productions typically consisting of vowel or consonant–vowel combinations. They are repeatedly associated with specific situations such as showing affect (emotion), indicating or pointing to aspects of the environment, or expressing a desire to obtain an object or event. Dore et al. observed that these PCFs seem to act as a transition to words wherein certain phonetic elements must be stabilized around a specific referent. Thus, it would be important in an evaluation of communicative function not only to determine which basic functions are present, but also to determine whether those functions manifest themselves on a gestural, vocal, or verbal level. Stark, Bernstein, and Demorest (1993) and Proctor (1989) report useful data on vocalizations produced for a variety of communicative functions and outline an orderly developmental sequence of vocal communication in the first 18 months of life.

According to Chapman (1981), the clinician may adopt an existing classification scheme or change these available systems so that functions that are of interest can be coded. Many systems might be useful clinically (Coggins & Carpenter, 1978; Dore, 1975; Folger & Chapman, 1978; Halliday, 1975; Tough, 1977). From examining the categories in these systems, it is clear that many of the terms overlap with respect to the functions they describe. McLean and Snyder-McLean (1978) have suggested that functions of language may be distilled into two basic uses. One use is to influence joint attention, and the other is to influence joint activity. These functions basically correspond to the imperative and the declarative in English. The clinician should select a system that contains at least some basic declarative and imperative operations so that the child's initiation of a response to communications can be coded.

Some additional general guidelines should be discussed. The assessment of communicative function should, in part, be carried out in a naturalistic situation. It is sometimes difficult to contrive situations in which a child will express a genuine communicative intent. The clinician should have present in the room a wide variety of toys and stimuli that would elicit a number of different expressions of need or declarations. If there are other children or adults in the situation, the clinician must remember that the functions expressed by the child are inextricably related to the behavior and utterances of other conversational participants. In addition, functions are only interpretable in light of the nonverbal context of communication.

Some authors have suggested using standard elicitation tasks for basic communicative functions. This has been done for imperatives and declaratives (Dale, 1980; Snyder, 1978, 1981; Staab, 1983; Wetherby & Prizant, 1993; Wetherby & Rodriguez, 1992) but not as widely for more specific functions of communication. Generally, declaratives seem to be elicited most effectively by presenting novel or discrepant events and objects in the sampling situation. The child may then comment on the novel stimulus. For example, a clinician can allow a child to remove unseen items from a bag. When the item is produced the child will often comment or name the object. Imperatives are more reliably obtained than declaratives since the clinician can maintain control over the stimuli and activities in the sampling situation. The child will ask for access to toys or will ask the clinician to assist in certain operations (winding of toys, etc.). Ideally, communicative intent should be sampled using a combination of spontaneous play and use of elicitation tasks.

Wetherby et al. (1988) have contributed research that practicing clinicians will find most helpful. These researchers studied normally developing children at the preverbal, single-word, and early multiword stages of development to describe their intentional communication. Rate of communicative acts increased predictably as the children increased in mean length of utterance. The children tended to move from gestural modes in the prelinguistic stage to verbal modes in the early multiword stage. Wetherby, Yonclas, and Bryan (1989) used similar procedures on children with language impairment, Down syndrome, and autism and indicate that some of these measures (e.g., rate of intentional communication) may have potentially useful clinical value in describing these populations. A rate of about one communicative act per minute seems to be related to the onset of single-word utterances (Wetherby et al., 1988).

Two standardized tools address gestural communication to some degree: the Communication and Symbolic Behavior Scales (CSBS) and the MacArthur-Bates Communicative Development Inventories, Words and Gestures (CDI). These are good starting points in the evaluation of gestural communication; however, it is recommended that less formal measures also be considered in assessment. For example, Crais, Watson, and Baranek (2009) suggest that we obtain measurements on the frequency of gesture use. Data on frequency of communication for children at 12, 18, and 24 months suggests that they should be communicating at 1 time per minute, 2 times per minute, and 5 times per minute, respectively (Wetherby, Cain, Yonclass, & Walker, 1988). Other measures such as the type of specific gesture used (e.g., distal point, reach, show, give) should also be inventoried as well as the communicative function of each gesture (e.g., imperative, declarative). Crais, Watson, and Baranek (2008) also recommend examining use of gestures in concert with eye gaze toward people/objects as well as the coordination of vocal/verbal productions with gestures.

More extensive normative data are available in the CSBS (Wetherby & Prizant, 1993). These scales examine the areas of communicative functions, gestural communicative means, vocal communicative means, verbal communicative means, reciprocity, social-affective signaling, and symbolic behavior. The data on this measure come from caregiver questionnaires, direct sampling, and some structured elicitation tasks. Standardization data on hundreds of children are available for use by the examiner. This test is a good example of how ecologically valid behaviors can be evaluated and put into a normative developmental framework. Standardized testing does not always have to be artificial. The "communicative temptations" used in the Communication and Symbolic Behavior Scales were piloted in the earlier work of Wetherby mentioned above and are excellent examples of how clinicians can elicit imperatives and declaratives from children in clinical settings. Videotapes are also available to demonstrate administration and scoring of the CSBS. This helps to increase reliability in the procedure.

In cases where the child is nonverbal or at the single-word level, it is feasible to analyze functions and target communicative functions in treatment (Wilcox, 1984). For example, the clinician may want to increase the number of regulatory attempts in a particular child or increase the verbal realizations of regulation in a client. Brunson and Haynes (1991) provide an example of an alternating-time sampling procedure that can be used in classroom contexts to monitor the use of communicative functions in naturalistic activities. This system can also track intentional communication of teachers for possible inclusion in the treatment program.

Use of Tests and Formal Procedures with Limited-Language Children

Only two decades ago there were few assessment instruments available to the SLP for use on children with limited language. This is not necessarily because SLPs were uninterested in preschool-age children, because we have always dealt with youngsters of this age. Several influences on test development have increased the construction of instruments appropriate for the preschool, or limited-language, population. First of all, passage of IDEA mandates that preschool children between the ages of 3 and 5 years will be dealt with by clinicians working in the public school setting. Many school systems are currently responsible for children between birth and age 3. With the enactment of federal legislation, test developers have increased their efforts in devising test instruments for preschoolers. The second influence on test development has been the significant strides that we have made in communication development research in the past 20 years.

We can divide the preschool tests that deal with communication into several categories. First, there are large test batteries that include language or communication as one aspect of assessment. These are standardized batteries that include sections on motor skill, cognition, personal-social behavior, adaptive behavior, and communication. The portion dealing with communication is necessarily incomplete and superficial since the entire battery must examine so many different domains. This general battery, however, could suggest that a child's communication development may be delayed in comparison to the norming sample, and herein lies one value of the test ("problem/no problem" issue). Certainly, the test could never tell a clinician specific aspects of communication that are delayed or that suggest treatment objectives. There are many large batteries that include language as a subpart.

On another level, there are tests that focus more specifically on language and communication. These instruments may be helpful to the SLP in providing direction toward areas in need of probing through nonstandardized methods. Some of these instruments are standardized, norm-referenced tests, and others may be criterion referenced. These measures should satisfy any administrative requirements imposed by work settings on obtaining scores in assessment. The measures also could prove useful as a beginning point for naturalistic evaluation tasks. Crais (1995) reviews many of these instruments and discusses issues related to early assessment.

This textbook does not devote significant space to listing or discussing the myriad standardized tests available on the market for early or later child language disorders. We feel that this approach is warranted to avoid two outcomes, Grim Scenarios 1 and 2.

GRIM SCENARIO 1: CARRYING COALS TO NEWCASTLE   At one time, the town of Newcastle provided virtually all of the coal for England. This led to the development of an expression for doing something that is clearly unnecessary: "carrying coals to Newcastle." We don't want to get our hands dirty in this chapter. Any speech-language pathologist who is a member of a professional organization is no doubt inundated with flyers, mailers, and brochures advertising the latest language tests. There are literally hundreds of standardized tests in the area of child language. When one considers all of the areas of language (semantics, syntax, phonology, morphology, pragmatics) and the age range from preschool to adolescence, it is no surprise that a plethora of assessment devices is available. If we add the areas related to language such as cognition, social skills, metalinguistics, and literacy skills (e.g., reading, writing), the number of tests increases exponentially. Certainly, it would be a challenge for a chapter in a diagnostic textbook to provide even a list of test titles, publishers, age ranges, and costs for all relevant tests due to lack of space. Even if we could provide a list of all the available tests, it would no doubt be inaccurate by the time our book is published, because tests are continually going off the market, being revised, and new ones are being developed. Some texts provide such lists of tests and a brief summary of selected tests in terms of their target population, domains tested, and perhaps some superficial data on psychometric adequacy (Nelson, 2010; Paul, 2007). It is our view that such summaries are helpful in locating particular tests that may be appropriate for child language assessment, but they list so many tests so briefly that they do not give enough detail for consumers to fully evaluate a test. Also, because most tests are very expensive, it behooves consumers to spend some time carefully examining these instruments at conventions or conferences before purchasing them. Professionals attending conferences have the opportunity actually to see test instruments and talk with publishing representatives about test development. There is no substitute for reading a thoughtful and lengthy review of a test, scouring a test manual, and fondling the examination materials themselves to really understand a test. The Buros Mental Measurements Yearbook Online (http://buros.unl.edu) provides in-depth reviews of most tests; however, there is a charge to access their information. Many libraries contain the *Buros Mental Measurements Yearbook*, and that can be examined at no cost. Finally, much test information is readily available on publishers' Web sites and in those multiple brochures that arrive in your mailboxes, and there is no need to replicate it here.

GRIM SCENARIO 2: LETTING THE TAIL WAG THE DOG We must also consider that this textbook is about the *process* of diagnosis and evaluation in speech pathology, not merely a list of tests. As stated earlier in this chapter, standardized tests represent only a very small part of understanding a child's language system; they confirm whether the child has a problem in comparison to his or her peers in a normative sample. This is the simplest level of diagnosis. Recall that the chapter on psychometric issues cautions against selecting treatment targets from standardized tests and says not to measure treatment progress with these instruments. Thus, while formal tests are a part of assessment, they are a relatively minor part of the process. Spending a multitude of pages dealing with such a crude measure of language use would be "letting the tail wag the dog." The standardized tests are the "tail," but the "dog" is probably best represented by nonstandardized tasks used by a clinician to determine what the child can do with language in real communication.

Assessment of Structure and Function in Early Utterances

So far, we have briefly sketched the development of cognitive and social prerequisites to language. The present section deals with formation of the linguistic code in communicative development. Our discussion will consider two general phases: single-word and early multiword. These stages are based on length of utterance (Miller & Chapman, 1981) and linguistic attainment (Brown, 1973; Lund & Duchan, 1988). Each stage has certain acquisitions associated with it that may indicate that the child is ready for transition to the next stage.

SINGLE-WORD UTTERANCES After a period of using no real words and becoming more consistent with the use of vocalizations accompanied by gestures, the child begins to use single words to code objects and events. The words are not adult productions, but typically CV or CVCV approximations of the correct production (Nelson, 1973). Nelson has found that children's early lexicons represent specific categories. Research has reported that subgroups of language-developing and language-disordered children are *referential* (word and object oriented) or *expressive* (social and conversation oriented). That is, the referential children use mostly nouns and refer to objects and events. They also like to play with objects and spend more time playing alone. The expressive children, on the other hand, enjoy talking to and being with people and use more personal-social words (Weiss et al., 1983). There are perhaps other ways to characterize early single-word productions, but the point is that children go through a period of talking, as Lois Bloom (1973) says, using "one word at a time." Toward the end of the single-word period, Nelson (1973) indicates that the child accrues an expressive lexicon of about 50 words and then begins to attempt word combinations.

Children in the single-word period can be examined both for the types of words they use and the apparent reasons they use them. Parent report measures are indispensable in this age of working closely with families. O'Neill (2007) has developed the Language Use Inventory (LUI) to evaluate pragmatic skills of early preschool children on variables such as use of gestures, vocabulary, and use of longer utterances to serve a variety of communicative functions. Most of the items require parents to answer yes/no or choose from options such as never, rarely, sometimes, or often. This inventory was found to discriminate between clinical populations and typically developing children with sensitivity and specificity ranges above 90%.

The form of single-word utterances has been viewed in different ways by various authorities. Nelson (1973), for instance, categorized single words as members of the classes in Table 4.2. Other researchers have found similar results (Benedict, 1975). Lahey (1988) provides a lengthy discussion and examples of a system for early-utterance analysis. Ideally, single words should be paired with functions such as those discussed earlier.

Parent checklists are especially useful in obtaining data on lexicon size and content. Fenson et al. (1993) developed the *MacArthur-Bates Communicative Development Inventories* that provide normative data on children from 8 months to 30 months of age in terms of gestures, words, and multiword utterances. Heilmann, Weismer, Evans, and Hollar (2005) found significant correlations between the MacArthur-Bates CDI and direct language measures in 38 late talkers at 30 months of age. In a sample of 100 children (38 late talkers and 62 normal language children), they found that the CDI identified children with low language skills up to the 11th percentile, and children with normal language were identified above the 49th percentile. Skarakis-Doyle, Campbell, and Dempsey (2009) found that the CDI total score coupled with chronological age effectively classified children studied into typically developing and language impaired groups with 96% accuracy. The CDI has also been shown to have excellent validity for children with cochlear implants who are in the early stages of language development, albeit at a more advanced chronological age (Thal, DesJardin, & Eisenberg, 2007). Benchmarks are beginning to appear in the literature for various groups of children on standardized test performance. For instance, Nicholas and Geers (2008) provide benchmark scores for children with cochlear implants on the Preschool Language Scale, the Peabody Picture Vocabulary Test III, and the MacArthur-Bates Communicative Development Scale. The three measures were significantly correlated and the researchers indicate that while these do not constitute normative data, they can be used as "benchmarks" to compare other children with cochlear implants who have similar histories to the subjects studied in the research.

TABLE 4.2	Percentage of First 50-Word Lexicon Accounted for by Grammatical Categories in Two Major Studies		
Category	**Nelson (1973)**	**Benedict (1975)**	**Example**
General Nominal	50	51	chair, kitty
Specific Nominal	11	14	person's name
Action Word	19	14	go, eat
Modifier	10	9	dirty, big
Personal-Social	10	9	hi, no, please
Function	0	4	that, for

Rice, Sell, and Hadley (1990) provide a system for online coding of children's verbal initiations and responses in natural classroom settings as a function of environmental and play variables. Although the system does not examine types of single words used, it documents whether the child is using single-word, multiword, or gestural communications. Rescorla (1989) developed the *Language Development Survey* (LDS) to screen children at the single/early multiword levels. The LDS is a checklist of communicative behaviors and lexical items to be completed by the parent. Rescorla has recommended the "Delay 3 cutoff" to determine which children should be recommended for a formal evaluation. Using this cutoff, a child who had less than 50 words or no word combinations at 26 months was effectively identified by the LDS as being at risk for language delay. Rescorla and Alley (2001) found the LDS to have excellent reliability, validity, and clinical utility as a screening instrument for expressive language delay in 2-year-old toddlers. Rescorla, Alley, and Christine (2001) also examined word frequencies in toddler lexicons using the LDS and extensive spontaneous samples. They found a high degree of consistency among vocabulary items reported on the LDS, words used in spontaneous samples, and words reported in diary studies of the first lexicon. Klee, Pearce, and Carson (2000) showed that supplementing the Delay 3 criterion with two additional questions (parental concerns about child's language ability and history of six or more ear infections) improved LDS specificity and predictive value while maintaining high sensitivity. Rescorla, Ratner, Jusczyk, and Jusczyk (2005) studied 239 children between 23 and 25 months of age and found that the LDS and CDI were highly correlated (>.90), and that both instruments can be used to rank order toddlers on the variables of vocabulary size and length of phrases based on parental report.

Prior to the first word combinations, Dore et al. (1976) noted another transitional phenomenon known as the presyntactic device (PSD). Dore stated that a syntactic utterance is one in which two words that have a meaning relationship are combined under the same intonational pattern (e.g., "Mommy go"). A presyntactic device is the combination of two elements under an intonation contour that do not have a meaning relation because one element is not a real word, or because the word combination is reduplicated or a highly learned "rote production." Thus, a child who says /WI KITI/ is combining a real word (KITI) with a nonword (WI) under an intonation contour. Other presyntactic transitional elements that have been reported are empty forms, which are consistently used productions that appear to be nonsense words (e.g., "wida," "gocking") (Bloom, 1973; Leonard, 1975). Bloom (1970) reports the use of two single words that have a meaning relationship, with a pause inserted between the two elements (e.g., "car . . . go"). All of the above presyntactic devices prepare a child to combine two meaningful language elements under an intonation pattern that is the essence of early multiword combinations. McEachern and Haynes (2004) conducted a longitudinal study of 10 normally developing children using single-word utterances. Children were sampled once a month from 15 months of age until they developed early multiword combinations. The study was designed to determine if certain types of gesture-speech combinations act as transitional phenomena preceding production of two-word utterances. Temporally synchronized gesture-speech combinations were analyzed over a 6-month period to describe whether they encoded one semantic element (pointing to a car and saying "car") or two semantic elements (pointing to a car and saying "big"). There was a significant increase in gesture-speech combinations encoding two semantic elements during the 6-month period, and the onset of these combinations preceded or co-occurred with the first productions of multiword utterances. Thus, the results support the notion that gesture-speech combinations encoding two elements may be a transitional period between single-word and the onset of early multiword combinations. Bain and Olswang (1995) point out the utility of using a dynamic assessment approach to examine readiness for learning early multiword utterances. This information would add a significant dimension to the assessment of a single-word communicator.

THE CASE OF "LATE BLOOMERS"   Children who reach the age of 2 years with significant delays in expressive language despite normal cognitive, auditory, structural, and language comprehension abilities have been the subject of much research. These children usually have less than a 50-word lexicon and no evidence of multiword combinations at age 2. Some authorities suggest that as many as 50% of these children will be at risk for the language delay's persisting beyond their third birthday, while the other 50% may catch up and exhibit near-normal communication at age 3. The latter group have been called late bloomers or late talkers. One challenge of the diagnostician is to be able to distinguish children who will persist in their language impairment from those who are simply late talkers. A series of studies suggests that there are some potent variables to use in making this distinction (Paul & Jennings, 1992; Rescorla & Goossens, 1992; Thal & Tobias, 1992; Weismer, Branch, & Miller, 1994). Olswang, Rodriguez, and Timler (1998) provide a useful review of the literature in this area and a chart of prognostic variables related to late talkers. The following are signs that research has suggested that may aid in discriminating late bloomers from those children whose language impairment will persist beyond age 3:

- Children whose disorders persist may have a family history of speech and language problems.
- Late bloomers tend to have a higher frequency of communication acts.
- Children whose disorders persist tend to have less mature syllable structure, for example, fewer consonants in their phonetic inventories.
- Late bloomers tend to have higher scores in language comprehension on measures such as the *MacArthur-Bates Communicative Development Inventories.*
- Late bloomers have higher levels of symbolic play and more evidence of combinatorial play as compared to children whose disorders persist.

Some recent research shows that there may be some caretaker and cultural variables that are predictive of children who do and do not resolve their language disorder. LaParo, Justice, Skibbe, and Pianta (2004) studied a national database of 73 children with preschool language impairment at age 3. Standardized assessment at age 4.5 revealed that 33 of the children had resolved their impairments, and 40 showed persistent language disorder. Maternal sensitivity and maternal depression contributed significantly to the prediction of group membership. Children who had greater comprehension deficits were also likely to be in the group that did not resolve their language problems. Caucasian children were over 13 times more likely to be in the resolved group as compared to African American children whose mothers also scored lower on depression and sensitivity measures.

The clinician should look for *patterns* of such signs and should not base a decision on one indication alone. It is notable that the majority of these symptoms are not typically addressed in most of our standardized tests for early language, and thus nonstandardized tasks can provide critical information to the well-informed clinician.

EARLY MULTIWORD UTTERANCES   Perhaps the most researched and reported period of language acquisition is the time when children begin to combine lexical items to form meaning relationships (semantic relations). There has been a long history of interpreting these early utterances as traditional parts of speech (e.g., noun, verb), telegraphic speech (Brown & Fraser,

TABLE 4.3 Semantic Relations Reported by Brown (1973)	
Nomination + X	"This ball"
Recurrence + X	"More milk"
Nonexistence + X	"Allgone egg"
Agent + action	"Mommy run"
Action + object	"Hit ball"
Agent + object	"Mommy shoe"
Action + locative	"Go outside"
Entity + locative	"Ball kitchen"
Possessor + possession	"Mommy skirt"
Entity + attribute	"Ball red"
Agent + action + object	"Mommy hit ball"
Agent + action + locative	"Mommy run outside"

1963), pivot/open classes (Braine, 1963), and underlying structures of transformational grammar (McNeill, 1970). Currently, most authorities support a semantic view of early multiword utterances using a case grammar (Fillmore, 1968) and have rendered interpretations of early utterances using semantic relations (Bloom, 1970; Bloom & Lahey, 1978; Bowerman, 1974; Brown, 1973; Leonard, 1976; Schlessinger, 1974). Some of the basic early multiword constructions are composed of the semantic cases (Brown, 1973) in Table 4.3. Note that these basic semantic relations code aspects of the world that the child has learned about during the sensorimotor period of cognitive development, which is one reason that some authorities have indicated the strong cross-cultural similarities in early utterances (Brown, 1973). There are many more "fine-grained" analyses of children's early multiword utterances (Bloom, Lightbrown, & Hood, 1975; Braine, 1976; Leonard, 1976), and the basic relation types in Table 4.3 are included in these analyses along with some other more subtle distinctions.

Semantic relations must always be interpreted in light of the nonverbal context surrounding the utterance. The main point here is that children begin to use word combinations that code various common relationships in their environments; and if we merely assign adult, syntactic categories (e.g., noun, verb) to the utterances, we miss some of the skill that children have in coding rather subtle relations that are cognitively understood in the sensorimotor period. This skill has been termed a "rich interpretation" by Brown (1973) and gives the child credit for being able to talk about various relationships that syntactic metrics do not. As in the single-word period, these semantic relations are used for various functions; that is, agent + action can be used as a comment/label (e.g., "Mommy run"—when a child points to mother jogging) or as a regulatory statement (e.g., "Mommy push"—when the child is trying to get mother to push the wagon). According to authorities, it is wise to always consider both the structure (form) and use (function) of early multiword utterances (Bloom & Lahey, 1978; McLean & Snyder-McLean, 1978). There is a more recent move toward not using a priori semantic relation categories and giving a child credit for a multiword relation only after he or she has demonstrated "productivity" of use (Howe 1976; Leonard, Steckol, and Panther 1983; Lund and Duchan 1988).

As mentioned previously, there are existing methods of viewing and analyzing early semantic relations in children's utterances (Bloom, 1973; Braine, 1976; Brown, 1973; Leonard,

1976; Retherford, 1993). There are also, as discussed above, a number of systems for examining communicative functions in children (Dore, 1975; Halliday, 1975). Few systems, however, exist that interactively analyze structure and function in early utterances. Lahey (1988) described an analysis system that takes into account structure and function. The system suggests that the clinician transcribe the child's utterances, the adult's utterances, and the nonverbal communicative contextual events that are relevant to the communication. Lahey (1988) prefers the use of videotape in recording a sample for use in the analysis, because all linguistic and contextual information can be preserved and reviewed. Lahey recommends that the beginning clinician start by gaining practice with a particular coding taxonomy through carefully scoring videotaped sessions. When speed and reliability are increased, then hand transcriptions may be easier and more accurate.

At the very least, we recommend that the clinician videotape the child in an interaction with caretakers, teachers, or children so that the former can transcribe the child's utterances and note the context of communication. We feel that the following assumptions are important in a basic early multiword assessment:

1. It is important to determine if there is a "basic" set of semantic relations or if the child uses just a few relations (Lahey, 1988; McLean & Snyder-McLean, 1978).
2. A child should be able verbally to code many relationships and aspects of the environment.
3. The clinician should obtain an inventory of communicative functions used by a child to determine if there is a "basic set" of uses of language (Wetherby et al., 1988).
4. Structure and function should be viewed interactively (Bloom & Lahey, 1978; Lahey, 1988; Muma, 1978).
5. The clinician may find it valuable to get a feeling for the percentage of time that a child initiates language versus the percentage of adult-initiated utterances (Bloom & Lahey, 1978; Wetherby et al., 1988).
6. The clinician must be able to analyze utterances from one to four words in length.
7. Early multiwords are analyzed in a way that is different from the analysis of later syntax (Bloom & Lahey, 1978; Bowerman, 1973; Brown, 1973; Leonard et al., 1983), typically using semantic grammars.
8. The clinician should be sensitive to later developing forms present with the early multiwords (e.g., word endings, function words) to project development into later stages (Lahey, 1988; Miller, 1981).

Appendix B contains a suggested transcription sheet for use with the analysis. The clinician should first write down the child's utterance either phonetically or orthographically, then follow this transcription with the immediate interpretation of a semantic relation and function. Thus, the first three columns can be filled out at the time of each utterance. The videotape can be rewound to replay problematic utterances. This procedure could be used as a preliminary part of an assessment to find out basic semantic relations and functions in a child's communication. It also can be carried forward as a means of monitoring treatment progress. From the data, later analysis can determine the percentage of child-initiated versus adult-initiated utterances as well as the percentage of the use of each function and semantic relation in the sample. A summary sheet is presented in Appendix C. The remaining columns (4–6) of the transcription sheet can be filled out by the clinician subsequent to the evaluation session and can be used to complete the summary sheet. When a child is leaving the early multiword period, he or she has reached a mean length of utterance of over 2.25. At this point, the acquisition of a variety of syntactic conventions begins to emerge.

Assessment of Children's Early Language Comprehension

CONFOUNDING FACTORS: NONLINGUISTIC CONTEXT.   Children's responses to language are multidetermined. That is, a child's correct response could be primarily in reaction to nonverbal contextual aspects of the situation. The following is a typical scenario:

> The mother says, "He can understand everything that we tell him. He just doesn't talk." The clinician leans forward and says, "Can you show me how you know he understands what you tell him?" The mother shifts uncomfortably in her chair and tells the child to "go turn off the light," as she points alternately between the light switch and the ceiling fixture. The child turns the light off and on several times. Later when the mother was told to provide only verbal stimuli, the child was not able to perform many one- and two-level commands if they were unaccompanied by gestures.

Thus, children and adults rely on the context in which language is used to aid in interpretation of what was said.

CONFOUNDING FACTORS: COMPREHENSION STRATEGIES   In 1978, Chapman discussed the notion of "comprehension strategies" exhibited by children. According to Chapman, a comprehension strategy is "a short cut, heuristic or algorithm for arriving at sentence meaning without full marshaling of the information in the sentence and one's linguistic knowledge. Thus, it sometimes yields the correct answer, although it may more usually give the appearance of understanding" (p. 310). Clinicians who attempt to assess early language comprehension should be wary of correct responses by children that could have been generated by attention to contextual stimuli or comprehension strategies. An example would be that many children process the name of an object and then act on the object in a habitual manner. This behavior gives the appearance of knowing an entire sentence (e.g., "Throw the ball"), when in actuality the child may understand only the word "ball" and simply throws it as he usually would. Chapman gives many other comprehension strategies, and we encourage clinicians to become familiar with these patterns.

We have suggested that comprehension is difficult to test without contaminating influences from the context and comprehension strategies. Understanding of single words in young children appears to us to be the easiest to test. The clinician should make sure that objects are maximally separated in the evaluation room so that it will be clear which item the child turns toward when the examiner names it. If the child directs his or her attention to or retrieves the appropriate object when its name is uttered by an examiner (with appropriate controls for contextual cues), the child probably recognizes the lexical item. We begin to run into trouble when we try to test two-word utterances and larger sentences. Edmonston and Thane (1992) point out the difficulty in assessing relational words because of comprehension strategies. Some attempts have been made to remove the effects of context and comprehension strategies by using anomalous commands in the testing of children (Kramer, 1977). This technique involves giving to children commands that they are not likely to expect from their past experience. A child may be told to "Sit on the ball" or "Kiss the phone." If the child performs, he or she is said to have comprehended both elements in the command. If the child does not perform (and this is where we run into the problem again), is it that he or she has not understood? Perhaps anomalous commands are "silly" to children and are disregarded. There may be a cognitive mismatch between the command and the child's knowledge of the object's typical use. At any rate, failure to perform an anomalous command may not really mean lack of comprehension. The clinician should also not avoid more naturalistic assessment methods such as engaging the child in play or conversation and evaluating the appropriateness of verbal and nonverbal responses. Several popular instruments rely on parental reports to gauge receptive lexicon size. For example, in *MacArthur-Bates Communicative Development Inventories* (Fenson et al., 1993), normative data are provided on lexical comprehension based on parental reports.

Chapter 5 outlines some additional considerations in assessing language comprehension in older children.

Assessment of Utterances Using Length Measures

One of the most common measures recommended for use in a basic language evaluation is the mean length of utterance (MLU) (Miller, 1981). Length measures are not new in speech pathology and were used historically as a mainstay of our clinical armamentarium. Early measurements included the mean length of response (MLR), in which the clinician segments the language sample into utterances, counts the number of words in each utterance, and divides by the number of utterances in the sample. This yields the average number of words per utterance. Later, clinicians began to use the MLU, which represents the average number of morphemes (free and bound) per utterance. The MLU gives the child credit for mastering bound morphemes such as plurals, possessives, progressives, and regular past tense, among many others. There are several reasons that authorities have continued to recommend computing a length measure on utterances obtained in a language sample. First, there is a general correlation between the MLU and chronological age in many groups of children up to age 4 (Miller, 1981). Thus, the MLU may be used as a very gross indicator of language development in children up to age 4, but the clinician cannot simply rely on length measures alone in an analysis. A second important reason for computing MLU on a child is that Brown (1973) has used this length measure to demarcate his five stages of language development. Allegedly, MLU is a much better predictor of language development than is chronological age. Brown (1973) has postulated that if two children are matched on MLU, a clinician may predict that the constructional complexity of their language will be similar. Brown (1973) and Miller (1981) provide suggestions for the computation of MLU. Miller (1981) recommends a distributional analysis to ensure that the MLU has a relatively normal distribution around an average length. The analysis is simply a listing of the number of utterances at each morpheme level (e.g., 1, 2, 3, 4). If the distributional analysis reveals an MLU with a small variation, perhaps an organic condition or sampling error has played a role in the length of utterance. Compared to normal-language children, Johnston et al. (1993) found that children with language impairments tended to respond to questions with higher proportions of elliptical utterances. This finding certainly could affect MLU measures by increasing sampling error. Table 4.4 shows the general relations among Brown's stages, chronological age, and MLU data taken from Miller and Chapman (1981). One obvious point in these data is that the variability, as reflected in the standard deviations, generally increases with age. Research on temporal reliability for older children has also been published (Chabon, Udolf, & Egolf, 1982). These investigators report that MLU has weak temporal reliability in older children, and its use for prediction of language level may be less sensitive than previously thought.

The data from Miller and Chapman (1981) were gathered on a relatively small sample from the Madison, Wisconsin, area. It is axiomatic that any data we gather will reflect the characteristics of the sample of people tested. Thus, we would not expect every study on MLU to agree exactly with one another. There have been more recent attempts to provide MLU norms for clinical use. Much of the data on mean length of utterance (MLU) that clinicians use in practice come from studies done over 30 years ago with relatively small samples. A more recent source of carefully gathered data comes from the Systematic Analysis of Language Transcripts (SALT)

TABLE 4.4	Relationships Among Language Development, Chronological Age and Mean Length of Utterance

Brown's Stage	Chronological Age (+/− 1 Month)	Predicted MLU and Standard Deviation (in Parentheses)
Stage I: relations or roles within the simple sentence (MLU 1.75)	18 months	1.31 (0.325)
	21 months	1.62 (0.386)
	24 months	1.92 (0.448)
Stage II: Modulations of meaning within the simple sentence (MLU 2.25)	27 months	2.23 (0.510)
	30 months	2.54 (0.571)
Stage III: Modalities of the simple sentence (MLU 2.75)	33 months	2.85 (0.633)
	36 months	3.16 (0.694)
Stage IV: Embedding of one sentence within another (MLU 3.50)	39 months	3.47 (0.756)
	42 months	3.78 (0.817)
Stage V: Coordination of simple sentences	45 months	4.09 (0.879)
	48 months	4.40 (0.940)
	51 months	4.71 (1.002)
	54 months	5.02 (1.064)
	57 months	5.32 (1.125)
	60 months	5.63 (1.187)

Adapted from Brown (1973) and Miller and Chapman (1981).

database (Miller & Chapman, 2008). This database has been developed since the 1980s and has been added to with each new version of the analysis software. The most recent MLU data come from Rice, Smolik, Perpich, Thompson, Rytting, and Blossom (2010) on 306 children, fairly evenly divided between those with language impairment and those that were typically developing. The data were very carefully gathered and the populations were meticulously described. The results for the typically developing children show, as in prior research, that MLU increases systematically with age, and that even the children with language impairment made gains as they got older, but never caught up to the typically developing sample. Interestingly, Rice et al. (2010) show fairly reliable changes in MLU even in older age groups, which may be at odds with earlier research. These new data will be of great interest and utility to practicing clinicians.

We should always remember that MLU is not an objective measure such as height or weight. It is hopelessly entangled with the type of sample that is obtained by the clinician. Muma (1998) has shown that while the typical language sample size in our field is between 50 to 100 utterances, sampling error rates are very high until one analyzes samples of 200 to 400 utterances. Clearly, the larger the sample size, the better and probably more stable the grammatical and length measures that are calculated. The norms for MLU are presently reported on a rather narrow population, and further data gathering is necessary for different socioeconomic and cultural groups. The use of MLU may presently be in a state of transition; but until more conclusive data and viable alternatives are provided, we feel that MLU should be routinely calculated in a language evaluation of limited-language children.

Infant, Toddler, and Family Assessment

The Individuals with Disabilities Education Act of 2004 mandates that the school speech-language pathologist assess and treat children between the ages of 3 and 5. Speech-language pathologists in many states are currently serving the birth to age 5 population, and this will no doubt progressively become the norm. The present section provides some references for SLPs faced with the assessment of infants and toddlers.

Many categories of infants and children are at risk for communication disorders. There is a host of syndromes (e.g., Turner's, 18Q, Down, Hurlers, Morquio, Goldenhar, Mohr, Treacher-Collins, etc.) with associated speech, language, and hearing problems (Clark, 1989). Also, communication disorders can result from a variety of other sources such as environmental toxins (mercury, lead, cadmium, fetal alcohol exposure), infections prior to birth (syphilis, rubella, congenital cytomegaloviris, toxoplasmosis), or postnatally acquired infections (herpes, otitis, streptococcus infections). Other groups such as premature infants and those suffering early respiratory distress or intracranial hemmorhages are also at high risk for communication disorders. In many cases, speech/language problems are not necessarily the result of some insidious syndrome that directly attacks communication skills, but more likely a condition that affects hearing or cognitive development (Paul, 2007). Children who have experienced maltreatment in the preschool years or prenatal alcohol exposure are especially vulnerable to manifold developmental delays across domains. Speech, language, and hearing are frequently affected, and communication disorders professionals will almost always be an important part of multidisciplinary teams working with these children and their families.

The good thing about early intervention is that children are being identified soon after birth, which allows the beginning of a dialogue between professionals and parents. Most states are now providing neonatal hearing screenings during the first weeks of life. Children who used to be identified as hearing impaired at 2 to 3 years of age when their speech/language development were delayed are now being found at birth. In many cases we can move to prevent or reduce the occurrence of secondary disorders such as speech/language problems if the early intervention is done effectively from the outset. The SLP is more frequently involved than ever before on evaluation and intervention teams working with high-risk infants and their families. Often, this population is intimidating to clinicians without experience serving infants and toddlers.

Assessment of infants and toddlers must involve several components: (1) assessment of the infant; (2) assessment of the family situation; (3) assessment of the primary caregiver; and (4) assessment of caregiver–child interaction patterns. Sparks (1989) provides some general guidelines for assessing the infant. First, the SLP should become intimately familiar with the child's prenatal and perinatal history. We must know the medical status of the child so that we can try to predict which types of communication disorders are likely to be associated with a particular syndrome or condition. This allows the SLP to take preventive measures against a variety of secondary impairments. Second, we should gain a general appreciation of the infant's ability to maintain homeostasis. This means learning how individual infants cope with handling, when they lose control, and how we need to help them to maintain respiration, thermal control, and proper nutrition (Sparks, 1989). Frequently used measures for this are the *Neonatal Behavioral Assessment* (Brazelton, 1984) or the *Assessment of Preterm Infant Behavior* (Als, Lester, Tronick, and Brazelton, 1982). Third, the child's oral-motor behavior is an important skill to evaluate. Often, these children have difficulty with feeding, and the speech-language pathologist is a primary participant in working with parents on evaluating and treating feeding disorders. Paul (2001) provides a useful overview of feeding assessment and intervention procedures for the SLP. Proctor (1989) provides an excellent description of vocal development and a detailed assessment protocol for use in evaluating infant oral/vocal skills. Finally, the infant's hospital environment should be examined in terms of available stimulation and opportunities for communication. Often, these children are in neonatal intensive care units (NICU) or in other hospital units, and these environments provide the child's only exposure to communication.

In terms of evaluating caregiver–infant interactions, a number of potential schemes are available (Cole & St. Clair-Stokes, 1984; Duchan & Weitzner-Lin, 1987; Klein & Briggs, 1987; Lifter, Edwards, Avery, Anderson, & Sulzer-Azaroff, 1988; McCollum & Stayton, 1985; Wetherby, Cain, Yonclas, & Walker, 1988). We are also interested in more basic issues, such as availability of the caregiver and caregiver expectations about communication. The actual analysis of caregiver–child interaction embodies many behaviors discussed earlier in this chapter. Examine some of the references listed above for specific procedures.

Some team member, perhaps the SLP if he or she is the case manager, will participate in a family strengths and needs assessment. Bailey and Simeonsson (1988) provide procedures and suggestions for family assessment. With infants and toddlers, the assessments of family status and interaction patterns are as important or even more significant than evaluation of the child. Without an intact family that functions adequately as a system, the planning and implementation of intervention cannot take place. Also, IDEA requires an Individualized Family Service Plan (IFSP), which specifies not only goals for the child, but objectives for the family as a unit. In most cases, the SLP will be an important part of a team of professionals that work with the family in assessing a child who is at risk for developmental delays. According to the the Individuals with Disabilities Education Act (IDEA) of 2004, and specifically Part C of this act, states must identify and provide early intervention services for children with established risks (e.g., hearing impairment), environmental risks (e.g., abuse, neglect), and biological risks (e.g., prematurity, respiratory distress) in the first 3 years of life. Working closely with the family, professionals must assist in developing an Individualized Family Service Plan (IFSP) that documents information in several important areas: (1) the child's status in terms of present levels of functioning in areas that include physical, cognitive, communication, social, and emotional; (2) information on the family's strengths, needs and concerns; (3) a list of measureable outcomes expected for the child/family; (4) a detailed description of early intervention services including frequency, intensity, methods, providers, and so on; (5) a description of any other services such as medical interventions; (6) a statement of projected duration of services; (7) a specification of who will be the service coordinator of the plan; and (8) a plan for transition from Part C services under the IFSP to IDEA services provided with an Individualized Education Plan (IEP) in the school system. We bring up the IFSP here because it is clear that evaluation and assessment are an integral part of this process. It begins with an in-depth interview(s) with family members in which the SLP listens to concerns and preferred goals of parents. In order to establish the child's present level of functioning in cognitive and communicative domains, the SLP must administer both standardized and nonstandardized assessments. The specification of measurable outcomes implies that assessment is ongoing and must continue through the intervention process to determine if progress is being made and if the goals need to be modified. Thus, it is not simply a clinician's arbitrary choice about what to do in early assessment/intervention, it is guided to a large extent by legal requirements.

Thus, assessing infants and toddlers typically involves a team approach, with the SLP working closely with social workers, psychologists, medical professionals, early childhood special educators, and others. As in many other disorders, the SLP spends a large amount of time with families and is often placed in the role of counselor. Families of high-risk babies are faced with many challenges such as shock, grief, guilt, confusion, information overload, anger, fear, uncertainty, financial concerns, and the intrusion of too many professionals. Sometimes the SLP is a major source of support for such families, who are going through perhaps the most difficult period of their lives.

One of the biggest challenges for the SLP is to train parents to recognize these various states in their child and to present communication stimulation at a time when it can do the most good. Stimulating language in a child who is too sleepy or too upset (e.g., crying) will only result in frustration for the parent and the child. Paul (2007) illustrates varying states of infant behavioral organization on a continuum ranging from (a) deep sleep, (b) light sleep, (c) drowsy, (d) quiet alert, (e) active alert, to (f) crying. It is important for parents and nursing staff to appreciate that the quiet alert state is optimal for language and communication and that infants can be moved from drowsy to quiet alert by gentle stimulation or from active alert to quiet alert by cuddling or consoling behaviors.

As a child matures, assessment must be continuous and ongoing because the goals during the first 6 months of life will differ from those in the following 6 months. As time goes on, the goals may shift from feeding to cognitive to social to linguistic. Therefore, the IFSP must be assessed and revised at regular intervals. Polmanteer and Turbiville (2000) provide many examples of how IFSPs can be written in a family-responsive manner with language and goals that are not only relevant to the family, but intelligible to them.

Assessment of Special Populations

COMMUNICATION IS THE MAJOR FOCUS   Because the nature of communication/language and the model to which we subscribe do not change with the client, the assessment of special populations should not be dramatically different from what we do with any child with a language disorder. That is, our business is still to assess the integrity of the communication system (cognitive, linguistic, social, pragmatic), and this process should be our focus, regardless of etiology. We feel, as do many others (Bloom & Lahey, 1978; Lahey, 1988; Paul, 2007), that the diagnostic group of which a child is a member contributes limited insight into his or her language impairment. Certainly, however, some characteristics are important to consider in evaluating specific populations. Paul (2007) and Nelson (2010) provide an excellent overview of the research on communication skills associated with mental retardation, sensory deficits (blindness, hearing impairment), psychiatric disorders, specific language disorder, maternal substance abuse, ADD/ADHD, pervasive developmental disorders (PDD), autism, traumatic brain injury, and acquired aphasia. The clinician should be familiar with this information because it helps in parent counseling as well as in knowing what to expect in an evaluation. Still, no matter what a child's etiology, the clinician's major tasks are to determine the child's linguistic capability and the status of cognitive/social/biological abilities, as well as to explore the child's use of language in the natural environment.

INCREASED PROBABILITY OF FOCUSING ASSESSMENT ON PRECOMMUNICATIVE AREAS
Dealing with special populations increases the probability of having to assess biological, social, and cognitive prerequisites to language. Some limited-language children arecognitively impaired

(Cosby & Ruder, 1983; Kamhi & Johnston, 1982; Rogers, 1977; Weisz & Zigler, 1979). The clinician must be certain that the child possesses the cognitive abilities necessary for learning a particular symbol system in terms of being able to deal with its abstraction level (objects, pictures, words, gestures, etc.). Many children with autism also have been reported to have cognitive difficulties, and the clinician should attempt to gain insight into this area in the evaluation (Clune, Paolella, & Foley, 1979; Curcio, 1978; Rutter, 1978). Children with autism are frequently reported to be socially withdrawn, and their general nonverbal social interaction may have to be modified as part of a treatment program if they are expected to use functional communication (Baltaxe & Simmons, 1975; Opitz, 1982). One of the earlier indicators of autism is the absence or reduced production of protodeclarative gestures such as pointing to regulate adult attention. Current research suggests that a diagnosis of autism spectrum disorder (ASD) can be made reliably at 24 months (Woods & Wetherby, 2003). Many variables appear to be predictive: Impairments in social interaction and impairments in communication are early signs, and these are observable by 24months. Use of restricted and repetitive activities/interests is usually not seen until closer to 36 months. Klinger & Dawson (1992) have found that children with ASD lacked the four following critical behaviors: pointing, showing objects, looking at the face of another, and orienting to their name. Woods and Wetherby (2003) suggested that failure to meet any of the following milestones should result in further evaluation: no babbling by 12 months, no gesturing by 12 months, no single words by 16 months, no spontaneous two-word combinations by 24 months, or any loss of any language or social skills at any age. These indicators are not just for ASD, but for any developmental disorder. For children with autism, Prizant and Wetherby (1988) recommend assessment areas that are highly similar to those previously advocated for any child with a language impairment. Thus, one implication of special populations is that they may involve the clinician in a more broadly based analysis of both precommunicative as well as communicative behaviors presented by the child coupled with a detailed analysis of the environment using the family as collaborators (Prelock, Beatson, Bitner, Broder, & Ducker, 2003).

INCREASED POSSIBILITY OF RECOMMENDING AUGMENTATIVE/ALTERNATIVE COMMUNI-CATION MODES   Another aspect involved in dealing with special populations is that the clinician has an increased probability of prescribing a nonverbal/nonvocal response mode or augmentative communication device. Research has shown that children with cognitive impairment or autism may benefit from training in nonverbal communication modes, and that using an AAC system may even increase communication attempts and speech production (Bondy & Frost 1998; Silverman, 1995). However, in a recent systematic review of research, Schlosser & Wendt (2008) found that while AAC speech treatments may result in more speech production, the gains were described as "modest," and we must be realistic in our expectations.

Thus, it may be incumbent on the diagnostician to determine the potential that a given client may have for learning a nonvocal system. Beukelman and Mirenda (1992) provide an excellent overview of the factors that should be considered in assessment and intervention with augmentative and alternative communication techniques. Clinicians who do formal evaluations in the area of augmentative communication should have specialized training and experience in this arena before prescribing a nonvocal mode for a client.

PROGNOSTIC IMPLICATIONS   Special populations, as a whole, generally have a poorer prognosis than language-impaired children without complicating difficulties. The prognosis worsens in proportion to the number of ancillary problems that the child exhibits (hearing impairment, neuromotor involvement, mental retardation, absent caretakers, etc.). Also, the existence of ancillary problems increases the likelihood that a larger multidisciplinary team will be involved in the evaluation. The assistance of special educators, audiologists, psychologists, and medical personnel is necessary and invaluable to the clinician in making treatment recommendations for children from special populations. As dictated by federal legislation, the speech-language pathologist has the opportunity to collaborate in staffings with other professionals to discuss the assessment and treatment of language disordered children. We have found this, in most cases, to be stimulating and in the best interest of all concerned, especially in early-language cases.

NOTING SPECIFIC CHARACTERISTICS   With certain types of children, the diagnostician should make an inventory of characteristic behaviors that may need to be modified in the treatment program. For instance, children with autism and/or cognitive impairments have been reported to engage in self-stimulatory behaviors (arm flapping, masturbation, rocking, etc.). Some authorities believe that new learning cannot effectively take place while the child is in a self-stimulatory state. Thus, one goal of treatment might be to reduce the occurrence of self-stimulation, and these behaviors should be catalogued by the diagnostician. In these populations there have also been many reports of self-abusive behaviors. These should also be noted by the clinician as potential considerations in planning treatment. Bopp, Brown, and Mirenda (2004) describe the process of functional behavior assessment. This includes functional assessment interviews where the clinician asks for descriptions of problem behaviors, contextual and antecedent factors that predict behaviors, and consequences following occurrence of problem behaviors. A second component of functional assessment is direct observation. A final component involves functional analysis of the behavior to determine the effects of various consequences on the occurrence of the behavior. While functional behavior assessment was historically the province of psychologists and other professionals, current practice involves teachers, parents, and SLPs in the process.

Consolidating Data and Arriving at Treatment Recommendations

To a certain degree, even if the diagnostician adheres to an integrative model of language, the assessment process tends to fragment the child and the information obtained in the evaluation. Before arriving at treatment recommendations, suggestions for further testing, or referral decisions, the clinician should pause and take stock of what has been done in the assessment process. We have found it useful and insightful to summarize the following areas (see Appendix D).

DATA OBTAINED IN THE EVALUATION   This section refers to the actual behaviors observed and procedures administered to a child in the evaluation. It does not include the different analyses of the data. For instance, a spontaneous language sample can be subjected to a variety of analyses (MLU, form-function analysis, phonological analysis, etc.). Often, at the end of an evaluation, a clinician will be struck by the need for additional data that may be obtained in the initial phase of treatment. We sometimes wonder why we cannot make clinical judgments about certain aspects of a child's language, and then we find that we did not gather all of the data necessary to make these decisions. Appendix D provides a checklist for clinicians to use in summarizing the data collected.

ANALYSES PERFORMED ON THE DATA   This section allows the clinician to summarize the analysis procedures performed on the data collected. On the surface, this procedure may appear to be rather simplistic; however, because language has so many aspects that may be important to assess, it is easy to forget to gather certain data or perform certain analyses.

AREAS OF CONCERN AND STRENGTH   By examining the data and analyses of the communicative process and language development stages, the clinician will be impressed with areas of normality, strength, and concern. The clinician should look for patterns in the data that are revealed when a judgment must be made about the overall effectiveness of each area in the language model. For instance, a clinician may have concerns in the biological prerequisite area over poor motor coordination and remarkable birth and developmental histories. The same child may have performed poorly on cognitive tasks, and the clinician questions whether the child needs work on the conceptual bases for language development. Similarly, on social areas of the model, the child is not operating according to age level and is not exhibiting optimal social prerequisites for communication. Adaptive behavior scales show a delay in all areas of development. In the language development area, the child turns out to be nonverbal. When the clinician checks the areas of concern and strength, the child will get a minus (−) under biological prerequisites for neurological areas and minuses for social areas of play partner and reciprocity. The child would also earn minuses on the cognitive prerequisites of play level, sensorimotor substage, and symbolic play as well. Finally, the child would receive minuses for most categories in single-word, phonology, and early multiword combination areas. By examining the summary statements, the clinician can develop a profile of areas of strength and concern for each case. If no clear-cut statement for concern or strength can be made, then the clinician should examine the data gathered and the analyses performed to determine if enough information has been accumulated. In most cases, an inability to make a general statement about areas of the model is due to insufficient information, poor-quality information, or insufficient analysis.

RECOMMENDATIONS   The areas that are covered in the recommendation section revolve around four topics. First, the child may require referral to other professionals to obtain further information. For instance, referral to a psychologist or special educator may be warranted to determine the child's cognitive ability and potential for learning. Audiometric referral may be another common need. Second, the clinician may have been unable to perform certain tests or analyses because of time constraints or lack of cooperation by the child. Before specific treatment recommendations can be made, it may be that more data are required. By examining the sections on data obtained and analyses performed, the clinician can determine this need.

Third, if enough data were obtained and analyses performed, the clinician is in a position to make treatment recommendations. By examining the child's areas of strength and concern, the clinician can consider intervention avenues that are the most appropriate. For instance, if a child is biologically, cognitively, and socially ready for communicative development and the clinician has located the child in the language development process, an appropriate goal might be to begin concentrating on the language forms that develop next according to the acquisition literature and the child's need to communicate. If the child is normal in most respects and the major concern is intelligibility, then this carries with it a phonological treatment priority. If the child has cognitive and social problems in addition to language delay, then some of the treatment goals might includethese areas (facilitating cognitive development; improving social nonverbal skills, etc.). The areas of concern and strength also carry with them prognostic implications. To date, we really have no certain method of computing a given child's prognosis for success in language treatment. There are so many variables that relate to the child's capacities, skills, motivation, environment, caretaker participation, time in treatment, and so forth. One approach to prognosis that will probably reflect reality is to regard the child who elicits fewer concerns in the major areas of the model as having a more favorable prognosis than one who has many deficiencies.

CONCLUDING REMARKS

We have attempted to show that assessment of limited-language children is no simple matter. It requires that the clinician learn a multitude of skills and read a disparate literature in order to perform it competently. The diagnosis of language disorder requires more than just a single test or procedure. It demands that the clinician examine the communicative process differently for children of varying communicative levels and cultures.

Assessment of School-Age and Adolescent Language Disorders

The model by MacDonald and Carroll (1992) that was presented in Chapter 4 dealt with specific competencies required for communication development. Specifically, we talked about becoming *play partners, turn-taking partners,* and the beginning of developing a role as a *communicative partner* through the use of communicative intent, single-, and early multi-word utterances. This chapter rounds out the last two components in the model by discussing the period when the child becomes a *language partner* through the use of semantic and grammatical rules. Finally, we will consider the child's becoming a *conversational partner,* as pragmatic rules are developed to regulate the social use of language in a conversational context.

This chapter focuses on children who are speaking at the sentence level but may have difficulty with syntactic rules and who may also have deficiencies in semantics, pragmatics, metalinguistics, morphology, reading, writing, cognitive abilities, and general language processing. Thus, the assessment targets, tasks, and measurements we discuss in this chapter differ dramatically from those mentioned in Chapter 4. As Figure 5.1 indicates, however, the process of assessment remains the same. We are still interested in evaluating biological bases of communication, obtaining background information, performing standardized and nonstandardized testing, and evaluating the environments relevant to the child's communication. The areas of nonstandardized testing and evaluating relevant environments address pertinent aspects of the World Health Organization ICF model presented in Chapter 1.

Table 5.1 lists some common symptoms of language disorders in school-age and adolescent students. One can see that these symptoms span all areas of language and include comprehension as well as production impairments. There are also phonological disorders in this population that are addressed more fully in Chapter 6. When assessing morphosyntactic development, it is especially important to perform a careful evaluation of not only linguistic skills, but phonological abilities as well. The ability to produce final consonant clusters is certainly related to adding bound morphemes; however, it has been found that children with phonological disorder in addition to language impairment are at risk for morphosyntactic difficulties whether they can produce final consonant clusters or not (Haskill & Tyler, 2007).

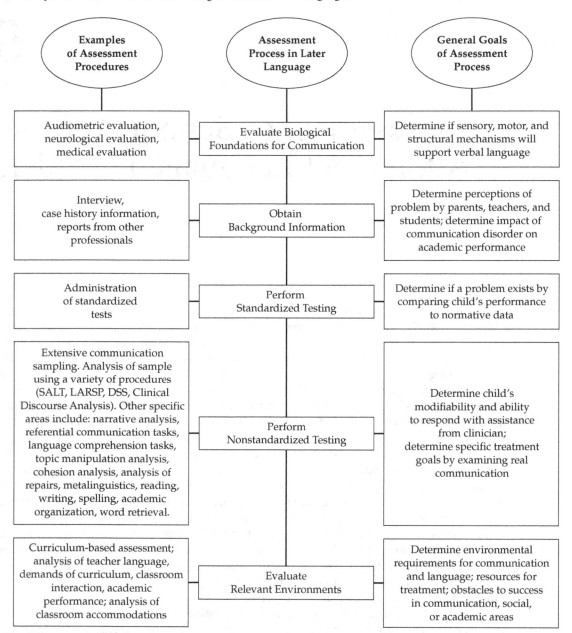

FIGURE 5.1   Critical assessment process in later language.

Some of the symptoms in Table 5.1 are rather gross linguistic errors that would be easily detected in conversation (e.g., syntactic rule violations), whereas other errors are rather subtle and discernible only with specialized communication sampling. Standardized tests may not reveal a subtle linguistic impairment in a school-age child (Plante & Vance, 1995). It is not unusual for an elementary-level student to pass many formal language tests and yet exhibit a

TABLE 5.1	Common Symptoms of Language Disorders in Older Students

Semantics

- Word finding/retrieval deficits
- Use of a large number of words in an attempt to explain a concept because the name escapes them (circumlocutions)
- Overuse of limited vocabulary
- Difficulty recalling names of items in categories (e.g., animals, foods)
- Difficulty retrieving verbal opposites
- Small vocabulary
- Use of words lacking specificity (thing, junk, stuff, etc.)
- Inappropriate use of words (selection of wrong word)
- Difficulty defining words
- Less comprehension of complex words
- Failure to grasp double word meanings (e.g., can, file)

Syntax/Morphology

- Use of grammatically incorrect sentence structures
- Simple, as opposed to complex, sentences
- Less comprehension of complex grammatical structures
- Prolonged pauses while constructing sentences
- Semantically empty placeholders (e.g., filled pauses, "uh," "er," "um")
- Use of many stereotyped phrases that do not require much language skill
- Use of "starters" (e.g., "You know . . .")

Pragmatics

- Use of redundant expressions and information the listener has already heard
- Use of nonspecific vocabulary (e.g., thing, stuff), and the listener cannot tell from prior conversation or physical context what is referred to
- Less skill in giving explanations clearly to a listener (lack of detail)
- Less skill in explaining something in a proper sequence
- Less conversational control in terms of introducing, maintaining, and changing topics (may get off the track in conversation and introduce new topics awkwardly)
- Rare use of clarification questions (e.g., "I don't understand," "You did what?")
- Difficulty shifting conversational style in different social situations (e.g., peer vs. teacher; child vs. adult)
- Difficulty grasping the "main idea" of a story or lecture (preoccupation with irrelevant details)
- Trouble making inferences from material not explicitly stated (e.g., "Sally went outside. She had to put up her umbrella." Inference: It was raining.)

significant linguistically based communication disorder. Many of these errors would only be seen in nonstandardized probing and conversational sampling. Similar difficulties have been found with some standardized language-screening instruments (Sturner et al., 1993). Interestingly, some surveys have indicated that the majority of public school SLPs routinely use a combination of formal (standardized) and informal (nonstandardized) methods of assessment (Hux, Morris-Friehe, & Sanger, 1993; Wilson et al., 1991).

Students with Language Problems: The High-Risk Groups

There are several specific groups of school-age students who have an increased likelihood of being diagnosed with a language disorder:

1. *History of Language Impairment as a Preschooler.* Longitudinal studies of children who had language delays as preschoolers have shown a strong tendency for the emergence of academic and language problems as these youngsters get older (Aram & Nation, 1980; Bashir et al., 1983; Hall & Tomblin, 1978; King, Jones, & Lasky, 1982; Strominger & Bashir, 1977). Many of these studies suggest that over 50% of preschoolers with a history of language difficulties are at risk for academic and language problems. This is not just because of their "weakness" in the area of language, but also because of increased academic difficulty and teacher language complexity as the child moves up the grade levels. Figure 5.2 shows the interaction of language ability, complexity of teacher language, and increased curricular demands as grade level increases. In the opinion of the present authors, the evidence suggests strongly that parents of preschoolers enrolled in language treatment, when they are dismissed from therapy, should be counseled about the possible reemergence of language-based problems as the child is faced with increasing academic and linguistic complexity after entering school. More recently, Johnson et al. (1999) followed 242 children into young adulthood over a 14-year longitudinal study involving 114 children with SLI and 128 children with typically developing language. They found high rates of continued communication difficulties in the children with SLI over the course of the study. They also found considerable stability of the language disorder over time. The outcomes were better for children with speech impairments only, and less favorable for those with both speech and language problems. Conti-Ramsden & Durkin (2008) followed 118 typically developing children and 120 children with specific language impairment into adolescence taking data using parental and self-report measures related to independence of function in daily life. They found that at age 16 the teenagers with a history of SLI were less independent than the typical group, and this was attributed to early language delay and poorer literacy skills in later years.

Johnson, Beitchman, and Brownlie (2010) followed a large sample of children identified as having language impairment at age 5 until they were 20 years old. They gathered data on family, education, occupation, and quality of life at four different time periods during the study. They

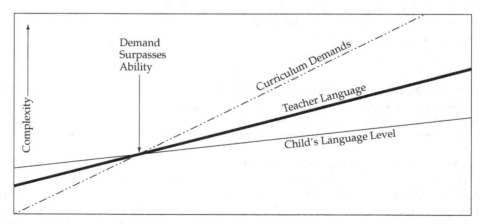

FIGURE 5.2   Interactions of language ability, teacher language, and curricular demands as grade level increases.

found that the group with language impairments showed poorer outcomes at age 25 compared to a typically developing group in communication, cognitive, academic, educational attainment, and occupational status. The authors suggest that this information might be useful in planning treatment goals to target these issues and in counseling with clients and parents.

2. *Students with Learning and/or Reading Disabilities.* The literature on learning disabilities has consistently supported the notion that the largest percentage of children diagnosed with reading and learning problems have either a history of language impairment or current linguistic difficulties (Maxwell & Wallach, 1984). Many recent publications have referred to this population as "language-learning disabled," emphasizing the pivotal role of language in their impairment. If a student is receiving services for reading problems or a learning disability, there is an increased risk that some form of language disorder may be present as well.

3. *Students Who Are "Academically at Risk."* Simon (1989) refers to a group of children who have "fallen between the cracks" of the educational system. These are students who have not been diagnosed as having a language problem but who are floundering academically on a consistent basis. Simon suggests that a significant percentage, maybe as many as 50%, of these students exhibit linguistic problems in addition to their academic difficulties. Simms-Hill and Haynes (1992) studied fourth-grade students who were rated as academically at risk by their teachers. These children consistently earned grades lower than C, were not receiving any remedial services in speech/language or in any other area, and had no history of language delay. Simms-Hill and Haynes (1992) found that over 50% of these students scored low enough on three different language tests to warrant clinical concern.

Thus, one mechanism of detecting school-age children with language disorders is to carefully examine students from the three high-risk groups mentioned above. This survey could be done through teacher referral, screening, or formal testing as part of a team evaluation of "at-risk" children.

USE OF STANDARDIZED TESTS WITH SYNTAX-LEVEL CHILDREN

As we indicated in Chapter 3, formal tests are best suited to comparing performance on a particular measure to the performance of same-age peers who took the test under similar conditions. Standardized tests address the issue of whether or not a problem exists. These measures are not particularly good at defining the nature of the problem or helping in the selection of treatment targets. We recommend that clinicians always use a standardized test to document the existence of a language disorder; most work settings require the use of such instruments as part of determining eligibility for services. However, even if a child "passes" a standardized test, a language-based communication disorder may still exist. Many children's language disorders are not exposed until a conversational sample is elicited by the clinician or until the child's language abilities are challenged by increased difficulty on academic tasks, narratives, or other activities that stress the communication system. In general, the symptoms of language impairment become more subtle with age; therefore, our assessment techniques must be more subtle as well.

No area in communication disorders has as many standardized test instruments as syntax-level language disorders. As we stated in Chapter 4, we will make no attempt to summarize the hundreds of tests available for this population, but we will focus on the process of assessment. Other sources provide general descriptions of many of these instruments (Nelson, 2010; Paul, 2007).

Wilson et al. (1991) surveyed clinicians in the state of California to determine which modes of assessment were used most in the public school systems. They also obtained data on specific standardized tests used by SLPs. Most clinicians used a combination of standardized and nonstandardized methods to test both comprehension and production in the public school population. As we stated in Chapter 1, assessment embodies elements of both art and science. It makes sense that working clinicians find they must go beyond formal standardized testing and probe behaviors in more informal ways to gain adequate insight into a child's language system. For example, historically we have only examined semantic deficits by measuring receptive and expressive vocabulary size. There are many other areas of difficulty in children who have semantic deficits such as (1) learning new words in indirect contexts, (2) using short-term memory to store phonological forms of new words, (3) creating/storing elaborate lexical representations, and (4) using known lexical items in expressive language that involves word retrieval (Brackenbury & Pye, 2005). Most of these areas can be tapped by nonstandardized testing and using subtests of existing examinations.

Most existing instruments focus on structural aspects of language (syntax, semantics, literal meaning of sentences), although there are several that deal with other areas as well (e.g., pragmatics, metalinguistics, concepts). Some of these tests may well be used by the SLP to gain *preliminary* insights into selected aspects of language performance, and the tests certainly can fulfill institutional expectations for obtaining scores on formal instruments. An example of an instrument that has excellent psychometric attributes is the Structured Photographic Expressive Language Test—Preschool, Second Edition. This examination was administered to groups of children with typical language development and those with language impairment, and the ability to discriminate the groups was impressive, with a specificity of 100% and a sensitivity of 90.6% using a standard score cutoff of 87 (Greenslade, Plante, & Vance, 2009).

NONSTANDARDIZED TESTING

Sometimes clinicians are interested in eliciting particular syntactic structures from a child, as opposed to administering an entire standardized test. This occasion would arise if the clinician wanted to probe the child's use of certain constructions, such as question forms in spontaneous speech. Mulac, Prutting, and Tomlinson (1978) suggest that a variety of tasks could be used to elicit a particular construction. They found that the most effective tasks for eliciting the "is interrogative" were those tasks that required intent, had contextual referents, and had some inherent structure to the activity. One example was a guessing game in which children had to guess what was in a bag (e.g., "Is it a ___?"). The notion of using several different informal elicitation tasks to evaluate certain syntactic structures has been supported by others as well (Eisenberg, 2005; Gazella & Stockman, 2003; Leonard et al., 1978; Lund & Duchan, 1993; Musselwhite & Barrie-Blackley, 1980; Paul, 2007).

The host of standardized tests that are available for examining the comprehension and production of language have more similarities than differences, because there are only so many ways that expressive and receptive language can be sampled. Although many formal tests of language demarcate linguistic ability into expressive and receptive modalities, some question the notion of a purely "expressive" language impairment. For instance, Leonard (2009) points out that the research shows that expressive language impairments are usually accompanied by difficulties in the processing of language input. He recommends that clinicians use the expressive language disorder classification with caution.

TABLE 5.2 Elicitation Procedures Used in Nonstandardized Assessment	
Comprehension	**Production**
Identification (pointing to, touching)	Elicited immediate imitation
Acting out (following directions)	Elicited delayed imitation
Judgment task (right, wrong, silly, polite)	
Conversation (requests for repair)	Cloze task (carrier phrase)
	Spontaneous evoked (naming, picture description, barrier)
	Story retelling (paraphrase)
	Narratives
	Conversation (legitimate)
	Free play

It is instructive to move from thinking about *tests* toward thinking about *tasks* that these instruments use to sample language. For example, many tests involve asking a child to point at pictures when the clinician gives a verbal stimulus (e.g., "Show me airplane flying"). When all tests are examined from the perspective of the types of tasks they use in assessing comprehension and production of language, the tests appear highly similar. Even language research projects use specific tasks to elicit responses to study the comprehension and production of language. Decades ago, Leonard et al. (1978) studied formal tests and research protocols to determine which types of tasks were used to gain insight into child language. Table 5.2 illustrates some of the common threads they saw running through tests and research projects. Clinicians who want to probe language comprehension and production in children informally have a relatively finite number of ways to do it. This is both comforting and disturbing at the same time. When clinicians use nonstandardized methods to assess language, they must design stimuli and tasks that will give them information beyond that provided by standardized instruments. The tasks in both comprehension and production fall on a continuum of "naturalness." In production, for example, elicited imitation and cloze tasks are further removed from real communication than legitimate conversation and free play. There is nothing wrong with using a combination of tasks to probe a child's capabilities with specific linguistic forms. Use of less natural tasks can even give us insight into how much support a child requires in terms of context or cues presented by the clinician. As stated in Chapter 3, just because nonstandardized methods are used, the clinician is not absolved from having to be systematic in the way data are gathered.

LANGUAGE SAMPLING: A GENERAL LOOK AT THE PROCESS

A common thread that has woven its way through the text thus far has been the notion of ecological validity. When done appropriately, language sampling of a spontaneous conversation is perhaps the closest we come to evaluating real communication. As Miller (1981) says, we must broaden our definition of what we mean by sampling. Perhaps a better name for this process would be *communication sampling* rather than *language sampling,* because a child can use flawless syntax and yet not communicate effectively if a pragmatic disorder is present. Spontaneous sampling is the only way to hold content, form, and use intact; thus, it is one of our most powerful tools.

Most SLPs have had the opportunity to sit in a small room with a child and attempt to record a representative sample of language. Most of us also have experienced the despair and humiliation (if we were being observed) of instead harvesting a string of one-word utterances and elliptical responses. Faced with this, we begin to put the pressure on the child for longer utterances and ask questions about the obvious. "What is in this picture?" we ask, when both the child and the clinician know the answer. "Tell me about what you did at school today," we cajole, and the child shrugs his or her shoulders, saying, "Nuthin." A very wise observation was made by Hubbell (1981) after he studied spontaneous talking in young children. When children feel they are being interrogated and there is a great deal of pressure for them to talk, they tend to clam up. One of the worst liabilities the clinician can have is a mother who says to her child in the waiting room, "Now we're here to get your speech evaluated. So be sure to talk." This is, in many cases, the kiss of death for a decent language sample. Children need to feel at ease and not pressured to talk. Clinicians also should try to resist the very strong urge to "interrogate" school-age children and, worst of all, to question them about the obvious. As we mentioned earlier, all communication is affected by the context in which it occurs, and language sampling is no different. Peets (2009) sampled four different classroom discourse contexts involving journal writing conferences, small group lessons, peer play, and sharing time. She found that there were significant differences among the four contexts in measurement such as language production, complexity, turn-taking, and self-monitoring. We have suggested that multiple samples in varied contexts will provide a more realistic view of a student's communication, and this study shows that even within a classroom situation there are different genres of communicative performance.

Since each sampling session is a product of an individual student, clinician, and communicative environment, it is impossible to provide guidelines that will work with all cases. All we can do is play the probabilities and provide some suggestions that may facilitate spontaneous talking in most cases.

For detailed treatments of language-sampling procedures, refer to the ample sources dealing with the topic (Barrie-Blackley, Musselwhite, & Rogister, 1978; Miller, 1981). Some general watchwords are as follows:

1. *Always record the sample.* We tend to subjectively fill in utterances that are incomplete if we transcribe during the sample. Additionally, it is distracting if you are attempting to carry on a legitimate conversation while scribbling on a tablet. Either we are engaging in a real conversation or we are not. We typically transcribe the communication sample so that a permanent record is available for comparison at a later date. Paul (2007) has suggested that some analyses can be done with less time commitment if the clinician simply listens to the taped sample while taking specific data on errors. This allows the clinician an opportunity to replay the tape in cases where the client's productions are less intelligible.

2. *Use a good digital recorder and position it for optimal recording.* This is one of the most often overlooked aspects of sampling language. It is a real disappointment when a clinician has done a masterful job of eliciting natural conversation from a child only to have the speech rendered unintelligible by a poor recording.

3. *Minimize your use of yes/no questions.* As soon as you ask these questions, you know the answer will be "Yes," "No," or "I don't know." Beginning clinicians typically bombard the child with yes/no questions, and the sample may be so loaded with single-word utterances that the child's MLU is severely underestimated because of sampling error (see Miller, 1981).

4. *Minimize questions that can be answered with one word.* (e.g., "What color is your dog?"). Although you have to ask some of these questions in the normal course of conversation, they do elicit single-word responses.

5. *Try to ask broad-based questions.* Examples include, "What happened?" "What happened next?" "Can you tell me about …?" "Why?" "How?" and so forth.

6. *Do not be afraid to make contributions to the conversation.* One of the most common errors made by beginning clinicians is that they want the child to do all the talking. This is not a natural conversational situation. Furthermore, the child's utterances are typically in the role of responder. Think back to the last language sample you took and ask yourself if the child had opportunities to initiate conversation instead of merely respond to your interrogations. In addition, ask yourself if you were a legitimate conversational participant. Did you tell the child some of your feelings and experiences? Did you talk mostly about things that were obvious or trivial? As Hubbell (1981) states, a facilitator of conversation is a good conversational model. It has been our experience that as soon as we stop the barrage of questions and begin to make some observations about what is going on in the session and what we think about things, the child begins to make some contributions to the conversation.

7. *As Miller (1981) says, try not to "play the fool" during a language sample, with an older child especially.* We have heard clinicians say, "I don't know what's in this picture, can you tell me?" Another example is a clinician who says, "Tell me how to make a sandwich. I don't know how." Give the child credit for the intelligence to know that you could easily describe pictures or that you know how to do simple, everyday tasks.

8. *Learn to tolerate periods of silence or pauses.* Beginning clinicians seem to feel that they have to fill up all the communicative space with verbalizations. Give the child an opportunity to initiate conversation.

9. *Stay on a topic long enough to converse about it.* Do not change topics after the child says one utterance on the issue. This approach encourages a series of "one-liners" from children, and the clinician is again placed in the position of having to interrogate. It also interferes with the clinician's ability to gather a sample that is appropriate for analyzing conversational mechanisms, such as topic maintenance.

10. *Finally, be aware of children's cognitive levels when you ask questions.* The clinician should be aware that children have differing conceptual frameworks from those of adults, as well as altered perspectives of time and space. We have heard clinicians ask 3-year-olds questions such as, "Why do you think the truck goes so fast?" Conversely, we do not want to ask questions that are cognitively too simple for older students.

There are variables that appear to affect the length and complexity of language samples obtained by researchers and examiners. First, the racial/cultural backgrounds of the participants could have a potential influence on a child's conversation. Several studies have suggested that some young African American children may engage in style-shifting or code switching when confronted with a white, adult examiner (Cazden, 1970; Labov, 1970). Cazden has stated that African American children speak in a school register for teachers and administrators and a street register for peers and family. Interestingly, the school register is different in content, has a shorter MLU, is less complex, and is more disfluent than the street register. Similarly, Harris (1985) reviewed the literature on assessing language in Native American children and reports that "Indian children tend to be nonverbal in totally teacher-directed activities, especially activities in which verbal responses are demanded of the participants" (p. 48). Of course, everyone style-shifts to some degree when conversing with another person from a different social, cultural, educational, or economic background. This certainly has implications for language sampling. Clinicians should realize that the samples they obtain from young children from a cultural group different from their own may underestimate linguistic abilities. Chapter 12 provides a more detailed treatment of this issue.

Verbalizations of the examiner also may affect language sampling. Lee (1974) suggests that the clinician attempt to speak with a variety of syntactic structures when sampling a child's language. The modeling literature has shown that children, in as little as a single session, can use language that is roughly similar in complexity to an adult model, whether the model uses extremely simple sentences or complex sentences involving embedding and conjoining (Haynes & Hood, 1978). Children are also sensitive to pragmatic aspects of a communicative situation. If they are placed in a play situation with younger children, their language will be simpler than it would be if they were talking to adults (Sachs & Devin, 1976).

Presupposition also may play a role in the length and complexity of samples obtained from children. Like adults, children will elaborate linguistically about objects and events that are not present in the current communicative context (Strandberg & Griffith, 1969). If a child does not share visual access to the stimuli with the clinician, he or she will tend to elaborate linguistically to a greater degree (Haynes, Purcell, & Haynes, 1979).

Several studies have shown that children provide longer and more complex language samples if they are engaging in conversation as opposed to performing picture description tasks (Haynes, Purcell, & Haynes, 1979; Longhurst & File, 1977; Longhurst & Grubb, 1974). Picture description tends to lend itself to the naming of elements in a picture rather than elaborating linguistically about a topic unknown to the clinician. These are typically single-word responses or elliptical answers. Most important, if the clinician views the picture with the child, the task becomes not one of conversing but of naming aspects of pictures. In the studies mentioned above, the children evidenced longer and more complex language samples when they were engaging in conversation than when they were describing pictures or objects. Conversation, of course, carries with it an element of presupposition because the clinician does not know what the child will talk about, and there is no contextual support for things removed in time and space. Thus, the child is forced to elaborate linguistically since the clinician is not aware of the conversational aspects that the child is attempting to convey. Picture description, however, is a viable method of sampling language for some children. Certainly, some children will not readily engage in conversation, and picture description is needed to elicit some language for analysis (Atkins & Cartwright, 1982). Evans and Craig (1992) have found an interview approach that elicits more language than a free-play scenario does. The topic of conversation may influence the productivity and syntactic complexity of a language sample. Nippold (2009) had school-age children who played the game of chess talk in three conditions: a general conversation, a conversation about the game of chess, and an explanation of chess. She found that the chess explanation task had significantly more length and complexity than the other tasks. This study highlights the possible effect of the interest and complexity of the conversational topic as it relates to the productivity and complexity of the language sample obtained.

Obtaining a language sample is a critical part of doing a language evaluation. A host of variables can affect the size and quality of the sample the examiner obtains. These variables, and their effect on sample size, may play a major role in the clinician's interpretation of the student's language sample and must be considered when analyzing the client's communicative ability.

It would be nice if language samples had the reliability and validity of physical measures such as height and weight. Unfortunately, they do not. Many researchers have reported that the size of language samples has a critical effect on their sampling error rates. Specifically, sampling error rates found by Muma (1998) dropped from 55% in samples of 50 utterances to 15% in samples containing 400 utterances.

Eisenberg, Fersko, and Lundgren (2001) reviewed the use of mean length of utterance (MLU) gathered from language samples. They caution against the use of MLU as a determiner of language impairment. First, it is not a measure of syntactic development, but is only one method of measuring utterance length. A child can have an MLU that is within normal limits and still have structural or pragmatic language difficulties. Second, the normative data on MLU are presently limited; especially in older children, the measure may also suffer from poor test–retest reliability. Finally, as mentioned above, there is considerable variability in the sampling of MLU, not only in the tasks and types of interactions, but in the sample sizes obtained. Eisenberg, Fersko, and Lundgren conclude that while a low MLU might be used as one piece of evidence for a language impairment, it should never be used as a sole measure.

Johnston (2001) found that MLU was affected by discourse variables such as answers to questions, imitation, and elliptical responding. Johnston studied differences between MLU calculated in the traditional manner and MLU computed without discourse variables and found that certain children were affected more than others by discourse variables. Johnston reminds clinicians of the complex nature of MLU and cautions them on any MLU-based decisions related to children with relatively advanced language and severe impairments.

Balason and Dollaghan (2002) found significant variability in both the obligatory contexts and grammatical morpheme production in 100 4-year-old children. They took 15-minute language samples obtained in caregiver–child play. The variability brings into question the reliability of findings used to distinguish between normal and abnormal morphological development, especially when relatively small sample sizes are used. This may underscore the need for supplementary elicitation procedures to augment the spontaneous sample, or the need to develop ways to make language sample analysis less time consuming. For example, Furey and Watkins (2002) sampled language from 22 preschoolers using a play-based sampling procedure that targeted 50 verbs. Target verbs were recorded by the examiner online and compared to a total language sample recorded on audiotape. There were significant correlations between verb repertoires in the online recording and in the total language samples. This suggests that online sampling of specific grammatical forms may be an accurate method of evaluation: Although the sampling time is the same as in traditional language sampling, the postsession time of transcribing a language sample is significantly reduced. Note that this method has not been validated on grammatical forms other than verbs.

LATER LANGUAGE DEVELOPMENT: EMERGING DATA

Structural analysis of a language sample can compare the child's production to the growing stockpile of normative data on youngsters between 9 and 18 years of age (Nippold, 1988, 1993). During the period from late elementary through high school there are slow but systematic changes in measurements, such as sentence length (Klecan-Aker & Hedrick, 1985; Loban, 1976; Morris & Crump, 1982), use of subordinate clauses (Scott, 1988), understanding of cohesive devices (Nippold, Schwarz, & Undlin, 1992), and use of the literate lexicon and figurative language (Nippold, 1993).

Scott and Stokes (1995) talk about the need for more relevant grammatical measures for older students. The measures that are used on younger children are not appropriate for older children. Evaluating older children requires quantitative measures such as sentence length (oral and written), clause density (degree to which a student uses subordinate clauses), measures of word structure (derivational morphology), phrase and clause structures, use of complex sentences, and the use of higher-level connectives, conjuncts, and disjuncts (e.g., *therefore, however, in addition, for example,* etc.). The authors make the case for building a normative base for these more complex structures so that the SLP can have a basis for comparing students during an evaluation. Also, normative data on pragmatics is limited (Norris, 1995). Children and adolescents are expected to adapt their communication across varied modalities in classroom, home, and social environments, and little is known about normative performance in these areas. As children move to more decontextualized contexts and are called upon to engage in more abstract discourse and semantic contexts, we know less about "normal" development. We also need to develop innovative methods of eliciting more complex sentence structures from students. For instance, Gummersall and Strong (1999) studied clinician support in the form of modeling specific complex language structures and the effect that practice with those structures had on children's production of complex language. They found that the assessment protocol was useful in eliciting a large and varied number of complex syntactic structures in a story context. Conversational samples, however, may not be the best vehicle to examine more complex syntactic development. Nippold, Mansfield, Billow, and Tomblin (2008) found that both typically developing and language impaired adolescents produced more complex language in an expository task as measured by mean length of T-units, use of clauses and subordination as compared to a conversational condition. We have maintained in the present text that gathering a narrative sample is an important part of any language assessment because narratives incorporate many complex aspects of linguistic ability. With older clients, we may want to include expository tasks as well to reveal use of linguistic complexity that may not be found in conversation alone. Nippold, Mansfield, Billow, and Tomblin (2009) studied groups of adolescents with typically developing language, specific language impairment, and nonspecific language impairment. They used a peer conflict resolution (PCR) task to sample language performance. This task involved solving a perceived conflict illustrated by a scenario presented by the researcher. The typically developing group had greater T-unit length and used more complex language than either group with language impairment. The PCR task seems well suited for use in gathering language samples from adolescent clients. Researchers are developing more databases on which we can compare performance on specific aspects of linguistic elaboration with development. For example, Eisenberg, Ukrainetz, Hsu, Kaderavek, Justice, and Gillam (2008) gathered data on 5-, 8-, and 11-year-old children to determine their ability to elaborate noun phrases in spoken narratives. They found a clear developmental progression that clinicians can use to determine expectations in typically developing children. At 5 years of age children use simple designating noun phrases, 8-year-olds used simple descriptive noun phrases, and the oldest group used postmodification.

Earlier we illustrated the interaction that takes place among a student's language ability, teacher language, and the demands of the curriculum. Essentially, as the grade level increases, the student is asked to do progressively more abstract and complicated things with language as well as thought. Clearly, the syntactic complexity of language increases as shown by progressively more use of conjunctions, subordinate clauses, and infinitives. The vocabulary becomes progressively more complex and technical with grade level. The use of figurative language increases in lectures and in textbooks as grade level increases.

Most educators are familiar with Bloom's taxonomy, which is a progressively more demanding series of levels that require a student to use language and thought interactively to learn more complex material and demonstrate knowledge (Paul, 2007). The tasks in the hierarchy begin with listing and identifying on the simplest level. Then a student must demonstrate his or her grasp of a concept by explaining, describing, and restating relevant material. Later the student must show how he or she can apply the learned information to solve problems, analyze a novel situation, or debate/defend a position using the information. Finally, a student must be able to compare/contrast and critically evaluate the information in relation to other perspectives. When we deal with students who have language impairment, we often are content to see them perform on the initial levels of Bloom's taxonomy (naming, listing, identifying). However, the classroom will stress their linguistic and cognitive systems much more using the higher levels of the hierarchy. Tests often ask students to compare and contrast, describe, explain, and apply learned information as the grade level increases. Thus, we must perform our language assessment on many levels to determine where the student has difficulty with using language in the service of cognition. If we find that a student cannot deal with higher levels of thought and language, these can be easily incorporated into the treatment program and result in communicative as well as academic payoffs. A good place to start is to determine what the classroom teachers expect of their students in terms of language and thought. This is part of what is sometimes called curriculum-based assessment.

TESTING LANGUAGE COMPREHENSION

Bransford and Nitsch (1978) point out that comprehension involves a situation plus an input. A human organism is not a static system but has a current state of excitation, a history, and background knowledge. A given input of language is placed in this situation along with the nonverbal context of communication. Many variables come to bear on the understanding of an input, not the least of which are the person's background, as well as the linguistic and nonlinguistic contexts. Rees and Shulman (1978) have written an article in which they indicate that most tests of language comprehension measure only the literal meanings of utterances. For example, if asked to point to a picture of a boy who is running, the child can choose the correct picture and not point to one of a boy who is standing. Thus, the child understands the notions of *boy* and *run* and can discriminate them from other literal meanings, such as *standing*. But comprehension involves so much more than the literal meaning of utterances. Miller and Paul (1995) provide several examples of other types of comprehension knowledge, as illustrated in Table 5.3. As another example, the skill of inferencing is used in almost every interaction and certainly many times during a school day. To fully comprehend an utterance such as "It's supposed to rain today, but I forgot my umbrella," one must infer that the person may get wet, although this is never specifically stated. Another broader notion of comprehension has to do with understanding the main point in a narrative, lecture, or conversation. If a child cannot comprehend the main point in a lecture, this is certainly as much of a comprehension problem as not understanding literal meanings. Comprehension of figurative language such as idioms and metaphors involves more than just literal meaning. If a teacher says, "This science project should really shine," the child should know that the teacher does not mean that the project requires lights (Simon, 1987).

We must go past the idea of assessing literal meanings when dealing with comprehension assessment. Most comprehension tests are quite artificial when compared to the richness of language comprehension in a natural situation. The typical comprehension assessment situation involves presenting a child with test plates containing pictures. The child is asked to point to the picture that best represents some verbal stimulus uttered by the examiner. The pictures are often line drawings, and the verbal stimuli are not discursively related to one another (in one case the child is asked to point to a "monkey," and in the next plate the topic is "shopping"). In these tests there is no temporal sequence of events that would allow a child to be able to predict what will be

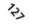

Selected Types of Comprehension Knowledge

Knowledge of literal meaning: "Show me the picture of the monkey."
A correct response would be to point to the monkey to show literal knowledge of the requested item.

- **Social knowledge:** "Do you want to be sent to your room without supper?"
This is not a question from a mother to a child. It is actually a threat and requires knowledge of the situation to interpret appropriately.
- **Knowledge of sincerity conditions:** "Is the Pope Catholic?"
When someone produces this question, we know that this is just another way of saying "Yes" in a conversation and is not a query about the religious affiliation of the pontiff.
- **Knowledge of cohesive devices:** "He fixed the car."
One cannot comprehend this sentence correctly unless information from outside the utterance is considered. The listener must be able to figure out who "he" is and whose vehicle was repaired.
- **Knowledge of presupposition:** "They managed to sell their house."
A listener must know not only that the people sold their home, but that it was done with some difficulty because of the word "managed."
- **General world knowledge:** "It's raining."
Miller and Paul (1995) give an example of poll workers who know that rainy weather often results in low voter turnout, and thus the above utterance takes on special meaning beyond simply talking about the weather.
- **Specific background knowledge:** "I'm the Michael Jordan of soccer."
Unless the listener knew about the prowess of this famous basketball player, it would be difficult to know that the utterance refers to playing soccer exceptionally well.

Source: Adapted from Miller, J., & Paul, R. (1995). *The clinical assessment of language comprehension.* Baltimore, MD: Brookes.

said, as in real language comprehension. Naturalistic situations also give the child the opportunity to ask for clarification or repetition in the face of information loss. The notion of comprehension monitoring implies that we are always scanning to determine if we are understanding someone's utterances; and if we do not understand, we initiate repair sequences that can clarify information that we do not comprehend. Skarakis-Doyle and Dempsey (2008) found that children with language impairment performed significantly lower than typically developing children matched for receptive vocabulary on a comprehension monitoring task. We do not afford children this chance in comprehension testing. In fact, we are often forbidden by the examiner's manual from presenting a stimulus a second time, even if the child asks for a repetition! The above statements are meant only to reinforce the notion that real language comprehension is a highly complex phenomenon and cannot be assessed easily.

Millen and Prutting (1979) studied three language comprehension tests for consistency of response on specific grammatical features. They found that on the *Northwestern Syntax Screening Test* (NSST), *Assessment of Children's Language Comprehension* (ACLC), and *Bellugi Comprehension Test* there was general agreement in the overall scores generated by the measures. There were, however, significant differences among the tests for more than half of the specific grammatical features evaluated. The investigators logically suggest that the tests are not equivalent and not clinically sound for generating specific remediation targets. Other stimulus, task, and subject variables have been studied in comprehension tests. Haynes and McCallion (1981) found that on the *Test of Auditory Comprehension of Language* (TACL), children with a reflective cognitive tempo, or long decision time, performed significantly better than impulsive children with a short decision time. Further, these researchers reported that scores on the TACL improved significantly over standard administration when the subjects were given two stimulus presentations or if the test was administered imitatively. Skarakis-Doyle, Dempsey, and Lee (2008) investigated the individual and combined effects of three comprehension measurements on preschool age children with typical and impaired language. The measurements (joint story retell, expectancy violation detection task, and comprehension questions) each classified children in their predetermined groups, but the combination of the three measures proved to be the most effective predictor (96%) of group membership. This study shows that comprehension impairments can be effectively detected in the preschool years using naturalistic tasks that take a total of about 20 minutes to administer.

Thus, it appears that variables other than language comprehension enter into test performance, and failure to do well on a comprehension test could be explained by other factors. Attentional set, hearing impairment, ambiguous pictures, test administration procedures (Shorr, 1983), cognitive style, and unrelated stimuli—all could account for poor performance on a standardized test of language comprehension. Additionally, Gowie and Powers (1979) showed that a child's expectations about what a sentence was going to say significantly influenced his or her performance on a comprehension task. Gowie and Powers observed that "knowing a word involves a set of expectations about the referents and about the types of messages in which the word is likely to occur" (p. 40).

We have suggested that comprehension is difficult to test in limited-language cases without contaminating influences from the context and the child's use of comprehension strategies. Further, we have said that failure to perform well on a test of comprehension does not necessarily indicate the presence of a comprehension disorder. Based on the current literature, about all we can say with some conviction is that adequate performance on a standardized test of language comprehension probably means that the child is capable of comprehending some language in a highly artificial situation. This does not necessarily represent comprehension ability in natural situations. Failure of a comprehension test, on the other hand, does not necessarily mean that the child is incapable of comprehending language either in the contrived testing situation or the natural environment.

Currently, language comprehension is tested in four ways by SLPs. First, there are a number of standardized tests of comprehension. Second, some researchers have tested comprehension by having children act out certain commands (Leonard et al., 1978). Third, several investigators have used a decision task in which the child makes judgments such as "good or bad" or engages in a preference task to say which of two sentences was the best. Finally, similar to the standardized tests, clinicians have used pictures or objects and have engaged children in an informal pointing task. Miller and Paul (1995) have developed an impressive series of nonstandardized comprehension assessment tasks for use with clients from under 12 months of age to those over 10 years old. Each task is directly related to a developmental level, and detailed instructions are provided for administration, scoring, and interpretation. Perhaps the "best" method of comprehension testing would be to examine it via several methods, both formal and informal. The clinician should utilize more naturalistic assessment methods such as engaging the child in play or conversation and evaluating the appropriateness of verbal and nonverbal responses. Observation in the classroom combined with teacher and parent interviews can provide valuable insight into comprehension in everyday situations. It also should be noted if the child uses requests for

Selected Evaluation Areas to Determine Source of Comprehension Breakdown

ıput Variables

- *Complexity of vocabulary (semantics).* Does comprehension break down when the vocabulary increases in complexity? Does the child lack knowledge of the literal meanings of words?
- *Syntactic complexity.* Does comprehension break down as sentences become more complex?
- *Sentence length.* Does comprehension break down as sentences become longer?
- *Context.* Does comprehension improve when there is a clear physical context to support the utterance? Does comprehension break down in decontextualized utterances?

Internal Variables

- *Auditory acuity.* Does comprehension break down because of hearing impairment?
- *Attentional abilities.* Does comprehension improve when a child is given a "set" to attend or when there is less distractions in the context?
- *Comprehension monitoring.* Does comprehension improve when a child is asked to judge continuously whether he or she understands utterances and to ask for repairs?

Specific Problems

- *Intersentence relations.* Does comprehension break down when meaning must be derived from analysis of multiple sentences?
- *Cohesion.* Does comprehension break down when the listener must derive the meaning of cohesive devices (e.g., pronouns) from prior discourse?
- *World or specific knowledge.* Does comprehension break down when the topic requires general or when it requires specific types of world knowledge?

clarification or repetition in conversation. Research has shown that these clarification/repetition requests can be successfully elicited by the clinician by using informal probes (Brinton & Fujiki, 1989). Gillam, Fargo, and Robertson (2009) illustrate the use of comprehension questions and "think-aloud" tasks to evaluate language comprehension beyond the typical tasks found on standardized tests. In their think-aloud tasks, expository stimuli are read by the clinician one sentence at a time and the child is asked what he or she knows about the story so far. Comprehension questions are also asked about the story.

When a child does not comprehend an utterance, the clinician should systematically determine where the process of understanding begins to break down. Unfortunately, no single test is presently available to solve this dilemma; however, several researchers have made progress in this area (Miller & Paul, 1995). For older children, clinicians can systematically experiment with the variables listed in Table 5.4 to determine where the breakdown occurs.

ASSESSMENT OF SYNTAX USING ANALYSIS PACKAGES

After the SLP has obtained a language sample, judgments must be made regarding the syntactic development of the child. Analysis of syntax can be conceptualized on a continuum. On the left end of the continuum is the administration of formal tests. These measures can give the clinician some insight into general syntactic development. In the middle of the continuum, the clinician can analyze a language sample in accordance with specific packaged assessment procedures (Lee, 1974) and obtain more precise information than is available from standardized tests.

Finally, on the right end, the clinician can analyze the sample by using knowledge of linguistics and language development and does not have to rely on a step-by-step package analysis procedure (Hubbell, 1988; Kahn & James, 1980; Lund & Duchan, 1993; Muma, 1973b; Retherford, 2000). The left end of the continuum requires less expertise than does the right end in terms of clinician experience and training. The left end of the continuum takes less time for the analysis than does the right, but also provides less clinically relevant information. Thus, the clinician must make a decision as to the time available for the analysis, training and expertise in linguistics, and the depth of information desired.

It is beyond the scope of this chapter to instruct clinicians in performing an analysis of a child's syntax. The best way to learn an analysis system is to obtain a sample and follow the guidelines provided by authors of complexity analysis packages. Typically, the authors provide explicit instructions for obtaining a sample, segmentation, and analysis. Beginning clinicians should realize that any syntactic analysis method requires practice in order to be used effectively. The most widely known analysis procedures are listed in Table 5.5.

Muma (1978) points out that descriptive procedures have greater power than normative ones do, because they help the clinician to describe individual differences. Descriptive procedures, because they are based on spontaneous language samples, also provide the clinician with more relevant intervention targets because these procedures do not fracture the integrity of the content-form-use model as imitative and standardized tests do. Thus, there are advantages to performing a descriptive analysis, and package systems provide the clinician with guidelines for completing such an analysis. We should, however, remember that each analysis procedure reflects the author's bias regarding language, and that most systems look at a language sample in only limited ways.

Consumers who intend to use an analysis package should be aware that the procedures differ importantly. These differences may determine whether or not a clinician finds it appropriate to use a particular package. We will use the Developmental Sentence Scoring (DSS) procedure in our examples because this methodology has been available for years (Lee, 1974), has been referred to in recent literature as being a potentially useful procedure (Hughes, Fey, & Long, 1992), and is included in recent computer-based language analysis programs (Long, Fey, & Channell, 2002). Using this procedure in our discussion is not meant to be a criticism or an endorsement of this particular approach.

TABLE 5.5 Selected Language Sample Analysis Procedures

- Assessing Children's Language in Naturalistic Contexts (Lund & Duchan, 1993)
- Assigning Structural Stage (Miller, 1981)
- Co-Occurring and Restricted Structures Analysis (Muma, 1973b)
- Developmental Sentences Analysis (Lee, 1974)
- Language Assessment, Remediation, and Screening Procedure (Crystal, Fletcher, & Garman, 1976)
- Language Sampling, Analysis, and Training (Tyack & Gottsleben, 1974)
- Linguistic Analysis of Speech Samples (Engler, Hannah, & Longhurst, 1973)
- Method for Assessing Use of Grammatical Structures (Kahn & James, 1980)

Source: Adapted from Owens, R. (2004). *Language disorders: A functional approach to assessment and intervention.* Boston: Allyn & Bacon.

1. Some package systems recommend obtaining a specific sample size before subjecting the language to analysis. For instance, Lee (1974) recommends using 50 subject-verb utterances for computation of the DSS. A later study, however, stated that a sample of 150 utterances may be more appropriate for reliable scoring. If the clinician does not have a large enough sample, perhaps a different procedure would be more appropriate.

2. The analysis packages vary considerably in the time required for completion. This may be due to several influences. First, some procedures are quite detailed and lengthy (Bloom & Lahey, 1978; Crystal, Fletcher, & Garman, 1976). Other procedures use very specific terminologies and vocabulary or have complicated scoring systems that require much time and practice in order for the clinician to use the procedure economically.

3. The procedures differ in terms of how they segment or separate utterances obtained in the sample. The DSS, for instance, analyzes only subject-verb utterances and does not score sentence fragments. Some clinicians, however, feel that there is much useful information in sentence fragments (e.g., elliptical responses) that may be important to analyze.

4. Some systems are recommended by their authors as ideal for use with particular treatment approaches. Lee, Koenigsknecht, and Mulhern (1975) use the DSS as an input to their interactive language teaching strategy and continue to monitor progress by using the system.

5. Another way that evaluation systems differ is in terms of the structures they do or do not analyze. For example, the DSS does not specifically analyze certain forms (e.g., prepositions and articles) and accounts for their presence or absence by assigning a "sentence point" to an utterance if it is grammatical. Other systems specifically analyze most structural elements of English, even structures that may not be of interest to the clinician.

6. Analysis packages differ in their provision of normative data. The DSS has normative data, while some other packages are purely descriptive and make no attempt to gather numerical scores on normal and disordered children.

7. Finally, the analysis procedures are not uniform in applying the results to a normal language development progression. That is, some procedures are designed to examine linguistic elements without locating the child on a language development continuum. Others apply their results to the normal developmental progression (Crystal, Fletcher, & Garman, 1976; Lahey, 1988; Lee, 1974; Miller, 1981). Research has shown that many aspects of syntactic and morphological acquisition in children with language impairments develop in an order similar to that found in normally developing children (Paul & Alforde, 1993).

Several investigations have shown that some of the package analysis procedures appear to be capable of documenting language changes in children, at least in a general way (Hughes, Fey, & Long, 1992; Longhurst & Schrandt, 1973; Sharf, 1972). Furthermore, any method that a clinician selects will require specific training and practice in order to use it effectively. It should be remembered that any method used depends to a significant degree on the quality of the sample obtained and typically analyzes only the structural elements of language, independent of pragmatics. Thus, any analysis package procedure will take the clinician time and practice to learn, and in the end will look at language only from a specific point of view (Miller, 1981). The present authors believe that if clinicians are going to spend time learning about analysis of the structural aspects of language, their time would be better spent learning linguistics and language acquisition instead of one specific analysis package that probably would not be appropriate for all clients. An analysis package could always be learned later to supplement the clinician's linguistic knowledge and would probably be learned more easily owing to the experience with

TABLE 5.6	General Guidelines for Syntactic Analysis of Language Sample

- Obtain a converstion sample.
- Transcribe the sample orthographically (or in phonetics if the client has misarticulations).
- Locate errors in sample:
  Find sentences containing errors and highlight them.
  Mark specific errors within the highlighted sentences (circle them).
- Make a list of forms/structures the child uses correctly.
- Make a list of forms/structures the child consistently misuses (never correct).
- Make a list of forms/structures the child inconsistently misuses.
- For inconsistently misused forms/structure, make a list of contexts:
  List contexts where form/structure is correct.
  List contexts where form/structure is incorrect.
- Common variables to consider regarding contextual influence:
  Syntactic complexity of sentence
  Semantic complexity of lexical items used in sentence
  Type of sentence (e.g., question, declarative)
  Phonological complexity of sentence
  Pragmatic variables (e.g., listener uncertainty; narrative)
- Look for possible patterns using above variables that account for when error occurs and does not occur.

linguistics. A knowledge of linguistics would allow the clinician to generally analyze samples for structures that are present, absent, and inconsistent and to still choose treatment targets that are relevant, instead of trying to find a package analysis procedure that is the "best fit" for the child. There are a number of fine textbooks that provide information on sentence structure (Hubbell, 1988; Quirk & Greenbaum, 1975). We feel that, ultimately, the clinician must determine (1) which structures the child appears to have acquired, (2) which structures are absent in obligatory contexts, (3) which structures are inconsistently used, and (4) which contexts seem to be associated with use and nonuse of the inconsistent structures. Muma (1973a) and Kahn and James (1980) have advocated such descriptive procedures that focus on determining present, absent, and inconsistent syntactic elements, and we view this as a commonsense approach to analysis that has direct clinical application. It also does not involve the clinician's commitment of time to learning one or two package procedures and their unique scoring systems. Tables 5.6 and 5.7 provide a hypothetical sample and analysis.

Recently, computer analyses of language samples have come to the fore. Software programs are available that provide detailed information about a language sample; however, the clinician must remember that some time is typically invested in coding the transcript into the computer. In some cases, this may take more time than a paper-and-pencil analysis, if the clinician merely wants to define treatment targets. In addition, the computer analyses may provide the clinician with more information than is really needed. The output from these programs is truly phenomenal.

We would like to provide a very brief overview of two computer programs that are currently available and are particularly useful in language analysis. Both programs are impressive

TABLE 5.7	Transcript Analysis Example

1. Grant got one of them.
2. Him go flop flop.
3. It go like that.
4. They have a wagon.
5. Jay is my brother.
6. Somebody drop a glass on the floor.
7. Him live at that house.
8. Him the boy that live next door.
9. They are going to town.
10. Him riding a bike.
11. It is at home.
12. Her going fast.
13. I don't know.
14. Smudge is a boy cat.
15. I four years old and I live in Eufaula.
16. It brown and brick.
17. Him go to the hospital.
18. Thats a hospital.
19. They are too big.
20. I running fast.
21. They boys are driving a car.
22. The cat is sleeping.
23. Her feed the baby.
24. Her have a cold.
25. We have to let him in car.
26. We ride in car and go fast.
27. A boy on the rocker and one in house.
28. They in parking lot while the boy sleep.
29. The cat is running up the drapes.
30. The girl is holding her ears.
31. Him carrying a box of apples.

Selected Forms Used

Proper noun
Irregular verb
Cardinal number
Plural pronoun
Verbs
Demonstrative ("that")
Adverbial of manner
Indefinite pronoun ("somebody")
Verb "have"
Nondefinite article
Nouns

Uncontractible copula
Personal pronoun ("my," "I")
Prepositions
Definite article
Auxillary ("are")
Present progressive
Auxillary ("do")
Adjective
Conjunctions ("and," "while")
Plural ("boys")

Errors

"him"/"he" (objective for subjective
pronominal case)
"go"/"goes"; "live"/"lives"; "feed"/"feeds";
"sleep"/"sleeps" (3rd person sing.)
"drop"/"dropped" (regular past "-ed")
Omitted copula "is"
Omitted auxillary "is"
Omitted copula "am"
"have"/"has"
Omitted definite article
Omitted copula "are"

Errors Consistently Misused

"him"/"he"
3rd person "-s"
Regular past "-ed" (1 instance)
Omitted copula "am"
"have"/"has"

TABLE 5.7   *(continued)*

Errors Inconsistently Misused

Omitted copula "is"
Omitted auxillary "is"
Omitted definite article
Omitted copula "are"

Context When Inconsistent Error Occurred

Copula "is":
   #8 high complexity, embedding,
     "him"/"he" substitution
   #16 complex, conjoining and deleting
   #27 complex, conjoining
Auxillary "is":
   #10 "him"/"he" substitution
   #12 "her"/"she" substitution
   #31 "him"/"he" substitution
Copula "are":
   #28 complex, conjoining
Definite article:
   #25 complex, embedding
   #26 complex, embedding
   #27 complex, embedding
   #28 complex, embedding

Context of Inconsistent Errors When They Did Not Occur

Copula "is":
   #5 simple, "Jay is . . ."
   #11 simple, "It is . . ."
   #14 simple, "Smudge is . . ."
   #18 "That is . . ."
Auxillary *is:*
   #22 simple, "The cat is . . ."
   #29 simple, "The cat is . . ."
   #30 simple, "The girl is . . ."
Copula *are:*
   #9 simple, *They are* . . .
   #19 simple, *They are* . . .
   #21 simple, *The boys are* . . .

Definite article:
   #6 simple
   #17 simple
   #21 simple
   #22 simple
   #23 simple
   #27 complex, conjoining
   #28 complex, conjoining
   #29 simple
   #30 simple

and are based on years of research and development. It would take many pages just to list the types of output from the programs. Thus, we cannot hope to do justice to either one in a couple of paragraphs. It is important, however, that clinicians move toward the use of computer analysis in language assessment. We have tried to make it clear in this text that conversational samples are the most valid target of a language assessment. Some clinicians have shied away from such analyses because of the time it takes to complete them and the expertise in linguistics required to make certain judgments. To some degree, these programs address both of these concerns and make language sample analysis more accessible to clinicians working in the field. Both programs have been developed with the cooperation of university faculty and clinicians working in school systems and other settings. These two programs represent somewhat different approaches to the input of data and analysis of language samples. One program has been characterized as a data retrieval program; it requires the clinician to code utterances, boundaries, segmentation, errors, and so on using codes specific to the software. Thus, the automatic part of the program is its summary of the data that has already been entered into the computer by the clinician. A second type of program uses a computer algorithm to actually parse the sentences and identify grammatical components for analysis, then summarizes the results. While the clinician still must type in a language transcript, certain decisions are made by the computer—such as the grammatical identities of sentence components, grammatical morphemes, and even the identification of phrases and clauses. Long and Channell (2001) analyzed 69 language samples using the grammatical analyses of MLU, LARSP, IPSyn, and DSS to determine if results using human coding and automatic computer analyses were in agreement. They found that: "Results for all four analyses produced automatically were comparable to published data on the manual interrater reliability of these procedures. Clinical decisions based on cutoff scores and productivity data were little affected by the use of automatic rather than human-generated analyses. These findings bode well for future clinical and research use of automatic language analysis software" (p. 180).

Both automatic analysis and data retrieval programs have significant value to the clinician attempting to analyze a language sample. We will give an example of each type of program. The first program, *Computerized Profiling* (Long, Fey, & Channell, 2002), which automatically parses utterances, can be downloaded from the Internet at no charge (http://www.computerizedprofiling.org) and thus is a resource available to all clinicians regardless of work setting. It has a variety of modules that are used to examine many linguistic areas. A module common to all analyses is the *corpus* module, which allows the user to create transcript files used by all other modules. In corpus mode the clinician can input samples, edit, print, and even convert files for export to the SALT program (which we discuss next). Computerized Profiling's PROPH module analyzes a child's phonetic inventory, syllable shapes, phonological processes, and percent of consonants correct using a traditional test or a conversational sample. The Profile in Semantics (PRISM) module examines the content of early and later vocabularies in children and provides a highly detailed lexical analysis based on semantic fields. It also has a submodule that analyzes semantic relations. There is a module for the Language Assessment, Remediation, and Screening Procedure (LARSP), which provides an age- and stage-based system for profiling a child's syntactic development. As a submodule in LARSP there is a Conversational Acts Profile (CAP), which examines a child's assertiveness and responsiveness in conversation. A prosody profile (PROP) is also included in Computerized Profiling for analyzing intonation patterns in grammatical structures. Finally, a module for Developmental Sentence Scoring (DSS) is included in the package. Channell (2003) found point-by-point agreement between computerized profiling's DSS and manual coding to be 78%, with a correlation of .97 between the two methods. Readers are encouraged to download the program, which is free of charge and has excellent help screens to guide new users in the analyses.

The second program we will consider is a data retrieval program called *Systematic Analyses of Language Transcripts* (SALT) (Miller & Chapman, 2008). Heilmann, Miller, and Nockerts (2010) provide an effective overview of the SALT database and how it might be used by clinicians. A long-standing use of these computer-based procedures has been to document clinical progress over time measured by naturalistic language samples instead of formal tests. The above researchers have shown that language sample analysis using the SALT program can even discriminate between typically developing children and those with language impairment with a fair amount of sensitivity and specificity, most values being between 80 and 89%.

This program allows the user to either type in a language transcript or import a transcript from a word processing program. Once the transcript is entered, the clinician must segment it and enter certain codes in the form of slashes, asterisks, and other symbols to define certain conversational or grammatical categories (e.g., bound morphemes, abandoned utterances, etc.). After the codes are entered, the program summarizes a series of standard analyses at the word, morpheme, utterance, and discourse levels. A particularly useful measure of SALT is its in-depth analysis of mazing (use of repetitions, fillers, etc.) in conversational samples. Another aspect of SALT that is extremely useful is its reference database of normative data on nearly 350 subjects, representing children from the ages of 3 to 13. There are norms for both conversation and narratives in the database. These norms are particularly useful because they indicate how many standard deviations away from the mean a child scores, compared to the reference database. Because the norms are based on conversational samples, they represent a source of normative data for many variables that we might want to examine in connected speech. Miller and Chapman (2008) show how particular patterns on the SALT may relate to specific subtypes of language impairment.

The advantage of the computer would appear to lie in the multiple analyses that can be performed once the sample is input. That is, a clinician can take the same transcript and analyze it for insight into the child's semantic system, phonological system, syntactic system, and occurrence of speech acts (if appropriately coded). An important point to emphasize is that these programs are only as good as the coding of the language sample that they analyze. Some programs automatically classify lexical items or grammatical forms based on internal algorithms. Most programs allow the clinician to change these a priori classifications of transcript items if they are incorrect. That is, sometimes a program will not identify a word or grammatical construction correctly, and the clinician needs to check how the computer has classified transcript items. There is no substitute for close clinician monitoring when using these programs. Just because the computer pumps out a profile or summary of a child's performance does not mean that the clinician should not at least spot-check the analysis for correctness. It is easy to be seduced into relying on complex summaries without checking on validity. Some excellent examples of how computer-aided language sample analysis can be used in clinical settings in initial assessment and measuring treatment progress are presented by Price, Hendricks, and Cook 2010.

No doubt we will learn much in the next decade from these procedures about patterns of error and subtypes of language disorder. No single procedure can tell a clinician all he or she needs to know about a child's language. Again, ultimately it is the clinician's judgment that must be applied to a particular case, whether it is a decision to choose among several package analysis systems, computer-assisted analysis, or to simply focus on a more specific descriptive linguistic analysis.

ASSESSMENT OF CONVERSATIONAL PRAGMATICS

Many reports exist in the literature that attest to pragmatic differences in children with language impairments. Some investigations report that these children have difficulty organizing narratives and staying on a topic (Johnston, 1982). Fey and Leonard (1983) have hypothesized that there may be subgroups of language-impaired children who exhibit a variety of pragmatic problems. There have been reports of children with language disorders who have difficulty taking listener perspective into account (Muma, 1975). Unfortunately, there are no tests that tap all relevant aspects of conversational pragmatics. Although there are some formal measures that focus on limited facets of pragmatic ability (Blagden & McConnell, 1983; Shulman, 1986), it would be difficult to develop a broader assessment device because of the many aspects included under the rubric of pragmatics. Conversational abilities are also difficult to tap by using artificial tasks, limited samples, or contrived topics of discourse. If the clinician is interested in conversational abilities, there is no substitute for legitimate conversation. When the clinician focuses on conversation and discourse, it is necessary to obtain a sample of the child's conversational performance and to transcribe both the utterances of the child and of the interlocuter. This transcription is a time-consuming task; however, if the clinician is to obtain data on the child's conversational performance, the contributions of both participants cannot be ignored. There are several measures that the clinician might elect to use to analyze conversation, depending on which aspects of the discourse are of interest. Some of these measures may overlap to a certain degree. We recommend beginning at a general level and then progressing to more specific analyses.

Evaluation of General Parameters: Identification of a Potential Problem

Damico and Oller (1980) noted that classroom teachers were easily able to make appropriate referrals of pragmatic disorders to the speech-language pathologist. In fact, some pragmatic problems are even more noticeable than morphological/syntactic difficulties. Ask a teacher sometime if there are children in his or her class that consistently have trouble carrying on a conversation because of inadequate information, listener perspective problems, and significant mazing. They often remember these children more easily than one who omits a plural morpheme.

Prutting and Kirchner (1987) developed a pragmatic protocol that gives an overall communicative index for children, adolescents, and adults. It includes 30 pragmatic aspects of language in the broad groupings of verbal, paralinguistic, and nonverbal skills. There are specific definitions for each parameter used in the system, and they provide preliminary data on both adults and children with normal and disordered language. This approach to evaluating a child's pragmatic abilities begins with a molar view of conversational performance to determine if certain types of errors are especially obvious to the clinician. Prutting and Kirchner (1987) rated children's conversation on the 30 parameters. The most inappropriate pragmatic parameters found in 42 children with language impairments involved turn-taking, specificity/accuracy, cohesion, repair/revision, topic maintenance, and intelligibility. Use of the protocol described above at the very least forces the clinician to consider the relevant parameters of pragmatics and to make a judgment regarding each. Then more concentrated evaluation tasks can be applied to the case that might define the nature of the conversational errors more specifically. Similarly, Damico (1985) has developed a screening tool that has been used successfully by teachers in identifying children with pragmatic disorders. This instrument includes a rating scale, to be completed by teachers, that focuses on common symptoms of pragmatic disorders as well as academic skills. Another more detailed system is recommended by Bedrosian (1985). Again, this type of approach moves from general to more specific in terms of evaluating language in older students. More molecular analyses can be initiated after a student is identified by a general procedure.

Another general area intimately related to pragmatics is the child's social skills. Humans develop social relationships largely based on our ability to communicate with others in a relevant and efficient manner. Some studies show that children with language impairment have social difficulties, compared to normally developing peers. Fujiki et al. (2001) studied the playground behavior of eight children with SLI and their age-matched peers and found that typically developing children spent more time interacting with peers on the playground, compared to children with SLI. Conversely, children with SLI demonstrated more withdrawn behaviors compared to the typically developing children. The authors suggest that including social interaction behaviors in the treatment program for children with SLI might be appropriate. This again illustrates how the SLP should extend assessment beyond formal testing and determine environmental effects of the the communication disorder and evaluate functional outcomes that extend beyond language. Fujiki, Brinton, and Todd (1996) studied 19 elementary school children with SLI and age-matched peers. They administered a number of measures to teachers and peers to determine a general measure of social skill and the quantity and quality of peer relationships. They found that the children with SLI had poorer social skills and fewer peer relationships than the age-matched controls. Also, the children with SLI were less satisfied with their peer relationships than the typically developing children. This again underscores the importance of evaluating the child's functioning in more than just language and of using teachers and peers as informants.

Narrowing the Focus: Assessment of Narrative Production

Narratives give an "account of happenings," as in telling a story, and adhere to some definable conventions or rules in the children's generation (Liles, 1993). Educational research has suggested that narratives are a bridge between oral language and literacy, since their structure resembles written text. Narrative skills have been shown to reliably predict academic success in children who are normally developing as well as those with learning disabilities and a specific language disorder (Paul, 2007). Narratives occur repeatedly in our daily discourse as we talk to others about weekend experiences, tell jokes, explain a process to a teacher, relate anecdotes, gossip, and describe our activities and possessions to impress our listeners. Thus, narratives are important academically as well as socially and communicatively. The narrative has been a topic of research interest over the past decade because it synthesizes a variety of abilities in order to be effective. For example, the ability to tell a story involves skill in sequencing events, creating cohesive text, use of precise vocabulary, nonreliance on contextual support, and understanding of universal story grammar to structure the narrative production. According to Liles (1993):

> There is a consistency across investigators regarding the structural limitations of young children's narratives and the apparent acceleration in development around age 5. Researchers analyzing the structure of narratives in older children have generally agreed that by age 6 children can produce an ideal (e.g., adult) structure, but development continues in 9- and 10-year old children. The development of narrative structure in older children is evidenced by both an increased number of episodes and the children's growing ability to link them together in complex ways (e.g., embedding one episode within another). More recent studies investigating narrative structure in older children . . . found that the number of complete episodes continued to increase in the narratives of children aged 8 to 16 years. (p. 875)

As narrative productions develop in children and become more complex, increasingly more elements of story grammar are incorporated into the narrative (Applebee, 1978; Johnston, 1982; Paul, 2007). For example, story grammar typically includes a description of the *setting,* which includes the environmental context as well as the main characters. Another component is the *initiating event,* which is some action, event, or change in the environment that affects the characters. This is often a "problem" of some sort (e.g., eruption of a volcano). Characters generally have an *internal response* to the initiating event, which may include emotions, goals, thoughts, and intentions leading to a plan of action. This plan of action leads to *attempts* or actions directed toward resolving the situation or attaining a goal. Next, the attempts will result in *consequences,* which will either result in the resolution of the problem or the attainment of the goal, or in the failure to deal adequately with the situation. Finally, the character will have a *reaction* to the consequence mentioned above, which includes internal states (e.g., feelings, thoughts). As narratives become more complex, the child will include more of the above elements in the production.

Studies of children with a specific language disorder have revealed narratives with some of the following characteristics (Merritt & Liles, 1989; Owens, 2004):

- Fewer total words
- Fewer different words
- Fewer story grammar components
- Fewer complete episodes
- Fewer protagonist plans and internal responses
- Fewer conventional story openings/closings
- Improper amounts of information (too much/little)
- Fewer successful repairs
- Fewer accommodations to listeners
- Fewer complete cohesive ties and more incomplete/erroneous ties

Clinicians who wish to analyze narratives in children with language impairments might look for some of the differences mentioned above. As children become older, their language disorders often take on more subtle characteristics. The impairment may not be revealed in structural errors, but may become obvious on a pragmatic-conversational level. Johnson (1995) points out that we need more information on the later development of narratives in school-age children and adolescents. Although we have information on early development, the establishment of norms on older children would be helpful to the diagnostician. Johnson also reviews information on situational variation and cultural diversity. Miller, Gillam, and Pena (2001) have developed a procedure for using principles of dynamic assessment to evaluate children's narrative production. An intervention program is coupled with this assessment procedure. Their assessment takes into account not only structural aspects of the narrative produced, but rating scales for clinician judgment as to a child's response to dynamic assessment and his or her modifiability. The degree of modifiability during dynamic assessment seems to be a better indicator in classifying children with language impairment as compared to pretest storytelling data (Pena, Gillam, Malek, Ruiz-Felter, Resendiz, Fiestas, & Sabel, 2006).

Paul (2007) talks about three major aspects of narratives that deserve assessment consideration. First, narratives include a basic plot and elements of story grammar that should be incorporated into the story; we briefly introduced story grammar elements in a prior section. Applebee (1978) characterizes narrative development in part as the progressive inclusion of more elements of story grammar with age and the existence of a defined plot as the child becomes older. For example, Applebee proposes five stages of narrative development that involve increased use of story grammar components and plot. Since looking for story grammar elements and basic plotting involve a general view of a child's narrative, these components are often referred to as narrative macrostructure.

A second assessment target for narratives according to Paul (2001) is evaluating cohesive ties in narratives. We have a later section in the present chapter on cohesive adequacy, but for now it is enough to say that certain elements in an utterance gain meaning only by searching outside a particular sentence. For instance, in the sentence "John hit him," we do not know who was hit unless we look at the prior sentence, "John was pushed by Mark." Now we know that Mark was the one that John hit. In narratives and conversation we can only use certain words if we have introduced them in a prior utterance. If you have done a good job of cohesion, a person can find meaning in an utterance by referring to other parts of the narrative to derive meaning. This is called a "complete tie," or the ability to effectively tie an ambiguous part of an utterance to some other part of the narrative. If you encounter a word such as "him" and you cannot figure out who "he" is, then the tie is incomplete. Paul suggests that kindergarten children have 85% complete ties in their narratives and children with language impairment have a few as 60% complete ties. She recommends a cutoff of 70% complete ties as an indicator of concern.

A third aspect of narratives to consider in evaluation is what has become known as "sparkle" (Paul, 2007). Although sparkle is a bit artsy in its interpretation, there are several important elements that are usually considered: richness of vocabulary, episode complexity, existence of a story climax, use of complex sentence structures, use of literate language style, and use of dialogue. The more of these elements included in the narrative, the more sparkle it has. Newman and McGregor (2006) found that teachers and laypersons noted differences between children with SLI and typically developing children after hearing a short oral narrative. The narratives of the children with SLI were judged to be poorer in quality. In addition to some quantitative variables such as utterance length and underdeveloped story themes, the laypersons also noted that "sparkle" was missing from the SLI narratives. A good place to start in a narrative analysis might be a standardized method of analysis such as the Test of Narrative Language (Gillam & Pearson, 2004). This test is one of the few measures that provides normative data on narrative production.

Narratives have been analyzed with regard to macrostructure and microstructure. Macrostructure has to do with inclusion of story grammar elements and the complexity of episode structure. One aspect of microstructure analysis is directed to the linguistic aspects of the narrative, including construction of noun phrases, use of conjunctions, and the inclusion of dependent clauses. Most authorities suggest that a thorough assessment of narratives includes both macro- and microstructural analyses. Justice, Bowles, Kaderavek, Ukrainetz, Eisenberg, and Gillam (2006) have developed the Index of Narrative Microstructure (INMIS) and provide preliminary normative data for 250 children between 5 and 12 years of age as they constructed narratives in response to a single picture stimulus. The authors found that microstructure analysis revealed two important factors of productivity (word output, lexical diversity, and number of T-units produced) and complexity (T-unit length, proportion of complex T-units). The procedure can be used in conjunction with macrostructural analyses to evaluate narrative development in children. Ukrainetz and Gillam (2009) studied 6- and 8-year-old children as they produced two imaginative narratives. They found that the younger typically developing children and those with language impairment produced narratives with less orientations to the story, less evaluations, and fewer abstracts and codas as compared to older typically developing children. The type of narrative used in language sampling may be important in assessment. McCabe, Bliss, Barra, and Bennett (2008) gathered fictional (wordless picture book) and personal (experience-based) narratives from children with language impairment between the ages of 7–9. They found that the personal narratives included more components required in adequate narrative production as compared to fictional narratives. Performance in one type of narrative did not appear to relate to the performance in the other genre. Heilmann, Miller, Nockerts, and Dunaway (2010) developed the Narrative Scoring Scheme (NSS), which deals with narrative macroscructure, but goes beyond basic story grammar to include higher level components such as cohesion, character development referencing, and conflict resolution. Each of the narrative components is scored using a 5-point scale ranging from minimal to proficient, and the clinician can obtain a total or composite score that represents a child's "overall narrative organization." Additionally, the narrative can be input into the SALT program and the child's results compared to NSS normative data. This is a relevant measure that can be used not only in diagnosis, but in monitoring treatment goals that focus on narrative production.

Narrative analysis is a valuable adjunct to our assessment repertoire and is regarded as an important diagnostic consideration by most current authorities (Owens, 2005; Paul, 2001; Swanson, Fey, Mills, & Hood, 2005). We must also remember that narrative production may vary according to a person's culture. Gutierrez-Clellen and Quinn (1993) indicate that narratives are influenced by a child's information and organization abilities, world knowledge/experience, the type of elicitation task, interactional style, and use of paralinguistic conventions. This will be discussed in more detail in Chapter 12. For certain disorder groups of children elicitation task may make a difference in gathering narrative samples. For instance, using pictures in eliciting narratives from children with Down syndrome resulted in longer utterances as compared to an interview technique (Miles, Chapman, & Sindberg, 2006).

Looking for Specific Errors: Clinical Discourse Analysis

Damico (1980, 1985) has taken a different approach and has advocated the analysis of specific discourse errors in children's language. He provides a list of nine discourse errors that can be detected in conversation and computed into a percentage of utterances containing pragmatic difficulties. He recommends obtaining 180 utterances over two sessions in conversational interaction about home and school activities. The goal of the analysis is to describe specific discourse errors that exist in the interaction. Damico has gathered data on many typically developing children and those with language disorders and proposes some error percentage ranges for determining very generally the existence and severity of a discourse problem.

Assessment of Topic Manipulation

Topics may use general knowledge shared by interactants, information physically present in the context, or previous discourse. According to Keenan and Schieffelin (1976), much conversational space is taken up by communicators to establish a topic. Once the topic is established, an interactant can use a turn to either maintain the topic (continuous discourse) or change the topic (discontinuous discourse). When speakers continue a discourse topic by corroborating a previous utterance with a related statement, or incorporating information in a prior utterance into their statement, the topic is maintained. When a speaker discontinues a discourse topic, it is either by introducing a topic that is unrelated to previous utterances or by reintroducing a prior topic ("Getting back to what we said about . . ."). Thus, topic-maintaining utterances corroborate a prior statement or incorporate it into a new statement that is still on the topic. Developmentally, the length of continuous discourse increases with age. In assessment, we need to determine how a child is able to secure the attention of a listener in order to initiate a topic (by crying, yelling, gesturing, and tugging; or with loudness, prosody, or an introduction such as "Know what?"). We can measure the length of the topic unit in terms of number of turns taken per topic. We also can measure the topic-maintaining and -shifting utterances used by a child. It is important in assessment to examine a child's ability not only to continue topics but also to initiate them. In sampling, as mentioned previously, we may not often provide for this. Some of the most productive work on in-depth analysis of topic manipulation has been done by Brinton and Fujiki (1984, 1989), who provide detailed procedures for evaluating all relevant aspects of topic manipulation in clinical work. We need further research to more specifically define the normal development of topic manipulation in both children who are typically developing and those with language impairments. Some language-impaired children clearly have difficulty with these skills (Prutting &

Kirchner, 1987), while other subgroups of children with linguistic impairment appear to manipulate topics normally (Edmonds & Haynes, 1988; Ehlers & Cirrin, 1983). Assessment of contingency (topic manipulation) may be important in documenting discourse problems in specific populations. For example, fragile X syndrome often co-occurs with autism spectrum disorders, and research has shown that boys with both of these disorders concurrently were significantly less contingent in discourse than those having only fragile X (Roberts, Martin, Moskowitz, Harris, Foreman, & Nelson, 2007).

We also need to know more about topic manipulation throughout the lifespan to determine changes in these skills in aging normal subjects, since there is some evidence that differences exist among age groups (Stover & Haynes, 1989).

Assessment of Repairs: The Contingent Query

Another major category of measurement of conversational competence is the contingent query. A number of studies (Garvey, 1977a, 1977b) show that contingent queries are used by adults and children to achieve cohesion in conversation. Children as young as 3 years use contingent queries. Basically, the queries serve multiple functions in conversation, many of which have to do with repair procedures that allow the conversation to continue. For instance, a contingent query can be used to request a general repetition ("Huh?"), a specific repetition ("A what?"), a request for confirmation ("A tape recorder?"), and elaboration ("We have to go where?"). There are more complex aspects of contingent queries that are explained in the above references. One can see, however, that these queries are important mechanisms of conversational competence and that a child who does not know how to ask for clarification, for instance, will have difficulty continuing a particular topic with an interactant. The term *conversational repair* has been used most often in association with contingent queries. Clinically, it would be important to determine if a child can both respond to and produce requests for conversational repair (Brinton & Fujiki, 1989). For example, we would like to see if a child can adjust an utterance to a listener's request for repetition, clarification, or elaboration. On the other hand, we would like to determine if a child would ask for clarification if a clinician asks for a *ferbis* or makes a statement violating truth constraints in a particular context. Brinton and Fujiki (1989) provide many helpful suggestions for both assessment and intervention with conversational repair mechanisms. Yont, Hewitt, and Miccio (2000) introduced a system for coding conversational breakdowns, called the *Breakdown Coding System* (BCS). This was piloted on typically developing preschoolers during natural interactions with caretakers. They found that the BCS had high interjudge reliability and was useful for profiling patterns of breakdowns in conversation. Further research on children with language impairment should be conducted.

Assessment of Cohesive Adequacy

Some children produce narratives or conversational turns that lack adequate *cohesion,* which refers to the relationships or ties between elements in discourse that are dependent upon one another (Halliday & Hasan, 1976). Stover and Haynes (1989) provide an example:

> Wash the *dirty dishes* that are in the sink. Dry *them* and then put *them* in the cabinet. In the second sentence *them* refers directly back to the *dirty dishes,* thus forming a cohesive tie. Of course, the cohesive marker may extend far beyond the immediately preceding sentence to an utterance produced earlier in the conversation. . . . In a complete tie, the referent to which a cohesive marker refers is easily found in a prior

utterance with no ambiguity as in the above example. In an incomplete tie, a cohesive marker refers to something not mentioned in prior utterances (e.g., I like ice cream. *He* does too). In this example *he* cannot be associated with a particular person mentioned previously in the sentence. In an erroneous tie, there is ambiguity or error in interpreting who a referent is (e.g., Tom and Jerry live in the city. *He* likes it.). In this example, we do not know if *he* refers to Tom or Jerry. (p. 140)

Liles (1985) provides specific procedures for cohesion analysis. One can readily see that this type of analysis would be useful in cases that do not take into account the listener's perspective in discourse and that are not aware of the requirements of conversational rules (Grice, 1975). Some recent studies suggest that there may be subgroups of children with cohesion difficulties. For example, Craig and Evans (1993) found that children with both receptive and expressive language impairments produced significantly more incomplete, erroneous, and ambiguous cohesive ties compared to children with disorders exclusively in expressive language. It is easy to see that measurements such as percentage of complete, incomplete, and erroneous ties could be used as an index of progress in treatment.

ISSUES OF MEMORY AND PROCESSING LOAD

Over time it has been noted by clinicians and researchers that children with language impairments seem to have difficulty processing linguistic material effectively. This is especially true when the processing load becomes less manageable with the addition of semantic, syntactic, phonological, or cognitive complexity. This quite possibly accounts for the phenomenon we referred to earlier when the child with SLI finds it progressively more difficult to cope with the increasing linguistic and cognitive demands of the educational curriculum. This is easy to see in studies that have used a "dual task" paradigm in which children are asked to complete two operations simultaneously. Johnston (2006, p. 54) summarizes this eloquently:

Other interpretations of dual-task findings stress the coordination of effort that is required, and argue that poor performance reflects inefficient deployment of knowledge, poor monitoring of performance, or difficulties in managing diverse responses. All of these interpretations rest on the assumption that the human mind functions as a limited capacity system. If there is a finite amount of mental energy available at any one moment, a task that requires great concentration or efficiency may use enough of this capacity that little remains for work on a second task. When the traffic is heavy, it's hard to talk and drive.

If children with SLI have a "weakness" in the area of language, they may use most of their processing capacity to just understand or produce an utterance and few resources are left for more complex activities such as inferencing, selection of novel vocabulary, or construction of complex sentences. Thus, the more we can help a child learn about language through therapy, the more processing capacity is freed up for use. Certain abilities such as "working memory" are necessary in order to hold critical information in mind from the beginning of a sentence, or a prior sentence while processing the rest of the utterance. Even in nonword repetition tasks (NRT), children with SLI seem to run into processing difficulty as the stimuli become longer. We mention some specific examples here because clinicians may want to probe these abilities as part of a thorough language assessment. Montgomery and Evans (2009) found that children with language impairment performed lower than typically developing children on tasks designed to tap working memory. Interestingly, the memory task scores in the language-impaired group corre-lated with scores indicating comprehension of complex sentences. Scores on a nonword repetition task correlated with comprehension of simple sentences. There were no significant correlations found between memory tasks and language comprehension for the typically developing group. Working memory has been found to be deficient in many studies of children with language im-pairment and is a skill that is required especially in a task requiring parsing of complex sen-tences. The processing load is significantly increased if a child is struggling to hold onto rapidly presented information while trying to make cognitive and linguistic judgments. Thus, compared to typically developing children, those with language impairment require more mental effort to process language whether it is simple or more complex. A recent factor analytic investigation suggested that 14-year-old students with specific language impairment may experience process-ing limitations in speed and working memory (Leonard, Weismer, Miller, Frances, Tomblin, & Kail, 2007). Montgomery, Magimairaj, and Finney (2010) provide an excellent review of the research on working memory as it relates to language impairment and a list of sources for tests and measurements that can be used by the SLP to measure processing speed, executive functions, working memory capacity, and short-term memory.

A recent meta-analysis of over 20 studies focusing on nonword repetition performance in children with language impairment found that this population exhibited significant impair-ments, performing an average of 1.27 standard deviations below typically developing children. The difficulties were on both short and long nonword stimuli; however, the problem became more significant on the longer stimuli. Also, the study found different effect sizes across stud-ies that used different sets of nonword stimuli, suggesting that the specific tasks may not be equivalent. Another example of a nonword repetition task for preschool children was developed in Britain by Stokes and Klee (2009). They found, as most nonword repetition tests do, that the longer syllable tasks were more difficult for the children in the study, and that the test could dif-ferentiate between late talkers and typically developing children with acceptable psychometric values for sensitivity and specificity. Chiat and Roy (2007) have developed a nonword repeti-tion test for preschool children. They have found the typical result of increased difficulty with increased item length and and more complex prosodic structure of the items. Children per-formed better with age between 2 and 4 years and the performance was not affected by gender or socioeconomic level. They also found that the test could accurately discriminate between children referred to a clinic for evaluation and typically developing children with high inter-judge and test–retest reliability.

Most tasks involving working memory and nonword repetition take little time to adminis-ter in an evaluation and may contribute one more piece to the picture of a child's total function-ing in the area of language. As you will see in Chapter 12, nonword repetition tasks have been used with bilingual children or those who speak dialects of English because nonwords do not de-pend on the rules of a child's first language. Thus, these have been promising tasks for use in nonbiased assessment.

EVALUATING LITERACY AND SCHOOL CURRICULUM

As we mentioned at the beginning of this chapter, several groups of youngsters are at high risk to develop a language disorder during the school years. First, children with a history of pre-school language delay are likely to experience subtle language disturbances throughout their school years and be at risk for academic problems (Aram & Nation, 1980; Bashir et al., 1983; Hall& Tomblin, 1978; King, Jones, & Lasky, 1982; Strominger & Bashir, 1977). These children were often dismissed from language treatment and then later rediagnosed as being reading or learning disabled. Most of these children exhibited low academic achievement throughout school, because the curricular demands increase significantly in terms of language and communicative expectations while the child's linguistic abilities may not improve to meet these challenges. A second group of children that is likely to demonstrate subtle language impairments consists of children diagnosed as being reading or learning disabled. The majority of learning-disabled students have experienced language delays and some of these problems continue into adulthood. Finally, children who are considered to be academically at risk because of poor school performance are also likely to have gaps in their ability to perform linguistic tasks (Simon, 1989). It is now clear that children with speech-language impairments tend to perform poorly on reading comprehension (Catts, 1993). Oral language skills are intimately related to reading achievement (Wise, Sevcik, Morris, Lovett, & Wolf, 2007). The SLP should carefully evaluate youngsters from the groups mentioned above, especially when referred by classroom teachers. Many of the specific language symptoms likely to be seen in these groups were listed in Table 5-1. One aspect that has not been emphasized, however, is specifically examining the types of language and communication abilities that are important for classroom success.

More than ever before, the speech-language pathologist is involved with literacy issues. This involvement may begin in preschool or early school age as early literacy screening programs are developed. Part of any thorough language assessment should address emerging literacy skills. If a child is lagging in literacy development the SLP can incorporate literacy activities into treatment. Even in typically developing children, literacy issues can have a significant impact on learning. For instance, Foster and Miller (2007) studied groups of children from kindergarten to third grade who represented low, average and high levels of literacy development upon kindergarten entrance. These children came from a pool of over 12,000 youngsters who were part of the Early Childhood Longitudinal Study. Students in the middle and high groups achieved good scores on phonics (decoding) by the end of first grade. The lower group did not meet such expectations until third grade. The lower group also manifested significant text comprehension difficulties. One can only speculate on the amount of information that these children had difficulty learning due to a struggle with literacy issues. Unfortunately, most children in the lower performing group came from lower socioeconomic levels and had an overrepresentation of African American and Hispanic students. Justice and Ezell (2004) provide a good developmental sequence of written language awareness achievements and their associated print-referencing targets for assessment and treatment. Justice and Kaderavek (2004) and Kaderavek and Justice (2004) outline a developmental model for emergent literacy development including phonological awareness, print concepts, alphabet knowledge, and literate language. Many literacy opportunities are available embedded in a child's natural environment and school setting, while other aspects may be approached explicitly by the SLP with small group, classroom, and individual activities. It is helpful to know the developmental progression in choosing assessment targets and intervention goals. Boudreau (2005) determined that experimenter-administered measures of rhyme, environmental print knowledge, knowledge of print conventions, letter name knowledge, letter sound knowledge, and narrative ability was strongly related to a parent questionnaire that tapped similar areas and parent literacy practices. The implication here is that such a questionnaire might be combined with assessment tasks to gain a broader view of emergent literacy. Never underestimate the contribution that parents and teachers can make to evaluation. Since many aspects of literacy (e.g., reading, writing, spelling, adequate narratives) are based on a child's oral language system, it is not surprising that many of our clients with language disorder also have poor literacy skills. In the beginning of this chapter we cited studies showing that children with language impairment are at high risk for reading problems and may have less academic success. Some more recent investigations address the relationships among language and metalinguistic abilities and reading. For example, Catts et al. (2001) studied more than 600 children in kindergarten and tested them again in second grade for reading ability. They found that letter identification, sentence imitation, phonological awareness, rapid naming, and mother's educational level uniquely predicted reading outcome in second grade. Gilbertson and Bramlett (1998) studied informal phonological awareness measures to determine if they could predict reading ability in first grade. Participants were 91 former Head Start students. Gilbertson and Bramlett found that the phonological awareness tasks of invented spelling, categorization, and blending were the best predictors of standardized reading measures at the end of first grade. The three phonological awareness tasks correctly identified at-risk students with 92% accuracy. The authors suggest that the SLP can play a primary role in identifying and remediating children with language-based reading disorders.

Catts (1997) provides a checklist for SLPs and teachers to use for early identification of reading disabilities. The checklist provides a number of language deficits often associated with reading difficulties. Boudreau and Hedberg (1999) studied 5-year-old children with SLI and normally developing language on a number of early literacy variables. The SLI children did not perform as well as normally developing children on tasks involving knowledge of rhyme, letter names, and print concepts. The SLI children also showed poorer performance on narrative measures of linguistic structure, recall of information, and total events included. Other research has examined literacy in terms of emergent readings in children with SLI. In emergent readings, a child who is not yet reading conventionally is asked to "read" from a familiar storybook, and the speech produced is analyzed for features of written language. Kaderavek and Sulzby (2000) studied SLI and normal-language children and found that children with SLI produced fewer language features associated with written language, and the SLI children had more difficulty with oral narratives. They suggest that emergent storybook reading may be useful as part of a language assessment protocol because it may provide insight into the relationship between language impairment and later reading difficulty.

Even in cases of late talkers who ultimately develop language in a relatively normal manner, there is concern expressed by some researchers. For example, Rescorla (2002) studied 34 children who were identified as late talkers as toddlers and followed them until the ages of 6 to 9 years. Most late talkers performed within the average range in most language skills by the time they entered school. Relatively few of the late talkers developed a reading disability, but the author regarded the early expressive language delay as a subclinical weakness in the skills that serve language and reading. Rescorla recommends providing extra exposure to activities for strengthening word retrieval, verbal memory, phonological discrimination, and grammatical processing. Thus, the speech-language pathologist should be involved in the early detection of literacy issues, because these are likely to be present in children with language impairment. We are learning more and more about the long-term effects of language delay. Rescorla (2009) studied typically developing and late-talking children with normal comprehension between the ages of 2 and 17 years. At age 17, the children who were late talkers had significantly lower vocabulary, grammar, and verbal memory compared to the typically developing children. It is important to note that the scores of both groups were within normal limits, but the late talkers were significantly lower in this range. Justice, Invernizzi, and Meier (2002) developed a protocol for early detection of children with high risk for literacy difficulties. The protocol is designed for use by a team of professionals in a school district and focuses on written language awareness, phonological awareness, letter name knowledge, grapheme–phoneme correspondence, literacy motivation, and home literacy. Guidelines are provided for designing and implementing an early literacy screening program and developing interpretive benchmarks for the protocol (passing scores, etc.).

As children get older, it should be the responsibility of the SLP to incorporate literacy issues into assessment as well as treatment activities. For example, Apel (1999) provides a rationale from the professional literature and ASHA-preferred practice patterns for assessing and treating reading and writing difficulties: ". . . speech-language pathologists should assess and facilitate reading and writing skills, in addition to oral language skills, if they have been identified as areas of concern" (p. 229). This can be an important facet of diagnosis and treatment even in older cases. For instance, Apel and Swank (1999) reported a case study of a 29-year-old university student with reading difficulties. They worked on phonological awareness skills, quality of visual orthographic images, decoding strategy, and morphological awareness and found that the client showed significant improvement in reading ability as measured in word attack skills, word identification, reading rate, and reading accuracy. Speech-language pathologists may also participate in assessments involving other literacy areas such as spelling and writing. Masterson and Crede (1999) discuss the development of spelling and factors that influence spelling performance. They provide a case example of how a thorough assessment and intervention for spelling problems can show improvement in both formal and informal measures of spelling performance. Graham and Harris (1999) illustrate how writing strategies can be assessed and explicitly taught in combination with procedures for regulating those strategies, working through the writing process, and eliminating undesirable behaviors that interfere with writing. As part of a comprehensive evaluation of the school-age student with a language disorder, we must remember that all modalities of language can provide important insights into the student's abilities and needs. A sample of the student reading several paragraphs aloud from one of his or her textbooks would allow the SLP to note miscues, comprehension ability, and decoding strategies that may indicate difficulty processing written information. Similarly, writing samples of stories or narratives can usually be obtained in less than an hour, including time for planning. Obviously, the younger the student, the less writing can be accomplished in a sampling period. Nelson (2010) provides a nice overview of analysis of reading and writing and additional internet and written resources for the clinician. Puranik, Lombardino, and Altmann (2008) provide a method for SLPs to use in quantifying writing abilities. The procedure can be administered individually or in groups. Specific measurements to be computed on a writing sample are illustrated and data are provided for school-age children between grades 3 and 6. This procedure can also be of value in quantifying writing growth over time.

If a school-age child has some subtle language impairments and shows poor academic performance, part of a thorough evaluation should include (1) assessment of the child's knowledge of successful strategies to perform well in the school culture, (2) an evaluation of the teacher's communication while instructing the child, (3) an assessment of the curriculum and materials that the child is expected to learn, and (4) assessment of literacy areas of reading and writing. You may wonder why an SLP would be interested in assessing these factors when they are peripheral to the child's abilities. A school-age child is part of a complex system that is constantly changing its expectations for academic performance. The child may have to deal with differing types of educational content and a variety of teaching styles throughout the school day. The school-age child must use language in both comprehension and production for a variety of academic tasks that often involve complex metalinguistic ability and the learning of abstract concepts presented verbally by a teacher. Teachers and SLPs should remember that metalinguistic abilities appear to be acquired in a general developmental order (Wallach & Miller, 1988).

Additionally, the child must be aware of the expectations of the school culture and must know how to study, memorize, and effectively learn classroom material upon which he or she will be thoroughly tested. If the child has no effective study skills or strategies for remembering and understanding information, failure will occur. Academic success requires self-discipline, prioritizing, organization, and time management, all of which are subsumed under the concept of executive function. Singer and Bashir (1999) describe executive functions as involving skills such as "inhibiting actions, restraining and delaying responses, attending selectively, setting goals, planning and organizing, as well as maintaining and shifting set" (p. 266). Self-regulation involves self-monitoring, self-evaluation, and behavioral adjustment. Both executive function and self-regulation are intimately involved in learning and implementing strategies for oral language, writing, and reading comprehension. In this article a case example shows how a client was taught to inhibit nonproductive responses and engage in systematic analysis of a situation, set goals for communication, and self-monitor. Executive functions and self-regulation are very important to evaluate and include in treatment programs.

The child's teacher could talk at a rapid rate during instruction or use figurative language and complex sentence types. The teacher could be quite adept at using audio and visual media as aids to instruction or could exclusively rely on the lecture modality. The reading curriculum could have a heavy emphasis on phonics or other metalinguistic tasks that may make the learning of reading extremely difficult or impossible for a child with metalingistic problems. Conversely, the curriculum might emphasize a whole language approach with little emphasis on phonics for a child whose phonological awareness is desperately in need of remedial work. In some cases, an alternative approach could help a child learn a particular skill. What we are saying here is that the diagnostician cannot fully understand the language-impaired child unless he or she is familiar with the child's learning environment. Sometimes, the most potent treatment recommendations include curricular, instructional, and learning strategy modifications. Without examining these areas in a thorough assessment, a clinician cannot hope to make effective suggestions for remediation. Obtaining input from teachers and the older child is an important factor in evaluation. Larson and McKinley (1995) and Paul (2007) provide examples of protocols to use in obtaining information from teachers and students with language impairments.

The rationale for using portfolios to evaluate students with language disorders is persuasive. It is important to examine these students from a variety of perspectives to determine the true impact of their communication disorders and abilities. First, portfolios provide a method of evaluation that is holistic and educationally relevant, as required by law. Second, traditional language testing is more related to labeling or placement issues and is not adapted to the development of treatment goals and strategies. Third, a portfolio represents a collection of a student's work across a variety of modalities and subject areas. Fourth, portfolios promote collaboration among team members in school settings. Finally, much of this information is readily available, and in school settings it is possible for the SLP to gather new information because he or she is working in the context. An important factor in using portfolios is that they should not simply be composed of random data but should be dictated by the clinician's questions and concerns. Kratcoski (1998) suggests that the clinician follow a four-step process: (1) define the student's problem; (2) form hypotheses about the causes and effects of the problem; (3) develop specific assessment questions; and (4) determine the specific items to be added to the portfolio that address the questions posed by the clinician. Kratcoski lists many potential items that could be included in a portfolio:

- Initial referral forms
- Language samples
- Story retell samples
- Referential communication sample
- Observational notes of class participation, work observation, and social interaction
- Work samples of tests, papers, assignments, speeches
- Teacher interviews
- Parent interviews, student interview
- Audiotapes, videotapes
- Writing samples, journal entries
- Peer evaluations
- Testing data
- Conference notes

Portfolio assessment is a broad-based and invaluable source of information to be used in language assessment with school age children.

Another area of interest is to assess the child's ability to deal with the types of communication and linguistic tasks typically encountered in the classroom. Some useful measures that focus on classroom communication abilities or metalinguistics in older students (e.g., upper elementary through junior high) are Evaluating Communicative Competence (ECC) (Simon, 1987), Classroom Communication Screening Procedure for Early Assessment (CCSPEA) (Simon, 1989), and Analysis of the Language of Learning (ALL) (Blodgett & Cooper, 1987). These procedures will provide insight into a child's ability to perform classroom-like tasks and will pinpoint specific difficulties. The clinician also can experiment with any facilitating procedures that make difficult tasks more easily accomplished and can mention these in the examination report for teacher use.

CONCLUSION

One can easily see that the diagnosis and evaluation of school-age and adolescent clients is a complex activity. The SLP must work closely with teachers, parents, and other professionals in successfully dealing with these cases. The interplay among linguistic, metalinguistic, conversational, and academic areas is great, and the work of the SLP can potentially reap benefits in a child's educational performance.

6

Assessment of Speech Sound Disorders

Historically, articulation was conceptualized by most researchers and clinicians as being primarily a motor act. This sensorimotor aspect of articulation was studied, and it was not uncommon for articulation treatment to emphasize almost exclusively the movements of the oral musculature through an emphasis on diagrams, models, and motoric drills. In these early years the disorder was known as an "articulation" impairment reflecting the importance of movements of the articulators in the vocal tract. Recent views on the use of nonspeech oral motor excercises in treatment for speech sound disorders suggest that such methods are not only controversial, but research evidence is insufficient to support their routine use in the treatment of developmental speech sound disorders (Powell, 2008a; Powell, 2008b).

In the mid-1970s SLPs became highly interested in the work of linguists (e.g., Ingram 1976) who examined sound production differences from the perspective of phonological theory. With the advent of greater attention to linguistics (e.g., phonology) it was noted that articulation had more components than simply motoric activity. It is now well accepted that linguistic activity contributes significantly to the articulatory process (Bernthal, Bankson, & Flipsen, 2009; Elbert, 1992; Fey, 1992; Schwartz, 1983; Shelton & McReynolds, 1979; Shriberg & Kwiatkowski, 1982a). During this period of studying linguistic theory an articulation disorder began to be referred to as a "phonological" impairment. Now that we are aware that both sensorimotor and linguistic factors can contribute to impairment, the current terminology has changed to "speech sound disorder (SSD)." The profession has a long history of terminological changes with fads and theories, and we are certain that it is only a matter of time until we change our nomenclature yet again. Until that time, clinicians who want to be viewed as "up-to-date" will use the term *speech sound disorders*. For us textbook writers, however, we will persist in using terms such as "articulation" and "phonological" disorder in this chapter because they may point more or less to a linguistically based or a motorically based difficulty. Since Bernthal, Bankson, and Flipsen (2009) vary their terminologies in this manner, we feel we are in good company.

MULTIPLE COMPONENTS CONTRIBUTING TO SOUND PRODUCTION

Many events contribute to the final motor act of articulating. First, the biological component provides the basic structures for articulation, such as the vocal tract and the articulators, as well as the intact nervous system, which allows us to perform the sensory (auditory, tactile, kinesthetic, proprioceptive) and the motor functions necessary for controlled movement. Second, there is a cognitive-linguistic component wherein the speaker conceives of "something to say." This thought then undergoes linguistic processing whereby semantic elements are selected, words are arranged in proper syntactic order, and the utterance is appropriately tailored to the communicative situation by the speaker, taking pragmatics into consideration. The selection of phonemic elements and their order is then accomplished by applying phonological rules of our language. The details of linguistic processing of an utterance are not fully understood. It is enough to say, however, that linguistic processing involving semantic, syntactic, pragmatic, and phonological areas must occur at some point prior to expressing an utterance. Third, there is a sensorimotor-acoustic component that includes motor programming and motor learning of actual sequences of physical movement in a wide variety of phonetic contexts. The motor production in the vocal tract then gives rise to acoustic vibrations that travel through a medium of air and arrive at the ears of our listeners. This brief sketch of the processes that result in articulatory production is highly simplified.

This gross division of the articulatory process into biological, cognitive-linguistic, and sensorimotor components carries with it several important implications. First, the diagnostician must be prepared to assess and treat any or all aspects of the process in a given client. Bernthal and Bankson (1988) indicate, for instance, that speech sound disorders can be "motorically based errors (the ability to produce a target sound is not within the person's repertoire of motor skills) . . . or cognitively or linguistically based (the client can produce a sound but does not use the sound in appropriate contexts)" (p. 3). They further state that differentiating a motoric from a linguistically based disorder is not always an easy task. Additionally, as Bernthal, Bankson, and Flipsen (2009, p. 279) indicate, "Even though a disorder may be perceived as relating primarily to either the motor or linguistic aspects of phonology, instructional programs typically involve elements of both." If the client exhibits primarily a linguistically based problem (e.g., a phonological simplification such as deletion of certain final consonants), we should be able to examine a sample of speech for patterns of error that represent these phonological reductions. Oral-peripheral, motoric, audiological, and ultimately medical/neurological evaluation procedures can pinpoint difficulties with the biological/sensorimotor foundations of articulation. The implication, then, is that a client can have difficulties with one or several parts of the process, and the diagnostician should be equipped to assess these. Bernthal, Bankson, and Flipsen (2009) point out: "Although it is convenient to dichotomize the motor/articulation and linguistic/phonologic aspects of phonology for organization purposes, normal sound usage involves both the production of sounds at a motor level and their use in accordance with the rules of the language. Thus, the two skills are intertwined and may be described as two sides of the same coin" (p. 278).

There are several ways of categorizing misarticulations. Historically, speech pathologists have used the traditional classifications of (1) substitution of one sound for another ("thoup" for "soup"), (2) omission of a sound ("kool" for "school"), (3) distortion of a sound (nonstandard production of a sound), and (4) addition of a sound ("puhlease" for "please"). These historical classifications have persisted because they do describe most articulatory deviations. If there is any fault with the categories, it is that they are not specific enough. The diagnostician must say more than "the child has substitutions and omissions in his speech." We need to know which sounds are substituted for others, how often, and in what contexts. The same could be said for distortions, omissions, and additions. Another example of the superficiality of the historical categories is that they do not imply what part of the articulatory process is affected. That is, we cannot discern from the category of "substitution" whether the error is related to deficiencies in the client's sensorimotor or linguistic/phonological systems. The traditional classifications, however, are a good place to begin the assessment of speech sound disorders. We can then assess further and attempt to determine the variability of performance in specific phonetic contexts as well as the ways in which misarticulation varies in utterances of different linguistic complexities.

Articulatory errors can also be divided into categories of *organic* (some physical cause for the misarticulation) and *functional* (no demonstrable organic cause). The latter term has come under criticism for quite some time. Powers (1971) has called the term *functional* a "diagnosis by default." This is because the diagnosis of *organic* requires some positive proof of organicity, while the diagnosis of *functional* requires no positive evidence. The classification of *functional* is made only when a lack of evidence of organicity exists. The words most frequently associated with the *functional* classification are "learned" or "habit." Thus, although the classification of *functional* has been justifiably criticized, it is still widely held that the vast majority of articulation disorders have no significant, maintaining, organic basis and that the treatment is behavioral in nature. However, future research may yet uncover subtle organic or behavioral differences in these individuals. Assessment of organically based articulation disorders such as dysarthria and apraxia will be dealt with in our chapter on motor speech disorders. This chapter focuses on misarticulations that have no obvious organic component. As mentioned earlier, we will use the term *phonological disorder* to refer to these functional cases that involve multiple phoneme errors presumably due to linguistic factors. The term *articulation disorder* will be reserved for clients that misarticulate only one or two phonemes and may be more related to learned motor patterns habituated over a long period of time.

Another implication of a multicomponent conception of articulation is that no single measure is currently capable of adequately examining all parts of this complex process. It is naive to believe that administration of a traditional articulation test and an oral-peripheral examination are all that is necessary to perform a complete assessment of articulatory behavior. The articulatory process is just too complex and the disordered population too heterogeneous to rely on one or two standard tests. We support the point of view stated by Stoel-Gammon and Dunn (1985) that both independent and relational analyses should be done to provide complementary perspectives on a child's phonological system. Independent analysis simply describes a child's productions in terms of features, segments, and syllable shapes that actually occur in the speech sample. Relational analysis attempts to gloss a child's productions and compare them to adult models, resulting in an assessment of "correct and incorrect" productions. Typically, the SLP dealing with infants and toddlers who may not be using language for communication will engage in independent analysis of vocal productions by the child. As children become older and develop a linguistic system, relational analyses are conducted to compare the child's productions to adult standards (Bernthal, Bankson, & Flipsen, 2009).

In this chapter, we are emphasizing the importance of knowing "where to go" and "what to do" to gain insight into aspects of articulation that are revealed to be problematic by the initial testing. As with any disorder area, no single chapter can possibly tell a student how to do everything well. Our goal is simply to make clinicians aware of the possibilities in assessment of speech sound disorders and refer the reader to the appropriate literature.

SEVEN IMPORTANT KNOWLEDGE AREAS FOR EVALUATION OF ARTICULATION AND PHONOLOGICAL DISORDERS

Before we discuss assessment of speech sound disorders, there are several important bodies of literature that the clinician should be familiar with. In actuality, there are more areas that could be considered, but these seven seem to us to be critical prerequisites to performing a diagnostic evaluation.

1. *Knowledge of the Anatomy and Physiology of the Speech Mechanism.* Before attempting to deal with an articulatory evaluation, the clinician should be fully familiar with the normal oral mechanism. Most students obtain this knowledge in their undergraduate training.

2. *Knowledge of Phonetics.* It is one thing to know about the anatomy and physiology of the vocal mechanism, but it is quite another to be aware of how that apparatus actually produces the variety of consonant and vowel sounds in English. Aside from knowing articulatory phonetics, the clinician must have well-developed skills in phonetic transcription. This expertise is important in order to record a client's productions accurately for later analysis. Reliable phonetic transcription abilities are especially important in order to accomplish phonological analyses (Shriberg & Kwiatkowski, 1980).

3. *Knowledge of Phonological Development.* A major goal in diagnosis is to compare a child's articulatory performance to the behavior of other children in the same age range. In this way we can tell if a child's misarticulations are developmental in nature or clinically significant. There are at least three interpretations of articulatory development that the clinician should be familiar with before doing an assessment.

The most abundant normative data available are traditionally oriented studies of children's phoneme production of words with the target sound in the initial, medial, and final positions (Poole, 1934; Templin, 1957; Wellman et al., 1931). Although the procedures and criteria for acquisition in these studies differ (Smit, 1986), they provide ages at which children master phonemes. More recent data (Irwin & Wong, 1983; Prather, Hedrick, & Kern, 1975; Sander, 1972; Smit, 1993a; Smit et al., 1990) suggest earlier development of speech sounds and provide age ranges of development of "customary production" (two of three word positions) and mastery. The data provided by Irwin and Wong (1983) deal with sound production in connected spontaneous speech as opposed to the typical single-word responses reported in other traditional studies. Figure 6.1 is an example of normative consonant development data. Most misarticulations in phonologically disordered children involve consonants, so only consonant development data are presented here. Vowels are typically developed by age three (Bernthal, Bankson, & Flipsen, 2009). This does not mean that vowels are never involved in phonological disorder or that vowels are easily acquired (Davis & MacNeilage, 1990).

Most preschool and school-age children seen by the SLP will have difficulty primarily with consonants, and this is reflected by the content of most articulation tests. However, if the child is very young or exhibits a severe speech sound disorder, clinicians will be interested in assessing the vowel system. Early intervention programs target infants between birth and 2 years, and these children are probably using more vowels than consonants in their productions. Thus, in such cases the clinician will want to perform a thorough assessment of vowels and dipthongs to determine the existence of vowel disorders (Ball & Gibbon, 2001).

In addition to developmental data on the development of singleton consonants, there are some studies on the acquisition of consonant clusters. For example, McLeod, Van Doorn, and Reed (2001) review acquisition literature over the past 70 years and describe the acquisition of

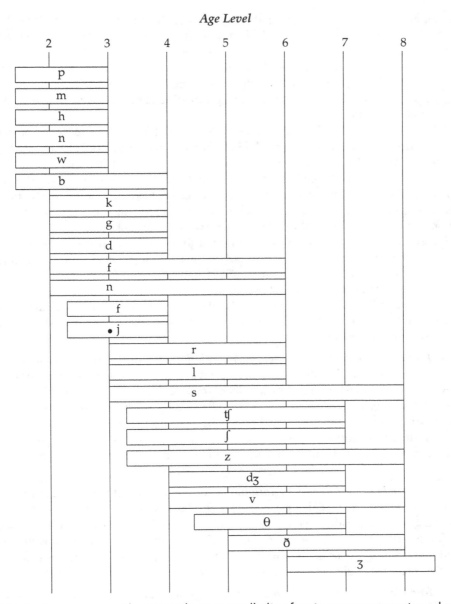

FIGURE 6.1   Average age estimates and upper age limits of customary consonant production. The solid bar corresponding to each sound starts at the median age of customary articulation; it stops at the age level at which 90% of all children are customarily producing the sound.

Source: Prather, E., Hedrick, D., & Kern, C. (1975). Articulation development in children aged 2 to 4 years. *Journal of Speech and Hearing Disorders,* 40, 179–191. Used with permission from the American Speech-Language-Hearing Association, Rockville, MD.

consonant clusters in childhood. The authors summarize this literature with 10 generalizations about the developmental progression, which may be useful to clinicians in assessment and treatment decisions.

A second type of developmental data involves distinctive feature acquisition. Several sources report a developmental order in distinctive feature acquisition (Blache, 1978; Singh, 1976). These data could be used when analyzing a child's distinctive feature system as opposed to more traditional norms.

Finally, data are available regarding the occurrence of phonological reduction processes or patterns of error in normally developing children (Ingram, 1976; Shriberg & Kwiatkowski, 1980; Smit, 1993b). These data provide some general age cutoffs for certain phonological processes and give the SLP a view of a child's error pattern not found in traditional norms. If a clinician sees a child who is deleting final consonants, for instance, the clinician cannot use traditional norms to determine when this tendency diminishes in normal children. Most studies have focused on children's phonological development between the ages of 3 and 8 years. More recent investigations have concentrated on children from 1 to 3 years in response to the emphases on early intervention and increased interest in early normal development (Dyson, 1988; Grunwell, 1988; Kahn & Lewis, 2002; Stoel-Gammon, 1987). Table 6.1 provides an example of normative data developed within the phonological process perspective.

A major point we wish to make here is that the clinician can look at an articulatory sample from a variety of perspectives. Traditional as well as phonological norms provide a reference point to use in assessment and treatment.

4. *Knowledge of Factors Related to Articulation Disorders.* Whenever undertaking a speech sound evaluation, the clinician can expect that parents will often ask questions regarding the etiology of the problem. The clinician, then, must be familiar with the pertinent literature dealing with research on etiological factors, as well as skills and abilities of children with speech sound disorders. Questions may be asked about language development, reading, spelling, educational performance, dentition, oral structures, gross and fine motor skills, intelligence, auditory abilities, and much more. Bernthal, Bankson, and Flipsen (2009) summarize this research handily, and this should assist clinicians in answering any questions.

5. *Knowledge of Dialectal Variation.* According to the American Speech-Language-Hearing Association, the clinician performing an evaluation of speech sounds must be able to differentiate a communication disorder from a dialectal variation (Battle et al., 1983). Since there are so few tests that take dialect into account, the clinician must become familiar with this material and must routinely consider it when evaluating misarticulations. We address this issue further in the chapter on multicultural issues.

6. *Knowledge of Coarticulation.* For at least 40 years, researchers have known that speech is produced in a parallel fashion as opposed to a serial, discrete manner (Winitz, 1975). This means that speech sounds are not isolated entities but that they overlap motorically and acoustically in time. Put simply, sounds are influenced by other phonemes that surround them. This influence of one sound on another is called *coarticulation* and is one of the most basic facts about the articulatory process. The phonetic environment or phonetic context in which a sound is produced influences the production of that phoneme. There are two major types of coarticulation that can be described in terms of the direction of the influence of one sound on another. Left-to-right coarticulation refers to a preceding sound's having an affect on a following sound (the "t" in *boots* is produced with some lip rounding because of the rounding /u/ vowel that precedes it). This type of coarticulation is perceived by some to be a type of "overflow" of movement from the first sound to the second. Thus, the left-to-right coarticulation is thought to be primarily the

TABLE 6.1	Most Common Phonological Processes Exhibited During Normal Development		
Process	**Description**	**Suppressed by Age 3**	**Persists After Age 3**
Weak Syllable Deletion	In polysyllabic words, the unstressed syllable is deleted (telephone → tephone).	X	
Final Consonant Deletion	The final consonant of a word is deleted (baet → bae).	X	
Reduplication	Two syllable words are produced by repeated the first syllable (bottle • baba).	X	
Harmony (sometimes referred to as "assimilation")	The manner, place, or voice characteristics of one phoneme changes to be consistent with another phoneme in the word (dog • gog). In this case the initial /d/ changed to be consistent with the final /g/.	X	
Cluster Reduction	Consonant clusters are reduced, usually to a single phoneme (stop • top).		X
Stopping	Continuant sounds (usually fricatives) are replaced by stops (see • tee).		X
Velar Fronting	Velar sounds such as /k/ and /g/ are replaced by alveolar sounds such as /t/ and /d/ (go • do).	X	
Gliding	Liquids such as /r/ and /l/ become glides such as /w/ and /j/ (run • wun).	X	
Context-Sensitive Voicing	Voiceless consonants preceding vowels are voiced, and voiced consonants at the end of words are produced as unvoiced (toe • doe; red • ret).		X

Source: Adapted from Haynes, Moran, & Pindzola (2011). Based on data from Grunwell (1988) and Stoel-Gammon & Dunn (1985).

result of mechanical-inertial factors. The other type of coarticulation is right to left. This means that a sound later in the speech sequence affects a sound earlier in the stream of speech. For example, the "t" sound in the word *tea* is produced differently from the "t" in the word *too*. The difference in the two situations is that in the word *tea,* the sound is followed by a vowel that is not produced with rounded lips. Thus, the "t" sound in *too* might be produced with lip rounding because the following vowel is rounded. Note that in both of these cases the sound that influences the "t" occurs after the "t" has been uttered. Researchers and theorists have suggested that the right-to-left influence is probably the result of articulatory preprogramming. That is, early sounds in a sequence are produced differently in anticipation of sounds that are yet to be said. This implies some sort of motor planning.

The implications of the existence of coarticulation for the assessment of speech sounds are significant. One implication is that testing sounds in isolation is an unrealistic and artificial enterprise. What a child can do with a sound in isolation may be totally different from the child's production in connected speech. Another implication has to do with testing in single words. When we speak, we typically do not put oral pauses or spaces between our words, as in the ones you are reading right now. The speech stream has been called an *unsegmentable whole* (Kent & Minifie, 1977). Research on coarticulation has shown that the effects of one sound on another can cross both word and syllable boundaries (Amerman, Daniloff, & Moll, 1970; Daniloff & Moll, 1968; McClean, 1973; Moll & Daniloff, 1971). Thus, sounds located in two adjacent words can have an effect on one another. This means that testing sound production on the single-word level may not be representative of sound production in spontaneous speech, because connected words may provide different coarticulatory effects as compared to single words alone (Faircloth & Faircloth, 1970). We have known for some time that specific phonemes are misarticulated less often in consonant cluster contexts as opposed to CV environments (McCauley & Skenes, 1987).

Yet another implication has to do with possible facilitating and sabotaging effects of phonemes surrounding a particular target sound. For instance, a misarticulated /r/ sound may be produced correctly by a child if it is preceded by a /k/ (e.g., /kræk/), perhaps because both sounds require grossly similar positioning of the tongue in the vocal tract (Hoffman, Schuckers, & Ratusnik, 1977). Conversely, an /r/ might be misarticulated as a /w/ if words surrounding the target sound contain a lip-rounded phoneme (e.g., /row/) (Winitz, 1975). Therefore, the effects of coarticulation can be either positive or negative, facilitating or sabotaging, and this finding is especially important for the clinician to consider in assessment and treatment.

Perhaps the most important implication of coarticulation is in accounting for articulatory inconsistency. Most misarticulations are notoriously inconsistent, and if the clinician analyzes these productions, he or she can find that this "inconsistency" may actually be quite consistent indeed. Phonetic context is often the common denominator among errors that appear inconsistent on the surface. We need not only think of the notion of phonetic context as a purely motoric phenomenon. In performing linguistic phonological analyses, a consideration of context is critical. In evaluating assimilation processes (e.g., nasal assimilation), the clinician may note than non-nasal sounds in the initial word position are changed to nasals only when there is a nasal phoneme in the final or medial position of the words.

7. *Knowledge of the Linguistic-Articulatory Connection.* An important postulate in discussing articulatory assessment is the intimate relationship between language and articulation. This connection has been shown in several ways in the literature.

- Phonology is a component of language. Theoretically, phonology has been considered a classical component of language models.
- Syntactic complexity affects misarticulations. Several studies have shown that misarticulations are affected by linguistic complexity (Haynes, Haynes, & Jackson, 1982; Panagos, Quine, & Klich, 1979; Schmauch, Panagos, & Klich, 1978). That is, more misarticulations will occur as syntactic complexity increases. Here is a clear relationship between articulation and language.
- Semantic complexity affects misarticulations. Shriberg and Kwiatkowski (1980) have suggested that even the word's syntactic class may affect sound productions. They found, for instance, that blends may be reduced differently in verbs as compared to the same blend in nouns. In early language development there appear to be more misarticulations

on action words as opposed to object words in the first lexicon. This observation has been made with normally developing as well as phonologically delayed children (Camarata & Schwartz, 1985).

- Pragmatics and communicative value affect misarticulations (Campbell & Shriberg, 1982; Leonard, 1971; Weiner & Ostrowski, 1979). This means that when there is a greater chance of being misunderstood, the child may articulate more correctly.
- Language and phonological disorders typically co-occur. A relationship between language and articulation can be inferred from the high co-occurrence of the two disorders in children. Generally, children who have speech sound problems are at high risk for language disorders and vice versa (Shriberg & Kwiatkowski, 1988).

The implications of the above connections between articulation and language are significant for assessment. First, routine assessment of articulation with an exclusively sensorimotor orientation is not appropriate. Language and articulation are hopelessly intertwined when a person speaks spontaneously (Locke, 1983). Second, when the speech pathologist is looking for sources of inconsistent phoneme production, he or she may find significant effects not only from phonetic context but also from semantic, syntactic, or pragmatic variables. Third, an evaluation that uses only single-word responses on which to base a clinical decision is incomplete, because there may be significant differences between a client's performance on the single-word and connected-speech levels.

There are several advantages of gathering a spontaneous speech sample in a phonological evaluation. First, the connected-speech sample keeps the actual process of producing utterances intact. Individual words are embedded within sentences and thus the effects of stress, intonation, rate, and syllable structure can influence productions. Second, you will recall that earlier in the present chapter we cited research that found the effects of syntax, semantics, and pragmatics can affect phonology. In conversation, all linguistic elements are present to allow such influences of language complexity on the sound system. Unfortunately, there are also disadvantages to conversational sampling. In cases where the client is unintelligible in connected speech, the clinician has little choice but to use shorter samples of single words or phrases in order to compare productions to an adult standard. Also, some children are reluctant to engage in conversation with an unfamiliar person. Finally, since a conversational sample is generated by the client, it may not include specific phonemes or syllable shapes of interest to the clinician. Single-word responses to picture-naming tasks offer a known target for the clinician to analyze. Many single-word tests suggest analyzing only one or two phonemes per word in accordance with their scoring sheets. We agree with Bernthal, Bankson, and Flipsen (2009) that much data are lost using this method. Clinicians should transcribe the entire word including both consonants and vowels in order to have a more robust corpus for analysis from single-word samples. One issue associated with single-word sampling is its fidelity to sound productions in continuous speech with all of its attendant influences. Many studies have shown that more errors occur in spontaneous connected speech (Morrison & Shriberg, 1992); however, there are also reported instances in which more errors occurred on the single-word level. In general, most authorities recommend both single-word and connected-speech sampling in gathering data for a phonological evaluation (Bernthal, Bankson, & Flipsen, 2009). We have made the point in this chapter that single-word tests may not reflect a child's productions in connected speech. Klein and Liu-Shea (2009) found that the substitutions and deletions children exhibited in a continuous speech sample were not predicted by their performance on a single-word articulation test. The authors suggest that in cases where a child may not qualify for remedial services based on single-word testing, a continuous speech sample should be evaluated to determine possible eligibility. They support the notion of including continuous speech sampling in every thorough phonological assessment.

The clinician can see that the most productive view would be to consider both sensorimotor and linguistic components in the assessment repertoire (Schwartz, 1983).

OVERVIEW OF THE ARTICULATION/PHONOLOGY ASSESSMENT PROCESS

As in other chapters, Figure 6.2 presents the critical assessment mechanisms in articulation/phonology. It should be noted that the same major areas of biological/linguistic foundations, background information, standardized testing, nonstandardized testing, and evaluation of the client's environment are relevant to a thorough evaluation. Note also that the figure

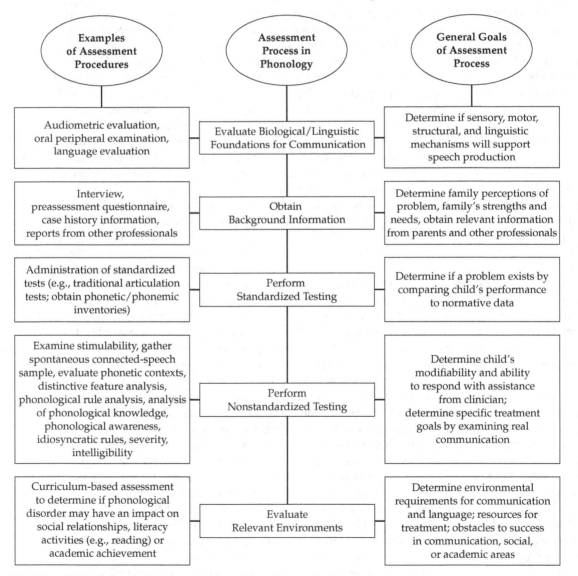

FIGURE 6.2 Critical assessment process in articulation and phonology.

covers all pertinent aspects of the World Health Organization ICF model presented in Chapter 1. The effects of the disorder are especially a focus when we perform nonstandardized testing and evaluate relevant environments.

SCREENING FOR SPEECH SOUND DISORDERS

One of the tasks performed by the SLP is screening for speech sound disorders. The purpose of a screening is to determine if a person should be referred for a formal diagnostic evaluation in which the phonological system is analyzed in detail. Although screenings typically take a short time (less than 5–10 minutes), evaluations can span an hour or two. Usually, if a clinician has any doubt about the normality of a person's phonological system in a screening, the client is referred for a more thorough evaluation. Thus, if a child did not talk during a screening or a large enough sample could not be elicited, it is better to err on the side of caution and refer the child for an evaluation. According to Bernthal, Bankson, & Flipsen (2009), screening is appropriate for preschool children as part of early intervention programs. In some school settings the SLP will screen third-grade children for speech sound errors since at this age, most phonemes should be produced correctly. In older clients, a screening is sometimes done to ensure that the person meets certain speech standards required for admission to a degree program (e.g., broadcasting, teaching.) Of course, screening is performed when a person is referred to a clinic or school SLP with a suspected communication disorder. Screenings can be done informally with the use of clinician-constructed materials such as pictures, a conversational speech sample, or a reading passage. Often informal screenings involve counting, saying the days of the week, or describing pictures. One disadvantage to informal screening is the lack of normative data and identifiable cutoffs indicating a passing or a failing performance. Often, school systems require a more formal method of screening to identify children for services. Some formal instruments that are often used for screening speech sounds are the Denver Articulation Screening Exam (DASE) (Drumwright, 1971), the Diagnostic Screen (Dodd, Hua, Crosbie, Holm, & Ozanne, 2006), the Fluharty Preschool Speech and Language Screening Test (Fluharty, 2000), the Speech-Ease Screening Inventory (K–1) (Pigott, Barry, Hughes, Eastin, Titus, Stensil, Metcalf, & Porter, 1985), and the Preschool Language Scale (Zimmerman, Steiner, & Pond, 1992). Most of these instruments have standard scores or cutoff scores to use in making screening decisions.

TRADITIONAL ASSESSMENT PROCEDURES

There are a variety of types of speech sound assessments that differ in their theoretical assumptions, method of sample elicitation, the type of information obtained, and their therapeutic implications. Perhaps the most common type of assessment is what we will call "traditional." The theoretical orientation of traditional testing is that each English consonant must be evaluated in the initial, medial, and final positions of words. These words are typically elicited from the client by means of pictures, word lists, sentences, or conversational sampling. Many studies examining articulation from a "traditional" perspective have shown that children tend to produce more singleton consonants correctly in single-word sampling contexts (Dubois & Bernthal, 1978; Faircloth &Faircloth, 1970; Healy & Madison, 1987; Johnson, Whinney, & Pederson, 1980; Kenney & Prather, 1984; Paden & Moss, 1985). On the other hand, when performance is examined from a phonological process perspective, some studies have shown no significant differences between single-word and connected-speech sampling conditions (Bowman, Parsons, & Morris, 1984; Dyson & Robinson, 1987; McLeod et al., 1994; Paden & Moss, 1985).

Masterson, Bernhardt, and Hofheinz (2005) found that there were few differences in the treatment ramifications between single-word and conversational speech samples. The conversational sample took three times longer to elicit and transcribe and still elicited less critical language targets as compared to single-word sampling. The single-word targets were "tailored" to the child's phonological system based on limited sampling. The authors still recommend conversational sampling to check on the representativeness of the single-word sample, and for judging intelligibility and prosody. Even though the data for the analysis might range from words to connected speech, the orientation of the clinician is to determine omissions, substitutions, and distortions of phonemes in differing word positions. Many tests are available for use in traditional assessment (Bosma-Smit & Hand, 1996; Edmonson, 1969; Fisher & Logemann, 1971; Fudala & Reynolds, 1993; Goldman & Fristoe, 2000; Lippke, Dickey, Selmar, & Soder, 1997; Templin & Darley, 1969). Some of these inventories include stimulus pictures for testing children and structured sentences for older clients to read. Several tests provide norms against which a child may be compared.

Traditional diagnostic procedures have other basic operations in common. Most traditional assessments accrue a phonetic inventory from the client. This is a list of all phonemes produced in the sample. One reason for obtaining a phonetic inventory is to compare to normative data on articulatory development the sounds produced correctly by a given client. As mentioned earlier, most normative studies are based on traditional notions and report phoneme productions of sounds in the three word positions (Poole, 1934; Prather, Hedrick, & Kern, 1975; Sander, 1972; Templin, 1957; Wellman et al., 1931).

Another traditional procedure is the testing of a client's stimulability, or response to stimulation. In other words, we evaluate the impact that the examiner's model has upon the client's production. Is there some modification in the direction of normalcy? Or is there no change in the articulatory behavior? Testing for stimulability is an extremely useful diagnostic procedure. If a client can produce the error correctly by imitating a standard model, either in isolation, in nonsense syllables, or in words, then there may be no serious organic obstacles that would prevent the eventual acquisition of the sound. Stimulability is also a useful prognostic sign; clients who can modify their articulation errors by imitating the examiner's standard production have a place to start the treatment process. Stimulability has also been implicated as a potential predicter of whether children will develop normal speech through maturation (Farquhar, 1961). Miccio, Elbert, and Forrest (1999) evaluated four normally developing children and four children with speech sound disorders to study training on stimulable and nonstimulable sounds. The investigators stated: "In both cases stimulable sounds underwent the most change and stimulability was related to the learning patterns observed. This study supports the hypothesis that nonstimulable sounds are least likely to change without treatment. The results also suggest that stimulability for production of a sound may signal that it is being acquired naturally" (p. 347).

Stimulability is frequently given short shrift by practicing clinicians and students in training. Sometimes it is totally omitted. Often, we see students hurry through the stimulability testing, frequently giving inadequate instructions and rather imprecise models to the client. The real spirit of stimulability testing is to see how the client performs under maximal, multimodality stimulation. This is why most tests recommend that the model be presented two or three times after the client has been given a strong attentional set. Students sometimes indicate that the client was not stimulable for error phonemes after rather cursory testing. Subsequent stimulability trials, done more intensively, may reveal that the client, in fact, can produce the target sound. Prior to making negative stimulability statements in a clinical report, the clinician should be certain that the stimulation task was administered effectively. A good example of providing systematic information to a client during stimulability testing is presented by Glaspey and Stoel-Gammon (2005) in which various elicitation cues and phonetic contexts are altered.

It is our contention that traditional testing is a good starting point in assessing speech sounds. In many cases, a traditional assessment may be all that is needed, especially when the client has only a few articulatory errors and is stimulable. In cases like this, the clinician knows what the errors are and how often they occur in a test and in spontaneous speech if analyzed traditionally. Further, the clinician has a place to start production of the target sound, since the client can make it correctly with stimulation. Probe tasks that focus on particular productions can also be used as a follow-up procedure. For example, specific probing techniques have been developed for use with consonant clusters (Powell, 1995). In the majority of cases, however, traditional testing does not go far enough. For instance, our discussion of coarticulation suggested that sounds will be produced differently in different phonetic environments. Most traditional tests examine only a limited number of these phonetic contexts. If a child or adult is not stimulable, the clinician may want to rely on experimentation with different coarticulatory transitions to determine if there is a facilitating context. Most traditional tests are just not equipped to do this. Another example is that traditional testing procedures are not directed toward detecting patterns of error in a client's speech. In order to define patterns of error, a phonological analysis is the most efficient method to use. Traditional analyses do not systematically examine the effects of stress, syllable complexity (Panagos, Quine, & Klich, 1979), linguistic complexity, and pragmatics on misarticulation. Finally, traditional analyses do not focus on certain parameters that may be relevant to certain cases, such as distinctive feature acquisition and use. In short, no one method can do everything, and so it is with the traditional approach. The traditional test, however, is a viable instrument to use generically. If other analyses are required, they should be done when appropriate.

It is far easier to describe the testing of speech sounds than it is to administer an articulation test. A student's first attempt is generally a confusing situation that requires careful listening, attention to visual cues, recording the client's responses appropriately, and maintaining a positive client–clinician relationship. We recommend that the beginning clinician listen for only one sound at a time. When possible, have the child repeat the test words a number of times. Audio-record, or better yet, videorecord the child's responses to assist in later scoring of the test. Experienced speech-language pathologists are able to save time by testing more than one sound simultaneously (Fristoe & Goldman, 1968).

It is especially true with speech sound assessment that the clinician is really the "test." Commercial articulation tests are nothing more than stacks of pictures bound together with metal or plastic. Since articulatory responses are so transient and fleeting, clinicians must listen carefully, practice frequently, and, above all, check their reliability. Studies have shown that speech pathologists are fairly reliable when the judgments they make are rather general, such as Correct or Incorrect (Winitz, 1969). When judgments become more fine grained, as in determining the nature of specific substitutions in certain word positions, our reliability tends to deteriorate. One can easily see that very complex analysis procedures such as those used in distinctive features and phonology are even more susceptible to misjudgments on the part of the clinician. The clinician must always strive to improve his or her reliability through practice and by rechecking results. A clinician's evaluation results are only as good as his or her ability to perceive the reality of the client's responses. No one, as an old professor said, has immaculate perception. Chapter 3 discusses interjudge reliability and provides a formula for its calculation.

TEST PROCEDURES THAT EVALUATE PHONETIC CONTEXT EFFECTS

After a traditional assessment, a client may be judged not stimulable. Procedures then need to be initiated to determine if a facilitating phonetic context can be found. As we mentioned in the section on coarticulation, phonemes are significantly influenced by other sounds that surround them. This phenomenon results in the existence of facilitating contexts that can encourage the correct production of a target consonant. The concept that certain phonetic environments can be facilitory of correct production was suggested in the early writings of Van Riper and Irwin (1958) where they indicated there were "key words" in which a phoneme could be produced more effectively. If certain key words were discovered for a nonstimulable client, then treatment could commence in these contexts. In 1964, Eugene McDonald devised the *Deep Test of Articulation* (McDonald, 1964), which, among other things, is based on the idea that phonemes will be produced differently depending on the sounds that precede and follow them. By systematically permuting a variety of consonants before and after a specific phoneme, the contexts in which correct production is observed can be noted by the clinician and can serve as a starting point for treatment. In the Deep Test of Articulation, each phoneme can be observed 40 or more times as the initiating or terminating sound in a syllable.

The evaluation of a variety of phonetic contexts provides an interesting contrast to the limited number of environments evaluated by traditional measures. Schissell and James (1979) compared the evaluation of articulatory abilities in children by using a more traditional test (Arizona) and the McDonald Deep Test. They found that the traditional test missed some of the children who did not have consistent control of certain sounds, and also that the traditional test failed children on certain sounds when in actuality the children performed the sound productions well in a significant number of contexts on the McDonald Deep Test. One interpretation of the disparity in results between these two measures is that the traditional test evaluated a limited number of phonetic contexts; for some children the environment happened to be facilitative, and for others it did not. The implication, of course, is that the more phonetic contexts examined, the more realistic the picture obtained of the clients' articulatory performance. In addition, we might find a place to begin our treatment. Other tests that systematically evaluate phonetic context effects are the Secord Contextual Articulation Tests (S-CAT) (Secord & Shine, 1997) and the Contextual Test of Articulation (Aase, Hovre, Krause, Shelfhout, Smith, & Carpenter, 2000).

Another way to examine phonetic context effects in children and adults is the use of sound-in-context sentences (Haynes, Haynes, & Jackson, 1982; Mazza, Schuckers, & Daniloff, 1979). These sentences can be read spontaneously by adults or imitated by children. Most work with these sentences has been done in research projects directed toward finding facilitating contexts for particular target consonants (mainly the /s/ and /r/ phonemes). The use of these sentence stimuli has shown that there are, in fact, facilitating contexts for /r/ and /s/ that occur for many clients. The essence of these sentences is that a clinician can ask the client to say any number of utterances that are constructed to determine phonetic context effects. For instance, if the clinician wants to evaluate the effects on /s/ production of a preceding /k/ sound and a following /p/ sound (e.g., /KSP/), a sentence can be constructed such as "The dress had a bla*ck sp*ot." In addition, phrases may be used instead of sentences. The clinician, then, can use knowledge of coarticulation and devise stimuli to probe phonetic context effects on a given client's articulation. Finally, Kent (1982) urges continued experimentation with phonetic context effects in clinical and research settings because there is much we do not yet understand about this phenomenon.

With a knowledge of the effects of coarticulation, the clinician may construct a variety of utterance types for a particular client and need not rely solely on instruments devised by others.

A thorough assessment could provide significant information that could be used at the outset of treatment if more attention were paid to ferreting out sources of error inconsistency attributable to phonetic context. The clinician should also be willing to experiment with a variety of segmental, suprasegmental, and linguistic complexity variables in the search for sources of inconsistency (Shriberg & Kwiatkowski, 1980).

ASSESSMENT OF SPEECH SOUNDS IN EARLY INTERVENTION

Historically, it has been a challenge to quantify the development of the sound system in children under the age of 3. Proctor (1989) provides an excellent developmental chart of consonant, vowel and syllable development in the first 2 years of life. These stages can be used to characterize a child's speech sound development in the early years and track development. Researchers have suggested several methods by which phonetic and syllable shape data can be quantified in a single score that can be used to monitor development over time. Two such methods, Mean Babbling Level (MBL) and Syllable Structure Level (SSL), were reviewed by Morris (2010) in terms of their clinical usefulness. While both measures were originally developed in the late 1980s and early 1990s, Morris reviewed investigations that had taken place over the past 20 years. The MBL is a measure of vocal or nonlinguistic productions in which each vocalization is assigned from 1 to 3 points depending on the occurence of phonetic elements and certain syllable structures. The more consonants included and the more complex the syllable structure, the higher the rating. Ultimately the ratings for individual vocalizations are averaged and a score (e.g., 1.54) obtained. You can see how an increase in the score suggests more complexity in the phonetic and syllable structure of a vocalization. The MBL was extended for use with productive lexical items and renamed the Syllable Structure Level (SSL) measure. Again, the SSL used a scoring system to quantify the phonetic and syllabic complexity of true words so that development could be monitored by a single value over time. After a thorough review of the literature, Morris concluded that both the MBL and SSL provided clinically valuable and reliable information with which to characterize change in phonological development in the early years. We mentioned the notion of an "independent analysis" of phonology as being comprised of an inventory of consonants and vowels and syllable structures. In the case of children who have not developed language for communication, such an analysis is all we have to work with regarding the phonological system. Samples of vocalizations can be obtained during normal caregiving activities and turn-taking during play and independent analysis conducted on the productions (Bernthal, Bankson, & Flipsen, 2009; Stoel-Gammon & Dunn, 1985).

THE PHONETIC AND PHONEMIC INVENTORIES

A most important source of information about a phonologically disordered client is the phonetic inventory. After gathering a representative sample, one of the first operations a clinician should perform is to inventory the client's sound system in several ways. The phonetic inventory is a summary of sounds the client has produced either correctly or incorrectly in the sample and represents the sounds that can be physically produced by the person. That is, if the client produced a glottal stop, this sound is part of the phonetic inventory. If the client produces an θ/s substitution and never produces the [θ] correctly when it is required to be, the [θ] is still included in the phonetic inventory. The phonemic inventory, on the other hand, includes sounds that are used contrastively and that are implemented to make a meaning difference in the client's language.

Thus, although an [θ] may be a part of the child's phonetic repertoire, it may not be part of the phonemic system.

As we will mention later, an examination of the phonetic and phonemic inventories is a critical part of assessing a child's possession and use of distinctive features of English phonemes. There are also some other ways to analyze data from a child's phonetic and phonemic inventories. Some authorities (Elbert, 1992; Elbert & Gierut, 1986; Maxwell & Rockman, 1984) have recommended searching for various types of rules that may or may not be operating in a child's system, and the phonetic/phonemic inventories are an important part of these analyses. For instance, static rules called "phonotactic constraints" (Dinnesen, 1984) may be operating to restrict the occurrence of certain sounds or phoneme combinations. Three types of phonotactic constraints have been reported. First, *positional constraints* are rules that allow the production of a sound in only certain contexts or word positions. Second, *inventory constraints* reduce the production of particular sounds because the phonemes are not included in the phonetic inventory. Finally, *sequence constraints* are rules that may not permit the child to produce sounds in particular combinations (e.g., the child can produce the phoneme as a singleton, but not in a cluster). One can see that examination of the phonetic and phonemic inventory is an important part of arriving at an appreciation of a client's phonotactic rule system.

There are a variety of systems for reporting a client's phonetic inventory. It would be most important for a phonetic inventory not only to reflect sensorimotor production of a sound but also to provide some indication of appropriate or phonemic use of the element. The phonetic inventory should also indicate failure to sample certain sounds so that the clinician does not assume the client cannot produce the sounds. The phonetic inventory in the Natural Process Analysis (Shriberg & Kwiatkowski, 1980) differentiates between a phone that is used correctly, appears in the sample, is glossed in the sample, and is never glossed. This analysis can tell the clinician if the phonetic element is phonemic (correct anywhere), whether it is used as a substitution for another sound (appears anywhere), whether it should have been in a word (glossed) but was not, or whether the sound was never expected to be produced in the sample. Other systems simply list the phones in the phonetic inventory from left to right in terms of place of articulation in the vocal tract (left = front, right = back) (Maxwell & Rockman, 1984). Another way to consider a child's phonetic/phonemic inventory might be to array the phonemes on the continuum of phonological knowledge, which we will discuss later. Elbert and Gierut (1986) provide an example of such a summary.

Whatever way the clinician decides to examine a child's phonological system, a phonetic/phonemic inventory is a good starting point because it can give significant insights into phonotactic rules (e.g., inventory constraints) and the child's overall knowledge of the sound system.

DISTINCTIVE FEATURE ANALYSIS

As we mentioned previously, neither traditional analyses or appraisals of phonetic context effects examine all pertinent aspects of a child's articulatory system. Researchers indicate that the most basic unit that speech can be reduced to is the distinctive feature, and the "reality" of features has been demonstrated both acoustically and physiologically (Singh, 1976). That is, as humans, we seem to pay attention to certain aspects of the speech signal both in perception and production. Phonemes are evidently made up of "bundles" of distinctive features that combine to produce a variety of different consonant and vowel sounds in a language. Singh (1976) states: "Children do not acquire phonemes one by one; rather, they acquire a feature that provides them with a basis for manifesting a number of phonemes distinctively in speech production and discrimination tasks" (p. 229). Features, then, are a "prerequisite" to phonemes, because without the knowledge of and ability to produce a given feature of language, certain sounds containing that feature will not be produced. For instance, if a child does not learn that the feature of "voicelessness" is important in differentiating certain sounds from each other, the phonemes with the − voice feature will not be produced (/s, f, p, k/, etc.). Distinctive feature theory attempts to specify the characteristics of phonemes according to the presence (+) or absence (−) of each feature that distinguishes or contrasts one speech sound from another.

One difficulty that is immediately apparent to a student studying distinctive features is the number of "systems" available (Singh, 1976) and the fact that no single system has received universal acceptance (Fey, 1992). Furthermore, these systems have been derived by different procedures and thus have disparate bases (acoustic, articulatory, perceptual). The feature systems also differ in the phonemes included in the scheme, the notation (binary, ternary, quarternary), and the number of features thought to be important. One source of solace to the clinician is the fact that most systems have some things in common. There are certain features that appear to be so significant and strong that they are included in the majority of systems. Specifically, the features of voice, nasality, some feature denoting duration, and a place feature are the most common. Many authorities simply use the traditional place, manner, and voicing features for assessment purposes (Stoel-Gammon, 1996).

Several investigations have suggested that there are at least two different types of feature problems exhibited by children: phonetic and phonemic (Elbert, 1992; McReynolds & Huston, 1971; Pollack & Rees, 1972; Ruder & Bunce, 1981). One type of distinctive feature difficulty is exemplified by a child who has not acquired the use of a feature at all. The child is not aware of the importance of the feature to differentiate English sounds and has difficulty producing the feature. The child might have one "aspect" or one half of the feature (+ voicing), but does not have the other half (− voicing). Features are rather like light switches; they are only useful when you know about both turning them on and turning them off. Thus, a child has not really acquired the feature of "voice" until both voiced and voiceless sounds can be produced appropriately and contrastively (Grunwell, 1988). If a child's phonetic inventory does not include voiceless phonemes used correctly or incorrectly, the child does not have contrastive use of the voice feature. A second type of feature error is shown in a child who has acquired the feature, but does not use it appropriately. Control of features, as with many things, is on a continuum. A child may be aware of the importance of a feature and be capable of producing both aspects (+ and −) of it, yet there are specific contexts in which the feature is not used appropriately. On the other hand, a child may not be able to produce the feature aspects without great difficulty in any context. Several authorities mentioned above have suggested that these two cases represent slightly different diagnostic groups. One child does not have the feature, and the other has it but is a feature misuser in certain contexts.

Currently, most authorities recommend the examination of distinctive features as part of the larger process of phonological analysis. That is, when we write phonological rules for a disordered child's system, we can use distinctive features to make our descriptions more specific and look for commonalities across different sound errors. Table 6.2 gives an example of how six individual sound errors can be construed as basically a problem with one distinctive feature (+ continuant). A phonological process analysis of the same errors would reveal a "stopping" rule, which is essentially a misuse of the + continuant. It would be important to determine if the child in the example ever produced the + continuant feature in the speech sample. One can easily see that using distinctive features is just another way to look at a client's misarticulations and can

| TABLE 6.2 | Example of Distinctive Feature Approach to Analyzing Articulation Errors |

Error	Features Used Correctly	Features in Error	
Substitution/Target		Target Phoneme	Substitution
d/s	vocalic, consonantal, high, back, low, nasal	− voice + continuant + strident	+ voice − continuant − strident
d/z	vocalic, consonantal, high, back, low, nasal	+ continuant + strident	− continuant − strident
d/sh	vocalic, consonantal, high, back, low, nasal	− voice + continuant + strident	+ voice − continuant − strident
b/f	vocalic, consonantal, high, back, low, nasal	− voice + continuant + strident	+ voice − continuant − strident
b/v	vocalic, consonantal, high, back, low, nasal	+ continuant + strident	− continuant − strident
d/th (*think*)	vocalic, consonantal, high, back, low, nasal	− voice + continuant	+ voice − continuant
d/th (*that*)	vocalic, consonantal, high, back, low, nasal	+ continuant	− continuant

Note: The features associated with phonemes are from Chomsky and Halle (1968). Compare the feature bundles of the target and error phonemes to determine features misused. One can easily see the most misused features are the voicing, continuancy, and stridency elements.

add some specificity to our descriptions as well as allow us to see relationships among individual sound errors. Elbert (1992) points out the importance of considering that a child can exhibit *both* phonetic and phonemic problems within the same disordered phonological system.

It was mentioned earlier that a major decision we must make in a distinctive feature analysis is whether a child has not acquired a feature or whether he or she is a feature misuser. This decision is typically quite easy for a clinician to make after looking at the child's phonetic inventory to see if whole classes of sounds and features are missing. An experienced clinician can examine a child's speech sample and accurately predict which features are the most in error. In many cases this may be enough to help the clinician to decide whether the treatment should be directed toward establishing a feature in a child's repertoire or altering the use of a feature that has already been acquired but is being used inconsistently in a child's system.

What are the advantages of considering distinctive features in our analysis of misarticulations? We see four advantages. First, considering distinctive features provides a model for understanding errors in many clients; an error on a given feature (e.g., voicing) that is shared by more than one phoneme accounts for the misarticulation of many phonemes by reducing the seemingly random errors to a simpler pattern. Second, considering distinctive features may provide one gauge of severity of sound substitution, in that the more feature differences between a target sound and its substitution, the more severe the problem may be. Third, it provides a basis for the selection of a target sound for therapy; the clinician can select the phoneme that shares features with many other misarticulated sounds. And fourth, it may provide a basis for more efficient therapy (Costello & Onstine, 1976; Ritterman & Freeman, 1974) by facilitating generalization to sounds not being directly treated. Therapy directed toward one sound often improves others that are phonetically similar. Considered within the framework of distinctive features, it makes sense that training in features common to many sounds would result in greater improvement in misarticulation than would specific training for each sound error.

Despite the many advantages, however, there are a number of factors that may limit the application of distinctive feature theory to clinical problems. A formal distinctive feature analysis may not even be necessary, as indicated by Grunwell (1988):

> The last few paragraphs have seriously thrown into question the clinical value of a formalised distinctive feature analysis procedure. This implication is intentional. None the less, the CONCEPTS of distinctive feature contrasts and natural classes are of major importance and considerable clinical applicability. The concept that phonemes are differentiated by their "content" of contrastive features enables the clinician to focus on the contrastive/distinctive feature that is in "error" and also to recognise similar "errors" in different phonemes, that is patterns in disordered speech. (p. 157)

We believe that whatever method the clinician uses to analyze distinctive features in a given client, the following are important:

1. The diagnostician should "think features" at some point in the analysis of a child with multiple articulation errors. In other words, one should at least be able to make the judgment as to whether or not all features are present or if error patterns reflect consistent, repeated misuse of specific features in certain contexts.

2. The clinician should determine if a child (a) has not acquired a feature or (b) is a feature misuser. If the child does not evidence a particular feature in his phonetic inventory, then treatment may best be directed toward basic introduction of the feature into the child's repertoire (McReynolds & Engmann, 1975; McReynolds & Huston, 1971; Pollack & Rees, 1972). If the child is a feature misuser, then further phonological analysis (which implies feature use) is indicated, and the clinician must determine the extent and loci of feature misuse. Phonological analysis techniques are more equipped to do this. More recent nonlinear phonological analyses include a feature level in their hierarchy.

3. Substitution errors especially should undergo a distinctive feature "substitution analysis" in which the feature bundles of the target and substituted sounds are compared and features that are misused are noted by the examiner, as in Table 6.1.

PHONOLOGICAL ANALYSIS

Another approach to analyzing a child's articulatory behavior is to perform a phonological analysis. In 1976, a landmark book by David Ingram entitled *Phonological Disability in Children* sparked an interest in a more linguistic approach to misarticulation analysis. Ingram cited many sources who reported that there were common patterns of articulatory simplification in children's speech (Compton, 1970, 1976; Oller et al., 1972; Smith, 1973; Stampe, 1969). That is, most children develop the ability to articulate gradually, and before perfecting an adult production they reduce the complexity of words in characteristic ways. Space in this chapter does not permit us to provide examples of each phonological pattern reported in the existing literature, and most training programs now include extensive exposure to phonological processes in course work. Refer to any of the sources discussed for myriad examples of phonological processes.

A phonological approach rests on certain assumptions. First, phonologists assume that there is a structure to every child's sound system and that even in the most unintelligible child there is a pattern of phonemic production. Sounds do not occur in random combinations. Second, a phonological approach assumes an underlying system that gives rise to the observable sound combinations that we hear from children. The implication is that a phonological error may be a product of the underlying system that organizes the overt sound combinations.

Earlier in this chapter we indicated that there can be both linguistically based and sensori-motor-based misarticulations. The linguistically generated errors could be construed as products of rules generated by the child's underlying phonological system. Rules, to a certain degree, imply patterns of performance, and phonological "rules" can be written to simply describe these patterns. Phonological rules, then, are descriptive of the way in which a child uses classes of phonemes. Many investigators have reported that, in development, it is commonly observed that children tend to simplify their word productions in comparison to the adult model. The simplifications are typically in the direction of producing physiologically easier sounds for more difficult ones. For reasons not presently known, some children appear to persist in using these simplification strategies; and if enough of these strategies are retained, the child is likely to be quite unintelligible. Most authorities report that many of the patterns of error found in disordered children are those observed in normally developing youngsters at earlier ages (Ingram, 1976; Shriberg & Kwiatkowski, 1980). Ingram (1976), however, also points out that deviant rules not typically found in normally developing children may appear in youngsters with phonological disorders. Phonological rules can describe these simplification techniques, and each rule implies a change in the use of distinctive features. That is, a child who substitutes stops for continuants is altering an important distinctive feature of the target phonemes.

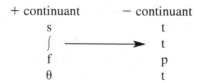

The clinician wishing to gain insight into phonological processes has at least two levels of analysis to choose from. First, there are instruments that are targeted toward discovering phonological processes in children (Bankson & Bernthal, 1990; Bosma-Smit & Hand, 1996; Compton & Hutton, 1978; Hodson, 1986, 2004; Kahn & Lewis, 2002; Lowe, 1986; Secord & Donohue, 2002; Webb & Duckett, 1990; Weiner, 1979). These measures provide picture or object stimuli and ask the child to give a single-word or connected-speech response. These responses are analyzed by the clinician for particular phonological simplifications.

Preliminary research suggests that traditional test stimuli can be used to aid the clinician in a gross analysis of phonological process use (Garber, 1986; Garn-Nunn, 1986; Klein, 1984; Lowe, 1986).

The measures mentioned above can be administered in a reasonable time period (under one hour); the scoring time will vary with the clinician's experience in using the test and the severity of the phonological disorder under evaluation. Most of the measures, however, do not evaluate spontaneous connected speech, and therefore the phonological rules obtained may only approximate those typically used by the child in conversation (Klein, 1984). Some research, however, suggests more similarities than differences between single-word and connected-speech productions. Andrews and Fey (1986) evoked the words from the Assessment of Phonological Processes in single-word and connected-speech contexts and found that most phonological errors, severity ratings, and clinical recommendations would be similar for either response mode. Bernhardt and Holdgrafer (2001a) point out the importance of sampling when attempting to complete an in-depth phonological analysis. The authors suggest that a given sample must adequately examine a variety of word shapes (e.g., CVC, CCV, CVCVC, etc.) and a variety of sequences of phonemes and features. That is, phonemes and features (e.g., place, manner) must have the opportunity to occur adjacent to one another and in more distant relationships. Clearly, it is difficult to predict if a spontaneous sample will provide many word shapes, phonemes, and sequences, so the case is made for supplemental sampling to determine the true nature of phonological errors. It is only with detailed and strategic sampling that we can effectively describe a child's phonological system and know the appropriate contexts to target in treatment. Some studies illustrate the notion that context may have important effects on a child's phonology. For instance, Kirk (2008) studied typically developing children between the ages of 1 and 3 to examine their production of word initial and word final consonant clusters in a picture naming task. While some prior investigations have shown that substitutions in clusters may be predicted by the errors made in production of singleton consonants, Kirk found that about one-third of cluster productions could not be predicted in this way. Furthermore, 70% of the unpredictable substitutions appeared to be the result of assimilation within the cluster itself, suggesting that "ease of articulation" may account for such errors.

Bernhardt and Holdgrafer (2001b) provide a nice overview of the advantages of both single-word sampling and connected-speech sampling for the analysis of phonology. The article also offers a conceptual summary of nonlinear phonology and states that both single-word and connected-speech samples are necessary to examine word/syllable structure, segments, distinctive features, and phrasal aspects of phonology. The case is made that in order to fully explain a child's phonological system, sampling must be strategic so that a variety of the above elements are available for analysis.

A second level of phonological analysis is to gather a spontaneous speech sample, transcribe it in the International Phonetic Alphabet, and attempt to discern patterns of error (processes) in the data. This is obviously more time consuming than the measures mentioned above, but it may also be more valid because the clinician is examining actual utterances that were generated by the client's cognitive-linguistic system. The analysis of a spontaneous speech sample is recommended by Shriberg and Kwiatkowski (1980) in the Natural Process Analysis (NPA). This procedure specifically targets eight processes for analysis and provides a unique and useful phonetic inventory. The Natural Process Analysis can provide valuable information for the practitioner and represents a well-planned procedure.

Ingram (1981) developed the Procedures for the Phonological Analysis of Children's Language (PPACL), which includes a phonetic analysis, homonym analysis, substitution analysis, and phonological process analysis. Twenty-seven specific processes are targeted. However, Ingram stated that the analysis is "open ended" and can continue "until all the substitutions in a child's speech have been explained" (p. 7).

Grunwell (1985) developed the Phonological Assessment of Child Speech (PACS), which provides a description of analysis procedures for a preferably spontaneous connected-speech sample of more than 200 words. The procedure results in phonetic analysis, contrastive analysis to determine which phones are used to make meaning differences, and a phonological process analysis. The Phonological Assessment of Child Speech also provides a developmental framework that is missing in many phonological analysis techniques.

There appears to be some agreement that certain processes are "high risk" in phonologically disordered children. Different authorities implicate specific phonological processes as being more important than others, at least in terms of focusing on them for assessment targets. Some preliminary evidence exists that suggests that similar phonological processes are detected whether one uses more involved, lengthy procedures (NPA, PPACL) or shorter tasks (APP) (Paden & Moss, 1985). This evidence, of course, does not indicate that in-depth phonological analyses and shorter procedures are equivalent, only that they both can identify basic phonological processes. Although there is considerable variation among the assessment techniques in the number of processes examined, there is also a high degree of agreement regarding processes that seem to be most at risk in unintelligible children. The actual number of processes targeted in an evaluation would seem to be related to the clinician's goals in the analysis (Ingram, 1981). If the clinician wanted to write a relatively complete generative phonology for a client, it would obviously focus on a larger number of rules than if the clinician's goal were to determine which major processes interfered most with intelligibility. In the latter case, the clinician may find that six phonological processes account for more than 80% of the child's misarticulations, and treatment targets might be selected from the processes having the most impact on intelligibility. For instance, if a child is exhibiting unstressed syllable deletion, final consonant deletion, and stopping, these will be initial treatment targets; rules such as epenthesis, vocalization, gliding, and so forth, which may have less effect on intelligibility, will not be of immediate concern. It should be noted that most of the evaluation techniques discussed above allow for the assessment of other processes as discovered by the examiner, even though the processes may not be specifically evaluated.

Recent work in the area of nonlinear phonology (Bernhardt & Stoel-Gammon, 1994; Schwartz, 1992; Stoel-Gammon, 1996) has pointed out the importance and utility of considering hierarchial relationships in child utterances. These relationships among words, syllables, segments, and features are illustrated in Figure 6.3. The initial consonant(s) in a syllable is/are called *onsets,* and *rhymes* are a vowel and any consonants following the onset. All English syllables require a rhyme, but the onset is optional, as in a vowel-initiated word such as *outside.* Segments in this model are similar to phonemes, and features can be viewed from a variety of

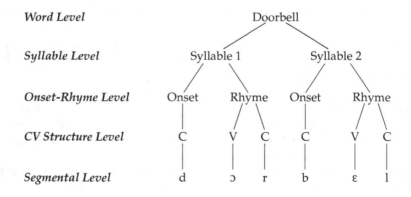

FIGURE 6.3 Hierarchical levels discussed in nonlinear phonology.
Source: Adapted from Stoel-Gammon (1996). Baltimore, MD: Brookes.

perspectives as simple as place-manner voicing and as complex as other distinctive feature systems mentioned earlier in the present chapter. The elegance of hierarchical models is that they allow analysis of syllable, onset-rhyme, CV structure, and segmental and feature levels and may account for misarticulations in a way not readily possible by traditional or phonological process modes of analysis. Stoel-Gammon (1996) provides excellent examples of using nonlinear phonology in the analysis of disordered phonology. Barlow (2001a) discusses how new phonological theories impact clinical aspects of assessment and treatment. One focus is optimality theory, in which "high-ranking markedness constraints, rather than rules or processes are responsible for children's simplified output forms" (p. 226). Also, traditional views of phonology have focused on segments or syllabic structures, and there is a move toward concentrating on larger structures such as words and beyond. Dinnsen and O'Connor (2001) also discuss newer theoretical approaches that have clinical relevance. They point out that prior explanations of children's phonological errors cited application of simplification rules that were independent of one another. Optimality theory has shifted the focus away from a priori rules to the notion that there are no rules at all. This theory further implies that error patterns, rather than being unrelated, are connected to one another in special ways, and one pattern, in fact, implies the existence of another in an "implicationally related" way. Rule-based, or derivational, theories imply underlying representations that are changed into phonetic productions through a series of phonological rules or processes. The authors state: "Optimality theory differs from derivational theories in several important respects. The central hypotheses are that there are no rules and thus no rule-ordering relationships, no serial derivations, no intermediate levels of representation, and no language-specific restructions on the set of available input representations (underlying representations)" (p. 261). They go on to state that traditional rule-based phonological process interpretations "have viewed children's error patterns as independent of one another. As a result, no one error pattern is expected to co-occur with any other error pattern. . . . On the other hand, the fixed ranking of certain constraints within optimality theory predicts that some error patterns will be implicationally related. . . . The general claim is that for error patterns in an implicational relationship, it will be the implying error pattern that is lost first. . . . Optimality theory offers a principled basis for targeting one error pattern for treatment over the other when the child presents with two (or more) implicationally related error patterns. For the most efficacious results, the recommendation in such cases is to treat that error pattern on which other error patterns are dependent" (p. 269). Barlow (2001b) demonstrates in a case study how optimality theory can be used to analyze several prototypical patterns of phonological errors. The analysis provides an account of variability in the child's productions that goes beyond the typical phonological accounts. The example also demonstrates implications for the selection of treatment targets based on this theory.

The Interaction between Phonology and the Lexicon

Barlow (2002) discusses the interaction between phonology and the lexicon, including relationships to morphosyntax and the use of morphophonemic alternations in assessment (e.g., pig/piggy). It is clear that recent theoretical and clinical approaches to phonological analysis are not "segment oriented" but rather "word oriented." That is, it is not reasonable to separate phonemes from lexical items in a child's phonological system.

Velleman and Vihman (2002) cite evidence that children enter language acquisition first from a word or phrase point of view. For example, children produce word approximations or primitive word combinations (e.g., "more juice") as formulaic structures. Velleman and Vihman say, "Only later, and construction by construction, does the child begin to decompose and creatively reconstruct such units, as evidenced by the very slow and graduate emergence of productivity, or the consistent use of specific forms for the expression of particular meanings across a wide range of different lexical contexts" (p. 9). This view that phonological development begins with whole-word learning has been gaining popularity since the 1970s. These authors indicate that children learn phonology through explicit learning (intentionally trying to replicate adult patterns) and implicit learning, which is incidental and unintentional and is a product of mere exposure to the language.

Ingram and Ingram (2001) advocate a whole-word approach because children acquire words, not individual phonemes. Early on, children have little awareness of segments and they differ in their acquisition patterns and phonological learning strategies. Whole words have been assessment targets for some time, as evidenced by the Whole Word Accuracy (WWA) measure developed by Schmitt, Howard, and Schmitt (1983). The WWA score increases between the ages of 3 and 7 years. The WWA is highly related to intelligibility. Ingram and Ingram (2001) compute the percentage of whole words correct (PWW). As children learn language, the complexity of their words increases in terms of syllable structure, number of phonemes, and complexity of sounds produced. Thus, Ingram and Ingram (2001) developed a measure called Phonological Mean Length of Utterance (PMLU), which focuses on the number of segments in words and the number of correct consonants in those words. According to Ingram and Ingram (2001), the PMLU is calculated by counting each segment (consonant and vowel) in the child's word and giving each segment a single point. Next, each correct consonant earns an additional point. The clinician then adds the total number of points for the words analyzed and divides by the number of words. In this article they propose some possible stages of PMLU development. Another measure proposed by Ingram and Ingram (2001) is the Proportion of Whole-Word Proximity (PWP), which is found by dividing the PMLU of the correct adult production of a target word list into the PMLU of a child's production of that list. Presumably, the closer the child's production is to the adult production of the word list, the higher the correlation with intelligibility ratings. Critical to Ingram and Ingram's (2001) assessment approach are four components: *whole-word analysis, word shape analysis* (syllables), *segmental analysis* (matches and substitutions of phonemes), and *phonological analysis* (determination of mastery of contrasts based on the acquisition of distinctive features).

If a clinician wishes to write phonological rules from a child's conversational sample, there are certain basic issues common to most procedures.

1. *Glossing and Segmentation.* The clinician must interpret the child's utterances and provide adult interpretations or "glosses" of what the child was trying to say. One cannot arrive at a phonological rule system unless the intended utterance is known. Several methods of segmenting or arranging the data have been reported. One method is to arrange correct and incorrect child productions and glosses word by word in phonetic transcription:

Child's Production	Adult Gloss
/ki/	/ki/
/bækI/	/bæskIt/
/pæ/	/fæn/
/go/	/go/

This allows the clinician the opportunity to compare productions with the adult model and hypothesize a phonological reduction pattern (e.g., final consonant deletion in the words "basket" and "fan"). Another method of segmentation is to retain spontaneous connected speech intact and divide the sample into utterances:

Child's Production	**Adult Gloss**
/tidəgɔgi/	/siðədɔgi/

This method of segmentation can sometimes help the clinician account for certain phonological reductions in a word that are influenced by sounds in previous words. Different authors (Ingram, 1981; Shriberg & Kwiatkowski, 1980) recommend a variety of methods for organizing segments once they have been glossed (alphabetically, by syllable shape, by consonant, etc.). The purpose of these varied organizational schemes is to aid in the retrieval and comparison of individual words and sounds when attempting to prove the existence of a phonological rule.

   2. *Hypothesizing a Natural Process.* After arranging the data from a sample, the clinician attempts to account for errors by hypothesizing a phonological reduction pattern. For instance, when comparing a child's production of a word to the adult gloss it may be noted that there is a deletion of the final consonant. The clinician may hypothesize the process of final consonant deletion. The "high-risk" processes listed in Table 6.1 should be ruled out before any "deviant processes" are suspected.

   3. *Finding Support for Hypothesized Rules.* It is not enough simply to postulate that final consonant deletion has occurred in a child's sample. Evidence must be obtained from the utterances to determine whether the process has, in fact, occurred. For instance, the child may have deleted the final consonant in a CVC word. The clinician should examine all other words in the sample that end in singleton consonants to determine the frequency of occurrence of the hypothesized phonological reduction. If there is widespread support for the occurrence of final consonant deletion, then the clinician may write the rule. If only certain final consonants are deleted consistently while others are produced normally, then the clinician must change the hypothesis to a rule that specifies particular kinds of final consonant deletion (e.g., stop and nasal deletion). This is where the use of distinctive features is helpful.

   4. *Specification of Frequency of Occurrence.* Authorities differ in their methods of specifying the frequency of occurrence of certain phonological rules. Some processes appear to be obligatory (occur virtually all the time), and others seem to be optional. In specifying optionality of a phonological rule, some authors recommend the three-stage system of "always," "sometimes," and "never" (Shriberg & Kwiatkowski, 1980). Other authorities (Ingram, 1981) recommend the use of percentage ranges such as 0–20, 21–40, 41–60, 61–80, and 81–100. Whatever method is used, the important thing is to indicate how often the process is occurring.

   5. *Writing the Rule.* After the clinician has gathered support for a rule from the transcript, the rule is written specifying the target phonemes, how they are changed, what context they are changed in, and how often the rule occurs. A phonological rule for final stop consonant deletion may look like this:

p
b
t $\rightarrow \varnothing$/ CV-# 80–100%
d
k
g

This rule says that the consonants *p, b, t, d, k,* and *g* are deleted in the context of the CVC word when the target sound is at the end. The slash stands for "in the context of," the blank represents the location of the target sound, and the # refers to a word boundary. Note that the percentage of occurrence is indicated after the rule.

6. *Recycling of 1–4.* As each rule is written and proof is gathered for each phonological reduction, the clinician repeats the process of examining the errors, hypothesizing a phonological process, looking for data to support the rule, and writing the rule. Soon, the clinician can account for the majority of the errors in the child's transcript with the exception of a small residue of words that the rules do not describe. At this point, the clinician may wish to hypothesize a phonological rule that is not normally seen in children's articulatory development. For instance, the child may delete initial consonants of certain types. The procedure, however, is still the same. The clinician must hypothesize the rule and find support for it before it can be written.

The detection of phonological simplification patterns can be a powerful tool in the hands of the well-trained clinician. A sample of speech that appears to have many unrelated misarticulations can be reduced to only a few phonological reduction patterns. The clinical implication of these processes is that the child does not need to work on a single sound, but may need to focus on the pattern of error. The assumption is that the observable error pattern is generated by an underlying rule; and if the rule is to be altered, then many of the segments that it affects should be targeted (Compton, 1976; Hodson & Paden, 1991; Ingram, 1976). Again, the only way to discover these patterns of misarticulation is to search for them through a phonological analysis technique. Traditional tests are not constructed for this purpose, although they certainly could be suggestive for further analyses and could provide hints for the clinician as to error patterns.

There are several cautions we might offer regarding phonological analysis of a child's misarticulations. First, a phonological approach requires that a clinician transcribe words and/or sentences of spontaneous speech. Although most speech clinicians have completed courses in phonetics during their undergraduate education, many of these courses did not offer students the opportunity to transcribe disordered speech from a variety of male, female, adult, and child speakers. Some clinicians may not have adequate experience to reliably transcribe connected speech. One clinician of our acquaintance remarked that "the only thing I have used my phonetics for in the past 10 years is to fill in the little blocks on the Goldman-Fristoe score sheet." It may be quite a leap, then, for some clinicians to transcribe words or connected speech in practice. Second, if our reliability is low in scoring phoneme errors, then we can only assume that reliability is even more of an issue in phonological transcription and analysis because we must construct rules from the data (Shriberg & Kwiatkowski, 1977). Interjudge reliability is important, but test–retest reliability should be considered as well. Earlier we mentioned the notion of "independent analysis" in evaluating the vocal productions of children. Recall that in such analyses we are not judging the accuracy of production, just the presence of phonetic elements and syllabic complexity. As we discussed in Chapter 3, reliability is an important variable in any type of measurement we use in clinical assessment. Morris (2009, p. 46) studied the test–retest reliability of independent measures of toddlers' speech and found: "Syllable structure level and index of phonetic complexity achieved high test–retest reliability. Word-final phonetic inventory and word shape analyses had moderate but not significant reliability. Word-initial phonetic inventory was not reliable." It is important to note that the data evaluated were 20-minute conversational samples. The researcher suggests that clinicians may want to use larger samples for use in assessment of young children.

A third concern is the compelling and captivating nature of phonological analysis. It makes an articulatory assessment rather like an interesting puzzle; and when the clinician reaches the "solution" and divines the phonological rules, it is tempting to view the child's problem from a linguistic-phonological perspective only and apply this type of treatment. Locke (1983) and Fey (1992) caution us about the utility of phonological rules. According to Fey (1992),

> Calling a pattern a phonological rule or process is only a descriptive exercise. The existence of the pattern does not necessarily explain anything; the pattern itself is in need of explanation. . . . We must be cautious that we do not stop our search for causal explanations of disorders simply because we have some elegant descriptive principles and terms that can be used to organize and label them. (p. 230)

Children of various etiological groups will demonstrate phonological regularities in their speech. Even if the disorder has a sensorimotor basis, phonological rules can be written and the child perceived as a phonological-linguistic case. Shriberg and Kwiatkowski (1982a) suggest that the clinician must examine linguistic, sensorimotor, and psychosocial aspects of a child's behavior and select appropriate treatment goals. Clinicians should not assume a linguistically oriented treatment simply because the child exhibits a systematic phonology. The treatment of choice for each child may require different emphases, which could include focusing on sensorimotor aspects of articulation. There is no doubt that phonological analyses are useful and constitute a major innovation in articulatory assessment; but the clinician must be careful to check reliability and should not apply a phonological linguistic interpretation to all errors without examining sensorimotor and social aspects as well.

ASSESSMENT OF PHONOLOGICAL KNOWLEDGE

Some researchers have considered the notion of phonological knowledge in children with speech sound disorders (Elbert & Gierut, 1986; Gierut, Elbert, & Dinnsen, 1987; Maxwell & Rockman, 1984). A basic question revolves around whether a child's phonological system is similar to or different from a typical adult system. It is possible that a child's underlying representation of a word is either similar to or different from an adult representation. Bernthal and Bankson (2004) illustrate this notion with final consonant deletion:

> One explanation for that process might be that the child misperceives the adult word, e.g., perceives [dɔg] as [dɔ]. A second explanation might be that the child's underlying lexical representation for dog is [dɔ]. A third possible explanation is that the child's perceptual system functions appropriately and the lexical match between what the child perceives and what he or she has stored is consistent with the adult standard, but he or she has a phonological production rule that calls for the deletion of word-final stops. A fourth possibility is that the child has a motor production problem; in this case the child may have the appropriate perception but does not possess the necessary motor skill to make the physiological gesture to produce the sound. (p. 243)

One might wonder how the clinician is to gain insight into a child's phonological knowledge. While we are just beginning to understand this area, some procedures have been used by researchers. Owing to difficulties inherent in assessing and interpreting a child's perceptual abilities (Locke, 1980) and the recent suggestion of independence between the perception and production systems (Dinnsen, 1985; Straight, 1980), most research has concentrated on data generated from a child's productive system. McGregor and Schwartz (1992) remind us that production data alone are not sufficient to describe the complexities of a child's phonological system. One example of a production analysis is provided by Maxwell and Rockman (1984):

> Evidence can be adduced that shows that Jamie does know or does represent these words underlyingly with the appropriate postvocalic obstruents, that is, that he represents them the same way we do, but that his pronunciation of these words is governed by a phonological rule of final obstruent deletion. . . . This evidence is available in his pronunciations of these words or morphemes in their inflected forms, that is, in morphophonemically related words. . . . These data reveal that for each morpheme the omitted consonant in question is not omitted when that consonant is in word-medial position. . . . For example, the morpheme meaning "duck" is pronounced [dʌ] without the final k in its uninflected form but as [dʌk] with the k when inflected with the diminutive morpheme [-i] as in [dʌki]. Morphophonemic evidence of this sort (e.g., k alternating with null) provides clear evidence that Jamie knows that the morpheme meaning "duck" must be represented underlyingly with a postvocalic k. (pp. 11–12)

Elbert and Gierut (1986) have suggested a procedure for determining a child's productive phonological knowledge on a six-level continuum from least to most knowledge. Gierut, Elbert, and Dinnsen (1987) summarize the six types of knowledge. It is recommended by Elbert and Gierut (1986) that the clinician gather an extensive sample that includes all phonemes of English in all word positions with a variety of canonical shapes that provide multiple opportunities for phonemic contrast. After examining the child's phonetic and phonemic inventories, phonotactic rules, phonological rules, and allophonic and neutralization rules, the clinician can categorize the types of phonological knowledge a child exhibits for individual sounds, sound classes, or the overall sound system. Gierut, Elbert, and Dinnsen (1987) found that the phonological knowledge continuum may relate to the amount of generalization to be expected in treatment. Basically, training of sounds with least phonological knowledge resulted in generalization across the entire phonological system, whereas training of sounds with most knowledge resulted in generalization to only the specific class of phoneme trained. Thus, the implication is that greater effects may be obtained by training phonemes for which the child has least knowledge. Gierut (2007) also has suggested that selection of more complex treatment targets rather than simple ones may result in more progress and generalization. This, of course, goes against the traditional view that treatment should begin on the earlier developing, simpler segments rather than those that are more compled. The research on this issue appears to be mixed. For instance, Rvachew and Bernhardt (2010, p. 34) found that "Children who received treatment for simple targets made more progress toward the acquisition of the target sounds and demonstrated emergence of complex untreated segments and feature contrasts. Children who received treatment for complex targets made little measurable gain in phonological development." These researchers do not view the clinician's decision as having to be dichotomous between simple and complex targets. They say (p. 48), "It is not that complex targets must be avoided—far from it. With horizontal and cyclical goal attack strategies there is no need to limit the treatment targets to simple or complex structures exclusively." More research needs to be done in this area.

OTHER TESTING

Six additional areas of examination relate significantly to a competent evaluation of a client with a speech sound disorder, depending on the type of case and its severity. The clinician should be prepared to assess the following areas as appropriate.

1. *Case History.* As in any evaluation, a complete assessment of speech sound disorders must include a thorough case history and interview with the parent/client. Bernthal, Bankson, and Flipsen (2009, p. 211) recommend the following important areas of information: "(1) possible etiological factors; (2) the family's or client's perception of the problem; (3) the academic, work, home and social environment of the client; and (4) medical, developmental and social information about the client."

2. *Language Assessment.* The clinician examining a child's articulatory system should expect the bulk of these cases to exhibit some language deviations as well. Many authorities report the high co-occurrence of articulation and language disorders (Paul & Shriberg, 1982).

In several chapters of the present text we have cited research on nonword repetition tasks as a means for screening children with language disorders. In most cases, children with language disorders also have some phonological involvement. One can see the dilemma of attempting to use a nonword repetition task when the child cannot produce certain phonemes or syllable structures. Shriberg et al. (2009) developed a syllable repetition task (SRT) for use with children who have speech sound disorders. The SRT includes one early developing vowel and four early developing consonants. Preliminary research shows that the task is valid and psychometrically sound for use with children who misarticulate.

The clinician should routinely gather a spontaneous language sample and administer standardized language tests for each client with a speech sound disorder.

3. *Audiometric Screening.* A second diagnostic procedure that should be routinely administered is an audiometric screening. It is critical that the possibility of hearing impairment be eliminated prior to beginning treatment. This becomes especially important if the parents report suspected auditory problems or if the child has a history of ear infections.

4. *The Oral-Peripheral Examination.* This is an integral part of the articulation examination (see Chapter 9 for guidelines in conducting this procedure). Oral-peripheral examination results may be important in distinguishing a sensorimotor from a linguistic disorder of articulation. Fletcher (1972) provides some normative data on diadochokinetic rates for children, and this should also be included as part of the examination for sensorimotor difficulties.

5. *Auditory Discrimination.* This area has been classically explored in articulation evaluation. Historically, many investigations have shown that children with speech sound disorders do not perform as well as normal speakers on auditory discrimination tasks (Bernthal, Bankson, & Flipsen, 2009; Powers, 1971; Winitz, 1969). Early treatment programs incorporated an obligatory module of auditory discrimination training (Van Riper & Irwin, 1958), and many authorities continue to believe that the assessment of auditory discrimination is an important part of an evaluation (Winitz, 1975). However, criticisms have emerged regarding clinicians' methods of auditory discrimination testing (Beving & Eblen, 1973; Schwartz & Goldman, 1974) and the efficacy of auditory discrimination training in treatment (Shelton et al., 1978; Williams & McReynolds, 1975). Recently, the most defensible position appears to be assessing the auditory discrimination of misarticulated sounds only (Bernthal & Bankson, 2004; Locke, 1980) rather than all phonemes and to evaluate it in a way that avoids the use of paired comparisons (mass-math). It is presently not clear if auditory discrimination testing needs to be a part of routine articulatory evaluations or if it should be embarked upon only when some suspicion of a discrimination problem is evidenced in trial therapy. The present authors would favor the latter option.

6. *Phonological Awareness.* Many children with phonological disorders have been shown to exhibit decreased levels of phonological awareness that relate to academic and literacy skills (Bernthal & Bankson, 2004; Bird, Bishop, & Freeman, 1995). Clinicians can examine these abilities with a variety of techniques (Ball, 1993; Robertson & Salter, 1997; Torgesen & Bryant, 1994; Wagner, Torgesen, & Rashotte, 1999). It is often recommended that preschool children with speech sound disorders be evaluated for phonological awareness skills prior to entering elementary school, and their articulation, phonological awareness, and literacy skills should receive ongoing monitoring (Ryachew, Chiang, & Evans, 2007). Larrivee and Catts (1999) studied 30 children with expressive phonological disorders and 27 children with normally developing phonology. They assessed expressive phonology, phonological awareness, and language ability in these children as they completed kindergarten. After 1 year, children were given tests of reading achievement. The group of children with phonological disorders performed significantly poorer than the normally developing children on the reading measures, but there was a great deal of variability; some of the phonologically disordered subjects had good reading outcomes. When the authors divided the group with phonological disorders into those with good and poor reading outcomes, they found that the children with reading difficulties had more severe phonological disorders, poorer phonological awareness, and poorer language skills than those with better reading outcomes. The authors suggest that the SLP consider the assessment of phonological awareness and incorporate phonological awareness goals and development of sound–letter correspondence into the overall treatment program. Peterson, Pennington, Shriberg, and Boada (2009) followed children with speech sound disorders and those with typically developing speech who were between the ages of 5–6 at the beginning of the study and between 7–9 at the end of the investigation. They found that the group with speech sound disorders had more reading difficulties, but that statistical analysis showed that lower literacy scores were not predicted effectively by speech sound disorder (SSD) alone, but by a combination of SSD and language impairment. Interestingly, phonological awareness scores were associated with the persistence of speech sound disorders, but did not predict literacy outcome effectively. Again, this study supports the many investigations that show children with both language and phonological involvement will be more at risk for literacy issues. Rvachew (2007) studied the relationship between phonological processing and reading in children with speech sound disorders (SSD) who were tested at preschool and again at the end of first grade. A group of typically developing children was also included. She divided the participants with speech sound disorders into groups that represented poor phonological processing skill and those with good abilities in this area. Specific aspects of phonological processing evaluated were speech perception, onset awarness and rime awareness. Other measures were taken on phonological awareness, receptive language, expressive language, speech production, and word reading efficiency. After first grade the groups with speech sound disorders performed at a lower level on the reading test as compared to the typically developing group, even in children with SSD who had language abilities within normal limits. The author recommends (p. 268): "Continued monitoring of reading development and the provision of appropriate interventions when required would be a prudent course of action for a child with a preschool history of SSD, especially if the child shows evidence of phonological processing difficulties and fails to achieve age appropriate speech and language skills prior to the onset of formal education."

Some researchers have studied the link between types of speech sound errors and/or the severity of the articulation disorder in relation to phonological awareness abilities. For example, Preston and Edwards (2010) studied preschool children with speech sound disorders and found that lower scores in phonological awareness were associated with more atypical articulation errors and lower scores on a measure of receptive vocabulary. The researchers note that while phonological awareness assessments are not routinely performed on children with speech sound errors, such evaluations should be recommended for children with such difficulties, especially in cases where the articulation errors are atypical in nature. In another investigation, Preston and Edwards (2007) compared adolescents with residual speech sound errors to typically speaking peers on a series of phonological processing tasks. Such tasks included repetition of multisyllabic words, spoonerisms, phoneme reversals, nonword repetition, and elision. They found that out of the six tasks of phonological processing the participants with residual speech sound errors performed more poorly on 5 of the 6 tasks. Also, the performance on phonological processing tasks was able to classify 85% of the participants correctly as having residual sound errors or normal speech. The authors recommend assessment of phonological processing even in adolescents who have residual speech sound errors, because they may have a weakness in this area. With the increased emphasis on assessing phonological awareness, programs have been developed to train such abilities both in children with speech sound disorders and those with poor phonological awareness skills. The rationale is that phonological awareness has been linked to literacy skills. Schuele and Boudreau (2008) provide an excellent tutorial on incorporating phonological awareness into an intervention program. Kirk and Gillon (2007) studied groups of children with speech sound disorders who received training in phonological awareness/letter knowledge and speech therapy versus a group who received speech therapy alone. Several years later the group who received the phonological awareness training performed better than the group who received speech therapy alone on decoding and spelling morphologically complex words. Research has shown that intervention targeting phonemic awareness can be effective in the preschool years. For instance, Koutsoftas, Harmon, and Gray (2009) performed a multiple baseline study showing that phonological awareness intervention conducted by SLPs and classroom teachers twice a week for a six-week period increased abilities for 71% of the children.

INTEGRATING DATA FROM THE ASSESSMENT

One issue of the *American Journal of Speech-Language Pathology* (Volume 11, Number 3, August 2002) was devoted to several clinicians outlining how they would orchestrate a 90-minute evaluation of a preschool child with a phonological disorder. Thus, each approach was constrained by time, ostensibly to mirror time limitations in the "real world." Most of the clinicians spent time doing a parent interview, language testing, hearing screening, oral peripheral exam, and taking a case history that consumed a large portion of the available time. Many of the clinicians administered a traditional articulation test or one of the phonological process instruments, and most also took a small language sample. At the end of the series of suggested phonological assessments, three reviews were presented that all pointed out limitations in the approaches suggested. Of course, it was not the purpose of the forum to outline the "ideal" phonological assessment, just one that could be done in 90 minutes. Let us first indicate that we are not of the opinion that time constraints should be a major determining factor in the assessment of a severe disorder. Certainly, some cases can be served well by applying a Band-Aid; however, others require major surgery. As speech-language pathologists we should be prepared to do more in-depth analyses spanning several diagnostic sessions for cases that require such attention. First, all children with phonological disorders will not require an intensive evaluation; in fact, the majority of children with articulation problems present relatively straightforward difficulties that are easily understood by traditional testing procedures. For children with severe problems and poor intelligibility, however, the speech-language pathologist possesses expertise that no other professional has to offer for an in-depth analysis of the child's phonological system and principled selection of treatment targets based on this detailed analysis. After all, the state of knowledge about phonological disorders in our profession is also part of the real world and should not be ignored. With all that we know about the significant co-occurrence of severe phonological disorders with language, social, reading, and academic difficulties, it is important for us to spend all the time necessary to fully understand the child's problem without arbitrary time constraints degrading the process. Skahan, Watson, and Lof (2007) conducted a national survey to determine methods used by SLPs in assessing speech sound disorders. They found that most clinicians administered a standardized articulation test, estimated intelligibility, engaged in stimulability, and performed a hearing screening. Also, most SLPs used nonstandardized procedures in addition to these measures. The authors conclude that while these measurements may be adequate to qualify children for entrance into a caseload to receive services, they may not contain sufficient information to develop a comprehensive treatment program.

It is reasonable that after an articulation evaluation, the clinician should, at the very least, be able to make statements on the following areas: (1) biological prerequisites (hearing, structure/function of the speech mechanism); (2) linguistic ability; (3) phonetic and phonemic inventories; (4) distinctive features acquired, used correctly, absent, or misused; (5) response to stimulation by sounds that the child should have acquired, according to normative data; (6) phonological processes evident in the sample; (7) an indication of facilitating phonetic contexts, if any, in cases where stimulability is unproductive; (8) a judgment of intelligibility; (9) a judgment of severity/prognosis.

There are a variety of ways to assess articulatory ability; and the broader the view taken by the clinician, the more realistic the picture obtained of the client. For instance, if only the results of a traditional articulation test are considered, the clinician may be able to summarize a phonetic inventory and make some preliminary judgments about distinctive feature acquisition; but perhaps an inventory of phonological processes may not be possible owing to limited sampling. Furthermore, the norms that might be used in comparing the child's phonetic inventory to other children (Sander, 1972; Templin, 1957) are not applicable to phonological processes. The nine areas mentioned above are simply different ways of looking at the child's articulatory system and should at least be considered in every case to the extent that the clinician can make a statement about each area. Then, further exploration might be undertaken in areas of concern, such as writing a phonology from a spontaneous speech sample if problems are indicated on single-word measures. If a child is noted to be missing entire classes of phonemes, then a more intensive distinctive feature analysis might be indicated. The point is, results from a variety of areas need to be considered and used as indicators for further analyses.

Shriberg and Kwiatkowski (1982a, 1994a, 1994c) have suggested that clinicians consider possible causal correlates of articulation disorders. They recommended gathering data on each client in the areas of cognition/language, speech mechanism integrity, and psychological/social parameters. Gathering specific data on children from different etiological groups could add further insight into differences in speech sound disorders and ways to assess them. For example, Barnes et al. (2009) found that children with fragile X syndrome, both with and without autism spectrum disorder, used similar phonological processes to typically developing children, but were less intelligible in connected speech. This suggests that further evaluation of other factors such as motor speech ability, prosody, rate, and fluency of connected speech may be important to include in assessing these populations.

Consideration of these areas helps to keep the clinician from becoming too narrowly focused in the conception of articulation assessment and treatment. It also forces the clinician at least to consider the possibility of a variety of single or interactive maintaining factors in the articulation disorder. If a clinician is enamored of phonology and a linguistic interpretation of most articulation problems, such an approach forces the clinician to at least gather some information on psychosocial and speech mechanism variables. Conversely, if a clinician has a sensorimotor orientation, the approach forces the evaluation of more linguistic aspects. The findings of such a broad-based analysis may provide the clinician with important information on prognosis and treatment goal that otherwise would not have been considered. Gathering this type of information has allowed Shriberg and Kwiatkowski (1994a, 1994b, 1994c) to construct short- and long-term outcome data on children with phonological disorders and to begin to define subgroups of this population.

SEVERITY AND INTELLIGIBILITY

Although traditional articulation tests can easily identify children with phonological disorders, the tests have difficulty clearly defining different levels of severity (Garn-Nunn & Martin, 1992). Several investigators have considered the problem of assigning a severity rating to children's misarticulation problems. We often hear clinicians rate a child's difficulty as "mild" or "moderate"; and when asked how this was determined, the clinicians sometimes have no empirical basis. Flipsen, Hammer, and Yost (2005) asked 10 highly experienced SLPs to rate 17 phonologically disordered children on the severity of their disorder. Severity ratings were correlated with common objective measurements (e.g., PCC, WWA), and it was found that the severity ratings by the "experts" were highly variable. The researchers concluded that "impressionistic rating scales" used even by highly experienced clinicians were so inconsistent that it raises questions regarding their usefulness. The more objective measures such as PCC tended to provide more consistent information. Shriberg and Kwiatkowski (1982a) suggest the use of the percentage of consonants correct (PCC) in a spontaneous sample as being a most reliable predictor of severity ratings. They had judges rank order variables that were thought to contribute to severity, and intelligibility was ranked first as an influencing factor. They also had clinicians rate tape-recordings of spontaneous speech on severity (mild, mild–moderate, moderate–severe, severe). Statistical analyses showed that the measure most predictive of severity rating was the PCC. Basically, the PCC is a calculation of the number of correct consonants divided by the numbers of correct plus incorrect consonants. The resulting number is multiplied by 100 to arrive at the PCC. Shriberg and Kwiatkowski (1982b) outline specific procedures and a worksheet for use in computation of the PCC. The point here is that the percentage of consonants correctly articulated relates to severity and severity relates to intelligibility. The number of errors a child has will obviously affect the PCC. Johnson, Weston, and Bain (2004) compared imitative sentence production with a conversational sample in computing the PCC to determine if severity ratings differed in the two elicitation methods. They found the PCC computed on imitated sentences was comparable to the PCC obtained from a conversational sample in children between the ages of 4 and 6 years. The imitative method took considerably less time to administer and complete. They still advocate caution in applying the imitative approach, and indicate that cases should be considered on an individual basis.

Hodson and Paden (1991) offered the Composite Phonological Deviancy Score (CPDS) as a measure of severity. The system considers age in the calculation as well as a number of phonological processes occurring in the Analysis of Phonological Processes. Edwards (1992) suggests the Process Density Index, which calculates the number of process applications per word, as a measure of severity and reports good reliability with listener judgments of severity. Shriberg (1993) has developed the Articulation Competence Index for use in genetic research. This index takes into account distorted productions that were not included in the original development of the

PCC. Gordon-Brannan and Hodson (2000) studied 48 prekindergarten children to measure intelligibility/severity. The measure used was percentage of words understood by an unfamiliar listener and correctly transcribed orthographically from a continuous speech sample. The authors found four groups of children, based on the percentage of words correctly understood. Children with adult-like speech had percentages between 91 and 100%. Children in the "mild" category had 83 to 90% understood. A third group, the "moderate" children, had 68–81% of their words understood, and a "severe" group had between 16 and 63% understood. The range of the top three groups was 68 to 100%, with a mean of 85%. According to the authors, if a child 4 years of age and older falls below 66% (2 SD below the mean), it could be an indicator of a phonological disorder. Recall also that Ingram and Ingram (2001) proposed the Proportion of Whole Word Proximity (PWP) as a measure that might logically correlate with intelligibility ratings. Although the above methods may have their critics, they are at least attempts to objectify severity in cases of articulation disorders and are available for use by practicing clinicians.

Another gauge of severity might be to have independent judges rate the severity of speech samples based on their perceptual judgments. Although this is not a quantitative measure, it certainly is an indication of society's reaction to a person's phonological disorder. Garrett and Moran (1992) compared the ratings of experienced (speech-language pathology majors) and inexperienced (elementary education majors) listeners to more objective measures such as the PCC and CPDS. They found all measures to be highly intercorrelated. The two objective measures appeared to be useful as clinical indicators of severity. This is especially interesting since the CPDS is derived from a single-word sample and the PCC from connected speech.

Of course, a clinician assessing the overall severity of a child's problem will also have to consider other variables in addition to phonology. For instance, if a child has a concomitant language disorder or hearing impairment, the severity level increases. Reliability is an important issue in making judgments of severity, and SLPs should become familiar with normative data, especially for younger children. Rafaat, Rvachew, and Russell (1995) found that phonological severity judgments by SLPs for preschool children were not adequate (40% agreement) for children under 3.5 years of age, but were adequate for older preschool children.

No matter how a child performs on an articulation test, a major concern of both the clinician and the parent is intelligibility in spontaneous speech. How understandable is the child in his or her daily interactions? Intelligibility is difficult to measure since it is affected by many variables (Kent, Miolo, & Bloedel, 1994; Kwiatkowski & Shriberg, 1992; Weston & Shriberg, 1992). For instance, variables such as utterance length, fluency, word position, intelligibility of adjacent words, phonological complexity, grammatical form, and syllabic structure may have an effect on intelligibility judgments for a particular word (Weston & Shriberg, 1992). Kent, Miolo, and Bloedel (1994) summarized 19 different intelligibility evaluation procedures and discussed the issues to be considered in testing intelligibility. They concluded that no single method would be adequate for assessing intelligibility and that a clinician should use some combination of assessment devices. Selection of a measurement should consider the child's age, language abilities, other disabilities, time available for assessment/analysis, and the purpose of intelligibility testing.

There are few data relating intelligibility to age, although we know that children become more intelligible as they get older. Generally, a child of age 3 should be generally intelligible to strangers, and inability to understand a child of this age is reason for clinical intervention (Bernthal, Bankson, & Flipsen, 2009). Bernthal, Bankson, and Flipsen (2009, p. 221) reviewed the literature on childhood intelligibility and said: "Commonly accepted standards for intelligibility expectations are as follows: 3 years, 75 percent intelligible; 4 years, 85 percent intelligible; and 5 years, 95 percent intelligible."

A child will be more intelligible to those who know him or her well because the latter have unconsciously decoded the child's "system" of substitutions and omissions. Kwiatkowski and Shriberg (1992), however, found that caregivers evidenced more difficulty than was anticipated in glossing their children's speech and overestimated their children's syntactic development. Another variable affecting intelligibility is the sound that the child misarticulates. Some sounds occur more frequently in the language than others; and if the child's error is on a sound that occurs frequently, intelligibility will be affected to a greater degree than when errors are on infrequently occurring phonemes. An obvious factor that could logically affect intelligibility is the number of phonemes that a child misarticulates, although Shriberg and Kwiatkowski (1982b) did not find high correlations between total number of errors and intelligibility. Another variable affecting intelligibility may be the consistency of the error in the child's speech. This would also affect the PCC calculation. A final factor that can affect intelligibility could be the type of error (omissions, substitutions) that the child exhibits (Shriberg & Kwiatkowski, 1982b).

At the very least, a clinician can rate the client according to a rating scale. Fudala and Reynolds (1993) recommend using a continuum for rating intelligibility similar to the following:

1. Speech is not intelligible.
2. Speech is usually not intelligible.
3. Speech is difficult to understand.
4. Speech is intelligible with careful listening.
5. Speech is intelligible, although noticeably in error.
6. Speech is intelligible with occasional error.
7. Speech is totally intelligible.

Every assessment of articulatory ability should contain some judgment regarding intelligibility. This is a factor that can be an important deciding variable in making treatment recommendations.

COMPUTER-ASSISTED ANALYSIS OF PHONOLOGY

Much of the work in phonological analysis is laborious and repetitive. Some of the major difficulties are keeping track of the data on a host of different worksheets, tallying up percentages and frequency counts, and cross-checking a variety of relationships found in different portions of the client's transcript. The nature of these tasks is ideally suited to computer analysis. The computer can take a corpus of language and the gloss of each utterance and produce more information than even the most zealous clinician would like to know about a child's phonological system. In some cases, computer analyses of human behavior are rather superficial, and the programs available are just in the early stages of development. In the case of phonological analysis, however, the computer programs are detailed, user friendly, and here to stay! An analysis that might take a clinician several hours to accomplish can actually be completed in less than a few minutes by most programs. The software is compatible with the most popular types of hardware available in the majority of school systems, universities, and even households of prospective users. The programs differ in their scope, ranging from those designed to analyze the responses from a particular test of phonology to those focusing on the assessment of spontaneous samples of connected speech (Hodson, 1985, 2003; Masterson & Bernhardt, 2001; Long, Fey, & Channell, 2002; Shriberg, 1986). Long (http://www.computerizedprofiling.org) maintains a website that offers a downloadable language analysis program including a detailed phonological analysis module at no cost to users. This program is an excellent resource for clinicians who want to gain experience with computer analyses of language and phonology. The program has ample help screens and even videos related to the analyses. There is no question that computer applications offer the clinician tremendous options for analysis (Louko & Edwards, 2001; Masterson, 1999). Ingram and Ingram (2002) advocate using computer-assisted methods for sampling, transcription, and storage. They suggest recording the sample directly onto the computer as a WAVE file so the clinician will have a digital copy of the sample. This allows for ease in transcription, since there is no need to rewind an audiotape, and the sample can be copied to a CD-ROM for storage and later comparisons. It is also possible to interface this sample with various speech analysis programs so that waveforms can be analyzed, if this will aid in interpretation of the sample. One example of such a program is provided by http://www.sil.org and is called Speech Analyzer. This program is freeware and can be downloaded for use in analyzing wave files and subjecting them to spectrographic analysis.

It would be ideal if the client simply talked into a microphone that was plugged into a computer and in a few seconds a miraculous printout appeared that revealed the secrets of the phonological system. Unfortunately, this is not the case. The clinician must still obtain the sample, transcribe the sample, input the sample into the computer through the keyboard, and in many cases do some other work, responding to menus and prompts produced on the screen. The tasks just described constitute a lot of painstaking work on the part of the clinician. Just transcribing a sample of connected speech can take hours of careful listening. The beauty of computer-assisted analysis is that the clinician does not have to spend several *more* hours of organizing data, scanning the transcript over and over again, and performing mathematical operations. The computer also provides elegant summaries of the data, such as phonetic inventories, canonical shape analyses, positional inventories, phonological process analysis, measures of severity (e.g., PCC, PDS), and even suggested treatment targets with some programs.

Thus, one misconception that some people might have is that computer analysis takes away all tedious work on the part of the clinician. The truth is, it takes away much of this work, but not all. A second misconception some people may have is that the computer will always come up with the "right answer" with regard to a client's phonology. Although the algorithms in most phonology programs are quite sophisticated, they have difficulty dealing with idiosyncratic processes and certain types of analyses. The one thing the clinician can expect, however, is output; it may not always be correct, but it *is* output. A clinician should be aware of the limitations of phonological analysis programs and practice by running phonological samples that have been done by hand, to see if there is general agreement between the two methods.

LONG-TERM IMPACT OF PHONOLOGICAL DISORDERS

Research has confirmed that many individuals with speech sound impairments, whether they receive treatment or not, experience academic difficulties. This, of course, could be related to the co-occurrence of phonological and language disorders in the majority of cases. Lewis and Freebairn (1992) found that subjects with a history of preschool phonological disorders performed more poorly than matched controls did on measures of phonology, reading, and spelling for age groups from preschool to adult. Subjects with a history of language disorder, in addition to the phonological problem, performed even lower on the measures. In a 28-year longitudinal study, Felsenfeld, Broen, and McGue (1994) followed a group of children who had phonological disorders. These children had phonological disorders as preschoolers, and the problems persisted through first grade. When the researchers interviewed these subjects in adulthood, they found, in comparison to matched controls, reports of lower grades earned throughout school, more academic remedial services required, and fewer years of formal education completed. The subjects with a history of phonological disorder also tended to choose more semiskilled or unskilled occupations than the controls did. The long-lasting effects of speech sound disorder can even be seen in parents who were treated for articulation problems as children. Lewis et al. (2007) found that such adults scored lower on multisyllabic word repetition, nonword repetition, reading, spelling, and language tasks when compared to parents without a history of speech sound disorder. Although these abilities did not affect educational or occupational outcomes, they do suggest that residual effects are seen in adults with a history of speech sound disorder. Bird, Bishop, and Freeman (1995) found that children with phonological disorders scored well below controls on measures of phonological awareness and literacy. These researchers felt that children who start school with severe phonological impairments are especially at risk for developing reading and spelling difficulties.

In view of the relation between phonological disorders and academic performance, clinicians should not underestimate the importance of early assessment, intervention, and counseling.

7

Disorders of Fluency

Stuttering is a curious, sometimes astonishing, and certainly a difficult way to talk. Why is the flow of speech, seemingly so easy and automatic for others, marred by tense interruptions? Unfortunately, the answer to that question still eludes clinicians and researchers—stuttering remains an enigma.

The puzzling nature of stuttering creates a dilemma for students. Confronted with a voluminous literature and a large number of treatment possibilities—each with its advocates—it is easy to give up in despair. Perhaps the negative attitude held by so many clinicians toward people who stutter stems, in part, from overwhelming confusion about the disorder and the paucity of solid academic training (Yaruss, 1999; Yaruss & Quesal, 2002). Yet, for some beginning clinicians, the dramatic nature of the disorder and even the confusion among experts have a fascinating appeal; they present a challenge.

We will assume in this chapter that the reader has a good foundation concerning the nature of stuttering. Books by Bloodstein and Ratner (2008), Conture and Curlee (2008), Gregory et al. (2002), Guitar and McCauley (2009), and Yairi and Seery (2011) provide excellent discussions of the many aspects of stuttering. We present the following list of "facts" about stuttering that have diagnostic implications and have been gleaned from the literature. For purposes of exposition, we have eschewed lengthy lists of references. Each item can be documented, however, even though some might disagree with our particular selection or interpretation.

1. The basic speech characteristics of stuttering consist of relatively brief part-word (phonemic, syllabic) repetitions and prolongations. These oscillations and fixations may be audible or silent and tend to occur more frequently at the beginning of an utterance and on words and phrases more complex motorically (such as long words and less frequently used words).
2. Stuttering is a disorder of childhood, generally having its onset in preschool years (especially 2–5); rarely does it begin in older persons, and when it does it may be a distinct subtype of the disorder (such as neurotic and neurogenic stuttering).
3. Stuttering (also known as developmental stuttering and in parts of the world stammering) is found more frequently among males.

4. Stuttering tends to run in families.
5. Multiple etiologies may account for stuttering.
6. Stuttering may be precipitated (and perpetuated) by certain environmental events, particularly the critical, demanding behaviors of significant others, usually parents.
7. Stuttering tends to appear more frequently in children described as "sensitive," who may be vulnerable or susceptible to stress. People who stutter may have a low threshold for autonomic arousal.
8. Stuttering tends to appear more frequently in children who were slow in acquiring speech or who manifest certain inadequacies of oral communication (articulation errors, language disturbances) other than fluency breakdowns.
9. Stuttering tends to exhibit cycles of frequency and severity in a given individual.
10. A significant number of individuals recover from stuttering (perhaps 80%), while others persist.
11. Stuttering tends to change in form and severity as the individual matures.
12. Stuttering is eliminated or markedly reduced in a variety of conditions: speaking while alone, choral speaking, singing, prolonged or slow speaking, talking in time to rhythm, or under masking conditions.
13. Stuttering, in its developed form, consists largely of escape and avoidance behavior; that is, much of the overt abnormality results from the individual's attempt to cope with the emission of the basic speech disfluency.
14. Stuttering is also characterized by speech and voice abnormalities other than disfluency (such as narrow pitch range, vocal tension, lack of vocal expression, muscular lags, and asynchronies) that can be detected in nonstuttered speech. These anomalies *may* reflect a basic impairment of phonation (difficulty in initiating phonation, making consonant-vowel transitions), respiration (abnormal reflex activity), neuromotor coordination, or cortical integration; they *may,* however, simply be effects of stuttering.
15. Stuttering, in its developed form, is often associated with an expectancy or anticipation of its occurrence.
16. Stuttering becomes personal; individuals who stutter report fear, frustration, social penalties, dissatisfaction with themselves, lower level of aspiration, and felt loss of social esteem. There is a tendency for problems common to all human beings to become associated with the speech disturbance. However, there is no particular "stuttering personality," nor is the disorder a manifestation of psychoneurosis.

Even though the fluency disorder of stuttering remains a tantalizing mystery, there is much that we can do to help persons who seek our services.

DIFFERENTIAL DIAGNOSIS

Speech is fluent when words are produced easily, effortlessly, smoothly, quickly, and in a forward flow. Speech is disfluent when one word does not flow smoothly and quickly into the next. Obviously, then, all speakers are, at times, disfluent and these so-called normal disfluencies should be of no consequence. The SLP needs to be able to differentiate normal from abnormal disfluencies; often this proves to be no easy feat with young children. If the clinician does identify a speaker's disfluencies as abnormal or clinically significant, the next decision is to distinguish the problem of stuttering from other conditions in which speech fluency is disrupted. A final aspect of the differential diagnosis process may be to identify subtypes within the stuttering population, so as to select the most appropriate form of treatment. Let us discuss these three aspects of differential diagnosis; we will do so in a different order.

Sorting Out the Types of Fluency Disorders

Assuming that the clinician has already identified a speaker as having abnormal amounts or types of disfluencies, the diagnostic task is one of deciding *which* disorder of fluency is exhibited. Along with a behavioral analysis of the disfluencies, the case history information will go far in suggesting the disorder type. We will provide an overview of some of the fluency breakdowns that can be confused with the common variety of stuttering, called developmental stuttering (or simply, stuttering).

EPISODIC STRESS REACTION   It is well known that most speakers exhibit some degree of disfluency—revisions, interjections, word and phrase repetitions, and occasionally even part-word repetitions and prolongations. Speech fluency is often considered a sensitive barometer of a person's psychological state. Stress tends to increase a speaker's disfluency, as seen in stage fright.

Fluency breakdowns owing to episodic stress show a number of consistent identifying features: an acknowledged source of intense or prolonged stimulation; tension overflow throughout the body (including the oral area), which may also produce a tremulous voice; an exacerbation of "normal" disfluency, including broken words, incomplete phrases, interjections, and repetitions of whole and part-words; and no avoidance but feelings of fear. Finally, the most crucial characteristic is that the disfluency decreases markedly or stops when (or shortly after) the stress terminates. These acute, or episodic, periods of disfluency are usually not clinically significant.

PSYCHOGENIC STUTTERING   Most persons who stutter, particularly confirmed adult cases, acquire a negative feeling about their speech. One of our clients summarized it succinctly when he said, "Stutterers are bugged because they are plugged." A few clients, however, show symptoms of a primary neurosis—they are "plugged because they are bugged." For these individuals, stuttering is a maladaptive solution to an acute psychological problem. Psychogenic stuttering has also been known as neurotic or hysterical stuttering. Referral to or a team approach with other health care professionals may be in order. The SLP is well equipped to diagnose and treatment the overt symptoms.

> Colleen, an eighth-grade parochial school pupil, began to stutter suddenly following the death of her parents in an automobile accident. She collapsed upon hearing the tragic news and remained mute, almost transfixed and catatonic, for several hours. During the planning for the funeral and extended period of the wake, she started to stutter—a monotonous repetition of the initial syllable of words. She showed no struggle, no avoidance behavior. She looked directly at the listener when she spoke and smiled bravely. We followed this case closely until the remission of stuttering two months later, and her disfluency was always the same; it never varied in form or severity from situation to situation. When she read a passage several times, she did not show the typical reduction (adaptation) in stuttering. School documents, as well as interviews with several relatives, indicated that Colleen had no prior speech difficulty. One maternal aunt whom we interviewed did recall, however, that the girl had several "spells" of uncontrolled weeping and laughing during her first menses the year before. The child had received an incredible amount of attention and solace after her parents' death, perhaps even more so because of her "stuttering," from sympathetic adults.

Psychogenic stuttering is a rare fluency disorder that is characterized by a sudden onset of rather severe stuttering. The onset may occur at any age, including adulthood, yet usually happens in an older child. Some severe (and lasting rather than episodic) psychological trauma, emotional upheaval, or stress seems to precipitate the occurrence of stuttering. In contrast to the exacerbation of "normal" disfluencies seen in episodic stress, the neurotic stuttering pattern is severe from the beginning, typically with unvoiced prolongations, laryngeal blocks, tension, or lengthy repetitions. Although highly aware of these sudden and severe disfluencies, the person may or may not be frustrated by them. The level of concern and motivation to change are important elements for the SLP to assess, as they may shape the prognosis for change and the direction of intervention.

NEUROGENIC STUTTERING   Stuttering, or a stutteringlike subset of fluency disorders, may occur following nervous system damage in adolescents or adults. Neurogenic stuttering may occur as a result of stroke, traumatic brain injury, infection, or tumor. Nervous system disorders like Parkinson's disease or Tourette syndrome are frequently affiliated with disfluencies and tic-like movements. The designation of neurogenic stuttering establishes these as fluency disorders. We also have observed disfluency in clients suffering from some types of cerebral palsy, apraxia of speech, and other neurological impairments. There are also reports of fluency disruptions in alcoholics, drug addicts, patients afflicted with AIDS and with dialysis dementia. Palilalia, perhaps a subtype of neurogenic stuttering, may be caused by bilateral subcortical brain damage. Individuals with palilalia repeat words and entire phrases, typically not sounds or syllables, and they do so with increasing speed and diminishing loudness.

Several patients with aphasia with whom we have worked, particularly those clients who show good progress in word finding but who have residual syntactic difficulty, exhibited fluency breakdowns superficially similar to stuttering.

> Mrs. Horn had suffered an aneurysm in the Circle of Willis, leaving her hemiplegic, apraxic, and with mild expressive aphasia. When we examined her, almost a year after the cerebral vascular episode, her speech pattern resembled clonic stuttering. She would begin a word, repeat a phoneme or syllable several times, back up, and try again; if blocked once more, a repetition might reverberate almost endlessly. She frequently pounded on the table as if to time her utterances. We could discern no evidence of fear or avoidance, just severe frustration. Interestingly, when she spoke or read swiftly her fluency increased dramatically; she also talked freely when distracted from closely monitoring the acts of speaking. Here is a sample of her speech taken from a tape recording during a group session: "I can't-I can't (sigh) . . . I-I-I-I have tr-trouble with my, ah, with my speech . . . and, ah, my leg is, is, you know is, stiff."

The disfluencies noted are rather typical: whole-word repetitions, revisions, interjections, broken words, and gaps in the flow of speech. This client had difficulty formulating messages and then programming the proper motor sequences to utter the thought. Unlike stuttering where the difficulty is getting started, Mrs. Horn's fluency breakdowns occurred at any point in a sentence.

The Stuttering Foundation (http://www.stutteringhelp.org) provides brochures on neurogenic stuttering that are useful with clients and families. The Tourette Syndrome Association maintains a home page at http://www.TSA-USE.org. Much research on neurogenic stuttering exists; one we recommend on disfluencies associated with stroke and traumatic brain injury is by Jokel, De Nil, and Sharpe (2007).

CLUTTERING   Cluttering is sometimes confused with stuttering, but it encompasses more than just a disorder of fluency. Cluttering has varied symptomatology and co-occurs with other speech, language, and behavioral disorders. Cluttering symptoms may include part- and whole-word repetitions (including repetitions of multisyllabic words), mazing disfluencies (too frequent to be within normal limits for false starts, revisions, and fillers or interjections), omissions of syllables and small words (telegraphic speech), excess speech rates (tachylalia), speech disrhythmia (spurts of speech), misarticulations, lack of awareness of how the speech sounds and poor monitoring of it, syntactic disorganization, short attention span, perceptual issues, poorly organized thinking, and possible motor disabilities (wise to assess diadochokinetic rate). Other academic difficulties, noted by clinicians, teachers, and researchers, include reading and writing disorders, difficulty with many language-dependent skills (owing to subtle language disorders), lack of rhythm and musical ability, and restlessness and hyperactivity (Daly, 1986). Of course, not all these symptoms need to be present in a child or adult for a diagnosis of cluttering. Excessive rate of speech seems to be the hallmark feature of cluttering along with poor intelligibility owing to some of the speech-language symptoms just cited. In addition to Daly, the information from the ASHA Forum (2009), Myers (1996), Myers and St. Louis (1996), and Van Zaalen-op't Hof et al. (2009) are particularly useful in understanding this fluency disorder and in making a differential diagnosis apart from that of stuttering. The Stuttering Foundation (http://www.stutteringhelp.org) offers a DVD and brochure on cluttering that may be useful to clients and clinicians alike. Information, resources, and support are available through the International Cluttering Association (ICA) online at http://associations.missouristate.edu/ICA/header.htm.

> Ralph was referred to us as a person who stutters by his industrial education supervisor during his semester of student teaching. When we examined him, he revealed no fears or avoidances, exhibited only a few short part-word repetitions, and had no fixations; he said that he enjoyed talking, did a lot of it, and that he was asked frequently to repeat himself, "especially when I talk fast." Ralph's difficulty seemed to take place on the phrase or sentence level; his interruptions broke the integrity of a thought rather than a word. In addition, he frequently omitted syllables and transposed words and phrases; he said "plobably," "posed," and "pacific" for "probably," "supposed," and "specific." Ralph's speech was sprinkled with spoonerisms (he said "beta dase" for "data base") and malapropisms (he described getting lost while hunting because the road he was following "dissipated" and told us he had a good "dialect" going with his roommate). His speech was swift and jumbled; it emerged in rapid torrents until he jammed up, and then he surged on again in another staccato outburst. In spontaneous talking, his message was characterized by disorganized sentences and poor phrasing. He gave the overall impression of being in great haste. When we asked him to slow down and speak carefully, there was a drastic improvement, but he soon forgot our admonishment and reverted to his hurried, disorganized style. By and large, Ralph was unaware and indifferent to his fluency problem. He was an impatient, impulsive young man, always on the go. His course work was characteristically done in a great, almost compulsive rush; he had difficulty reading, and his handwriting was a scrawl.

Distinguishing among Subtypes of Stuttering

Are there different kinds of developmental stuttering? Although there is no conclusive answer to that question, clinical opinion is that there must be—if only to explain the wide variety of clients, symptomatologies, and responses to intervention programs. Possibilities that come to mind include interiorized and exteriorized speaker characteristics; predominantly clonic (repetitive disfluencies) and predominantly tonic (with tension, prolongations, and blockages) persons who stutter; clients who feature escape techniques; those who are addicted to avoidance; and those who can predict an occurrence of stuttering and those who cannot. Perhaps there are even variations in stuttering that stem from cultural influences. These distinctions may be useful in planning treatment and are explored in Chapter 12.

Differentiating Stuttering from Nonstuttering Disfluencies

We saved this aspect of the differential diagnosis for last, although the clinician must determine it first. It is a vast topic. The literature shows good agreement regarding the general principles for distinguishing between stuttering and nonstuttering types of disfluency. All speakers are disfluent from time to time. Where to draw the line segmenting typical from atypical types and amounts of disfluency is still a matter of clinical debate and philosophy. Some maintain that persons who stutter and persons who do not stutter commit the same sorts of disfluencies initially, but that parents and others in the immediate environment react negatively and cause the child's speech to spiral unacceptably—with more fragmentation and tension the by-product in speech. In contrast, and based on considerable research evidence, the current philosophy holds that young nonstuttering and stuttering children's disfluencies are categorically divergent. Let us begin our discussion with the various types of speech disfluencies. A nonexhaustive list of some types of disfluencies includes the following and, as we will see, some types pose more concern than other, innocuous types.

1. Whole-word repetition: "My, my ball went under the car."
2. Part-word repetition (either easy or with tense; fleeting or with multiple interation): "My i-i-ice cream is melting."
3. Phrase repetition: "I want, I want some ice cream."
4. Sentence revision: "It went—My ball went under the car."
5. Filled pause/Interjections (fillers include *uhm, ah, uh):* "I want some . . . uhm . . . ice cream."
6. Unfilled pause (either relaxed hesitation or tense silence/inaudible block): "Daddy, I want (relaxed pause before next word) some ice cream." "Daddy, I (lips in posture for /w/ but blocked and unable to flow forward in audible speech) want some ice cream."
7. Sound prolongations: "SSSSSSally took my ball."
8. Broken word (same as numbers 5 and 6)

Some of these types of disfluency overlap by definition, and frankly, some of these types of disfluency are of more concern than others. Keeping track of so many types of disfluency can be clinically cumbersome and imprecise.

The often-cited works by Yairi's research team at the University of Illinois segmented stuttering-like disfluencies (SLDs) from other disfluencies (ODs) (Ambrose & Yairi, 1994; Ambrose & Yairi, 1999; Yairi & Ambrose, 1992, 2005; Yairi, Ambrose, & Niermann, 1993; Yairi & Lewis, 1984). The types of disfluencies that characterize SLDs and ODs are shown in Table 7.1. By describing only three types of stuttering-like disfluencies, Yairi simplifies the multitude of descriptors that have been used. Disrhythmic phonations encompasses events such as within word disruptions of air flow, sound prolongations, blocks (whether audible or inaudible), instances of noticeable stress, as well as unusual patterns of intonation.

TABLE 7.1	Stuttering-Like Disfluencies (SLDs) as Compared to Other Disfluencies (ODs)

Three SLDs	Example ODs
Part-word repetitions	Interjections
Single syllable word repetitions	Polysyllabic word repetitions
Dysrhythmic phonations	Phrase repetitions
	Revisions

What types of disfluencies and other factors represent early signs of concern for the onset of stuttering? How should a speech-language pathologist proceed? There are many opinions in answer to these questions. There also are many tools available to the SLP for appraising developmental stuttering near onset in the preschool years as well as for adolescents and adults with persistent stuttering. Gordon and Luper (1992) reviewed six often-used protocols for identifying beginning stuttering. Two of these will be mentioned here. Adams (1977) provides a clinical strategy for differentiating the normal-speaking child from one beginning to stutter; his criteria and guidelines for clinical interpretation are summarized in Table 7.2. Also useful is the Protocol for Differentiating the Incipient Stutterer (Pindzola, 1988; Pindzola & White, 1986).

In making decisions about common disfluency versus stuttering disfluency, the clinician should be guided by information available in the literature. The clinician then pulls together a vast array of information collected on and about the client to arrive at a diagnosis. We admit this is a judgment call on the part of the clinician, but if the evaluation is done thoroughly, it is an "informed" judgment call. Overt features we like to assess include:

- Predominant type of disfluency (SLDs versus ODs)
- Frequency of disfluency

TABLE 7.2	Adams's Guidelines for Distinguishing between the Normally Disfluent Child and the Incipient Stutterer

	Guidelines for Interpretation	
Criterion	Nonstuttering Disfluent	Incipient Stutterer
Total frequency (all types)	9 or fewer disfluencies per 100 words	10 or more disfluencies per 100 words
Predominate type	Whole-word and phrase repetitions, interjections, and revisions	Part-word repetitions, audible and silent prolongations, and broken words
Unit repetitions	No more than 2 unit repetitions ("b-b-ball")	At least 3 repetitions ("b-b-b-ball")
Voicing and air flow	Little or no difficulty starting or sustaining voicing or air flow; continuous phonation during part-word repetitions	Frequent difficulty in starting or sustaining voicing or air flow; heard in association with part-word repetitions, prolongations, and broken words; more effortful disfluencies
Intrusion of the schwa	Schwa not perceived ("ba-ba-baby")	Schwas often perceived ("buh-buh-buh-baby")

- Duration of the disfluencies
- Speech rhythm and rate
- Presence of any learned behaviors and physical involvement

We have discussed various types of disfluencies, but now a few words about how to get a frequency count since it is an important diagnostic measure. The clinician first must determine what to count, meaning that the SLP must adopt an acceptable system of types to include or exclude. Yaruss (1998) described a real-time analysis method of counting fluent and disfluent words (or syllables) from a speech sample. On graph paper or a page marked with small blocks for marking words (or syllables) spoken, instances of disfluent words (or syllables) are coded as R for repetition, P for prolongation, B for block, lowercase p or - for long pause, rv or x for revision, and F for filler/starter. A percentage of disfluency can then be calculated (number disfluent divided by total disfluent + fluent). Totals per type of disfluency can also be analyzed for pattern trends.

Yairi and Ambrose (2005) illustrated how to track and tally information about stuttering-like disfluencies from a speech sample. The number of times a unit is repeated is marked for duration analysis. Frequency is calculated using the SLD notation as follows. DP indicates disrhythmic phonation, PW indicates part-word repetition, and SS is a single-syllable word repetition. The following is provided:

"Mmmmake a snake" (1 DP)

"Sitting on the the the couch" (1 SS with 2 units)

"Lllllike th- th- th- th- that" (1 DP and 1 PW with 4 units)

In this example from a 100-syllable speech sample, the client demonstrated a total of 4 SLDs. The percent of stuttered syllables, then, is 4% (total of 4 divided by 100 syllables).

It should be obvious to the reader by now that the type of disfluency that predominates in a client's speech and the size of the speech unit affected by the breakdown influence society's judgment of fluency normalcy. For example, repetitions of whole phrases are quite common in all speakers; whole-word repetitions are disfluencies typical of both persons who do and persons who do not stutter. Yet the predominance of part-word repetitions distinguishes stuttered from nonstuttered speech (especially if done frequently) and this is true in preschool children and adults. Hesitations or pauses before phrases or before words may, likewise, be less worrisome than such gaps within words (i.e., preceding syllables or sounds) or when accompanied with tension. The rule of thumb is that the smaller the speech unit affected, the more abnormal the disfluency.

The frequency with which disfluent behaviors occur has long been recognized as important in the diagnosis of stuttering. As we have shown, there are various types of disfluenceis and ways to measure them for use clinically. A host of normative data is also available for the different systems. A clinician needs to be careful in applying similar systems and interpretative data. Dissimilar information is not interchangeable. Using the popular and straightforward distinction between stuttering-like disfluencies (SLDs) as opposed to other disfluencies (ODs), norms reported by Yairi and Seery (2011) are summarized in Table 7.3.

As part of the assessment, the clinician will gauge the duration of the client's disfluency. This is often expressed as an average number of reiterations of the repetition or as an average amount of time stuck in an audible or silent prolongation (disrhythmic phonation). If the typical duration of prolongations exceeds 1 second, or if repetitions involve numerous reiterations—say, three to five or more—then these behaviors may be interpreted as signs of concern, perhaps

TABLE 7.3	Percent Syllables Disfluent in Preschool Children Who Do and Do Not Stutter	
Disfluency Type	**Mean Percent Disfluent for Children Who Stutter**	**Mean Percent Disfluent for Children Who Do Not Stutter**
SLDs (part-word repetitions, single-syllable repetitions dysrhymic phonations)	over 11%	under 2%
Other disfluencies (ODs)	over 5%	under 5%

stuttering. Audible effort while speaking is not typical and therefore when noticed may be indicative of stuttering. There are many signs of audible effort; some examples include disrupted airflow, hard contacts (explosive, crisp articulation), effort or tension heard in the voice, and a pitch rise during a moment of stuttering.

Clinicians over the years reported perceiving the presence of the neutral schwa vowel, rather than the appropriate vowel, in the part-word repetitions of persons who stutter, regardless of age, and that this was not heard in the occasional part-word repetition of a nonstuttering person. An example in the word soap is "suh-suh-soap" as compared to "so-so-soap." This has been confirmed by some acoustic research. Another audible insight into differentiating stuttering from nonstuttering may be the overall impression and speech naturalness. When adults or children who do not stutter have speech repetitions, those disfluencies preserve the normal rhythm and rate of speech. Not until the tempo of the multiple reiterations speeds up or the rhythm becomes irregular and choppy is there substantial reason for concern. The SLP, then, should subjectively judge the client's rhythm, tempo, and speed of disfluencies when trying to make a differential diagnosis.

The presence of learned behaviors, also called secondary characteristics, is strongly suggestive of stuttering, rather than other innocuous disfluencies. The clinician therefore should determine whether the client uses concealment devices (such as word substitutions or talking around a word, which is called a circumlocution), postponement devices, starting tricks, and so forth. Visually, the clinician may note physical involvement of the facial, head, and body regions. Frequently observed contortions are eye blinks, wrinkling of the forehead, distortions of the mouth, overt mandibular tension, head jerks, and the more subtle head turnings to divert eye contact.

Once the SLP has made a differential diagnosis and determined that the client is stuttering, the next issue to be resolved is the developmental progression or severity of the disorder. In actuality, the information gathered to differentiate normal from abnormal speech is part of the same kind of information needed to determine the level of severity. Assessment instruments guide the SLP in determing the severity level (mild, moderate, and severe). Following that, the next decision that confronts the clinician is the recommended course of action. Is treatment warranted? If so, the assessment information should help the SLP decide on the direction of intervention and treatment goals.

THE APPRAISAL OF STUTTERING

In our discussion of making a differential diagnosis, we glossed over the details of how to obtain the information necessary to make such a decision. What information is necessary? What published appraisal instruments are available to help collect and make sense of this information? What less tangible factors need to be judged, albeit subjectively, by the clinician? We will now try to answer these questions. Bear in mind, however, that the answers may differ for different clients, depending on their age, intelligence, reading abilities, and so forth.

Case History Information and Parent Materials

We will discuss two forms of the case history intake: one done with the parents of a child who stutters or is beginning to stutter and one done with a teenager or adult who stutters.

INITIAL INTERVIEW WITH THE PARENTS   The initial interview with the parents of a child beginning to stutter is of critical importance. We must establish our professional competence, demonstrate our genuine interest, and convince the parents that we can be trusted. In short, our primary task in this initial contact is to build a relationship for subsequent counseling sessions. We also listen carefully to the parents' presenting story: How do they see the child's problem? In their view, what might have caused it? What do they identify as their role in the onset of the child's stuttering? What expectations and apprehensions do they have regarding the nature and the outcome of treatment?

  We like to regard the initial interaction between parents and clinician as a time for information gathering and information sharing. As we said, we first want to hear the presenting complaint—and encourage the telling of their child's speech story. We may opt to be more or less directive in our style with the parents; it does not matter, so long as the information we need unfolds. A parent's careful review of the many factors involved in the child's problem tends to foster objectivity. It also shifts the focus away from a general impression of "trouble" to the observation of specific behaviors. Here are some questions we use as guides in assembling information from parents:

1. When did the child begin exhibiting disfluencies?
2. What were the circumstances under which the disfluencies were noted?
3. How long has the child been exhibiting the disfluencies?
4. What changes have been noted in the frequency or form of the disfluencies?
5. What factors seem to increase or decrease the child's disfluency?
6. In what ways has the family tried to help the child?
7. What is the child's reaction to the family's efforts to help?

Additional items to assess in obtaining a case history include (1) a specific review of the familial incidence of stuttering; (2) the impact, if any, of siblings, relatives, teachers, or babysitters upon the child; (3) a description of how the child spends a typical day; and (4) a description of any prior professional treatment.

  The case history interview can be done either before or after the child has been seen and evaluated by the clinician. Consequently, this initial meeting may, in fact, involve several points of interaction or separate sessions. We try to refrain from being influenced by the parent's push for us to provide too much information prematurely; naturally, they want to know what caused their child's disfluency and what can be done (quickly) about it. We, however, do enlist the parent's help in collecting observations of the child's behavior in the home environment.

  What things at home seem to promote fluency and what seems to promote disfluency? Is it all right for the parents to remind the child to "slow down" (as advocated by Cooper & Cooper, 2004; Shine, 1988; and Yairi & Ambrose, 2005), or is that counterproductive and something to be considered taboo (owing to earlier philosophies)? We do not know the answers to these questions for a *particular* child; the parents must find out. Parents' recording of home behaviors is a clinically useful assignment.

We often find that simply asking parents to monitor the antecedents and consequences of their child's speech disfluencies is sufficiently motivating to engender change. Enviromental events that disrupt a child's flow of speech typically become obvious when parents begin to chart. The work of Ratner (2004) is recommended to the reader as she dispels some commonly held beliefs on caregiver-child interactions that have clear implications for counseling and treatment.

Even though there is much information that we simply cannot give the parents early on (often because we do not yet know the information), clinicians have a responsibility to help educate the parents. That is to say, clinicians need to provide a good understanding of stuttering and its many ramifications. In addition to what clinicians say, they like to provide the parents with reading materials; some are of their own preparation, while others are brochures and booklets from published sources such as the Stuttering Foundation (http://www.stutteringhelp.org) and the American Speech-Language-Hearing Association (http://www.asha.org). Videos and printed matter available from these sources are invaluable in helping parents understand how they can help children.

The clinician may wish to have one or both parents complete a checklist or questionnaire that may prove useful in identifying parental perceptions, attitudes, and topics in need of exploration at subsequent counseling sessions. Most texts on stuttering guide the clinician in such areas, as does the Parent Attitudes Toward Stuttering Checklist in the program by Cooper and Cooper (2004).

It is important that parents obtain some closure from these initial interviews. Let us demonstrate a typical conversation, showing how we relate our diagnostic findings to the parents of a client named Stephen.

> Stephen does indeed have some breaks in speech, more than normal for a child of his age. He is doing some stuttering, but it is still the "good kind": He is not struggling or avoiding and, most important, he doesn't seem to be very aware that talking is tough (we drew a rough sketch of the stuttering gauge depicted in Figure 7.1 and showed them that Stephen exhibited only the first three early danger signs of stuttering). We want to prevent the disorder from developing further and cannot do anything without your help. We need to find out why he is having speech breaks; we need to know when he does it, under what circumstances. In short, we have to start looking at behaviors, at what he *does,* not a condition he *has.* In many cases like this, if we identify and alter certain enviromental situations, the child stops stuttering. You were very wise to bring him in now, before the fear and frustration have a chance to develop. Let's plan on meeting again tomorrow, and together we can begin to review Stephen's background and then decide how to gather information on what is happening now.

CASE HISTORY INTERVIEW WITH OLDER CLIENTS   The case history and initial interview with an older client who stutters are obviously different from those we just described. Prior to undertaking formal observation and testing, clinicians like to perform an intake interview. This brief preliminary discussion is designed to accomplish four objectives: (1) to inform the client what to expect in the diagnostic session, (2) to determine why the client is coming for treatment at this particular time, (3) to assemble historical information, and (4) to establish a working relationship.

Because the clinician wants the client to be a partner in the exploration of the problem, it is important for the client to know *what* the clinician intends to do and *why* the clinician proposes to do it. The clinician also likes to determine why the client is coming (or being sent) to an SLP

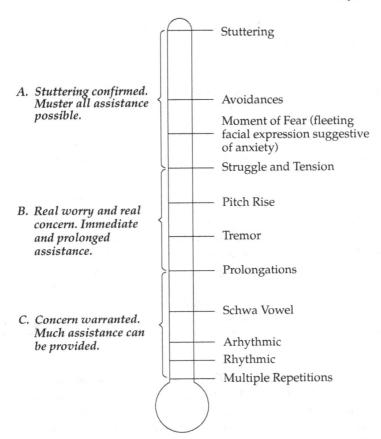

FIGURE 7.1 Signs of concern depicted vertically.

at this particular point in time. Has the individual undergone a "bottoming-out" experience, a severe crisis in his or her social, occupational, or educational life? What does he or she expect from treatment? What do others expect? Answers to these questions are useful in determining the client's motivation and in making a prognosis. All in all, the initial contact with a client is of inestimable importance in establishing a working relationship.

Differentiating and Predictive Scales

As we discussed earlier in this chapter, one of the clinician's major responsibilities is differentiating normal speakers having usual disfluencies from persons who are stuttering. This may be obvious in the evaluation of some clients, but it may be quite difficult with others—particularly young children.

Complicating the issue further with young children is the notion of spontaneous recovery. Estimates are that as many as 80% of the children who begin to stutter recover after a transient period of stuttering. The transient period is believed to conclude within the first 18 to 24 months after onset for reasons that are not well understood (Finn, 1998; Mansson, 2000; Yairi et al., 1996; Yairi & Seery, 2011). Although clinicians are far from being able to precisely differentiate children who will recover from stuttering from those that will not, SLPs do have some help. The

TABLE 7.4 Child Risk Factors Believed to Be Important in Prognosing Recovery versus Persistence of Stuttering

Of Top Importance

Frequency of disfluence	stable or increasing amounts over time suggestive of persistence
Gender	boys are at higher risk
Family history	persistent stuttering more likely when relatives stutter
Time elapsed since onset	after 3 years of stuttering the chance of natural recovery diminishes to about 15%

Of Importance

Types of disfluencies	SLDs rather than ODs
Stuttering severity	more severe may or may not be more persistent
Phonological skills	coexisting disorder is complicating factor
Language skills	coexisting disorder is complicating factor
Motor coordination	coexisting oral motor abilities (diadochokinesis) may be complicating factor
Environmental	parental/society assistance, not ridicule, may aid recovery

Stuttering Chronicity Prediction Checklist (Cooper & Cooper, 2004) and the Stuttering Prediction Instrument for Young Children (Riley, 1981) are examples of published and available prediction instruments, though with poor predictive validity as reviewed by Biddle et al. (2002). In the hands of an experienced clinician, all assessment indices provide information useful in "projecting" who will and who will not recover from stuttering. Table 7.4 summarizes important symptoms and risk factors helpful in projecting stuttering recovery as opposed to persistence (Yairi & Ambrose, 2005). Those that do not recover—with or without intervention—may be said to have persistent stuttering that can be managed or improved in therapy but not likely eliminated.

Geetha and colleagues (2000) report differentiating normal childhood disfluencies from stuttering using a computer program termed ANN, Artificial Neural Network. With 92% predictive accuracy, the computer program relies on input from historical, attitudinal, behavioral, and general development information as garnered from traditional clinical interviews and from a variety of published instruments.

Clinicians have at their disposal, either commercially or in research publications, an assortment of tools that guide the assessment and interpretative process. The assessment of overt, observable features of stuttering is more straightforward than covert features that tend to be less observable, hidden, and subjective. Table 7.5 lists many of the available assessment instruments, useful for a variety of overt purposes.

Severity Scales

The clinician's primary mission in the evaluation of a person who stutters is to perform a careful analysis of the individual's speech disfluency behavior. Not only is this necessary for differential diagnosis, but also for the appraisal of the severity of the disorder. With regard to treatment, the disfluency assessment also accomplishes two basic purposes: It delineates the behaviors to be

TABLE 7.5	Some Available Instruments for the Assessment of Overt Features of Stuttering, Including Diagnostic, Severity, and Predictive Scales

A Protocol for Differentiating the Incipient Stutterer
   (Pindzola, 1988; Pindzola & White, 1986)

A Stuttering Chronicity Prediction Checklist
   (Cooper & Cooper, 2004)

Assessment Form: Systematic Fluency Training for Young Children
   (Shine, 1988)

Client and Clinician Perceptions of Stuttering Severity Ratings
   (Cooper & Cooper, 2003, 2004)

Concomitant Stuttering Behavior Checklist
   (Cooper & Cooper, 2003, 2004)

Self-Rating of Stuttering Severity
   (O'Brian & Packman, 2004)

Stuttering Frequency and Duration Estimate Record
   (Cooper & Cooper, 2003, 2004)

Stuttering Interview (Forms A and B)
   (Ryan, 1974)

Stuttering Prediction Instrument for Young Children
   (Riley, 1981)

Stuttering Severity Instrument for Children and Adults (SSI-4)
   (Riley, 2009)

altered, and it provides a base measure to which the clinician can refer when monitoring the impact of treatment. The majority of published assessment instruments help the clinician determine the extent of the speech problem. We will call these instruments *severity scales,* whether or not the score from the test yields a severity modifier, such as "mild" to "very severe."

Table 7.5 listed some of the available instruments that assess the overt features of stuttering. By using a variety of these instruments, many aspects of the stuttering problem can be tapped, including the frequency of disfluency, the duration of the disfluency, the physical behaviors that accompany speech attempts, and so forth. Judging from the length of this (nonexhaustive) list, there are many severity scales from which to choose. We will highlight a commonly used scale of severity. In wide use is the Stuttering Severity Instrument for Children and Adults, which is now in its fourth edition (Riley, 2009). This SSI-4 is useful with both children and adults and has provisions for testing those who can and cannot read. The number of syllables stuttered and the number of total syllables spoken are computed by the SLP as the client reads or is engaged in conversation. Frequency, expressed as percentage of stuttered syllables, is then computed. The clinician also monitors the duration of the longest stuttering events and rates the presence and conspicuousness of physical behaviors concomitant with the speech attempts. Frequency, duration, and physical concomitant task scores are then combined for a total score. The fourth edition also includes an assessment of the individual's speech naturalness, though this does not contribute to the severity score. The severity of the client's stuttering can be ascertained by comparing the total score to the normative data provided in the test manual. Stuttering severity may be described as very mild, mild, moderate, severe, or very severe in this manner. The SSI-4 kit includes optional computerized software for assistance in scoring. This recent edition also addresses its reliability and validity, a weakness that was previously raised.

Though probably the best referenced and most widely used assessment tool for overt stuttering, Biddle at al. (2002) determined that the third edition of the SSI met stringent validity criteria but not reliability criteria. Despite norms being available with the published commercial tool, independent normative data from other sources were lacking in the literature.

The appraisal of the overt symptoms of stuttering need not require administration of a commercial test. The clinician's analysis, whether using a formal published test or an informal look at a speech sample, should include a thorough description of the stuttering pattern (topography) and measures of the relative frequency with which various features of the pattern occur. Starkweather and Givens-Ackerman (1997) believe that the assessment can even be reduced to a bare minimum so long as three aspects of fluency are measured. These are the client's speech rate (usually, total number of syllables divided by total number of seconds talking), articulatory rate (number of syllables per second—with disfluencies excluded), and speech continuity (the extent to which speech flows without interruptions, such as repetitions, filled pauses, or broken words).

Some clinicians prefer to measure speech rate at the word level; others measure at the syllable level. The average conversational rate of normal-speaking adult males is 168 words per minute (wpm) and 221 syllables per minute (spm). Adult females tend to speak slower and use longer but fewer words. Their conversational speech rates an average 151 wpm or 204 spm (Lutz & Mallard, 1986). Clinicians often assume that it is possible to convert between word and syllable counts for basic clinician measures, but be cautious. The existing conversion factor of approximately 1.5 syllables per word derives from adult speech samples. Slower speaking rates of 3–5-year-old children generally range between 119–183 syllables per minute (Pindzola, Jenkins, & Lokken, 1989). If counting words, young children produce fewer multisyllabic words than do adults. Yaruss (2000) demonstrated that a conversion factor of 1.15 syllables per word is more accurate and stable for children ages 3 to 5.

The Assessment Process

We will now walk the reader through our assessment process as shown in Figure 7.2 in a stylized form. We often begin with the discussion of the presenting complaint and with nonstandardized testing to obtain a disfluency analysis of a representative sample of the client's speech. The operative word here is *representative;* stuttering is an intermittent disorder, and the amount of difficulty an individual has is contingent on the speaking task, the situation, and other variables. If it is possible, there are obvious advantages to collecting samples of the client's "real" communication in naturalistic settings—the playground, informal group situations, the family dinner table. Generally, however, clinicians rely on data obtained from speaking tasks, such as reading aloud a standard passage, giving a monologue, or conversing. Be sure to tape-record, or, even better, videotape, the session and note the time elapsed for each segment of the total sample: It will then be easier to specify rather precise frequency and severity values. We always ask the client to discuss both neutral topics (hobbies, sports, vacations) and threatening topics (family, school, dating) to ensure that we obtain a range of speaking difficulty. It is important to know what produces stress and how the individual responds to it; we experiment in the session with things like hurrying the client, feigning listener loss, and asking the client to repeat.

AN OVERALL DESCRIPTION   We begin the analysis with a global description of the individual's speech behavior. What is his or her typical speech like in terms of rate, rhythm, degree of tension, articulation, and voice? What are the salient features of the stuttering pattern?

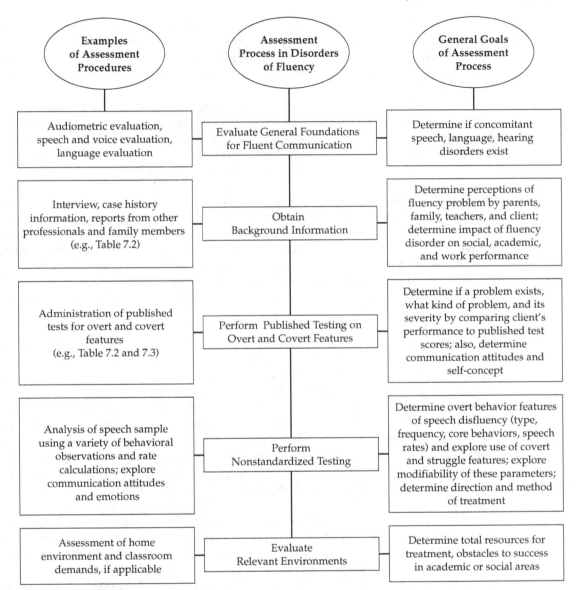

FIGURE 7.2   Critical assessment process in disorders of fluency.

CORE BEHAVIORS   The lowest common denominators of the problem of stuttering seem to be repetitions (oscillative phenomena) and prolongations (fixative phenomena). Although other overt disfluencies and related behaviors are part of stuttering, most individuals have either predominately repetitive or predominately tense disfluency patterns—with a dose of variability thrown in. A key feature of the disfluency analysis, therefore, is a precise description of these core behaviors. The methods of counting, presented earlier, need to be decided upon for a thorough description and comparison to norms.

With respect to *repetitions,* the clinician wants to identify the size of the unit (phrase, whole-word, syllable), the duration or number of oscillations per unit (e.g., b-boy vs. b-b-b-b-boy), their tempo and degree of tension involved, and how they are terminated. Are there silent oscillations of articulatory postures? Does the client have difficulty finding the proper vowel during the course of the repetitions?

In terms of *prolongations,* the clinician is interested in the anatomical site of the fixations, whether they are silent or audible, how long they last, the degree of tension involved, and how they are terminated. *Disrhythmic phonation* is an umbrella term for a collection of SLDs such as within-word disruptions of air flow, sound prolongations, blocks (whether audible or inaudible), instances of noticeable stress, as well as unusual patterns of intonation.

STRUGGLE-TENSION FEATURES   Very rarely does a client exhibit *only* repetitions and prolongations. Anyone who has observed persons who stutter knows that they appear tense and often make irrelevant sounds and movements while attempting to speak. Persons who stutter display a wide variety of these physical mannerisms, which may vary in frequency of occurrence and degree of involvement in particular clients; some individuals manifest an astounding array of eye blinking, head jerking, postponement rituals, and other behaviors, whereas others appear relatively quiescent, at least overtly. The clinician should take note of these "accessory features." Several scales listed in Table 7.5 can be used as well.

COVERT MEASURES   In developed stuttering, the overt symptoms may be only the tip of the problem. After years of difficulty in speaking, especially since the amount of difficulty varies with the speaking situation, it is only natural that the person would develop hidden feelings and attitudes about speech. Vanryckeghem et al. (2001) show evidence that mal-attitudes and negative emotions are evident in even young children who stutter. Yairi and Ambrose (2005) have similar evidence. The negative feelings may be generalized but are often directed toward particular speaking situations, conversational partners, and even particular word and phoneme combinations. Following on the heels of apprehension, dislike, and fear of these events come the avoidance of them. Therefore, measuring the covert side of a client's stuttering problem is often part of the diagnostic process. This approach is consistent with the World Health Organization's Classification of Functioning, Disability and Health (WHO, 2002) as depicted in Figure 7.3. Furthermore, it is consistent with the recent shift in treatment from behavioral fluency approaches to cognitive, comprehensive lifestyle integration approaches (Blood & Conture, 1998). The impact of stuttering can affect one's quality of life, regardless of age. Early on, perhaps in the initial session, we attempt to discuss with the client his or her feelings, attitudes, fears, and experiences. This helps us "get to know" the client and better understand the depth of the disorder. Counseling may need to be part of the treatment program for some clients; Manning (2010) is a good resource for counseling strategies and techniques. In addition to discussions of feelings, the clinician can utilize published instruments. Sentence completion tasks and adjective checklists help to identify attitudes and personality traits. Several of these instruments are listed in Table 7.6; some of the dated items are now classics and are still in use.

We would be remiss if we did not acknowledge that some behavioral clinicians opt not to measure, or clinically deal with, covert feelings and attitudes. The focus of intervention may, indeed, be to train fluency and let the covert aspects drop out of the client's repertoire on their own, in due time. Likewise, the clinician may use an attitude scale as a baseline measure, proceed with a behavioral approach that focuses only on the overt side of stuttering, and then probe for attitudinal change as a consequence of successful fluency. Evidence-based practice often uses such an approach.

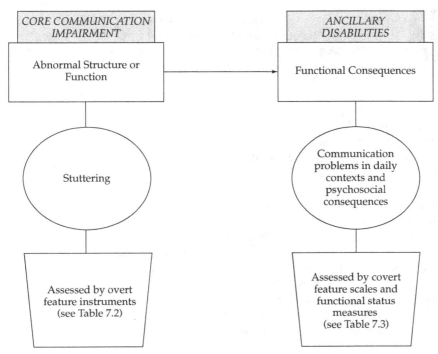

FIGURE 7.3   Assessment of stuttering using the World Health Organization's classification of functioning, disability, and health (ICF).

The clinician *is* interested in avoidance behaviors that the client exhibits. We feel that, clinically, avoidance behavior is an important feature to deal with because it tends to reinforce and compound the speaker's difficulty. Rather than diminish, fears tend to incubate and grow when a person recoils from them; avoidances cause apprehension to increase and the problem to expand.

Avoidance is characterized by reduction or cessation of communication: The person who stutters retreats from the act of talking. The clinician can discern the types of speaking situations and listeners who increase or decrease the client's stuttering. This evaluation can be accomplished by interviewing or by having the client fill out a checklist. The clinician can devise a form for recording data (simply listing different speaking situations, topics of conversation, and so forth) or use a published inventory. Table 7.6 lists assessment instruments useful with the covert side of stuttering. We admit they lack reliability and validity measures; still, they remain classics.

The Speech Situation Checklist (Brutten & Shoemaker, 1974) is still in use clinically and in research (Ezrati-Vinacour & Levin, 2004). The checklist has the client rate his or her degree of emotional response and severity of speech disruption in 51 life situations. Although no formal instrument is supplied, various circumstances (audience size, specific people, different talking situations) may be useful in sampling actual speech. In addition to listing the conditions under which stuttering is increased or reduced, the clinician may ask the client to rank-order the items in terms of speech difficulty and emotional impact. The Communication Attitudes Test (CAT) is another self-report tool that has stood the test of time and is still used as a research and clinical attitude scale, even with grade-school children (Brutten & Dunham, 1989; Vanryckeghem et al., 2001).

TABLE 7.6	Some Available Instruments for the Assessment of Covert Features of Stuttering, including Situation/Avoidance Checklists, Perception/Attitude Scales, and Quality of Life Impact Scales

A-19 Scale for Children Who Stutter
 (Guitar & Grims, 1977; see also Guitar, 2006)

Assessment of Child's Experiences of Stuttering (ACES)
 (Yaruss, Coleman, & Quesal, 2006)

Communication Attitude Test (CAT)
 (Brutten & Dunham, 1989; see also Guitar, 2006)

Culture-Free Self-Esteem Inventory
 (Battle, 1992)

Iowa Scale of Attitude Toward Stuttering
 (Ammons & Johnson, 1944)

Modified Erickson Scale of Communication Attitudes (S-24)
 (Andrews & Cutler, 1974; see also Guitar, 2006 or Manning, 2010)

Overall Assessment of the Speaker's Experiemce of Stuttering (OASES)
 (Yaruss & Quesal, 2006; see also Manning, 2010)

Perceptions of Stuttering Inventory (PSI)
 (Woolf, 1967; see also Guitar, 2006 or free online, see text)

Self-Efficacy for Adolescents Scale (SEA-Scale)
 (Manning, 2010)

Situation Avoidance Behavior Checklist
 (Cooper & Cooper, 2003)

Speech-Related Anxiety Questionnaire
 (Dietrich & Roaman, 2001)

Speech Situation Checklist
 (Brutten & Shoemaker, 1974)

Stutterer's Self-Ratings of Reactions to Speech Situations (ARSF Scale)
 (Shumak, 1955; see also Guitar, 2006)

Stuttering Attitudes Checklist
 (Cooper & Cooper, 2003)

Subjective Units of Distress Scale (SUDS)
 (Marks, 1987)

Wright and Ayre Stuttering Self-Rating Profile (WASSP)
 (Wright & Ayre, 2000; see also Manning, 2010)

In addition to situation fears, many who stutter report that they have particular difficulty with certain words and speech sounds. We make a list of these items and then examine the speech sample to determine if in fact there is more stuttering on some sounds or words. During attempts at trial treatment, we like to show the client ways of ameliorating the stuttering and often use his or her most feared words as stimuli.

Any assessment of stuttering should also include the client's own perceptions of the magnitude and impact of their stuttering. This includes both severity self-assessment and quality of life impact measures; both are useful as pre- and post-treatment measures to document change. The clinician can obtain such information from many of the instruments listed in Tables 7.5 and

7.6. In particular, we like to administer the Perceptions of Stuttering Inventory (PSI) (Woolf, 1967); it is available free online at http://www.speechpathways.com/PerceptionsOfStuttering. aspx. The PSI is devised to assess three dimensions of stuttering behavior: struggle, avoidance, and expectancy, as perceived by the person who stutters. It yields a profile that the clinician can then compare to scores obtained by a reference group of stutterers. With renewed clinical research emphasis into daily functioning and disability impacts by the World Health Organization (2002), this area of assessment is again becoming popular.

Having now discussed the predictive instruments, severity scales, and a myriad of covert measures typically used in the evaluation of stuttering, let us turn our attention to some general evaluation principles and special considerations for clients of various ages.

EVALUATION AT THE ONSET OF STUTTERING

Experienced clinicians agree that the problem of stuttering is much easier to prevent or manage in children than to treat in chronic adult clients. Indeed, the early detection and management of children beginning to stutter is one of the most significant contributions a speech clinician can make. The SLP must seek answers for a great many questions: Is the child stuttering? If so, how far has the disturbance progressed? When did it begin? What factors were associated with the onset of the problem? How aware is the child of the speech disturbance? How do listeners attempt to help, and how does this affect the child's efforts? How can the SLP alter the child's environment to prevent the problem from getting worse?

Throughout this book, we have repeatedly suggested that diagnosis and treatment are not separate undertakings. The careful assessment of a client's speech-language is often therapeutic; only by working with an individual (and his or her parents) for a period of time does the clinician truly come to know the dimensions of the disorder. This is particularly true in the management of children beginning to stutter.

In many cases, a physician is the first professional to be consulted by parents. The clinician is wise to enlist the support of local pediatricians in the early identification of children beginning to stutter.

The onset of stuttering is a crisis situation in which swift intervention is absolutely essential. In planning for the evaluation, we delineate several objectives that will guide the clinician's efforts:

1. Determine if the child is stuttering (problem/no problem determination).
2. If so, identify to what developmental extent the disorder has progressed (factors include overt and covert severity).
3. Obtain the parent's perception of the onset and current status of the disorder.
4. Sample the child's general level of functioning in regard to auditory, motor, social, articulatory, and cognitive-linguistic abilities.
5. Commence the development of a counseling relationship with the parents.

We have already discussed most of these objectives. Various assessment instruments are available to help the clinician make a differential diagnosis, determine the severity of the speech difficulties, appraise the home situation and parental attitudes, and begin a healthy dialogue with the parents of the child who is beginning to stutter. What remains to be discussed are the ancillary areas that need to be assessed in the young child.

Several authorities recommend assessing the child's rate of speech, as well as the parents' rates (Peters & Guitar, 1991; Starkweather, Gottwald, & Halfond, 1990) but others do not

(Ingham, 2005). Speech rate is a basic element of fluency and therefore warrants assessment, as explained earlier in this chapter. The rate at which parents talk may be demanding of fluency in the child and also merit assessment. Speed and coordination of repetitive oral movements may be tested using norms for diadochokinesis, which, among other places, can be found in the Oral Speech Mechanism Examination (St. Louis & Ruscello, 2000). Phonological disorders seem to co-occur frequently with stuttering (about 16% of the time), as do language disorders (about 10% of the time). Some 7% have concomitant learning disabilities and about 6% have reading disabilities (Arndt & Healey, 2001; Blood et al., 2009; Conture, 2001; Yairi & Seery, 2011).

Recent literature suggests the need to assess and monitor lexical and word retrieval skills (Hall, 2004; Silverman & Ratner, 2002), pragmatic competencies (Weiss, 2004), linguistic utterance length and complexity—especially as related to fluency breakdowns (Ryan, 1974; Weiss, 2004), and in general to assess language skills and phonology.

Various articulation and language tests should be used as part of a thorough fluency evaluation. Information contained in Chapters 4, 5, and 6 certainly pertains. The presence of speech and language disorders concomitant with stuttering may affect the planning of an appropriate treatment program.

Along with these areas of assessment, we routinely screen the oral mechanism, voice, and hearing. We advocate referral for additional testing of cognitive, motoric, and psychological status, as needed, with particular clients.

A Direction for Treatment

Even though it is beyond the scope of this chapter to discuss the myriad of treatment programs available, we do wish to point out that different philosophies exist regarding the treatment of young persons who stutter, such as those between the ages of 2 and 9 years. In addition, although many preschoolers continue to receive intervention services in clinics and through private practitioners, with the implementation of PL 94-457 more and more are being treated by the public school SLP. School systems serve children ages 3 to 5, and many are responsible for the birth-through-age-2 population. Four treatment options may be considered.

In the first option, environmental treatment, the SLP determines that the most prudent course of action is to work through the significant others in the child's life—parents and teachers—to modify the daily environment. The goal is to structure the child's environment to make it more conducive to fluency. The child is not seen for treatment; typically, parents and teachers meet regularly with the clinician to discuss environmental modifications and results. Opting for only environmental treatment is commonly done for the child "at risk" for developing stuttering or for the child beginning to stutter who displays early developed symptoms. Modifying parental and teacher reactions to disfluencies; altering the pace and organization of home and school; and generally educating significant others about fluency, disfluency, and the modeling of good speech habits are beneficial. Reduction in communicative pressures that the child is vulnerable to are a necessary and important aspect of treatment.

A second treatment option is to combine the environmental treatment with direct, but modified, therapy for the child. Sessions may be individual but are often in groups. The treatment is considered modified as it does not focus on specific symptoms of stuttering. Rather, treatment may emphasize the concept of rhythm by having children sing, speak to a rhythm, practice rhymes, use choral speaking, and just generally experience much success in easy, fluent speech. Modified treatment often involves language treatment. The language skills of a child who stutters may be somewhat delayed. The length and complexity of utterances affect the likelihood of even normal speakers having a disfluency. By shoring up weak language skills, and by systematically controlling the linguistic output of young clients (e.g., sentence length and syntactic complexity), SLPs are able to reduce or eliminate stuttering. Additionally, some SLPs may include in the modified program mention of "smooth" and "bumpy" speech and train the children to identify samples of each. Altering the "bumpy" speech, however, is not done in this form of treatment.

A third option of treatment for the young child who stutters is to combine the environmental approach with direct intervention. The child attends individual or group treatment sessions (depending upon the severity of the problem) with the purpose of modifying specific stuttering symptoms. A variety of therapeutic emphases are possible. The student may be taught a new, fluent way of talking by learning patterns such as "slow speech," "breathy speech," "stretchy speech," the "easy speaking voice," "slow, easy speech," and other similar strategies for fluency. Discussions of feelings and attitudes are often a component of the treatment program for children ready to address personal issues surrounding their speech difficulties.

The fourth option of direct stuttering modification alone expands the details involved in mastering strategies, techniques, or targets for fluency. The absence of co-occurring environmental treatment may be a function of (1) the setting in which services are provided (parents may not be available to participate fully in the intervention program); or (2) the child's stuttering symptoms may have progressed beyond the level where environmental manipulations would be expected to have much effect. In such cases, efforts need to be focused on direct treatments using greater specificity.

Prognosis with Young Children

We are very impressed with the efficacy of treatment for young children who are beginning to stutter. When the clinician can intervene before the child develops fear and avoidance reactions, and if the parents are amenable to counseling, the prognosis for recovery is excellent—remember the 80% recovery rate discussed earlier. The reader also is encouraged to review the recovery factors presented in Table 7.4. It is worth reiterating these and other intuitive factors that the clinician must consider when estimating a client's prospects for recovery:

1. How long has the child been stuttering? Time is an enemy of recovery.
2. What is the frequency of disfluency?
3. What are gender and familial factors that may shade the prognosis?
4. What types of disfluency are exhibited and their severity?
5. What co-existing speech-language and other disorders exist?
6. What type and intensity of enviromental reactions has the child been exposed to? In our experience, children who have been slapped or have suffered other forms of physical abuse have the worst problems.
7. Is the child aware of speaking difficulties? The more heedful the child is of speech interruptions, the less positive the prognosis. (This may be argued as evidence of the progression of the disorder; hence the less favorable prognosis.)
8. How amenable are the parents to counseling? An all-out concerted effort at the home front is ideal, perhaps essential, for amelioration.
9. What is the child's level of intelligence? We have had more limited success with "slow" children.
10. Are there organic or neurotic factors that figure in the onset of stuttering? Chances for recovery are more limited if either is present.

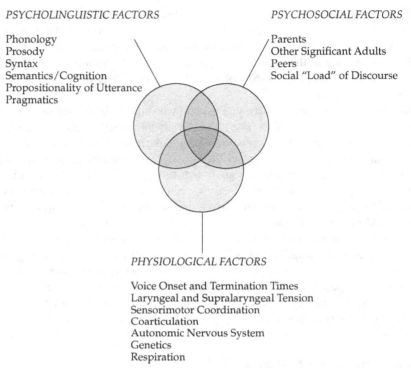

PSYCHOLINGUISTIC FACTORS

Phonology
Prosody
Syntax
Semantics/Cognition
Propositionality of Utterance
Pragmatics

PSYCHOSOCIAL FACTORS

Parents
Other Significant Adults
Peers
Social "Load" of Discourse

PHYSIOLOGICAL FACTORS

Voice Onset and Termination Times
Laryngeal and Supralaryngeal Tension
Sensorimotor Coordination
Coarticulation
Autonomic Nervous System
Genetics
Respiration

FIGURE 7.4 Factors influencing early childhood stuttering.

Our clinical success or failure with children who are beginning to stutter is also related to the characteristic pattern of factors present at the onset of stuttering. We find it important to synthesizing diagnostic information and making a prognosis about a young disfluent child. The many variables that may be involved in the onset of stuttering are organized into three major categories: physiological, psycholinguistic, and psychosocial (Figure 7.4). Note how the three categories overlap. For example, a child delayed in language development and deficient in motor skills could be particularly susceptible to high parental standards or communication competition with siblings.

One question continues to nag clinicians who work with young children. Would the children have gotten better without the clinicians' help, owing simply to the passage of time and some internal recovery potential in the child? Although we cannot answer that question with any authority, we do see that in most instances, the child's recovery from stuttering occurred too swiftly after the initiation of treatment (two weeks to several months) to be attributed to spontaneous recovery.

EVALUATION OF THE SCHOOL-AGED STUDENT

Elementary Students

Appraising and treating elementary school students who stutter is particularly challenging. This group of children, approximately 7 to 12 years old, is no longer beginning to stutter; they are not simply repeating and hesitating. They struggle noticeably when speaking and attempt to avoid or disguise their difficulty; they are frustrated, and it is now necessary to deal directly with the stuttering.

The clinician is faced with several thorny problems when planning an examination of a young person who stutters: (1) Young children frequently lack the insight and cooperation necessary to analyze their problem objectively and rationally. (2) Children are reluctant or unable to verbalize their internal feelings freely. (3) The speech clinician is associated in the child's mind with the teaching personnel, who may in some cases be penalizing or disturbing listeners. In addition, the clinician may be identified with authority figures; this tends to undermine a trusting relationship. (4) Last, and perhaps most significant, the child usually has no choice about entering treatment; most likely the student is brought for evaluation by the parents, referred by a teacher, or identified in a screening by a speech clinician.

The clinician may find that these students respond to an honest, straightforward clinical approach. With early elementary school children, we use descriptive language, such as "tensing" or "getting stuck," to inquire about their speaking difficulty, not out of any fear of the word *stuttering,* but simply because the term either doesn't mean much to the child or, in some cases, is too negatively charged. With older elementary school children, we use a frank, direct style. Establish trust and confidence by showing the client that the clinician is competent and *knows* about the problem of stuttering.

The evaluation of a student does not differ greatly in substance from an assessment of an older individual except that with young children, enviromental, parental, and school factors are more important. In order to reveal the range of information generally sought, Figure 7.5 outlines an assessment plan prepared by a diagnostic team composed of a faculty member and graduate students. The plan was compiled for the evaluation of a 10-year-old child referred to a university speech clinic by a public school clinician.

Junior and Senior High School Students

The assessment and treatment of stuttering in older students is even more challenging than with the youngsters. Denial of the problem, lack of cooperation, and lack of motivation seem typical in the teenagers we have seen. The assessment outline does not differ much from the example shown for Alan Schlicher. The process, however, is very adultlike; environmental and parental factors are downplayed.

Direction for Treatment

The treatment of stuttering among some older children, adolescents, and adults is of the direct type. Obviously, programs differ in complexities and emphases for these disparate age groups. As negative feelings and attitudes develop late in the evolution of stuttering, treatment for the older student often involves explorations into these psychological topics. The emotional crisis of stuttering escalates during the teenage years when social interactions become so critical. (Students may benefit from reading *Do You Stutter: A Guide for Teens,* published by the Stuttering Foundation, http://www.stutteringhelp.org.) Physiological modifications of speech are often components in adolescent and adult fluency programs. Physiological targets may include breath, voice onset, and rate, as well as a host of others. Computerized instrumentation may help in the training of these speech targets. Much practice is necessary to habituate new speaking patterns, and support from family, friends, and school personnel can be critical to success. The book by Hegde (2006) provides treatment protocols for clients of all ages.

I. Identifying Information

Obtain all the usual information regarding address, grade level, and so on. This can be obtained from Mrs. Hronkin, the referral source, or in the parent interview. Be sure to inquire about living arrangements: Ms. Hronkin mentioned that a parental grandfather may reside with the family, and apparently he is a dominant force in the family (reportedly, he is against Alan receiving speech therapy and insists he overcame stuttering by eating mashed potatoes!).

II. Description of Stuttering

A. *Global description.* What are the salient descriptive features of Alan's stuttering behavior? Is it basically fixative or oscillative? Are there long silent periods of internal struggle, or does he exhibit a more overt pattern?

B. *Core behaviors.* Make an analysis of the repetitions and prolongations observed—the number of oscillations per unit, tempo, duration, and so forth.

C. *Tension-struggle features.* Note the occurence and location of any ancillary behaviors.

D. *Frequency.* This analysis will serve as our baseline for reevaluation of Alan, so we need to be especially precise. Collect data (count repetitions, prolongations, other salient features of his moments of stuttering) on at least three types of speech samples—reading, paraphrasing, and spontaneous speech. We can compute the relative frequency of stutterings per minute, or per total syllables uttered, by analyzing the videotape later.

E. *Severity.* We will use the Stuttering Severity Instrument-4 (Riley 2009); this instrument employs the three dimensions of frequency, duration, and physical concomitants and yields a score that can be converted to a percentile. A severity measure like this (particularly when it allows the examiner to score a client on a common scale of 0 to 100) is useful when communicating the results of the evaluation to the parents, teacher, even the child himself.

F. *Variations in frequency/severity.* Explore with the child and his parents whether his stuttering comes and goes in cycles, which situations or listeners provoke variations in his speech, and whether there are any words or sounds that are particularly difficult. Determine what impact delayed auditory feedback and masking noise have on his speech, and the impact of a rhythmic metronome. Probe fluency changes as a function of linguistic length and complexity, while both answering and asking questions, and while following a model of easy onset speech and stretched (slow, prolonged) speech.

G. How does the child try to control his stuttering? What techniques has he devised for coping with speech interruptions? How effective are they? Additionally, we need to identify which speech-altering strategies—slowing, easy onset, and so forth—induce fluency. Use Cooper and Cooper's (2004) Disfluency Descriptor Digest as a checklist to record observations.

H. Can the child predict when he is about to stutter? Ask him if he can; but also have him underline words he thinks he might stutter on as he reads silently a simple passage. Have him read it aloud and determine the degree to which he can accurately predict his stuttering.

I. What is the client's poststuttering behavior? Does he continue talking, give up, become angry, or cry? Does he appear indifferent?

III. Attitude Dimension

This is the most difficult and least reliable aspect of the evaluation. Some information can be obtained through observation of Alan and his parents and by what they say about the problem. We can also administer several self-inventory scales such as the A-19 Scale (Guitar, 2006). What is the child's attitude toward treatment? How much does he know about stuttering? Has he been teased at school or home because of his problem?

FIGURE 7.5   Assessment plan for Alan Schlicher.

IV. Case History
We will want to obtain background information with respect to four basic areas: history of general development (motor, language, social), onset and development of stuttering, medical history, and family history. These areas can be explored in the parent interview.

V. Present Functioning
A. *Personality.* Describe the child's personality in general terms (shy, aggressive, and so on) and identify any special features (fears, tics, nail-biting, and the like) that may apply to him. Ascertain his special interests or hobbies.
B. *School.* Obtain information relevant to his academic and social adjustment in school.
C. *Related testing.* Is a psychological or medical referral indicated? Perform screening evaluations on the child's motor behavior, hearing, voice, phonology, and language ability. The latter two are particularly important, as we have discussed in this chapter. Select tests accordingly.
D. *Diagnostic session.* How did the child behave during the diagnostic session? What could be discerned about his level of motivation? How did he respond when put under communicative stress? How did he respond to trial therapy?

FIGURE 7.5 *(continued)*

Prognosis

What factors are crucial for improvement with students? What variables should the clinician consider when making a prognosis? We believe that the most significant improvement in treatment is noted in cases with the following operative factors:

1. No prior record of unsuccessful treatment (An absence of treatment seems more conducive to success than a history of therapeutic failure.)
2. Cooperative parents, willing to participate meaningfully in a program of counseling
3. More severe stuttering pattern (Mild stutterers typically show little improvement.)
4. A predominantly clonic stuttering pattern featuring struggle and escape (Students adept at avoidance generally have more difficulty.)
5. Cooperative teachers and other school personnel
6. No other significant problems (reading difficulty, a scholastic problem independent of stuttering, and so on)
7. Other available resources (expertise in scouting, athletics, music)
8. A schedule of intensive therapy (at least three, preferably four, contacts a week)

ASSESSMENT OF THE ADULT WHO STUTTERS

The disorder is fully developed in the adult client: Speech interruptions are more complex and characteristically compulsive; fears and apprehensions become chronic; avoidance, disguise, and negative attitudes hamper and distort the individual's relationships with others. At this stage, a speech breakdown is not simply a response, it is also a stimulus—the problem has become cyclic and self-reinforcing. Clinicians agree that the treatment of stuttering at this advanced stage is complicated—but far from impossible. There is a bewildering array of treatment approaches (and indexes of their successes); we, however, will not attempt to summarize them here but refer the reader to works by Bothe (2004), Guitar (2006), Hegde (2006), Ingham (2003), Manning (2010), and Onslow (1996).

Prognosis

Making a prognosis about success and failure in stuttering is an inexact science. As noted earlier, recent research efforts have tried to delineate some factors that may be involved in determining successful outcomes. We present an incomplete and heuristic list of factors that help in making prognoses. The items are presented in random order, for at present we have no data that would allow us to assign weight to them.

1. *Severity.* Paradoxically, persons with more severe stuttering, other factors being equal, seem to make better progress than do milder cases.

2. *Motivation and Attitude.* Motivation to change is, of course, a most significant variable in all intervention programs. The better the client's pretreatment attitude, the more successful the outcome of treatment is likely to be.

3. *Timing.* A client's motivation for treatment is often related to crucial life experiences. Persons who have reached a critical stage and feel blocked by their disordered speech, barred from job advancement, education, or marriage, and who voluntarily seek treatment have a more favorable prognosis.

4. *Age.* Adolescents, particularly between the ages of 13 and 16, are especially resistant to treatment. Similarly, clients over 40 tend to do poorly in treatment.

5. *Sex.* Women seem to be more difficult to treat than men.

6. *Nonstuttered Speech.* The more well integrated the client's nonstuttered speech is, in terms of prosody, the better the prognosis.

7. *Type of Stuttering.* Those with predominantly repetitive stuttering make more rapid progress than do those with predominantly fixative disfluencies; clients who feature escape reactions are easier to work with than chronic avoiders. Interiorized stutterers—especially those manifesting laryngeal blocking—are very resistant to treatment.

8. *Concomitant Problems.* Clients presenting with organic complications (e.g., sensory, intellectual, or motor impairments) or psychological symptoms require more prolonged treatment and do less well than clients without concomitant problems.

9. *Prior Treatment and Intensive Treatment.* Clients with a history of therapeutic failure have a poor prognosis. Token treatment may be worse than no treatment at all. When intensive treatment (minimum daily contact of at least 1 hour) is available and the client can participate in a comprehensive program, the prospects for recovery are more favorable.

To conclude this chapter we wish to echo the preferred practice patterns of ASHA (2004) with regard to expected outcomes of a fluency assessment. These include identification and description of the person's:

- Type of fluency disorder (the diagnosis)
- Characteristics of the fluent, disfluent, and covert behaviors
- Effects of fluency impairments on the individual's daily activities
- Contextual factors that act as barriers to or facilitators of communication
- Co-occurring communication disorders, if any
- Prognosis for change
- Recommendations for intervention and support

8

Assessment of Aphasia and Adult Language Disorders

When an adult suddenly loses the easy use of language, it is a devastating experience for the individual and for the family. Aphasia and other adult language disorders affect that which makes us uniquely human—our ability to communicate with each other by a system of language symbols.

THE NATURE OF APHASIA

Aphasia is the most common disorder of communication resulting from brain injury. Damage occurs in the hemisphere of the brain that is dominant for language; for most of us, this is the left hemisphere. An adult with aphasia has a basic interference with *comprehension* and *use* of language in its many forms. More specifically, aphasia is a syndrome of language deficits resulting from destruction of cortical tissue and is characterized by one or more of the following symptoms:

1. Disturbance in receiving and decoding symbolic materials via auditory, visual, or tactile channels (Although the individual can still hear and see, there is difficulty deciphering the learned associations of messages.)
2. Disturbance in central processes of meaning, word selection, and message formulation
3. Disturbance in expressing symbolic materials by means of speech, writing, or gesture

Aphasia may result from trauma, brain tumors, certain inflammatory processes, and degenerative diseases. The vast majority of aphasias, however, are the consequence of a cerebrovascular accident (CVA), commonly called stroke or brain attack.

The cerebrovascular accident is a relatively common illness that affects approximately a half million persons each year. In the United States, CVA now stands as the third leading cause of death (outdistanced only by heart disease and cancer). No one knows precisely how many surviving stroke victims are left with language impairment; estimates suggest at least a quarter of the victims present some degree of aphasia that warrants treatment. It is an exciting time to be an aphasiologist—an SLP who specializes in the diagnosis and rehabilitation of adult language disorders. There is an explosion of new technologies to aid in understanding the brain's biology. There are new and promising approaches to pharmacology to aid the brain's recovery immediately following CVA. And medicines are becoming more effective in aiding cognition.

Etiology can influence the onset, progress, and type of aphasia symptoms. The onset of symptoms is likely to be insidious when caused by tumor, and abrupt when due to CVA. Further, improvement is more likely if the aphasia is caused by a CVA than by a tumor, and patients with tumors may have wide differences in abilities across modalities (reading, writing, listening, speaking). Such large differences are less likely from a CVA. Aphasia resulting from trauma is often accompanied by a greater variety of cognitive deficits, but it shows a faster recovery than does aphasia resulting from CVA.

There is a host of other disorders that may resemble aphasia and have brain damage as their basis. These include the language of confusion, language of intellectual deterioration (dementia), communication deficit subsequent to a nondominant lesion (usually right hemisphere damage), language associated with psychosis, and motor speech disorders. These disorders will be discussed later in this chapter as part of the differential diagnosis process.

The severity of aphasia can vary greatly, from minimal, temporary language dysfunction to almost total and permanent inability to use and comprehend language. It is important to remember that the impoverishment of language observed in aphasia is *not* due to loss of mental capacity, impairment of sensory organs, or paralysis of the speech apparatus. These problems, however, can co-occur with aphasia, making differential diagnosis important. And current research is starting to acknowledge cognitive aspects within aphasia (Chapey, 2001; Raymer & Rothi, 2001).

Classifying a patient as to the *type* of aphasia displayed can be an important feature of diagnosis and treatment planning. Many labels and classification systems have been put forth through the years for this purpose. Three methods are currently in wide use: (1) fluent–nonfluent dichotomy, which is based on the patient's length of utterance; (2) the "Boston" classification system by Goodglass et al. (2000); and (3) the Western Aphasia Battery (WAB) taxonomy by Kertesz (2006). The Boston and WAB systems are quite similar and use fluency, auditory comprehension, repetition, and naming abilities for arriving at a diagnostic label. Table 8.1 lists characteristics of each of the major types of aphasia.

Although there is some controversy as to our ability to localize language functions in the brain, there is fairly good agreement with site of lesion information and the language character-

---

TABLE 8.1   Neurolinguistic Features of the Major Types of Aphasia

Broca's Aphasia	**Transcortical Motor Aphasia**
Impaired fluency; limited verbal output	Preserved ability to repeat
Relatively good auditory comprehension	Nonfluent
Impaired articulatory agility	Some auditory comprehension impairment, similar to Broca's aphasia
Stereotyped grammar	Superior naming ability compared to spontaneous speech
Telegraphic and agrammatic (especially reduced use of articles, prepositions, auxiliaries, copulas, and derivational endings)	
Prosodic alterations	

| **TABLE 8.1** | *(continued)* |

Global Aphasia

Severe loss of all receptive modalities

Severe loss of all expressive modalities

Almost totally absent speech

Stereotypic utterances (perhaps with normal melody and intonation)

Wernicke's Aphasia

Fluent; copious verbal output

Impaired auditory comprehension (often severe)

Frequent paraphasias (especially semantic types)

Neologisms and jargon, if severe

Normal articulatory agility

Normal prosody

Normal or supranormal phrase length

Full range of grammatical forms

Preserved syntax

Impaired naming and repetition abilities

Transcortical Sensory Aphasia

Preserved ability to repeat

Conversation resembles symptoms of Wernicke's aphasia

Extreme difficulty with nouns

Excessive paraphasias

Impaired auditory comprehension, resembling Wernicke's

Conduction Aphasia

Poor repetition ability

Fluent speech; good articulation and phrase length

Frequent paraphasias (especially literal types)

Some auditory comprehension impairment

Acute awareness of errors

Anomic Aphasia

Severe word-finding deficits

Frequent circumlocutions

Minimal paraphasic errors

Fluent speech; good articulation and phrase length

Appropriate grammatical forms

Good auditory comprehension

istics seen in individual patients. Lobes of the brain and primary language areas of the left (dominant) hemisphere associated with various types of aphasia are shown in Figure 8.1. As can be seen, anterior lesions generally produce nonfluent aphasia, such as Broca's and transcortical motor aphasias. Posterior lesions are associated with the fluent aphasias, such as Wernicke's, conduction, and transcortical sensory aphasias.

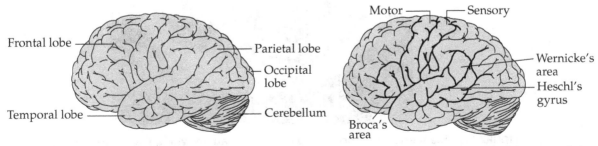

FIGURE 8.1 Lobes of the brain (left figure) and areas of the left hemisphere associated with some of the types of aphasia (right figure).

Source: L. Justice (2010). *Communication Science and Disorders: A Contemporary Perspective.* Pearson Allyn & Bacon.

Site of lesion (anatomical areas affected) and type of lesion (tumor, CVA, and so forth) can usually be determined by modern methods of brain imaging such as computerized tomography (CT), positron emission tomography (PET), and magnetic resonance imaging (MRI). An example of an MRI scan is shown in Figure 8.2. These methods have contributed greatly to aphasiology. The emerging role of single photon emission computed tomography, or SPECT, might aid in the prediction of recovery (Mimura et al., 1998). Although anatomical evidence supplied by the neuroradiologist is diagnostically valuable, the speech-language pathologist may be wise to focus on carefully describing what the individual can and cannot do with respect to language. The clinician must first and foremost delineate the patient's ability to talk, listen, read, and write.

In our zeal to identify the neurolinguistic dimensions of aphasia, it is possible to forget that brain injury is a grave health problem. The individual has suffered a major life crisis that has profound medical, psychological, and social consequences. In addition to the language impairment, the patient may present paralysis or paresis of the extremities (generally the right

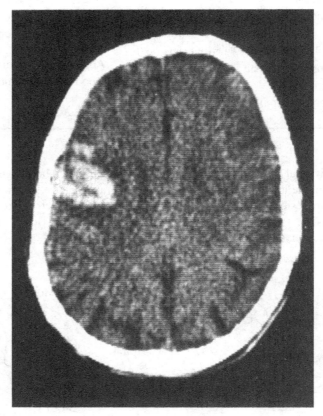

FIGURE 8.2 Magnetic resonance image (MRI) of a patient with aphasia subsequent to a left hemisphere lesion.

Source: Image courtesy of E. Plant and P. Beeson (2008). *Communication and Communication Disorders: A Clinical Introduction.* Pearson Allyn & Bacon.

side, sometimes including the face), sensory abnormalities, and behavioral disturbances. There seems to be little, if any, relationship between these difficulties and the extent of the language impairment. Above all, the clinician must remember that aphasia is both a personal catastrophe and a family crisis.

CASE HISTORY

It is wise for SLPs to remember that they work with *persons* who have aphasia, not aphasia. Language treatment for an adult with aphasia has to be very personalized. Therefore, SLPs need to know as much as possible about their clients when planning a rehabilitation program. What sort of people were the clients before the strokes? How did they meet their problems? What educational levels were achieved? What were their occupations? Their avocations? What changes in behaviors, if any, have occurred following the brain injuries? The style, pace, and content of treatment will be based on the answers to these and many other questions.

Unfortunately, the aphasic patient is often in no position to provide the kind of detailed information we seek. In some instances, official records (educational tests, military records) and personal documents (diaries, letters) are helpful. Usually, however, we must rely on the accuracy and veracity of informants who are familiar with the patient. The most common method of assembling information about the language-impaired individual is a case history form that is filled out by a spouse or other close relative. Sample questions from a typical case history form are listed in Table 8.2. Ideally, the clinician also interviews the respondent to clarify any ambiguities in the written information and to permit additional questioning. Keep in mind, however, that a long-term marriage partner typically sees the patient as less impaired than objective language testing may show. On the other hand, acontextual tests of language do not measure communication and so the client may, in fact, perform better in a "real" setting.

Health history of the patient is ascertained, in part, during the case history interview (recall Table 8.2), but medical records provide greater specificity. Information concerning the current medical episode is particularly useful in differential diagnosis and treatment planning. At a minimum, the following medical data should be collected:

1. Major and secondary medical diagnoses (e.g., thrombosis of left middle cerebral artery, organic brain syndrome, diabetes, CVA with right hemiparesis, and the like)
2. Date of onset as regards etiology of communication disorder
3. Localization of brain damage (hemisphere and lobes affected) and source of data (e.g., CT, MRI, and other techniques)
4. Previous CNS involvement (type and date of onset)
5. Brain stem signs (e.g., facial weakness, extraocular movement, dysphagia, other bulbar signs)
6. Limb involvement
7. Vision (acuity, corrective lens, visual field deficits, etc.)
8. Hearing (acuity, discrimination, amplification, etc.)

Access to the patient's medical chart is therefore essential to the SLP. In addition to the physician/neurologist report, entries by the neuroradiologist, social worker, nurse, and other health care professionals are enlightening. Important information can be gained from this telegraphic chart note entered by a neurologist:

> This alert, oriented adult male suffered a CVA on 3-19-11. Expressive-receptive
> aphasia. Right hemiplegia. Babinski sign on the right. Gross motor functioning of

TABLE 8.2   Sample Questionnaire Topics for a Case History

Personal

Marital status

Name and occupation of spouse

Names and locations of children

Information about grandchildren

Amount of education

Occupation

Current employment status (retired?)

Hobbies and special interests

Preferences in reading material, television entertainment, and use of writing

Preferred hand

Native language, knowledge of others

Description of personality

Description of involvement in group activities (e.g., bowling leagues, church fellowships)

Description of any changes since the injury in mood, personality, ability to care for self, and the like

Medical

Date of injury

Cause of injury (accident, stroke, disease)

Length of unconsciousness, if any

Description of paralysis, if any

Complaints of dizziness, faintness, headaches, if any

Description of any visual or hearing problems

Description of any other problems, illnesses, or injuries

Communicative

Description of the patient's speech at the onset of the problem

Description of how the speech has changed

Check the appropriate column as it applies to the patient *now:*

Can	Cannot	
_____	_____	indicate meaning by gesture.
_____	_____	repeat words spoken by others.
_____	_____	use one or a few words over and over.
_____	_____	use swear words (often).
_____	_____	use some words spontaneously.
_____	_____	say short phrases.
_____	_____	say short sentences.
_____	_____	follow requests and understand directions.
_____	_____	follow radio or television speech.
_____	_____	read signs with understanding.
_____	_____	read newspapers, magazines.
_____	_____	tell time.
_____	_____	write name without assistance.
_____	_____	write sentences, letters.
_____	_____	do simple arithmetic.
_____	_____	handle money, make change.

involved leg is returning; arm and hand are doubtful. CT scan revealed a focal lesion in the left parietal-temporal region. Right side astereognosis. Right homonomous hemianopsia.

This brief report told us several important things about the patient: The neurologist observed that the brain damage was apparently localized and was not widespread; he also observed that the aphasia was probably not transitory, as lesions in the region cited generally result in more persistent language impairment; the patient could not identify objects by touch when they were placed in his right hand; and he could not see in the right field of vision. This last anomaly would require that we present testing materials from the patient's left side. Information assembled by the neurologist is, of course, very useful to the SLP. In addition to the size and locale of the lesion, the nature of the injury may be pertinent diagnostically. (For example, patients incurring traumatic brain injury often experience a different course of recovery from persons suffering vascular episodes.) The chart note also underscores the importance of being familiar with pertinent medical terminology.

After garnering case history information, the SLP should have a rather detailed description of the salient aspects of the patient's premorbid personality, health history and current status, and social orientation. But what impact would this sudden illness have? How much change could be expected, and in what areas? Would the patient's responses to the language impairment and physical disabilities merely be an exaggeration of earlier behavior patterns?

There are only limited answers to these questions. We suspect, however, that the nature of the illness, the treatment the patient receives, and premorbid factors are all crucial in determining the impact of the problem upon the individual. Impact measure and quality of life scales may be done at a later point in intervention. In summary, any and all information about the individual that can be pulled together is important and may shape our course of assessment and treatment.

DIAGNOSIS AND FORMAL TESTING

A comprehensive evaluation of an adult with aphasia includes several clinical tasks: (1) a review of pertinent medical information and the sequence of events leading up to the referral; (2) a preliminary interview with the patient's spouse or other close relatives; (3) a case history, including information about the impact of brain injury on the patient and how much natural or spontaneous recovery has taken place; (4) an inventory of the client's language/communication performance; (5) observation and related testing (including informal assessments, oral peripheral examination, hearing test, and the like); and (6) a diagnostic determination with recommendations as to the nature of treatment and a judgment about the individual's prospects for recovery. This process is shown in Figure 8.3. In arriving at a diagnosis, the clinician first determines whether or not a communication problem exists and, if it does, what kind of problem. This involves sorting out among various possible conditions and among subtypes within specific conditions.

Having discussed the first three tasks in the list, let us now turn our attention to the fourth and see how the evaluation process leads to a diagnosis. The SLP may need a quick idea of the client's language abilities and disabilities in order to determine the need for further testing and to better choose the most appropriate standardized tests to employ. A screening test, therefore, may be administered.

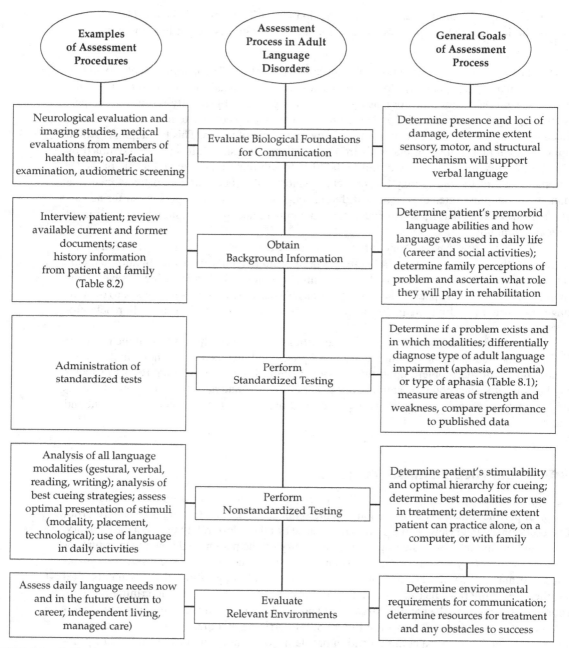

FIGURE 8.3 Critical assessment process in aphasia and adult language disorders.

Screening for Aphasia

When a patient is referred in a medical setting, the SLP may begin with a *bedside consultation*, the term reimbursement agencies prefer to *screening* (Hallowell & Chapey, 2001). A screening instrument is designed to swiftly evaluate a patient's language abilities before the administration of a more thorough (and lengthy) examination. One reason for using a screening instrument is that it allows the SLP quickly to advise relatives and health care professionals about the best means of communicating with the patient. Additionally, patients' symptoms change rapidly during the first days and months following brain injury; screenings allow for frequent reassessments to document the patient's progress (or lack of progress) and to modify suggestions as to how best to communicate with the patient. Frequent readministrations of formal, standardized tests—many lasting 1 to 6 hours—would not be practical. Table 8.3 lists some of the available screening tests for aphasia.

Some experienced clinicians design their own screening device—usually one that is more cursory than published tests. In some work settings, for example, the SLP must quickly (in five minutes or so) interview and screen all newly admitted patients to determine if a communication problem exists and to decide whether to suggest that the physician order a speech-language consult. This is done because third-party reimbursement agencies require that evaluations be medically necessary and physician ordered. Typically, the SLP will elicit spontaneous conversation and judge it for contextual accuracy, topic maintenance, length of utterance, syntactic variety, facility with word selection, and fluency. Limited or absent conversation may lead the SLP to quickly assess more basic skills, such as naming and pointing to objects in the room, repeating, following commands (nonverbally), and responding to yes/no questions (verbally or gesturally). Such a quick, albeit incomplete, screening permits the clinician to judge (1) whether or not a communication problem exists on a gross level, (2) the need for further testing (and hence the need for a physician-ordered consult), and (3) which formal tests would be best suited to the patient's level of functioning.

TABLE 8.3	Some Screening or Bedside Tests for Aphasia

Acute Aphasia Screening Protocol (AASP)
  (Crary, Haak, & Malinsky, 1989)
Aphasia Language Performance Scales (ALPS)
  (Keenan & Brassell, 1975)
  (also available in Spanish)
Aphasia Screening Test (AST)
  (Whurr, 1996)
Bedside Evaluation and Screening Test of Aphasia, 2nd ed. (BEST-2)
  (West, Sands, & Swain, 1998)
Bedside Western Aphasia Battery-R
  (Kertesz, 2006)
Frenchay Aphasia Screening Test (FAST)
  (Enderby, Wood, & Wade, 2006)
Multimodal Communication Screening Test for Persons with Aphasia (MCST-A)
  (Garrett & Lasker, 2007) (available online)
Quick Assessment for Aphasia
  (Tanner & Culbertson, 1999)
Sheffield Screening Test for Acquired Language Disorders
  (Syder et al., 1993)
Sklar Aphasia Scale (SAS)
  (Sklar, 1983) (also available in German)

Standardized Testing

To devise a plan of treatment, as well as to predict the probable course and outcome of treatment, the SLP needs a comprehensive appraisal of the patient's present language abilities. Where is the patient having difficulty? Which modalities are working best? How are errors made and are there discernable patterns to the errors? To answer these and other questions, we inventory the patient's language.

The SLP has many published tests from which to choose; Table 8.4 lists some of the more commonly used tests of aphasia. Only a cursory discussion of the more popular—and different—tests will be presented here. Beginning clinicians often ask which aphasia test they should select for examining patients. We prefer not to advocate any particular instrument but instead ask the clinicians to specify their purposes in testing. What do they want the test to show? If prediction of the course of the patient's recovery is important, the PICA (Porch, 1981) or the Western Aphasia Battery—Revised (WAB-R) (Kertesz, 2006) are the instruments of choice; if the clinician is more interested in the site of lesion, the Boston Diagnostic Aphasia Examination (BDAE-3) (Goodglass et al., 2000) or the WAB-R are indicated; if the clinician wants to know how the patient performs on basic-to-complicated language functions, then the classic Minnesota Test for Differential Diagnosis of Aphasia (Schuell, 1973) is a good choice. To sample a patient's communication ability in natural settings, the Functional Assessment of Communication Skills for Adults (Frattali et al., 1997) or the Communicative Abilities in Daily Living (Holland et al., 1998) would be the instrument of choice.

TABLE 8.4 Commonly Used Tests for Aphasia and for Measures of Treatment Outcomes

Aphasia Diagnostic Profiles
  (Helm-Estabrooks, 1993)
Boston Diagnostic Aphasia Examination, 3rd ed. (BDAE-3)
  (Goodglass, Kaplan, & Barresi, 2000)
Boston Assessment of Severe Aphasia (BASA)
  (Helm-Estabrooks et al., 1989)
Communicative Abilities in Daily Living, 2nd ed.
  (Holland, Frattali, & Fromm, 1999)
Examining for Aphasia, 4th ed.
  (Eisenson, 2008)
Functional Assessment of Communication Skills for Adults (ASHA FACS)
  (Frattali et al., 1997)
Minnesota Test for Differential Diagnosis of Aphasia (MTDDA)
  (Schuell, 1973)
Multilingual Aphasia Examination (MAE)
  (Benton & Hamsher, 1989)
Porch Index of Communicative Ability (PICA)
  (Porch, 1981)
Western Aphasia Battery—Revised
  (Kertesz, 2006)

In the hands of a skilled and perceptive clinician who is thoroughly familiar with the materials, *any* of the published tests will provide a detailed description of an aphasic patient's language disturbance. As we pointed out earlier in this book, a test is only a tool, a way to help the clinician make relatively precise observations of a particular individual. With this in mind, let us comment further on a few popular, even classic, tests with regard to assessment philosophy and content coverage.

THE PORCH INDEX OF COMMUNICATIVE ABILITY   Better known as the PICA (Porch, 1981), this is a psychometrically well-constructed test that assesses verbal, gestural, and graphic responses to common objects. Although now infrequently used as an aphasia test, the PICA features a multidimensional scoring system that is necessary in the administration of other instruments, such as the still popular Revised Token Test (McNeil & Prescott, 1978). The multidemsional scoring system uses 1 to 16 categories that allow the clinician to make precise observations of the patient's responses. Scores with percentile norms, performance plots, and recovery curves are generated through data manipulation. Speech-language pathologists have found the overall score (as a single index of communication ability) and the recovery predictions extremely useful information to share with physicians.

On the other hand, we find that administration of the PICA is time consuming and that starting the examination with the most difficult task often overwhelms the aphasic person and disturbs his or her subsequent performance. The PICA offers only limited information about a patient's verbal ability: Only 4 of the 18 subtests elicit verbal behavior; only one of the four, "describing how objects are used," affords any insight into how the patient talks.

THE BOSTON DIAGNOSTIC APHASIA EXAMINATION   The BDAE-3 (Goodglass et al., 2000) operates on the localization premise that test scores and profiles correspond to specific types of aphasia. We particularly recognize as a strength the conversational and expository speech section that rates six features: melodic line, phrase length, articulatory agility, grammatical form, paraphasia, and word finding. Subtests cover a wide variety of skills and modalities, making it a well-rounded examination. Supplementary tests are included for use with related disorders. We, however, do find that the BDAE is a lengthy test and one that may frustrate low-level patients. The Computerized Boston (Code, Heer, & Schofield, 1989) is a computerized scoring program for the BDAE.

WESTERN APHASIA BATTERY-REVISED   The WAB-R (Kertesz 2006) is based on neurolinguistic and neuroanatomic models of language. With an efficient administration time of 1 hour, the Western Aphasia Battery assesses various language abilities through subtests such as information content, fluency, auditory comprehension, repetition, and naming; it taps the auditory modality but also the communicative modalities of reading, writing, and calculation. Analysis of the patient's performance yields an Aphasia Quotient that enables the clinician to classify the patient's type and severity of aphasia. The test battery provides data on language functioning that is useful in establishing a prognosis, designing treatment, and tracking progress.

COMMUNICATIVE ABILITIES IN DAILY LIVING, 2ND EDITION   Holland et al. (1999) designed the CADL-2 to sample the patient's functional communication skills in naturalistic situations. It is to supplement traditional tests of aphasia, not replace them. As such, it does not lend itself to differential diagnosis. The content of the CADL-2 is unique; it includes categories such as role-playing, utilizing nonverbal context, and analyzing speech acts. All in all, it is a test that measures what it purports—communication in daily activities.

Regardless of the test used, the evaluation process permits the clinician to identify islands of communication ability the patient retains. In many instances, however, the SLP will want to do additional, more extensive testing in particular areas. Some specialized tests follow.

1. *Auditory Comprehension.* Almost every comprehensive aphasia battery has at least one section that evaluates auditory comprehension. Since the integrity of the auditory modality is so crucial in predicting recovery, we urge thorough, standardized testing. We acknowledge that some focused auditory comprehension tests were published in the 1970s and that some current audiology tests can be adapted for nonstandardized explorations.

2. *Expressive Abilities.* Early aphasia batteries have been criticized for not evaluating the spontaneous speech of patients. The Boston Diagnostic Aphasia Examination is a well-known exception. Discourse analysis with adult patients has shown clinical promise, albeit time-consuming, with contextual, syntactic, and semantic assessments of expressive output. On a syntactic level, the Sentence Completion Test, available in journal form (Goodglass et al., 1972), is useful in assessing sentence construction abilities and the patient's use of derivations. The many psychology-based sentence completion tests are less useful.

3. *Word-Finding Abilities.* Word fluency and naming difficulties (*anomia*) are a common sequela of adolescent and adult brain damage, such as from stroke or traumatic brain injury. Specialized testing might include the Boston Naming Test (BNT) (Kaplan, Goodglass, & Weintraub, 2000), the Test of Adolescent and Adult Word Finding (German, 1990), and the neuropsychological Test of Verbal Conceptualization and Fluency (Reynolds & Horton, 2007).

4. *Reading Ability.* The Reading Comprehension Battery for Aphasia (RCBA-2) (LaPointe & Horner, 1998) and subtests of aphasia batteries are useful measures of reading ability.

5. *Neuropsychyological/Neurolinguistic Analysis.* Batteries that assess aphasia from this different perspective include the Psycholinguistic Assessment of Aphasias (PALO) (Caplan & Bub, 1990) and the Psycholinguistic Assessments of Language Processing in Aphasia (PALPA) (Kay et al., 1997).

6. *Others.* Additional special testing almost surely includes an oral-peripheral and motor examination and a test of hearing acuity, as well as others deemed necessary for particular patients.

Finally, we do not feel that a clinician should abrogate his or her personal clinical responsibility for judgment by deferring to a test or the numerical scores it generates. A combination of clinical intuition, patient observations, lesion information, and test scores and performances should shape our diagnoses and predictions.

Differential Diagnosis

The SLP must often distinguish between aphasia and a number of other conditions involving abnormality in language or speech. A variety of special tests may be needed to supplement standard aphasia batteries in order to facilitate differential diagnosing. Table 8.5 lists some tests useful in differentiating aphasia from other adult language disorders, as gathered from the literature

TABLE 8.5	Useful Tests for Cognitive-Communicative Assessments and in Tracking Outcomes

Arizona Battery for Communication Disorders of Dementia (ABCD)
  (Bayles & Tomoeda, 1993)

Assessment of Communicative Effectiveness in Severe Aphasia (ACESA)
  (Cunningham et al., 1995)

Boston Naming Test
  (Kaplan, Goodglass, & Weintraub, 1983)

Cognitive Assessment of Minnesota
  (Rustad et al., 1993)

Funtional Independence Measure and

Functional Assessment Measure (FIM + FAM system)
  (Hall, 1992)

Functional Linguistic Communication Inventory (FLCI)
  (Bayles & Tomoeda, 1994)

Galveston Orientation and Amnesia Test (GOAT)
  (Levin, O'Donnell, & Grossman, 1979)

Global Deterioration Scale of Primary Degenerative Dementia (GDS)
  (Reisberg, Ferris, & Crook, 1982)

Mattis Dementia Rating Scale (MDRS)
  (Mattis, 1976)

Mini-Mental State Examination (MMSE)
  (Folstein, Folstein, & McHugh, 1975)

Revised Token Test
  (McNeil & Prescott, 1978)

Ross Information Processing Assessment-Geriatric
  (Ross-Swain & Fogle, 1996)

Scales for Cognitive Ability for Traumatic Brain Injury (SCATBI)
  (Adamovich & Henderson, 1992)

Test of Nonverbal Intelligence (4th ed.) *(TONI-4)*
  Brown, Sherbenou, & Johnsen, 2010

(Adamovich, 1998; Bayles & Tomoeda, 2007; Davis, 20074; Holland & Thompson, 1998; LaPointe, 2005). Special tests delineate patient's strengths and weaknesses beyond the realm of language; areas such as intelligence, cognition, perception, mood, and behavior need to be tapped.

We present the following brief discussion of some disorders that might be confused with aphasia. Keep in mind, however, that impairment of symbolic functioning can coexist with any of these conditions.

Psychosis

Although it is rather easy for the professional to distinguish *aphasia* from *psychosis,* it is understandable why laypersons are often confused. The aphasic may say yes when he or she means no, use obscenities and other antisocial language or gestures freely, laugh or cry often, lapse into euphoria, deny his or her symptoms, or withdraw into severe depression and despair. The distinguishing features of psychosis are, however, rather obvious: severe personality decomposition—

not just frustration or emotional overflow when trying to comprehend or speak—and distortion of, or loss of contact with, reality. The vast majority of aphasic patients do not show evidence of mental deterioration or gross disturbances in processing reality. Additionally, the person with aphasia will generally try hard to communicate with others; for the psychotic, interpersonal contact is irrelevant.

Considering all the frustrations that persons with aphasia encounter, we have often wondered why they do not behave in a more abnormal manner than they do. Indeed, their demeanor and social interaction, aside from the language impairment, are remarkably normal. Nevertheless, some individuals with aphasia do experience psychotic episodes and periods of severe depression.

Language of Confusion

The *language of confusion* describes patients with irrelevant and confabulatory language, cognitive confusion and unclear thinking, reduced recognition of the environment and other perceptual issues, faulty memory, and disorientation to time and place. Syntax, word retrieval, auditory comprehension, and ability to repeat are usually not impaired. The patient's relatively good language is, therefore, unlike aphasia.

The onset of confusion typically is sudden, owing to a traumatic injury. In persons who exhibit the language of confusion, the injury to the brain is widespread and perhaps affects the hemispheres bilaterally. The following case example illustrates the irrelevance and confusion:

Tom Snively, a 20-year-old college junior, suffered a closed head injury in a skiing accident. He was in a coma for two weeks. Now, two months post onset, he is an inpatient in the Marquette Rehabilitation Center. When evaluated with a standard test of aphasia, Tom showed no disturbance of vocabulary or syntax; he did have some limited word-finding difficulty. The examiner noted, however, that the young man had trouble attending and staying in touch with the test situation. The patient tended to give responses that, although syntactically correct, were often irrelevant. Additionally, Tom was disoriented and particularly in response to open-ended questions gave rambling, fabricated answers. Here is a portion of an interview conducted by a medical social worker that reveals the patient's disorientation and tendency to confabulate:

WORKER: Where are you?

   TOM: Ah, in training camp. Colorado Springs. And tomorrow we do time trials for the giant slalom.

WORKER: But, what is this place?

   TOM: A training center. I had a hamstring pull and need whirlpool treatments.

In addition to language confusion and other cognitive symptoms, patients may show changes in personality as well. Areas to be assessed include orientation, memory, reasoning, story retelling, and verbal explanations, to name but a few. The SLP may wish to select from tests presented in Table 8.5. Regarding prognosis, the confusion may range from mild and temporary, such as in concussion or hypothermia, to profound and chronic, as in head injury or drug overdose.

Language of Generalized Intellectual Deterioration

The *dementias* are a group of disorders that feature generalized cognitive declines; speech-language declines figure prominently in the dementias but there can be a host of other symptoms. Depending on the type of dementia, causes may include infectious diseases, tumor, and multiple strokes. The area of brain affected is diffuse and may be cortical, subcortical, or both. While Alzheimer's disease is a well-known type of dementia, other examples include Parkinson's diseases, advanced Down's syndrome, and vascular dementia stemming from repeated strokes, to name but a few (Bayles & Tomoeda, 2007). Unlike the language of confusion, the dementias often have a gradual, insidious onset.

Before a clinical diagnosis of dementia can be confirmed, several key features must be present:

1. A sustained deterioration of *memory,* plus a disturbance in at least three of the following areas: (a) orientation in time and place; (b) judgment and problem solving (dealing with everyday situations); (c) community affairs (shopping, handling finances); (d) home and avocations; and (e) personal care
2. A gradual onset and progression
3. A duration of at least six months or longer

Generalized intellectual decline and cognitive dysfunction are hallmarks of the dementias that are evident in the patient's overt language. Table 8.6 highlights differences between dementia and aphasia (Bayles & Kaszniak, 1987; Rosenbek, LaPointe, & Wertz, 1989).

TABLE 8.6	Cognitive and Communicative Differences between Aphasia and Dementia	
Variable	**Aphasia**	**Dementia**
Progression	There is rapid onset; improvement is typical.	There is slow onset and progressive deterioration.
Cognition	Cognition is generally intact.	Cognition is mildly to profoundly impaired; it worsens with the condition; problem solving is poor.
Memory	Memory is generally intact.	Memory ranges from mildly forgetful to profoundly impaired or amnesic; it worsens with the condition.
Emotionality	Mood is typically appropriate with occasional periods of depression or frustration.	Person is typically labile; is apathetic and withdrawn; intermittently shows agitation; and can exhibit depression or mania.
Pragmatics	Socially appropriate skills are evident despite some comprehension failures; communication efforts typically show relevance.	Social skills are mildly to severely affected; inappropriate behaviors and irrelevant comments are typical; thought processes are disorganized.
Repetition ability	This ability is slightly to severely impaired.	This ability is generally intact unless the condition is severe.
Semantics	Word retrieval difficulties can be mild to severe; semantic and literal paraphasias may be used.	Impairment ranges from mild word-retrieval difficulties to visual misrecognitions to severe vocabulary reductions.
Syntax	Syntax is affected to varying degrees; it can be classified as fluent or nonfluent based on length of utterance.	Syntax is intact when disorder is mild; there is reduction of syntactic complexity as the disorder progresses.
Phonology	Phonology is impaired in nonfluent aphasia; it may be present as literal paraphasia in fluent aphasia.	Phonology is generally intact unless the condition is severe; dysarthria is possible.

To illustrate the salient behavioral and communicative symptoms observed in dementia, we include a portion of a diagnostic report on a patient in the second phase of Alzheimer's disease (Powell & Courtice, 1983):

This 64-year-old patient manifested the following behaviors: lowered drive and energy level; memory loss; slow reaction time; and difficulty making decisions. Her personality has changed in the past year so that now she typically is dull, bland, and unresponsive socially.

Mrs. Davis's language abilities are only mildly impaired at this time. She can match objects; point to and name pictures; and repeat words, phrases, and short sentences. Phonologically and syntactically, her speech is within normal limits. She does have limited output, however, and restricted usage. The patient's speech performance is slow and often, after trying to respond to a task, she will say, "I don't know."

The patient's language disturbance was more evident on tasks requiring greater intellectual effort and abstraction. For example, Mrs. Davis was unable to find and correct semantic errors in sentences ("My sister is an only child") or discern the ambiguity in sentences ("Visiting relatives can be a nuisance").

The Arizona Battery for Communication Disorders of Dementia (ABCD) (Bayles & Tomoeda, 1993) profiles patient performance along the subtests of mental status, linguistic expression, visuospatial construction, episodic memory, and linguistic comprehension. The ABCD is a popular test and can be used to document disease effects over time, as with Alzheimer's. Dementia scales are also provided by Mattis (1976) and by Reisberg, Ferris, and Crook (1982), as well as others. Whichever test is selected, the SLP assesses cognitive and communicative areas such as memory, orientation, associative thought, intelligence, reasoning (both verbal and nonverbal), story retelling, object descriptions, explanations, and vocabulary. Many of the tests listed in Table 8.5 would be appropriate to use.

Right Hemisphere Impairment

Most individuals are left hemisphere dominant for language; yet, injury to the right hemisphere can cause communication deficits. Typically these patients exhibit deficits in visual perception, attention, cognition, and complex communicative events (both verbal and nonverbal). The communicative inefficiencies resulting from right hemisphere damage do not resemble aphasic symptoms. Table 8.7 summarizes deficits typically seen in patients with right hemisphere damage. The interested reader is referred to works on right hemisphere communication disorders (Myers, 2001; Thompkins, 1995; Thompkins & Lehman, 1998).

Only in recent years have tests of right hemisphere communication impairment been marketed. Typically, SLPs and neuropsychologists form a test battery using selected subtests from standard tests of aphasia, learning aptitude tests, perceptual tests, and others (recall Table 8.5). Informal test items also are often part of the assessment battery. Of particular importance are the patient's abilities and disabilities with visuospatial perception, prosody, judgment, and high-level communication. Nevertheless, some of the cohesive tests in clinical use are presented.

The Right Hemisphere Language Battery (RHLB) (Bryan, 1995) consists of subtests such as metaphor-picture matching, written metaphor choice, inferred meaning comprehension, humor appreciation, lexical semantic recognition, emphatic stress production, and discourse production. Rating scales for scoring the discourse sample along 11 parameters are used.

| **TABLE 8.7** | Sequelae of Right Hemisphere Damage |

General Symptoms

Denial of illness

Impaired judgment

Impaired self-monitoring

Poor motivation

Memory problems

Disorganization

Problem-solving deficits

Visuospatial Deficits

Visual field deficits (especially neglect of left half of space)

Visual memory and imagery problems

Facial recognition difficulties (disorientation to person)

Geographic and spatial disorientation (to place)

Visual hallucinations

Visuoconstructive deficits (constructional apraxia)

Deficits in Affect and Prosody

Indifference reaction

Reduced sensitivity to emotional tone

Impaired prosodic production and comprehension

Linguistic Deficits

Problems with figurative language (interprets literally)

Impaired sense of humor

Linguistic deficits, including

Comprehension of complex auditory material

Word fluency

Word recognition and word–picture matching

Paragraph comprehension

Higher order communication deficits, including

Difficulty organizing information

Tendency to produce impulsive answers with unnecessary detail

Insensitivity to contextual cues and pragmatic aspects of communication

---

The Mini Inventory of Right Brain Injury (MIRBI) (Pimental & Kingsbury, 2000) is a 27-item screening tool that assesses visual scanning, integrity of gnosis, body image/body schema and praxis, visuoverbal processing, visuosymbolic processing, affective language, higher level language skills, emotion and affect processing, and general behavior/psychic integrity.

The Rehabilitation Institute of Chicago Evaluation of Communication Problems in Right Hemisphere Dysfunction (RICE) (Halper et al., 1996) has sections focusing on assorted aspects of this disorder. Included are general behavioral patterns, visual scanning and tracking, assessment and analysis of writting errors, assessment of pragmatic communication violations, and metaphorical language.

Motor Speech Disorders

Motor speech disorders often coexist with language disorders, particularly aphasia. The presence of a speech disorder certainly affects the language treatment goals and procedures. For example, facilitative articulation techniques must often be incorporated into the total management program. The evaluation of a patient with brain damage, therefore, should include tasks to determine the existence of either *apraxia of speech* or one of the *dysarthrias.* We will discuss these disorders, and the process of differential diagnosis, in Chapter 9.

Summary

What is aphasia and what is not aphasia remains controversial, even among the experts. Many definitions of aphasia exist—some broad and all-encompassing and others quite specific and limiting. Speech-language pathologists will be wise to keep this in mind as they seek to differentiate aphasia from other speech and language disorders. In the final analysis, labels we use reflect speech-language diagnoses, not medical diagnoses. The evaluation process is likened to taking an inventory of the patient's communicative strengths and weaknesses; this can be done informally as well.

THE ART OF INFORMAL ASSESSMENT

Regardless of which standardized test the clinician administers, for treatment planning it is important to examine *how* the patient made the errors. Did the patient seem to perseverate? At what level of complexity did responses break down? Did the patient give synonyms or associations for words when asked to name pictures or objects? For example, when asked to name a picture of a dollar bill, a patient who says, "Put it . . . pocket . . . wallet . . ." is making a "better error" than a response of "soup" or "don't know." Was the patient attempting to correct the errors? Are responses significantly delayed? How did the patient respond to various cueing techniques? What strategies, if any, were used to assist in word retrieval—using gestures, writing, semantic, or phonetic cues? Answers to these questions are based more on clinician observations during the testing process than on test scores. Informal assessment with activities that probe treatment levels and cueing needs may be most insightful.

In evaluating a patient, it is not *necessary* to use a "test" at all—though tests do lend scores some degree of statistical validity and reliability important for evidenced-based practice. Functional communication skills exhibited by the patient are relevant to designing treatment. Questions that should come to the mind of the clinician include the following: Which of the patient's strategies should be capitalized on and reinforced? Which can be made more effective? Which strategies are counterproductive and interfering? Should alternative modes of communication be employed to develop functional responding? The evaluation provides an excellent time to observe *patient-generated facilitation strategies,* such as gesturing an action to aid in word retrieval, finger tapping to pace speech production, requesting repetitions or using a delay to gain extra processing time, and the like. In addition, before designing a management program, the SLP must consider *characteristics of the stimulus* and which *cues and prompts* may be presented to the patient to increase the likelihood of response accuracy. Treatment probes to determine these things may be initiated during the evaluation stage but should continue to be used throughout the management program to maintain efficiency. (Patient progress is often uneven, and "steps" in the program may be skipped from time to time.)

Characteristics of the stimulus affect the patient's ability to respond. The prevailing clinical assumption is that parameters of the stimulus can be hierarchically arranged to produce a level of responding that is not only continual but also correct (appropriate) more than half of the time. Some general guidelines can be summarized here; the clinician may want to probe the patient's needs regarding the following stimulus characteristics:

1. Presentation of a stimulus through more than one modality increases the likelihood of a correct response. This also provides more contextual information.
2. Salient and nonambiguous stimuli affect performance positively—for example, large pictures without distracting backgrounds, or intense auditory stimuli with a favorable signal-to-noise ratio.
3. Reduced length and complexity of presentation, such as using short words or short and grammatically simple sentences, improves comprehension and production accuracy.
4. Presentation of stimuli at reduced rates for longer periods of time and with an imposed response delay affects performance favorably.

Various cues and prompts may be presented to increase the likelihood of response accuracy. These may be provided by the clinician initially and later, through training, may be faded from use or become self-generated cues, thus helping the patient become a self-sufficient, functional communicator. Cueing can also be part of computer software programs (Katz, 2001). Cueing characteristics and optimal hierarchies are an often-researched area in aphasiology. Table 8.8 lists a 10-level cueing hierarchy, which is useful in assisting patients with word retrieval problems. Cue the patient at the highest step possible to initially aid in word recall and back down the steps, supplying more assistance, as needed. Table 8.9 explains strategies that might prove helpful during the informal assessment and that later can be integrated into treatment. We have often used such stop-and-go strategies to elicit optimal, elaborate, on-target responses from our patients in both assessment and treatment situations.

TABLE 8.8   A Hierarchy for Word Retrieval

Step 1.   Ask patient, "Say (<u>word</u>)." (Patient imitates.)

Step 2.   Ask patient to complete sentence with first and second phonemes supplied (e.g., "You sleep in a be _____.").

Step 3.   Ask patient to complete sentence with first phoneme supplied (e.g., "You sleep in a b _____.").

Step 4.   Ask patient to complete sentence with first phoneme silently articulated (e.g., "You sleep in a . . . [form /b/ on lips]").

Step 5.   Ask patient to complete sentence (e.g., "You sleep in a _____.").

Step 6.   State function, demonstrate function, and supply a carrier phrase (e.g., "You sleep on it . . . motion sleep . . . it's a _____.").

Step 7.   State function and supply a carrier phrase (e.g., "You sleep on it; it's a _____.").

Step 8.   Direct the patient to demonstrate the function (e.g., "Show me what you do with it.").

Step 9.   Direct the patient to state the function (e.g., "What do you do with this?").

Step 10. Request the name (e.g., "What's this?").

TABLE 8.9   Compensatory Strategies for Aphasia

Comprehension Strategies

- Repeat the utterance for the patient; later ask the patient to assume the responsiblity of requesting repeats.
- Augment verbal material with the same information in writing; patient eventually should ask for material to be written if this modality aids comprehension.

"Stop" Strategies

These strategies are useful with patients who have fluent aphasia. These strategies assist in controlling fluency and monitoring empty speech or paraphasic errors.

- If desired, model a slow rate of speech and monitor the patient's pace, stopping to correct when needed.
- Encourage the patient to listen to him- or herself. Frequent verbal reminder to "listen" may be employed.
- Actively stop the patient's speech output, if necessary. This can be done by touching the lips, saying "Stop," using a gesture signal (such as hand up) or any combination of these that successfully terminate the jargon. Fading of the stop cue should be incorporated into the treatment plan.
- Encourage self-correction in the patient. Direction to use another strategy, such as a word-retrieval technique, may be helpful.

"Go" Strategies

These strategies are useful with patients who have nonfluent aphasia. "Go" strategies encourage the patient to keep communication going by using telegraphic speech, gestures, or graphics on which to expand.

- Get the patient started; the clinician can suggest a gesture or "key word" to initiate a telegraphic response.
- Keep the patient going; the clinician can replay or feed back to the patient what was said initially and encourage expansion or elaboration.

SUMMING UP THE FINDINGS

Patient abilities and disabilities are determined through the formal and informal evaluation process. Such information permits the SLP to diagnose the type of aphasia (or other communication disorder), if any. The diagnostic label is useful as a "summary statement." The information collected is used in determining the patient's prognosis for recovery. Furthermore, it shapes the direction that treatment will take. Of course, the ultimate goal of evaluation and diagnosis is to ensure that the patient's symptoms are managed appropriately.

Prognosis

Selecting patients for treatment who have the best chance of recovery from aphasia is an unsettling task. Rather than abandon anyone, the clinician's impulse is to attempt to work with every person, even though prospects for improvement in cases of severe language impairment are dim. When there is little real progress, the patient's labors are like those of Sisyphus.

How, then, can the SLP identify patients with the best potential? A list of interrelated factors that we have found helpful for making a prognosis is presented here; however, we trust the reader's forecasting will be guided by four important maxims: (1) Do not make a final prognosis on the basis of a single evaluation session—a period of trial therapy is always highly informative; (2) do not make a prognosis solely on the basis of a single measure of behavior (such as one test); (3) do make evidence-based decisions (such as knowing the poor relationship between a patient's motivation and improvement potential); and (4) be sure you understand the value of predictors— they can be potent self-fulfilling prophecies.

1. *Initial Severity.* Initial severity of aphasia is the single best predictor of recovery. The more severe the patient's language impairment at the time of assessment, the poorer the prognosis. Three aspects of language functioning are particularly important in predicting recovery:

- *Auditory recognition.* Patients who make errors (even a few errors—two or three out of 10 items—are significant) when identifying pictures or common objects named by the examiner have an unfavorable prognosis; an impairment at this level is apparently irreversible.
- *Comprehension.* Patients who have marked difficulty in comprehending verbal messages make poor candidates for treatment. In fact, a reliable index of the severity of language impairment in aphasia is the degree of disturbance in comprehension.
- *Speech fluency.* Patients who speak more fluently seem to make better recoveries. But the presence of jargon, especially when it is coupled with lack of self-monitoring, euphoria, or denial, is a poor clinical sign.

2. *Time Elapsed since Onset.* Many studies have concluded that patients who receive language treatment before six months has elapsed since the cerebral insult show the most significant gains in treatment. The longer the time elapsed since onset of aphasia and the beginning of treatment, the poorer the prognosis. Habits of dependence, withdrawal, and possible secondary gains accruing from a nonverbal role tend to defeat therapeutic intervention.

3. *Type of Aphasia.* Recovery of aphasia seems to follow a pattern of evolution. Progress in global aphasia is often poor, but when improvement occurs it is toward the symptoms of Broca's aphasia. Broca's aphasia typically shows fair-to-good recovery; when symptoms diminish, the patient usually retains word-retrieval difficulty and dysfluency. Wernicke's aphasia carries a split prognosis, with some patients doing fairly well and others poorly. Although the symptoms of Wernicke's aphasia often persist, recovery can occur with symptoms evolving toward conduction or anomic types of aphasia. Conduction aphasia improves toward symptoms of anomic aphasia or may recover completely. Anomic aphasia also shows complete recovery or recovery with only the persistence of mild word-retrieval difficulties.

4. *Etiology.* Depending on the location and extent of the lesion, patients who have suffered traumatic brain injury tend to make better recoveries than do individuals who have had thrombotic or other vascular episodes and tumors.

5. *Age.* The importance of age as a prognostic variable is not clear, as it often overlaps with factors such as etiology. For example, trauma patients tend to be younger than CVA patients. However, it can generally be said that younger patients recover faster and more adequately than do older patients. Presumably this is because younger brains show more plasticity, and older patients may have more widespread cerebral damage due to arteriosclerosis. In addition, aphasic patients in or near retirement may lack the energy and motivation to persist in a treatment program.

6. *Presence of Other Health Problems.* In our clinical experience, aphasic patients presenting health problems in addition to the brain injury (such as diabetes, systemic vascular disease, or kidney disease) often do poorly in treatment.

7. *Family Response.* Patients whose families provide supportive understanding and appropriate stimulation and who permit the individual to regain his or her role within the family unit have a more favorable prognosis. Said another way, patients who are discharged to home have a better language outcome than do those discharged to long-term institutional care.

8. *Extent of the Lesion.* The more extensive the brain injury, the poorer the prospects for recovery. However, there is evidence that CT scan data per se are not predictive of patient outcome.

9. *Location of the Lesion.* This variable overlaps with type of aphasia. In general, damage occurring posterior to the fissure of Rolando, especially at the junction of the parietal and temporal lobes, tends to result in more persistent aphasia.

10. *Premorbid Personality.* The more outgoing, flexible individual generally responds better to treatment than does an inhibited, introverted person. Personality and temperament are often said to have altered as a result of brain damage. Behavior patterns seen in some aphasic patients have been labeled "egocentricity," "catastrophic response," "concretism," and the like. Despite the tremendous frustration and alteration in self-concept that aphasia produces, most of our clients have not exhibited much change in their basic personality traits.

11. *Intelligence and Education.* The more intelligent, better educated patients make better candidates for treatment. Although this is generally true, a few of our most highly educated patients were so vividly aware of the discrepancy between their premorbid abilities and their present condition, they simply withdrew in futility.

12. *Self-Monitoring.* Patients who are aware of their errors and attempt to correct them have a more favorable prognosis than those who do not. Related, patients who are attentive and cooperative during initial testing tend to be those whose outcome includes independent daily living.

13. *Handedness.* Left-handed patients have better prognoses than right-handed ones. However, it may be that left-handed individuals are more likely to become aphasic regardless of which hemisphere of the brain is damaged, suggesting that left-handers show bilateral language representation.

As we near the end of this chapter, let us remember that aphasia and other adult language disorders impact the daily lives of our patients. It behooves us as clinicians to assess such functional impact at the beginning, middle, and end of our intervention. Only in this manner can we objectively collect functional status measures and track the communicative impacts and improvements in daily living—or lack thereof. The World Health Organization's ICF classification focuses attention on the patient's functioning and disability, rather than the disorder per se, and so is a useful schema for thinking about health outcomes (WHO, 2002). This is depicted in Figure 8.4.

Throughout the chapter and its many tables we have mentioned various instruments for the functional assessment of communication. One's level of communication competence and the ability to participate in social activities are inextricably linked. In general, there is a direct relationship between a person's quality of life and the severity of the persisting aphasia or other adult language disorder. One to three years after a stroke or brain episode, the person's quality of communication is related to the presence or severity of depression: the more severe the communication disorder the more severe the depression. Holland and Thompson (1998) reviewed the literature on aphasia and concluded that treatment indeed improves both the quality and quantity of language than if no treatment was received. The knowledge and skill of the SLP, however, is the

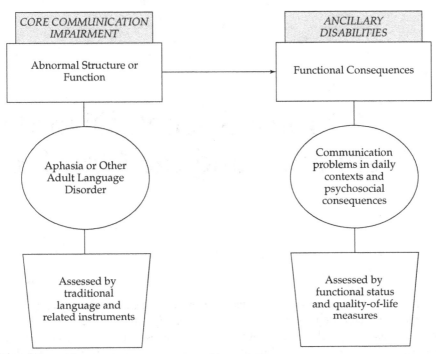

FIGURE 8.4   Assessment of aphasia and adult language disorders using the World Health Organization's classification of functioning, disability, and health (ICF).

foundation upon which diagnosis, ongoing evaluation, and treatment are built. Information presented in this chapter therefore is consistent with ASHA's preferred practice patterns (2004) wherein the SLP is expected to:

- Assess the individual's underlying strengths and deficits related to spoken and written language factors
- Appraise effects of the language disorder on the individual's activities and participation in ideal settings and in everyday contexts
- Explore contextual factors that serve as barriers to or facilitators of successful communication and participation

9

Motor Speech Disorders, Dysphagia, and the Oral Exam

Motor speech disorders is an umbrella term that includes many diverse, neurologically based problems. Those that may come to mind first are the many adult dysarthrias. The cerebral palsies originate in infancy, and the speech impairment that may coexist with the movement disorder is also considered dysarthria. Neuromuscular difficulties may result in swallowing disorders or dysphagia, which may or may not co-occur with speech disorders. Then, there are the apraxias that may affect various parts of the body, in particular the control of oral muscles, leading to oral (nonverbal) apraxia or apraxia of speech (verbal apraxia). All in all, we have our work cut out for us in this chapter. To adequately cover evaluation and diagnosis of such a broad spectrum of motor disorders, we will discuss each in individual sections of the chapter. This chapter also provides the logical place for discussion of "how to do an oral-motor examination" of a patient. Information important to the diagnosis of motor speech disorders will come, in part, from the oral exam. We will, however, attempt to be generic in our discussion of the oral examination to make it applicable for clients of any age (child to adult) or with any speech-language disorder (e.g., articulation, cleft palate, dysarthria). With our territory now laid before us, let us begin our journey with the oral exam.

THE ORAL PERIPHERAL EXAMINATION

An examination of a client's oral cavity and surrounding area is a routine part of every speech-language evaluation. Regardless of the client's particular communication impairment, the findings of the oral peripheral examination may help shape a theory of etiology, diagnosis, and prognosis for change and provide a direction that the treatment should take. In order to avoid repetition in the chapters of this book, we thought it best to consolidate our discussion of the oral peripheral examination into one place. Since the oral peripheral examination not only looks at structures but also assesses the function of those structures from a motoric point of view, we thought it most appropriate to include it in our discussion in this chapter on motor speech disorders. Indeed, the oral peripheral examination is often called the oral-motor exam, a reflection of the importance of motoric integrity for normal speech production.

As we said, it is common practice to inspect a client's oral region to determine its structural and functional adequacy for speech. To provide an example of typical data gathered during an oral peripheral examination, we have included notes hastily scribbled during an evaluation of a 9-year-old boy with a hoarse voice and several articulation errors:

> Lips look okay. No asymmetry of face. Slight open bite; poor dental hygiene (lots of cavities and tartar build-up). Tongue has good mobility, no paralysis or sluggishness; can protrude, wiggle from side to side swiftly, and touch the alveolar ridge; can even curl and groove. Hard palate seems OK, no scars. Soft palate has good tissue supply; elevated fine, no asymmetry. Palatine tonsils are *really* enlarged, filling the whole isthmus between the fauces. Pharynx looks inflamed (possible postnasal drip?). Good gag reflex. Wonder why he has mandible thrust to left side on /ʃ/ and /tʃ/?

Note the systematic nature of the inspection. Although the period of observation was relatively brief—an oral examination is generally completed in less than 2 minutes—the clinician has a sound basis for making a referral to a laryngologist. Now we shall present a rather detailed procedure for conducting an oral examination.

Tools You Will Need

You will need a light source; a small flashlight is good (we avoid the head mirror because it makes us look like a physician). Next, we obtain a supply of wooden tongue depressors; the individually wrapped ones are best for sanitary purposes. Since we are living in the age of AIDS and other contagious diseases, the prudent clinician will wear sterile gloves, or at least use a finger cot, when palpating the roof of the client's mouth. Finally, your kit might include several pads of cotton gauze (for holding onto tongues), a few candy suckers, and a mirror. For more elaborate or specialized examinations, additional materials may be needed. These might include cotton-tipped applicators, various flavor vials for taste sensation, oral stereognostic forms, bite blocks, a syringe of water, some cookies or crackers, and the like. Beach (2002) offers an Oral-Motor Toolbox complete with some 25 items, not only handy for the oral-motor evaluation but also for phoneme cueing and other treatment elicitations.

Areas to Be Assessed

It is important to be *systematic* and *swift* when conducting an oral examination. This demands considerable practice. Use every opportunity to scrutinize normal-speaking persons of all ages, not only to perfect your technique and observational skills but also to establish a frame of reference on the range of normal structural and functional variation. The following outline is presented as a guide for conducting a typical oral peripheral examination:

1. *Lips and Lip Movement.* Inspect the lips first for relative size, symmetry, and scars. Can the client smile, pucker the lips, and retract them? Can she or he close the lips tightly for the sounds /p/, /b/, /m/? Can the client utter the nonsense syllable "puh" at least once per second?

2. *Jaws.* Scrutinize the client's jaw in a state of rest; observe for symmetry. Can he or she open and close the mandible at least once per second? Does the mandible deviate to the right or the left on opening? Assess mandibular strength by having the client attempt to open or move his or her jaw laterally against resistance.

3. *Teeth.* Inspect the client's bite during a state of rest. A normal dental bite is characterized by the upper incisors overlapping the lower incisors by not more than one half of their vertical dimension. Is there an open, under-, or overbite? Does the client have cavities, jumbled teeth, gaps between teeth, or more than the normal complement of teeth? Does he or she wear a dental prosthesis?

4. Tongue. Note the size of the tongue relative to the oral cavity (macroglossia may suggest an endocrine disorder). Observe for symmetry of structure and during movement (in hypoglossal nerve palsy, the tongue deviates to the side of the palsy). Is there any scarring, atrophy, or fasciculations? (Fasciculations suggest motor neuron disease.) Can the client protrude and retract the tongue, wiggle it from side to side, and touch the alveolar ridge without random movement or extraordinary effort? Inspect the tip of tongue and the frenulum for any evidence of tongue tie (see Kummer, 2005; Messner & Lalakea, 2002, for discussion of ankyloglossia and speech). Some clients, especially those presenting with neuromuscular problems, may find it difficult to elevate the tip of their tongue to the alveolar ridge on command. We use a sucker, placing the moistened candy behind the upper incisors and encouraging the client to go after it. (A spot of peanut butter or a tiny paper wedged high between the central incisors can also be used.) Can the client trill his or her tongue when the mandible is stabilized? Test for diadochokinesis by having him or her utter "tuh"; can he or she say at least one per second? Can the client say "pattycake" swiftly and repeatedly? Be sure to look for regularity as well as rate in any tongue movement task. This is important in patients suspected of motor speech disorders. Table 9.1 provides

---

TABLE 9.1 | Diadochokinetic Rate Assessment

Definition and Purpose

Diadochokinetic rate (DDK) assesses the client's ability to make rapid alternating speech movements. It is a maximum repetition rate task that is a form of alternating motion rates (AMR), a term often used among neurology professionals. The speed of movement, along with the observed rhythm and coordination, are indicators of neuromuscular integrity. The premise is that DDK increases as a child ages and the neuromotor system matures, and that there are expected declines in speed among the elderly. DDK rates outside the expected norm and patterns of any discoordination are helpful in the differential diagnosis of certain disorders.

Types of Stimuli Used

Single, double, and/or triple syllabi may be used as in "puh-puh-puh," "puh-tuh, puh-tuh," and "puh-tuh-kuh, puh-tuh-kuh," respectively. The later rapidly changes place of articulation from anterior to posterior (bilabial, lingualveolar, linguavelar). Alternative stimuli for use with clients include words such as "pattycake" or "buttercup."

Method of Measurement

Provide instructions, stressing the importance of doing the task "as fast as possible"; allow practice. Use a stopwatch or similar instrument. For measuring DDK rate, it is typical to average 3 trials per type of stimulus (single, double, triple syllabi). Two methods of measurement are used clinically. Select one method, taking care to compare the client's results to normative data using the same method.

(1) *Count-by-Time Method:* Count the number of syllables repeated by the client within a predetermined number of seconds. Example: the number of "puh" syllables uttered within 15 seconds.

(2) *Fletcher Time by Count Method:* Time the number of seconds necessary for the client to repeat a predetermined number of syllabi. Example: the number of seconds needed for the client to produce 20 repetitions of "puh."

Norms

Use published norms appropriate to DDK method used. Selected sources include the following.

For children: Canning and Rose (1974), Fletcher (1972), St. Louis and Ruscello (2000), Yaruss and Logan (2002)

For adults: Dabul (2000), Prathenee (1998), Sonies at al. (1987)

more information on diadochokinetic rate testing. Is there any evidence of tongue thrust? (An open bite in a child might alert you to this possibility.) When the person swallows, does he or she have an exaggerated lip seal? Does his or her tongue protrude beyond the incisors? Is there no apparent bunching in the masseter muscle? (If the answers to these last three queries are positive, then the client may be a tongue thruster.)

5. *Hard Palate.* Note the shape (is it flat? high and arched?) and width of the hard palate. Are there any scars present? Is there any blue coloration to the palate (suggestive of a submucous cleft)? Can you palpate solid bone under the tissues at the palatal midline? Can the client produce /r/ and /l/?

6. *Soft Palate and Velopharyngeal Closure.* Inspect the velum for total size, scars, and symmetry of movement. Is it bifid? Look carefully for any variations in color, such as bluish borders or striations. Does the soft palate move back and up toward the posterior pharyngeal wall? What is the size of the velum relative to the depth of the pharynx? Can you visualize lateral movement of the velum? Can the client whistle or puff up his or her cheeks? (Chapter 11 presents details of assessing velopharyngeal competency as it relates to hypernasality and nasal emission.)

7. *Fauces.* Inspect the pillars for scars, the status of the palatine tonsils, and the width of the isthmus. Check the general condition of the oropharynx.

8. *Others.* Observe the client's breathing during speech and at rest. Is there an obstruction of the nasal passages? Is the client a mouth breather? Observe the facial muscles: Is a nasolabial fold flattened? Does an eyelid droop (ptosis)? Is one side of the face smooth and devoid of normal creases? Is there anything unusual about the appearance of the individual's head or spacing of the facial features?

The preceding outline is typical of the methodical process that clinicians do, albeit swiftly, with all clients. Indeed, the oral peripheral examination can be done with the basics of a light, gloves, and tongue depressor and the clinical knowledge just outlined. Free outlines also are available online (such as http://www.speechfriends.com), though the problems with such checklists are the lack of guidance as to what constitutes normal and how observations are to be rated or scored. An excellent journal article regarding adult oral-motor functioning is the following. Sonies et al. (1987) developed a scale to assess three areas: oral anatomy, physiology, and speech. There are 10 categories covering these three areas, and each is rated on a 4-point severity scale (1 = normal, 2 = mild, 3 = moderate, 4 = severe). Some weighting of measures is done to obtain a profile of performance. Anatomy ratings include assessment of the appearance of facial bones, tissues, and oral facial symmetry. Physiology ratings include assessment of range of motion, strength, precision, and speed of lingual, labial, palatal, velar, and facial muscles along with assessment of oral sensation. Swallowing function, a subcomponent of the scale, is assessed from a questionnaire, an ultrasound visualization of the swallowing act, mealtime observations, and a medical history. Speech ratings include articulation, voice, fluency, and diadochokinetic rate.

A popular commercial product for use with clients between the ages of 5 to 77 years is the *Oral Speech Mechanism Screening Examination* (OSME-3) by St. Louis and Ruscello (2000). By using the scoring form and the audiocassette training that is provided in the kit, the SLP may make more reliable judgments. Being a screening tool rather than a detailed diagnostic assessment, the OSME-3 provides little to no guidance for planning treatment.

Another oral motor screening tool with the same limitation is the *Screening Test for Developmental Apraxia of Speech* (2nd ed.) (Blakeley, 2001). The STDAS-2 is appropriate for children between the ages of 4 to almost 8 years. As it is a screening test, the reader is cautioned against diagnostic decision, especially as regards the complex disorder of apraxia.

It now may be obvious to the reader that some assessment scales are more detailed than others and that some seem to weigh heavily certain aspects of the total oral peripheral examination. This certainly is the case. Specific oral examination protocols exist for individuals with cleft lip and/or palate, childhood apraxis, pediatric feeding/swallowing difficulties, stuttering, various adult neurogenic disorders, and so forth. Specific oral-motor diagnostic examinations are covered later in this chapter and in other chapters of this book.

To conclude our discussion of the oral peripheral examination, we would like to say that at some point in the not-too-distant future, the diagnostician may have instruments that measure tongue, lip, and other movements very precisely. Remember, though, one swallow does not make a summer, and one deviancy in the oral area does not necessarily cause disordered speech.

APRAXIA OF SPEECH IN ADULTS

The Greek word *praxis* means action. The performance of action can go awry with damage to the central nervous system, and the resulting disruption of movement control can affect various body parts and abilities. Limb apraxia, constructional apraxia, and a myriad of apraxic conditions have been reported; we will focus our discussion on apraxia of speech in adults with brief mention of its close cousin, oral (nonverbal) apraxia.

Cortical damage to the inferior-posterior region of the frontal lobe in the left (dominant) hemisphere can impair oral movements and speech production. This condition has been called by many names, but is generally known as *apraxia of speech* (AOS). Prevailing opinion, though not without controversy, and the perspective of this chapter, is that apraxia is a nonlinguistic speech disorder. It can coexist with other disorders, and it is frequently observed in concert with aphasia and/or dysarthria. The differential diagnosis of a patient's motor speech deficit is important in shaping the appropriate management program. This view of AOS as a motor planning and control disorder is reflected in its definition provided by McNeil et al. (2008):

> Apraxia of speech is a phonetic-motor disorder of speech production caused by inefficiencies in the translation of a well-formed and filled phonological frame to previously learned kinematic parameters assembled for carrying out the intended movement, resulting in intra- and interarticulatory temporal and spatial segmental and prosodic distortions.

The Characteristics of Adult Apraxia of Speech

The hallmark of AOS in a patient is articulatory groping and searching for articulator placements. Speech output may sound struggled, even stuttering-like, or speech may mimic errored word selection (saying something sounding like "chicken" when intending to say "kichen"). Individual symptoms vary. The motor speech output may well be a distortion rather than a pure articulatory substitution. This needs to be remembered, even when most writings about apraxia of speech differentially diagnose it from dysarthria on the basis of articulatory distortion. Our overview suffers this fate as well, but it is an acceptable way to learn about both these motor speech disorders. Another hallmark of apraxia of speech is the impact on volitional productions of articulation and prosody. These articulation and prosodic disturbances do not result from muscle weakness or slowness (as in dysarthria), but from inhibition or impairment of the central nervous system's programming of oral movements. Auditory comprehension, in pure cases of apraxia, is not affected and is "relatively unaffected" in typical cases of this motor speech disturbance. Probably for this reason, most individuals with apraxia of speech have good monitoring skills and are aware, even frustrated, by their motor speech attempts. The most frequent speech symptoms associated with acquired apraxia of speech in adults are (in no particular order):

1. Perceived substitutions and distortions
2. Perceived omissions and additions
3. Effortful articulation
4. Trial and error groping
5. Slow speech; dysprosody
6. Difficulty imitating
7. Excess and equal stress; dysprosody
8. Part-word repetitions
9. More errors on polysyllabic words
10. Inconsistent errors
11. Islands of error-free speech
12. Severe cases may be nonverbal

Oral, nonverbal apraxia can be described as problems in making volitional oral movements in the absence of significant paralysis or paresis. For example, the patient may have great difficulty when asked by the clinician to "pucker your lips" but may have no difficulty kissing his or her spouse as they part for the day. Apraxia of speech and this oral, nonverbal form of apraxia may coexist or may occur independently of each other.

Case History and Prognostic Factors

As with any evaluation, we collect case history information on the patient suspected of having apraxia of speech. Rarely do we know ahead of time that we are going to evaluate a patient with apraxia. More often than not, we are asked to evaluate a patient who sustained brain damage, and a language assessment is of foremost importance. During the testing for aphasia, we may become aware of a motor speech impairment and may test further to diagnose the specific nature and extent of the impairment.

As far as case history information is concerned, marital status, place of residence, social networks, and the like may influence treatment. Prognostic significance has been attributed to some biographical data, such as age, education, premorbid handedness, occupational status at onset and highest occupational level achieved, and premorbid intelligence.

Medical information helpful in making a differential diagnosis includes localization evidence of damage to the third frontal convolution and the presence of right hemiplegia. Medical data suggestive of a favorable prognosis are damage from a single episode (no previous history of brain damage), a small lesion confined to Broca's area, recent onset, and absence of coexisting medical or health problems.

The Evaluation of Apraxia

As mentioned, seldom do we know ahead of time that a patient is apraxic. The speech-language referral merely mentions a brain-damaged adult, so a multitude of coexisting problems *could* be present: aphasia, intellectual impairment, dysarthria, apraxia, and other possibilities. The job of the SLP is to thoroughly evaluate the patient to identify problem areas as well as strengths. In this way, a diagnosis will be arrived at based on the patient's characteristics. The clinician should plan a battery of measures but maintain flexibility so that as the patient's performance unfolds, planned tests can be altered, and additional items can be added to the battery. A typical starting

TABLE 9.2	Typical Assessment Battery for the Evaluation of Adult Apraxia of Speech
Aphasia test	Intelligence, cognitive, memory tests, as needed
Apraxia battery	Oral peripheral examination
Articulation test	Spontaneous speech sample

point is elicitation of a spontaneous speech sample and the administration of an aphasia test (see Chapter 8 for possibilities). As hints of motor problems emerge in the patient's speech attempts, the clinician alters testing plans to investigate in detail the possibility of a motor disorder. Both formal and informal measures can be used. Table 9.2 lists areas to include in a thorough evaluation. Diagnostic questions should unfold in the mind of the clinician: Is there a clinically significant motor speech problem? If so, is it an apraxia or a dysarthria? Which type of apraxia does the patient have? Does the patient have mixed types of apraxia? Which kind of dysarthria is present? Are coexisting motor disorders present?

Several of the aphasia tests evaluate the articulatory agility, melodic line, phonemic difficulties, and oral-nonverbal skills of patients. The inclusion of a word fluency test is good. The Boston Diagnostic Aphasia Examination (Goodglass et al., 2000) and the Western Aphasia Battery (Kertesz, 2006) are examples. A spontaneous speech sample should be analyzed, and an articulation test may be given as well. Of extreme importance is the oral-motor examination. The general oral peripheral examination is supplemented with motor and articulatory tasks to reveal volitional programming deficits. Such tasks or tests should address oral, nonverbal apraxia, and apraxia of speech.

Let us now walk through this evaluation process as it relates to apraxia. Although several so-called tests of apraxia exist, few have adequate psychometric properties and normative data. These tools, therefore, should be considered informal yet insightful, rather than formal, standardized tests. Some tests available for evaluating apraxia of speech are listed in Table 9.3. Let us highlight the components of a few.

Early, modern attempts to evaluate oral and limb apraxia assessed rudimentary skills like instructions to "Stick out your tongue," "Whistle," "Show how you would kiss someone," and the like. Groundbreaking work at the Mayo Clinic in the 1970s advanced the understanding of all motor speech disorders, yet assessment was refined very little. Many research clinicians published informal test protocols with rudimentary scording procedures without norms. Patients were instructed to say lengthening words and phrases to stress the articulatory system. Now-famous assessment stimuli included "gingerbread," "statistical analysis," "zip–zipper–zippering." Some also included tasks of vowel prolongation and imitation of syllable sequences, as well as

TABLE 9.3	Differential Diagnosis of Conduction Aphasia and Apraxia
Conduction Aphasia	**Apraxia**
Repeated trials, attempts self-correction	Groping, inconsistent trials
High proportion of sequencing errors	Low proportion of sequencing errors
Frequent and unpredictable substitutions	Frequent and predictable substitutions
Difficulty linked to "planning load"	Difficulty associated with word length
Intact prosody	Abnormal prosody
Easy speech initiation	Difficult speech initiation, often struggled
Association with posterior brain lesion	Association with anterior brain lesion

the production of words and phrases. Responses were scored and analyzed for phonemic and prosodic errors. Informal testing for apraxia of speech using these classic stimuli is still done by many speech-language pathologists. Commercially available instruments include similar stimuli and are making strides at standardization.

Dabul (2000) designed the popular Apraxia Battery for Adults (ABA-2) to measure AOS and to rate its severity. As apraxia of speech is an acquired condition following brain damage in a specific area, it is worth noting that the ABA-2 is reported to be useful with adolescents and adults. The battery includes six subtests: diadochokinetic rate, increasing word length, limb apraxia and oral apraxia, latency time and utterance time for polysyllabic words, repeated trials, and an inventory of articulation characteristics of apraxia. A variety of methods are used to score these subtests; scores are then used to complete a checklist of apraxia features and to rate the severity on a Level of Impairment Profile.

The Motor Speech Evaluation (Wertz, LaPointe, and Rosenbek, 1984) is useful in detecting the presence of apraxia of speech or dysarthria and in rating the severity of the condition. The evaluation includes the following tasks: conversation, vowel prolongation, rapid alternating movements, repetition of multisyllabic words, repeated production of the same word, repetition of words that increase in length, repetition of monosyllabic words that begin and end with the same phoneme, repetition of sentences, counting forward and backward, picture description, and oral reading. Several methods of scoring are suggested by the authors; however, severity is rated on a 1–7 scale, with 1 being equivalent to mild and 7 to severe.

The Apraxia Battery for Adults (Dabul, 2000) and the Motor Speech Evaluation (Wertz, LaPointe, and Rosenbek, 1984) are probably the most widely used instruments for assessing apraxia of speech. In using evaluation tools to diagnose a patient, we need to remember the important maxim: A test does not make the decision; a clinician does. The clinician has a responsibility to evaluate and interpret the patients' efforts competently.

Differentiating Apraxia from Other Disorders

As we stated earlier, apraxia of speech often coexists with other disorders of communication. Differential diagnosis of the many components of a patient's problem is of paramount importance.

Apraxia is often differentiated from aphasia on the basis of the patient's relatively normal auditory comprehension as compared to oral expression difficulties. In actuality, this differentiation is clear-cut for some forms of aphasia but is quite muddled for others.

On occasion, patients with apraxia of speech have sufficient phrase length and grammatical form to appear somewhat "fluent," despite their prosodic and articulatory difficulties. Errors may mimic literal paraphasias. Table 9.3 summarizes symptoms that differentiate apraxia from fluent, conduction aphasia, as discussed by McNeil et al. (2008).

Apraxia is differentiated from the language of confusion and generalized intellectual deterioration on the basis of more intact orientation, memory, and learning abilities. The reader should refer to Table 8.5 from Chapter 8 for examples of cognitive tests that might be used to make such a differential diagnosis.

Apraxia, classically, is differentiated from dysarthria by the preponderance of phonemic substitutions compared to distortion errors and intact neuromuscular functioning with the exception of facial weakness and hemiplegia. Current thinking is that this substitution versus distortion dichotomy is less straightforward than once thought; still, Table 9.4 provides information useful in making a differential diagnosis of dysarthria and apraxia of speech.

Patients with apraxia of speech can generally anticipate their errors and can also recognize them once emitted. Perhaps this explains, in part, the many retrials and false starts heard

TABLE 9.4	Differential Diagnosis of Dysarthria and Adult Apraxia of Speech	
	Dysarthria	**Apraxia**
Definition	There are distinct patterns of speech owing to weakness, slowness, and uncoordination of speech muscles. Oral movements are disrupted and reflect different types of neuropathology.	There are articulation errors in the absence of muscle slowness, weakness, uncoordination, owing to disruption of cortical programming for the *voluntary* production of speech sounds.
Oral peripheral examination	There is obvious defectiveness: slow, weak, and uncoordinated. *Vegetative* functions (sucking, chewing), as well as speech movements, are disturbed.	There is no obvious dysfunction except when person is asked to execute *voluntary* movements. Vegetative functions are performed adequately.
Articulation	There is simplification: a. Distortions b. Substitutions Errors are consistent. More complex units (clusters of consonants) are more difficult. There are more errors in final position. Errors are consistent with neurological record. Severity is related to extent of neuromuscular involvement.	Complications are: a. Transpositions, reversals b. Perseverative and anticipatory errors c. Fewer distortions, more substitutions, intrusive additions Errors increase proportionate to word weight (grammatical class, difficulty of initial consonant, position in sentence, and word length). There are fewer errors in spontaneous performance. Inconsistency is key sign.
Repeated utterance	Same performance obtains.	Person makes repeated attempts and may achieve correct performance. Person appears to grope or struggle for correct production.
Rate	There is deterioration of performance with increased rate. There is slow rate of speech.	Performance improves at faster rate. There are disturbances of prosody: stuttering-like struggle reactions; slow, labored speech during voluntary attempts.
Response to stimulation	Person may alter performance slightly to match auditory-visual model. Best response is to demonstration of specific articulatory gestures.	Best performance obtains if person sees and hears model. Person does better if provided one stimulation and given several chances to match the model.

in the speech of apraxics. The effortful articulatory groping and repetitive attempts may, at times, be reminiscent of stuttering secondary behaviors. This raises the question of a relationship between neurogenic stuttering (see Chapter 7) and apraxia of speech. Although we do not know the nature of this relationship, if any, it is worth considering in making a differential diagnosis.

Mr. Nils Elander was referred to the hospital-based speech-language pathologist for testing. Evidence from the neuroradiology department showed a left hemisphere thromboembolic infarct. Speech and language improvement was rapid during the two weeks postinfarct. A predischarge reevaluation was performed by the clinician. Mr. Elander presented with mild Broca's aphasia and a moderate coexisting apraxia of speech. Numerous techniques were tried on a trial and error basis to see what stimulation and assistance aided Mr. Elander in initiating difficult words that occurred randomly, as well as at the beginning of utterances. The clinician was able to refer Mr. Elander for outpatient treatment at another facility. The report forwarded to that facility included specific recommendations as to the future direction of treatment. These recommendations included multimodality prestimulation, first phoneme cueing, and use of baton gestures or finger-tapping to impose rhythmical fluency.

CHILDHOOD APRAXIA OF SPEECH

Childhood apraxia of speech (CAS) is the preferred term for a perplexing disorder that previously was termed developmental apraxia. Children with CAS typically have little or no intelligible speech. Childhood apraxia may seem to have core motor speech impairments in common with adults who have apraxia of speech, yet these are distinct disorders. The key difference seems to be that the motor programming deficits are not acquired, rather they are present from infancy and impact linguistic processing as well as phonological development. Emerging information on CAS points to genetic and/or neurological underpinning—even relationships to food allergies. This had recently led some researchers to think of childhood apraxia of speech as a syndrome of issues in much the same manner as is current thinking on attention deficit disorders and autism spectrum disorders (ADVANCE, 2010).

ASHA's ad hoc committee on childhood apraxia of speech (ASHA, 2007) offers the following working definition of CAS.

> Childhood apraxia of speech is a neurological childhood (pediatric) speech sound disorder in which the precision and consistency of movements underlying speech are impaired in the absence of neuromuscular deficits (e.g., abnormal reflexes, abnormal tone). CAS may occur as a result of known neurological impairment, in association with complex neurobehavioral disorders of known or unknown origin, or as an idiopathic neurogenic speech sound disorder. The core impairment in planning and/or programming spatiotemporal parameters of movement sequences results in errors in speech sound production and prosody.

The ad hoc committee further states that there is no valid list of diagnostic features that comprise childhood apraxia of speech. Differentiation of CAS from some childhood dysarthrias or even severe cases of phonological disorder (presumably in the absence of programming deficits) is problematic.

Differential Diagnosis

There is a growing consensus of the presence of three cardinal features in childhood apraxia of speech. According to ASHA (2007) these are:

1. Inconsistent errors on repeated productions of consonants and vowels in syllables and words
2. Lengthened and disrupted coarticulations between sounds and syllables
3. Inappropriate prosody

A host of other symptoms can characterize childhood apraxia of speech and "signal early and pervasive problems in speech, expressive language, and phonological foundations of literacy as well as the possible need for augmentative and alternative communication."

Classic information provided by Yoss and Darley (1974) remains helpful in recognizing childhood apraxia of speech as opposed to other forms of defective articulation. These predictors are as follows:

1. Neurologic findings, such as difficulty in fine motor coordination, gait, and alternating motion rates of the tongue and extremities (often manifested as a generalized dyspraxia)
2. Two- and three-feature articulation errors (for example, /p/ for /ð/ involves an error in place, voicing, and continuancy), prolongations and repetitions of sounds and syllables, distortions, and additions in repeated speech tasks
3. Distortions, omissions, additions, and one-place errors in spontaneous speech
4. Slower than normal rate on measurements of oral diadochokinesis
5. Poor maintenance of syllable sequences and shapes; polysyllabic words altered by addition, omission, or revision of syllables

Crary (1988) elaborates on the symptomatology, stating that children with apraxia exhibit slow and irregular alternating motion rates (diadochokinesis). They possess a reduced sound inventory, including vowels, and have obvious prosodic deficits, including slow rate, excess stress, prolonged sounds and pauses, postural/articulatory groping, and unusual intonational contours.

Other authors have cited nasal resonance and nasal emission as characteristics of developmental apraxia of speech (Hall, Hardy, & LaVelle, 1990). Presumably, the velopharyngeal mechanism performs inadequately during complex, rapid, sequential speech. Nasality, then, is more pronounced with conversational speech as opposed to single-word utterances.

In the diagnostic session of a child with the potential of CAS, the speech-language pathologists should determine, to the extent possible, the child's etiological factors through a case history and should thoroughly assess the child's oral-motor development, speech, language, and prosody so that the presence or absence of CAS signs and markers can be determined.

Case History Indicators

Square and Weidner (1981) reviewed case history information from cases diagnosed with childhood apraxia. They found commonalities. Parents reported that auditory responses of the infants seemed normal but that early vocal patterns were suspect. The parents reported that little, if any, babbling occurred. If babbling was done by the infant, parents expressed that its phonetic pattern was undifferentiated. The infant was often described as a "quiet baby." Feeding differences were also reported by the mothers. Babies were said to prefer liquids and soft foods. Some were described as "lazy chewers." As regards general motor development, reports suggest clumsiness, developmental immaturity, and possible "soft" neurological signs. As a toddler, there remained little or no attempt to imitate sounds or words.

From this we can conclude that in a case history interview, the SLP must inquire about the child's health (and hopefully results from neurological testing), history of infant babbling, prosodic patterns of early vocalizations, a description of the infant's temperament (quiet versus fussy), and history of any feeding difficulties. These sorts of historical questions are repeated in the interview to collect the current status of the child. A full description of the child's speech, prosody, language, cognitive status, and general motor coordination (speech and nonspeech) are in order. This is the type of child that can benefit from an interdisciplinary team approach. Certainly, input from a neurologist, neuropsychologist, and speech-language pathologist is at the core of a diagnostic work-up. Additional questions regarding motor coordination, health/neurological issues, and any chewing or eating concerns need to be raised (and the textures and types of food the child prefers). Some commercially available CAS assessment instruments provide case history suggestions as well.

Assessing Childhood Apraxia

Recognizing the ill-defined nature of childhood apraxia of speech, it is not surprising that the assessment of CAS is a process of excluding other disorders and including, or identifying, apraxic signs and symptoms. The medical evaluation will seek to exclude other causes of the motor impairment, such as neoplastic disease, degenerative conditions, cerebral palsy, acquired CNS damage, and the like. The neuropsychological evaluation will exclude general intellectual deficits, autism (along with the SLP), and behavioral-emotional problems (however, it is recognized that behavioral problems are often a consequence of the child's apraxia). The primary sensorimotor evaluation will exclude problems of muscular tone, strength, speed, and sensation.

Instruments are commercially available for the SLP's communicative assessment, but the evidence on which most are based is still emerging. Earlier in this chapter we mentioned a screening test entitled the Screening Test for Developmental Apraxia of Speech (Blakeley, 2001). It screens expressive language discrepancy, vowels and diphthongs, oral-motor movement, verbal sequencing, motorically complex words, articulation, transpositions, and prosody. A screening instrument, though, is not adequate for diagnostic assessment and for treatment planning. Crary (1988) and Square and Weidner (1981) suggest areas important for the SLP to tap in the assessment of childhood apraxia of speech. We have summarized these areas in a list, displayed in Table 9.5, while Table 9.6 lists some suggested nonspeech oral movements for the child to perform.

It is highly desired, however, that the SLP use diagnostic tests with standardized norms and indexes of reliability and validity. McCauley and Strand (2008) reviewed various diagnostic tests of childhood nonverbal oral and speech motor performance for psychometric properties and content characteristics. All examined tests were found to be in need of refinement; reliability

---

TABLE 9.5   Four Key Areas for SLP to Assess in Childhood Apraxia

Motor Assessment

Facial/limb praxis

Oral apraxia on simple and complex tasks

Lingua-mandibular and labial-mandibular synkinesis

Velar function

Oral reflexes

Facial mimicry tasks

Motor-Speech Assessment

Diadochokinesis

Nasal resonance (and further tests, if noted)

Standard articulation tests

Phonological analysis (distinctive features and phonological error processes)

Prosody Assessment

Stress patterns

Intonation patterns

General fluency and articulatory flow

Language Assessment(s)

Auditory memory assessment

TABLE 9.6	Nonspeech Tasks for Assessing Childhood Apraxia

Volitional Oral Movements

Stick out your tongue.

Try to touch your nose with your tongue.

Try to touch your chin with your tongue.

Bite your lower lip.

Pucker your lips.

Puff out your cheeks.

Show me your teeth.

Click your teeth together.

Wag your tongue from side to side.

Clear your throat.

Cough.

Whistle.

Show me that you're cold by making your teeth chatter.

Smile.

Show me how you would kiss a baby.

Lick your lips.

Sequenced Volitional Oral Movements: Two Items

Puff your cheeks, then smile.

Pucker your lips, then wag your tongue.

Sequenced Volitional Oral Movements: Three Items

Puff out your cheeks, show me your teeth, then pucker your lips.

measures were particularly lacking. We would like to conclude this section with a brief mention of a few of the well-known diagnostic tests for CAS; see Table 9.7. But because of the complex and multifactorial nature of childhood apraxia of speech, we caution SLPs that no single test score should be used to diagnose childhood apraxia of speech. The decision rests with information for an entire team of professionals and with the skills of an experienced clinician. Only then can the overdiagnosis of CAS be curtailed (ASHA, 2007).

TABLE 9.7	Some Diagnostic Tests for Childhood Apraxia of Speech

Verbal Motor Production Assessment for Children (Hayden & Square, 1999)
    For children 3–12 years

The Apraxia Profile (Hickman, 1997)
    For children 3–16 years

Verbal Dyspraxia Profile (Jelm, 2001)
    For children of unspecified age

Kaufman Speech Praxia Test for Children (Kaufman, 1995)
    For children 2–6 years

THE ADULT DYSARTHRIAS

Dysarthia, or more accurately the dysarthrias, is a collection of motor speech disorders due to neurological abnormalities in strength, speed, range of motion, steadiness, tone, or accuracy of movement (Duffy, 2005). Dysarthria, particularly in adults and adolescents, may be due to trauma (e.g., automobile wreck, stroke, near poisoning) or disease state (e.g., muscular dystrophy, myasthenia gravis, tumor invasion, multiple sclerosis, encephalitis, inherited degenerative disorders). The same may occur in children, but also cerebral palsy from infancy is a typical cause of dysarthria. Regardless of the cause or age of onset, damage or disease can affect the neuromotor system and impact the processes of respiration, phonation, articulation, and resonation. More specifically, the dysarthrias are neuromuscular speech disorders arising from motor pathway damage at singular or multiple sites from the cortex to the muscle. The entire speech production mechanism, including respiratory, phonatory, articulatory, and resonatory processes may be affected (as in Parkinson's disease). Likewise, disruption may be confined to specific musculature (as in Bell's palsy of the face).

Differential Diagnosis

Novice clinicians often have difficulty differentiating the two motor speech disorders: apraxia and dysarthria. The underlying neuromotor impairment is clearly different and site of lesion knowledge will go far in sorting out the two possibilities. Yet, going only on clinical (behavioral) signs that the patient displays, the diagnosis is not nearly as clear-cut as many textbooks imply. Review Table 9.4, which lists distinguishing characteristics of patients with apraxia of speech and dysarthria. Complicating the differential diagnosis is the fact that the two disorders can co-occur.

Differential diagnosing also involves categorizing the patient's symptoms by type of dysarthria. Again, this often proves to be a difficult task for many clinicians, not just the novice student. The type of dysarthria demonstrated will depend upon the site of lesion within the motor pathways. The landmark investigation that delineated the types of dysarthria, prominent speech dimensions, and neurological disruption was conducted at the Mayo Clinic in the 1970s. This expertise continues through the writings of Duffy (2005). An understanding of the types of dysarthria is paramount to the assessment process and the differential diagnosis. We present a synopsis of the characteristics of each type of dysarthria but are assuming that the reader has an understanding of the nervous system and neuroanatomical terminology. In addition to Duffy's other texts on motor speech disorders, we recommend those by Freed (2000), Love (2000), or Yorkston et al. (2010).

FLACCID DYSARTHRIA Flaccid dysarthrias result from disorders (or lesions) of the lower motor neuron system. The muscle-movement problem may be progressive, as in myasthenia gravis, or may affect the bulbar motor units, as in the bulbar palsies. In bulbar palsy, a common form of flaccid dysarthria, the muscles are weak, hypotonic (flaccid), and hyporeflexive and may be atrophied. Spontaneous twitches or dimpling of the skin over the muscle may be noted (fasciculations and fibrillations). Often the bulbar palsy is due to damage of one cranial nerve, and the muscular problems are confined to the body region or group of muscles served by that nerve. For example, in facial palsy (also known as Bell's palsy), the damage to one of the facial nerves (cranial nerve VII) results in a drooping facial expression, inability to raise the corner of the mouth during a smile, infrequent blinking, lowering of the eyebrow, and inability to wrinkle the forehead on the affected side. In hypoglossal palsy, there is damage to cranial nerve XII, and the tongue becomes flabby, atrophied/shrunken, and wrinkled. The client will be unable to perform many of the tongue maneuvers asked during the oral peripheral examination. Damage may be due to multiple cranial nerve involvement as well. This type of flaccid dysarthria is known as generalized bulbar palsy. It would not be uncommon in this condition for the lips, tongue, jaw, velum, pharynx, and larynx to be affected in varying degrees.

Speech abnormalities that are often observed in the bulbar palsies include hypernasality, imprecise articulation of consonants, breathiness, monopitch, and nasal emission. Other characteristics are certainly seen in these patients. We have only attempted to highlight some of the most prominent.

SPASTIC DYSARTHRIA   Spastic dysarthrias result from disorders of the upper motor neuron system—in particular, the pyramidal system. As a result, there can be whole extremity damage (as in cortical lesions) or generalized damage (as from lesions of the internal capsule). The damage may be unilateral, as often seen following a stroke where the patient has aphasia and hemiparesis, or the damage may be bilateral. If bilateral, we often use the classification *pseudobulbar palsy,* as the bulbar system is affected indirectly. Muscular symptoms include spasticity, weakness, limited range of motion, slowness of movement, and hyperreflexia.

Deviant speech dimensions include imprecise consonant articulation, monopitch, reduced stress, harsh voice quality, monoloudness, low-pitched voice, and slow speech rates. Again, we have only attempted to list some of the more prominent and severe symptoms.

ATAXIC DYSARTHRIA   Disease or damage to the cerebellum can result in ataxic dysarthria. In ataxia, there is inaccuracy of movement (affecting force, range, timing, and direction of movements), slowness of movement, and hypotonia (flabby muscles). Speech characteristics include imprecise consonant articulation, use of excess and equal stress patterns, and irregular articulatory breakdowns, among others.

HYPOKINETIC DYSARTHRIA   Disorders of the extrapyramidal system, such as in the basal ganglia complex, often result in hypokinesia, a reduction of movement. A commonly encountered disease causing hypokinesia is Parkinson's. There seem to be six characteristic signs of hypokinetic dysarthria: (1) slowness of movement; (2) limited range of motion; (3) paucity of movement, where the patient may have difficulty initiating a movement and may experience false starts, arrests of movement, or even immobility; (4) rigidity or hypertonicity (may be intermittent); (5) loss of automatic aspects of movement; and (6) presence of rest tremors. Deviant speech dimensions often seen in patients with Parkinsonism highlight the movement difficulties of the hypokinetic dysarthrias. The most deviant are monopitch, reduced stress patterns, monoloudness, imprecise consonant articulation, inappropriate silences, and short rushes of speech. Other, less deviant characteristics exist as well.

HYPERKINETIC DYSARTHRIA   Hyperkinetic dysarthrias result from disorders of the extrapyramidal system. The hallmark of these disorders is the presence of abnormal involuntary movements—some are quick movements and others are classified as slow. In the short space we have in this textbook, we cannot completely describe the numerous forms of both quick and slow hyperkinesias. The interested reader is urged to study further. We will, however, summarize some of the most distinguishing and deviant speech characteristics, averaged over the various subtypes. These include imprecise consonants, variable (or perhaps slow) rate, monopitch, harsh or strained voice quality, inappropriate silences, distorted vowels, and excess loudness variation.

MIXED DYSARTHRIAS Mixed dysarthrias, as the name implies, result from involvement of several motor systems. Often mixed dysarthrias are associated with syndromes or particular diseases, such as amyotrophic lateral sclerosis, multiple sclerosis, and Wilson's disease. Owing to the mixed nature of these dysarthrias, it is almost impossible to summarize characteristic speech disturbances.

The Appraisal of Dysarthria

As evident from the various speech characteristics associated with the types of dysarthria, the patient may have difficulty with any or all of the speech production processes. Consequently, the clinician must assess features of respiration, phonation, articulation, and resonation.

Such an appraisal follows along the lines of a voice evaluation. This topic will be dealt with more thoroughly in Chapters 10 and 11. Suffice it to say that we need to take note of any inhalatory noises, poor breath support, poor management of the airstream, abnormal vocal loudness and stress patterns, abnormal vocal pitch and inflectional patterns, and abnormal vocal-resonatory qualities. Of particular interest is analysis of the sustained phonation during the "ah." With proper instrumentation, detection of irregularities in shimmer and jitter may be quite suggestive. Tanner (2001) notes that progressive neurological diseases such as amyotrophic lateral sclerosis, multiple sclerosis, and Parkinson's can be detected early and monitored through minor changes in voice irregularities. Respiratory/phonatory dysfunction often is a hallmark of speech dysarthria, an area for perceptual and instrumental assessment, and a focus in behavioral management. A systematic review of evidence-based practice for respiration/phonation dysfunction is provided by Yorkston, Spencer, and Duffy (2003).

Regarding the articulatory impairment that is often present in the dysarthrias, the clinician should analyze a sample of spontaneous speech and/or have the patient read aloud. Standard articulation tests, either single-word or sentence versions, are also useful in documenting phoneme errors. Distortion is the most common articulatory error in dysarthric speech. Unlike the difficulties seen in apraxia of speech, the imprecision of consonantal articulation is fairly consistent in dysarthria. In essence, intelligibility is a key speech measure in the diagnosis and continuing evaluation of a person with dysarthria. An evidence-based practice review of oral motor exercises is provided by McCauley et al. (2009).

In addition to the voice test (which includes appraisal of respiration, phonation, and resonation) and the articulatory assessment, a thorough evaluation of a patient with dysarthria should include an oral peripheral examination and a special "dysarthria test," which involves appraisal of both speech and nonspeech motor functions. Published tests of dysarthria are helpful in assessing the severity of the disorder, as well as the type of dysarthria. We will mention a few.

The Frenchay Dysarthria Assessment (FDA-2) (Enderby & Palmer, 2008) profiles oral-motor performance for the various diagnostic categories, such as spastic—upper motor neuron, flaccid—lower motor neuron, extrapyramidal, cerebellar, and mixed neurological lesions. Clinicians may find this helpful in differential diagnosis decision making. Normed on patients aged 12 to adult, performances are rated on eight functions: reflexes, respiration, lips, palate, larynx, tongue, intelligibility, and other influencing factors.

The Assessment of Intelligibility of Dysarthric Speech (AIDS), first published in the 1980s, is one of many dysarthria assessment tools described by Yorkston et al. (2010). The AIDS has the patient read words and sentences. Several measures can be derived, including intelligibility for single words, intelligibility for sentences, speech rate, rate of intelligible speech, rate of unintelligible speech, and a communication efficiency ratio. Classification by type of dysarthria is also possible with this test. Also available from these authors is the Computerized Assessment of Intelligibility of Dysarthric Speech. The software provides for efficient quantifying of single-word intelligibility, sentence intelligibility, and speaking rates without tedious stimuli selection or computation.

The Dysarthria Examination Battery (DEB) (Drummond, 1993) evaluates responses to 23 tasks spanning the areas of respiration, phonation, resonance, articulation, and prosody. Responses are rated on a 1 to 5 scale. Administration of the DEB requires the use of a stopwatch, audiotape recorder, dry spirometer, laryngeal mirror, bite block, and a few other more standard items.

One diagnostic task to which many authorities attribute importance is that of diadochokinetic testing; refer again to Table 9.1. The rhythm and speed with which alternating motion rates can be performed are helpful in sorting out the various types of dysarthrias. Differential diagnosis may be difficult from only a conversational sample of speech. DDKs, on the other hand, seem to "stress" the motor system and, consequently, reveal the difficulties of movement more clearly. The instructions to the patient should stress this notion of "fast and even." Information that is important to the clinician includes the rate, regularity, and duration of the alternate movements of the articulators.

A slow, regular diadochokinetic rate is highlighted in spasticity. For ataxia, alternate motion rates underscore the irregular breakdowns in articulatory precision. It is characteristic to hear fluctuating changes in the intervals between syllables, as well as variations in their duration and loudness. Rate of syllable production varies from normal to slow. In hypokinetic Parkinsonism, alternate motion rates may begin at a slow rate and then accelerate to a rapid, yet usually regular, rhythm. Imprecise articulation due to limited excursions of movement (i.e., hypokinesia) may produce the sound of a continuous blur. Hyperkinetic dysarthrias take on many different forms; AMRs are usually irregular, slow, and perhaps interrupted by arrests of speech.

We offer one final note about appraisal. The patient with dysarthria is not expected to have language, cognitive, intellectual, memory, or learning deficits unless such deficits are associated with the disease process that produced the dysarthria. The clinician, however, should be alert to deficits in these areas and should include appropriate language-cognitive tests in the assessment battery, if necessary.

CEREBRAL PALSIES AND DYSARTHRIA IN CHILDREN

Brain damage sustained before, during, or shortly after birth can produce movement disorders, known as *cerebral palsies*. Movement can be mildly affected or severely crippled. When the muscles underlying speech are affected, we may say that the person has dysarthria (a motor speech disorder) subsequent to the cerebral palsy. Cerebral palsy is a static encephalopathy, meaning it does not worsen by spreading. The causes of CP may include anoxia (lack of oxygen to the brain at any time), trauma during delivery, faulty genetics, maternal infection, infectious disease during childhood, and a traumatic injury during childhood.

Although various classification systems for cerebral palsy have been proposed through the years, most typical is to classify CP accourding to both distribution and type. Terms describing distribution include the following:

- *Hemiplegia*—is the most common form of distribution; an arm and leg (and perhaps speech muscles) on the same side of the body are affected but not necessarily to the same degree.
- *Paraplegia*—is where both legs are affected (speech muscles not affected unless in the torso/respiratory area).

- *Quadriplegia*—results from widespread brain damage where both arms and legs are affected (and probably many speech muscles as well).

Often the types of cerebral palsy are classified into six principal symptoms:

1. Spasticity is characterized by hyperactivity of the stretch reflex. It is secondary to a lesion in the cerebral cortex that causes a loss of control and differentiation of fine voluntary movements with increased muscle tone.
2. Athetosis is involuntary writhing or squirming movements that are irregular, coarse, relatively continuous, and somewhat rhythmic. It is secondary to damage in the extrapyramidal system, often the basal ganglia complex.
3. Cerebellar ataxia is incoordination and poor balance owing to cerebellar dysfunction.
4. Rigidity is a "lead pipe" characteristic of affected muscles and often resembles a severe form of spasticity.
5. Tremors, either athetoid or rigid, involve generalized trembling of the extremities.
6. Flaccidity, as a form of cerebral palsy, is due to damage to the sensorimotor cortex. Affected muscles are unable to contract except reflexively. Perhaps 90% of the cases of cerebral palsy are of the first three types, with spasticity overwhelmingly being the most common.

The Assessment of a Child with Cerebral Palsy

All authorities on cerebral palsy strongly advocate the multidisciplinary approach to assessment, diagnosis, and intervention. Certainly the SLP will not assess motor function and abnormal reflexology without the aid of a physical therapist or other health care professional. Such information, however, is necessary to shape the feeding and prespeech stimulation programs that the infant may need, the handling and positioning techniques that need to be applied, and the facilitating and inhibiting techniques that might be incorporated in the speech rehabilitation program. The Gross Motor Function Classification System (GMFCS) is a simplistic but commonly used five-level classification schema based on walking and gross-motor movements (Palisano et al., 1997).

The child with cerebral palsy typically presents with a host of impairments—orthopedic, sensory-perceptual, intellectual, feeding/swallowing, socioemotional, and so forth. Of interest for this chapter is the assessment of communication skills and deficits. A review of the literature clearly documents that children with cerebral palsy (particularly athetosis) have higher auditory detection thresholds, poorer speech reception thresholds, and poorer speech discrimination than do normal children. A complete audiological evaluation, then, should be part of every evaluation session.

About 50 to 60% of the cerebral palsied population show some degree of mental retardation, while the rest possess normal intellectual capabilities. Impaired language development, learning difficulties, and academic problems often occur in children with cerebral palsy. Etiological reasons may be numerous. Certainly, the SLP must assess cognitive development and linguistic attainment in a cerebral palsied client. Procedures discussed in Chapters 4 and 5 should be utilized.

Speech is a dynamic process requiring highly skilled coordination of the articulatory movements for the production and sequencing of sounds into utterances. It is of no surprise, then, that speech impairments are common among children with cerebral palsy. About 70% of cerebral palsied children exhibit speech disorders; athetoid and ataxic forms seem to be particularly deleterious to speech. However, there appears to be insufficient evidence for the notion that these speech impairments are so distinctive as to justify the concept of *cerebral palsied speech.* This myth was laid to rest in Chapter 6 when we discussed articulatory and phonological speech disorders. The assessment tools discussed in that chapter are certainly applicable to the child with cerebral palsy. Respiration, phonation, and rhythm are likely to be affected as well and must be assessed by the clinician. The ultimate measure of speech effectiveness is its intelligibility; a severity rating scale may be one aspect of the assessment battery. Last, we would remind the clinician that an oral peripheral (oral-motor) examination should be done. The SLP may also need to consider the need for augmentative or alternative communication, a vast topic of its own. The client's feeding and swallowing abilities may warrant assessment. How to do this is the subject of our next section.

DYSPHAGIA

The role and scope of practice in speech-language pathology includes the burgeoning area of evaluation and treatment of swallowing disorders, or *dysphagia.* Clinicians tend to specialize their practice into adult or pediatric swallowing issues based on employment setting. Swallowing difficulties emerge as a consequence of many neurologic conditions. In order of frequency these are stroke, traumatic head injury, spinal cord injury, and brain tumor (Cherney, 1994). Dysphagias also can result from progressive neurologic diseases, head and neck cancers, vocal fold paralysis, and various conditions of the upper aerodigestive tract. The area of pediatric swallowing and feeding disorders is also one of tremendous growth for the SLP. While considerations for assessment and treatment of infants and children with dysphagia can be quite different from adults, a good place to start is with normal anatomy and physiology.

Normal Deglutition in the Adult

The purpose of swallowing is to transport food and other materials from the oral cavity to the stomach without allowing entry of substances into the airway. Safe swallowing entails precise coordination of neuromuscular events including those in the brain, brainstem, cranial nerves, and muscles of the oral cavity, pharynx, larynx, and esophagus.

Swallowing is considered a three-phase process by most authorities although the first phase may be subdivided for clinical utility into the preparatory stage and transport stage. Normal feeding begins with the *oral phase,* specifically the oral preparation stage, which is under volitional control and so may be manipulated in a therapeutic regime. Oral preparation reduces food to a consistency appropriate for swallowing. Lips are closed, the tongue manipulates the food in the mouth as muscles of mastication move the jaw, the teeth tear and crush the morsels, and saliva is mixed with the mass of food forming a cohesive *bolus.* Duration of oral preparation is highly variable, depending on the consistency of the food and the time spent tasting it. Oral preparation provides much of the pleasure from eating, and so it is an important psychological consideration when working with a patient with dysphagia. Liquid diets bypass this pleasurable subphase.

When readied, the bolus is manipulated to the back of the oral cavity, near the faucial pillars. This transport stage is the second part of the oral phase, and it too is considered under volitional control by way of the hypoglossal cranial nerve XII. Tongue muscles nestle the bolus, then elevate and retract to propel the bolus to the back of the oral cavity. The swallowing reflex is believed to be triggered by tongue action as the bolus passes the anterior faucial pillars, although little is understood of this elicitation. Triggering of the swallow is crucial to a safe swallow, but the importance of healthy tongue manipulation cannot be underestimated. Logemann (1998) explains that with impaired tongue action

> the food will spread through the oral cavity as the patient attempts to move it backward. Some food drips down into the pharynx as the patient struggles to control the food and initiate the swallow. The food dripping into the pharynx prematurely may be aspirated before the swallow, or may come to rest in the valleculae and pyriform sinuses. Where the food lands will depend on the patient's posture, the amount of food and the consistency of the food. (p. 6)

From this, the astute reader will discern areas of behavioral assessment and variables to systematically manipulate in the evaluation and treatment of a person with dysphagia. Worthy of mention is that the oral phase of swallowing lasts approximately 1 second, regardless of the person's age, gender, or the consistency of the food being swallowed.

As the swallow is triggered, there is a pharyngeal response. Events in this *pharyngeal phase* are automatic and mediated primarily by the glossopharyngeal (IXth) cranial nerve and the brainstem. Logemann (1998) identifies four sequential, split-second neuromuscular activities in the pharyngeal phase: (1) velopharyngeal closure to separate breathing from swallowing; (2) peristaltic action of the pharyngeal constrictor muscles to clear food from the pharynx; (3) elevation and closure of the larynx to protect food from entering the airway; and (4) relaxation of the muscles encircling the top of the esophagus. Each event lasts a fraction of a second with the total pharyngeal phase occurring in 1 second. This duration does not vary with age, gender, or food consistency. Potential to reestablish a patient's normal pharyngeal phase is a key assessment/prognostic feature of a dysphagia evaluation: In the pharyngeal phase, food is propelled into the esophagus and the airway is protected.

Once the bolus has entered the esophagus, it cannot be controlled volitionally and does not respond to exercise programs. This *esophageal phase* of swallowing begins when the bolus enters the esophagus and ends when the bolus passes through the lower esophageal valve and into the stomach. Duration of this phase varies from 8 to 20 seconds and often lengthens with age.

Bedside Assessment of Adult Swallowing Disorders

The patient suspected of dysphagia warrants assessment and management by a team of medical professionals. Team members may include not only the SLP but also the physician (perhaps a laryngologist, gastroenterologist, and/or neurologist), radiologist, nurse, dietician, occupational therapist, pulmonologist/respiratory therapist, and others (especially in pediatric cases). The bedside evaluation of an adult in a hospital, or the initial assessment in a related setting, begins with a thorough review of the patient's medical chart. What were the presenting complaints and medical diagnoses? What has the physician noted? What insights about feeding and swallowing are in the notes from the nurse, dietician, and social worker? What is the current method of nutrition?

Bedside, the SLP methodically ascertains as much history as possible directly from the patient. Spouses or caregivers can help complete the history intake. Ask questions about the patient's eating habits, duration of feeding, diet, frequency of meals, weight changes, and the like.

According to Schindler and Kelly (2002), patients with feeding problems secondary to cognitive difficulties may eat sporadically and for short periods and so lose weight. Patients with primary dysphagia often require longer feeding periods (and may use compensations like multiple swallows, smaller bites, and prolonged chewing) and may feel self-conscious about their slow feeding or be fearful of coughing or choking. There is even the likelihood of weight gain, as such patients gravitate to more processed and high-caloric foods (e.g., milkshakes and dietary supplements). Question further about any differences noted among solid, semisolid, and liquid swallowing. Patients with fixed obstruction (such as webs, strictures, or neoplasms) often complain of solid rather than liquid dysphagia. Patients who complain of difficulties with liquids are more likely to have neurological conditions that weaken the pharyngeal musculature or result in discoordination of the swallowing reflex. Associated symptoms of nasopharyngeal regurgitation and dysarthria may point to the level of the lesion. Breathy hoarseness may suggest glottic incompetence (and a risk for aspiration), so check for a poor cough. Although wet vocal quality is commonly thought to be a symptom of swallowing incompetence, controversy exists over its importance. (Wet quality alone often reveals adequate swallow in imaging studies, but wet quality with onset after stroke is a likely warning sign.)

All in all, the case history interview leads the SLP methodically into a perceptual voice assessment (see Chapter 10) and into a very thorough oral examination, as presented earlier in this chapter. Additional attention should be directed at observing the integrity of the oral mucosa, the quality and quantity of saliva (which helps form the bolus and trigger the swallow), tongue control and mobility, and other observed oral movement abilities. The ability to gag when stimulated is of questionable importance. Compare any oral exam findings with the neurological exam results that should have been noted in the medical chart. Information on cranial nerve integrity for V, VII, IX, X, and XII is particularly relevant.

Ask about current medications, as these may point to other conditions affecting appetite, feeding behavior, or swallowing. Puntil-Sheltman (2002) warns that polypharmacy may also interfere; medications she indicates that may affect swallowing are shown in Table 9.8.

In evaluating the dysphagic patient, the most important determination is the risk of aspiration. This determines the patient's feeding method (bolus unrestricted, bolus restricted, some alternative to oral intake). Of course the evaluation also strives to determine the need—or not—for swallowing treatment and what compensatory strategies might be brought to bear to improve the safety of the patient's swallow. The book by Groher and Crary (2010) provides

---

TABLE 9.8   Partial List of Medications That May Affect Swallowing

Decreased Saliva (Dry Mouth)	**Impaired Cognition and Attention**
Oxybutynin (Ditropan)	Diazepam (Valium)
Diphenhydramine (Benadryl)	Lorazepam (Ativan)
Gastroesophageal Reflux and Esophageal Dysmotility	**Distorted Taste**
Nifedipine (Procardia)	Chemotherapeutic drugs
Albuteral	Tetracycline
Impaired Chewing and Swallowing	**Improves Ability to Focus on Tasks Such as Eating**
Haldol	Ritilan
Thorazine	Provigil
Risperidone	

sample questionnaires and recording forms. It is critically important to assess the patient's danger of aspiration from food particles, liquids, or the patient's own saliva. Aspiration refers to the inward flow of suction of food or liquids into the airway and lungs. Aspiration pneumonia in patients with dysphagia can be life-threatening. The serious reader is referred to Groher and Crary for discussion of procedures such as the water test (a 3-ounce sip; see also Swigert, 2009), the oxygen saturation test (a 2% drop in SpO_2), and the modified Evan blue dye test (as observed radiographically).

Many protocols for assessing adult dysphagia are available. Five protocols will be highlighted in this chapter.

SAFE: The Swallowing Ability and Function Evaluation (Ross-Swain & Kipping, 2003) guides the SLP through the three stages of evaluation identified as (1) the evaluation of general information relative to swallowing, including cognitive and behavioral factors; (2) examination of the oropharyngeal mechanism; and (3) a functional analysis of swallowing with attention to the oral preparatory, the oral, and the pharyngeal phases of the patient's swallow. The SAFE seeks to provide "a definitive diagnosis or label of dysphagia" in adolescents to adults as well as to provides suggestions for treatment planning.

The BELZ Dysphagia Scale (Longstreth, 1986) rates 12 categories on a 0–3 scale. The rating categories include a clinical swallowing evaluation, otolaryngology examination, cognition/communication status, physical status, pulmonary function, chest x-ray, videofluoroscopic evaluation of swallowing physiology, tracheostomy tube status, diet consistency, tube feeding, respiratory tract treatments, and gastrointestinal function.

The Fleming Index of Dysphagia (FID) (Fleming & Waver, 1987) is a computerized index. Responses to questions and prompts are input; each item is assigned an impact score, and these scores are combined with severity ratings and problem codes to determine the severity of dysphagia, the urgency for treatment, and suggestions for patient management.

The Clinical Evaluation of Dysphagia (CED) from the Rehabilitation Institute of Chicago (Cherney, Pannelli, & Cantiere, 1994) outlines the areas to assess for the SLP. Typically, a prefeeding evaluation is first done when a patient is at high risk for aspiration (e.g., patients who are not yet eating orally or those with tracheostomies).

The evaluation of prefeeding skills on the CED includes collecting a complete history of the problem and observing oral, pharyngeal, and laryngeal structures and functions. From this, the SLP decides the patient's potential for oral intake and the need for further evaluation and referral. The CED's prefeeding evaluation form guides the clinician in the collection and documentation of the following relevant information:

1. Medical/nutritional status (Inquire about diseases, surgeries, medications, and swallowing complaints.)

2. Respiratory status (Ascertain rate [normal = 12–16 breaths per minute] and note any chronic coughing or shortness of breath.)

3. History of aspiration

4. Type and size of tracheostomy, if any

5. Level of responsiveness (Assess ability to follow directions.)

6. Behavioral characteristics

7. Current feeding methods (Describe type of feeding [oral, nasogastric tube, gastrostomy tube, percutaneous endoscopic gastrostomy], when tube was placed, and the frequency and amount of food intake.)

8. Positioning (Note habitual body, head, and neck positions and any motor control problems; determine the best feeding position without giving food [maximal airway protection is upright at 90 degrees with head tilted forward] and what is needed to achieve that position comfortably [use of wedges, pillows, other supports].)

9. Observation of oral motor, pharyngeal, and laryngeal functioning (Perform a thorough oral motor examination, include observations on quality and strength of the voice.)

10. Cough (Note the presence or absence of both involuntary and elicited coughs.)

11. Gag reflex (Elicit reflex and note its strength bilaterally.)

12. Voluntary swallow (Assess ability to perform a dry swallow on command; feel and watch for laryngeal elevation.)

13. Other observations (Observe presence of drooling, mouth odors, and abnormal reflexes that may affect feeding.)

14. Response to stimulation (Note adequacy of lip closure, lip protrusion, response to touching by a spoon, and the like.)

15. Recommendations and goals

Although it may be determined after this assessment that a patient should remain "NPO" (nothing per oral; nutrition must be accomplished through other means), treatment may be recommended to improve prefeeding skills with the anticipation of improvement and future reassessment.

Next, a clinical or bedside evaluation of dysphagia can be performed on patients who can tolerate at least one food consistency. The nature of this evaluation differs substantially for patients of differing levels; Cherney, Pannelli, and Cantiere (1994) provide guidelines for patients with severe dysphagia, those with a tracheostomy, and those receiving an oral diet.

The CED guides the SLP in observing (or inferring) behaviors during swallowing, from the oral phase through the pharyngeal phase. Six different food consistencies can be evaluated; Table 9.9 lists sample foods. The clinician documents his or her observations and rates the performance (ranging from adequate to nonfunctional) for each structure (lips, tongue, mandible, and so forth) and for each phase of swallowing.

The Northwestern Dysphagia Patient Check Sheet (Logemann et al., 1999) is available free online at the American Dysphagia Network (http://www.americandysphagianetwork.org). The check sheet is a 28-item screening test useful in differentiating patients who do or do not aspirate, have an oral stage disorder, a pharyngeal delay, or a pharyngeal stage disorder. The screening procedure covers five categories with individual items rated as "safe" or "unsafe." These are (1) medical history, including items on history of pneumonia or length of intubation; (2) behavioral variables such as the patient's awareness and ability to manage secretions; (3) gross motor function such as posture and fatigability; (4) oral motor test results covering nine areas like physiology, voluntary cough, and saliva swallow; and (5) specific observations. In this fifth category the clinician records observations made during trial swallows of small but varied consistencies.

In a national survey of dysphagia clinicians, the top preferences of clinical/bedside methods in current use were discerned (McCullough et al., 1999). Table 9.10 lists the top seven methods per area. And, on a cautionary note, Martino et al. (2000) state that only two bedside findings have been proven to help in predicting aspiration, as seen by videofluoroscopy. These are (1) reduced unilateral pharyngeal sensation, and (2) coughing with the 50 mL water swallow procedure. Consequently, an imaging study should follow the bedside examination of any patient. The patient's performance on various diagnostic tasks serves as a dynamic assessment. What tasks

TABLE 9.9	Foods and Food Consistencies Used in Evaluating Dysphagia	

Thin Liquids	**Ground Foods**
water, apple juice	rice, scrambled eggs, tuna, ground chicken, hamburger
Thick Liquids	
tomato juice, cream soups, yogurt	**Chopped Solids**
	tender bits of meats, vegetables
Pureed Foods	**Regular Solids**
applesauce, pureed canned fruit, pudding	(usual table foods)

were difficult or unwise for the patient? What tasks facilitated improved swallowing? What, if any consistencies, positions, and techniques were revealed in the assessment that might be the basis for treatment? Some of these same clinical questions need further exploration using objective instruments to best judge improved and safe swallowing. And it bears mention that some cases do not warrant oral feeding and swallowing, a topic that is beyond the scope of this book.

INSTRUMENTAL ASSESSMENT   A range of technologies is useful in studying various aspects of the swallow. Ultrasonography involves the use of transducers to observe structural movements (e.g., of the tongue, hyoid, or to study an infant's suck and oral transit). Surface electromyography records electrical activity of various muscles involved in swallowing, scintigraphy (also referred to as radionuclide milk scanning in the pediatric population), and others. Some of the more popular methods allow dynamic visualizations, such as videofluoroscopic and endoscopic assessments of swallowing.

TABLE 9.10	Dysphagia Clinicians' Top Seven Preferred Methods in Bedside Evaluations

History	**Trial Swallows**
Patient reports	3-oz swallow
Family reports	150-mL test
History of pneumonia	Other thin liquid
Neurological insult	Thick liquid
Nutritional status	Pudding
Gastrointestinal	Puree
Structural (nonsurgical)	Ice chips
Oral Motor	**Voice**
Rapid alternating speech	Variations in pitch/loudness
Tongue strength/range	Breathiness
Lip seal/pucker	Harshness
Jaw strength/lateral	Wet/gurgly
Soft palate movement	Strained/strangled
Palatal gag	Dysphonia/aphonia
Pharyngeal gag	Resonance

The traditional barium swallow concurrent with radiography is useful in visualizing upper airway anatomy and perhaps observing lesions and neoplasms. But to see a swallowing sequence of motions, the barium consistency is modified and a videofluoroscope is used. A modified barium swallow provides a dynamic view of swallowing from the oral cavity through to the lower esophageal sphincter. The SLP and radiologists need to work cooperatively. The patient swallows puree, liquid, and/or solid food consistencies that have been mixed with barium for fluoroscopic image. For the oral/pharyngeal portion of the exam, liquid barium may be given and the patient asked to hold it there for 10 seconds before swallowing. Any incidence of leakage before the swallow is observed for insight into oral-pharyngeal muscle coordination. Observations also include volume of the swallow, leakage into the nasal cavity, and entry into the laryngeal vestibule. The modified barium swallow is useful in assessing the patient's ability to protect the airway versus penetration and threat of aspiration.

The flexible endoscopic evaluation of swallowing (FEES) also provides the SLP a dynamic view of swallowing and, some would argue, a more thorough view of the entire swallowing process. In FEES, the flexible nasopharyngoscope is passed thought the nose and into the nasopharynx to visualize the anatomy and function of the palate, pharynx, larynx, saliva pooling, and sensation. It is good to observe the patient during phonation such as saying "ka-ka-ka" and singing a vowel up and down the scale. Then swallowing is assessed with varying consistencies of food (such as a bit of cracker or applesauce) and with a small amount of liquid (grape juice aids visualization). It is very important to observe any pooling of secretions in the piriform sinuses, vallecula, and laryngeal vestibule as this can indicate an aspiration danger.

Regardless of which imaging technique is used, it is essential to notice any penetration of food and liquid the patient is having (often "silently") so as to best judge the patient's potential for aspiration. Clinical research is underway to establish reliable *penetration–aspiration (PA)* scores.

Pediatric Feeding and Swallowing Disorders

Voluminous literature exists on disorders of sucking, feeding, and swallowing in infants and children, much of it focusing in speech pathology on the optimal handling of infants with cerebral palsy. In addition to neuromotor feeding difficulties evident from birth, as may be the case in cerebral palsy, other forms of dysphagia become evident with the passage of time. Neurologic conditions of childhood associated with feeding disorders are cited in Table 9.11 (Ichord, 1994). Additionally, the anatomy and physiology of suckling, sucking, chewing, and swallowing in the pediatric population differs from that in adults. The SLP is referred to Arvedson and Brodsky (2002) or Groher and Crary (2010) to better understand these developmental aspects and for discussions of body tone and oral motor reflexes, which have implications for treating the young.

Pediatric assessments vary widely depending on causative factors but also on the child's age, development (including reflexes, muscle tone, posture), cognitive ability, and such. A team approach, as discussed previously, is ideal. The ultimate goal of a feeding and swallowing assessment is to develop a management plan that enables safe and efficient feeding that is enjoyable for both the child and the caregivers. Adequate nutrition and hydration goals must be achieved without compromise of airway safety. The writing of Groher and Crary (2010) further elaborates on the goals of a clinical evaluation. The case history ascertains a possible cause of dysphagia and current status of the child. A key focus will be the SLP's assessment of the child's ability to protect the airway and the practicality of oral feeding versus the need for alternative

TABLE 9.11	Neurologic Conditions of Childhood Associated with Dysphagia

Dysfunction of Cortex or Basal Ganglia

static encephalopathy (e.g., in utero intoxications, chromosomal defects, CNS infection, cerebrovascular accidents, trauma)

progressive encephalopathy (e.g., Wilson's disease, HIV, multiple sclerosis, drug-induced movement disorders)

Brainstem

congenital CNS anomalies

tumors of brainstem or posterior fossa

trauma

brainstem encephalitis

Cranial Nerves

trauma (asilar skull fracture)

motor neuron disease (poliomyelitis, progressive bulbar paralysis of childhood, spinal muscular atrophy)

tumors (schwannoma, neurofibromatosis)

toxins (diphtheria, heavy metals)

Neuromuscular Junction

myasthenia gravis

drugs/intoxications (e.g., tetanus, streptomycin, bacitracin, beta blocker, phenothizines)

Muscle

congenital (e.g., muscular dystrophy)

errors of metabolism

endocrine (e.g., hyperthyroidism, hypothyroidism)

Esophageal Motility

associated with CNS dysfunction

induced by reflux esophagitis

drug induced (e.g., beta adrenergics, muscle relaxants associated with myopathies)

methods of nutrition. Another purpose of a feeding/swallowing assessment is to establish baseline clinical data. The Oral-Motor Feeding Rating Scale (Jelm, 1990) may be useful in tracking the progress and skills from 1 year of age through adulthood. Also of interest for clinicians working with dysarthria among school-aged students is the 2-hour audio CD and manual provided by ASHA (Bailey & Staskowski, 2009).

To accomplish these goals, pediatric feeding and swallowing evaluations should include four primary components: a careful history, examination of the oral motor mechanism, observation of a trial feeding, and specialized imaging studies as clinically indicated. An overview of each component is presented.

CASE HISTORY Medical records help identify medical, neurological, developmental, and etiological factors that predispose the child to dysphagia. Likewise, knowledge of medications, syndromes, and systemic problems (e.g., cardiopulmonary and respiratory distress) that increase demands on pharyngeal function and boost nutritional requirements is necessary.

The mother or primary caregiver/feeder can provide details of the feeding history. The SLP needs to know the child's current oral feeding patterns: types of food and liquids tolerated, manner of presentation, feeding position, duration of meals (10 to 30 minutes is best), frequency of meals, total intake, and the like. If the client is tube fed, the SLP needs details on the type of feeding tube, when it was initiated, formula amount per feeding, feeding schedule, position during feeding, and use of and response to oral stimulation.

Oral Motor Examination

The SLP should observe the child at rest, noting body tone and posture. If in an acute care setting, baseline respiratory rates, heart rates, and pulse oxygen levels can easily be obtained (changes in these physiologic patterns during feeding may indicate general intolerance or airway compromise). Look for clinical signs of oral or pharyngeal dysfunction, such as drooling, coughing, and upper aerodigestive tract noises. As discussed earlier in this chapter, a thorough oral motor examination is performed. The lips, tongue, and velum are evaluated for precision, strength, range, and symmetry of movement. Cranial nerves screened for oral phase function include V, VII, X, and XII. The pharyngeal phase of deglutition is dependent on muscles innervated by cranial nerves IX, X, and XI. Oral sensations and laryngeal functions are also assessed.

OBSERVATION OF A TRIAL FEEDING   The SLP should observe a regularly scheduled mealtime. As Lefton-Greif (1994) states,

> The parent should feed the child using foods, utensils, special adaptations (e.g, thickening formula or cutting a large hole in the nipple), and positioning equipment used at home. The child is monitored for clinical signs associated with aspiration, including: cough, choke, and/or gag episodes; changes in vocal quality or upper aerodigestive tract noises; episodes of oxygen desaturation; and episodes of apnea or bradycardia. (p.106)

Observation of a trial feeding allows the clinician to define patterns of oral intake, positioning, and optimal stimuli for feeding (i.e., bolus characteristics of size, texture, and temperature). Specific forms have been developed to guide the clinician through the case history intake and other prefeeding observations. The Rehabilitation Institute of Chicago provides a Parent/Caregiver Questionnaire and a Pre-Assessment Form with excellent details (Perlin & Boner, 1994). Other resources include Lefton-Greif's form for Assessing Nutritional Patterns and Methods of Feeding (1994) and Arvedson's Oral-Motor and Feeding Evaluation (1993). Arvedson (2009) has a 2-hour DVD and manual entitled Evaluation of Pediatric Feeding and Swallowing that is offered through ASHA (http://www.asha.org) as continuing education.

Other assessment scales merit mention. The Neonatal Oral-Motor Assessment Scale (NOMAS) (revised by Case-Smith, 1988) yields semiquantitative information for the identification of oral-motor dysfunction by 40 weeks' gestational age. The scale rates tongue and jaw responses during nonnutritive and nutritive sucking. The Multidisciplinary Feeding Profile (MFP) is a comprehensive feeding disorder assessment package for patients who are dependent feeders (Kenny et al., 1989). Scaled numerical ratings are made on physical/neurological factors (posture, tone, reflexes); oral-facial structure, sensation, and motor function; ventilation/phonation; and a functional feeding assessment.

INDICATIONS FOR SPECIALIZED STUDIES   When to proceed with special tests and imaging procedures is a decision reached by the multidisciplinary team. The child must be medically stable (and able to risk an episode of aspiration); usually there is some prognosis for change in the current feeding regime. As discussed in the adult section, modified barium swallow, FEES, and other instrumemtal measures are feasible, even with children. Visual assessment of swallowing function is common to better understand the child's oral and pharyngeal phases of the swallow. Many factors affect oral and pharyngeal performance, including the rate and manner of food presentation (which can be mixed with barium for image enhancement). The evaluation itself often manipulates bolus characteristics (texture, amount, temperature), manner of presentation (bottle, spoon, cup), and special adaptations (positioning, specific modifications of feeding devices). Test protocols and assessment forms are available in the literature, including those provided by Benson and Lefton-Greif (1994). Other instrumental assessments in the pediatric population include endoscopy, ultrasonography, scintigraphy, manometry, and electrography, as mentioned previously.

We leave the reader with one sobering note of caution when working with the multiply handicapped population. Rogers et al. (1994) conducted a study of 90 infants with cerebral palsy and multiple disabilities. Videofluoroscopic swallow examinations showed that almost all patients had abnormalities of both the oral and pharyngeal phases of deglutition. In particular, tongue control abnormalities and oral phase delays were present, along with delayed, multiple swallows and pharyngeal pooling. In addition to these observations, some 38% of the children aspirated in the absence of coughing or choking (silent aspiration). The clinician's work with dysphagia patients of any age is both dangerous and rewarding. The SLP should seek indepth training in this area of specialization.

Summary

This chapter covered the waterfront of motor speech disorders, including the oral exam, adult apraxia, childhood apraxia, adult dysarthria, childhood dysarthria (including cerebral palsy), as well as adult and pediatric feeding/swallowing disorders. We have but scratched the surface of information available to the SLP. Yorkston et al. (2010) remind us all that clinicians can be guided in their decision-making processes by following a model of disablement that provides a framework for understanding the broad range of motor speech disorders. The World Health Organization's ICF model is a disablement model (WHO, 2002). Figure 9.1 presented this model for motor speech disorders as discussed in this chapter.

The ASHA (2004) preferred practice patterns for assessing motor speech is not only consistent with the framework provided by the World Health Organization, it is a concise conclusion to our chapter. It states that motor speech assessment is conducted to identify and describe:

- Underlying strengths and deficits related to structural and physiologic factors that affect motor speech and swallowing performance
- Effects of the motor speech and swallowing disorder on the client's activities, both capacities and performance, in everyday contexts
- Contextual factors that serve as barriers to or facilitators of successful communication (and swallowing) in individuals with motor speech disorders.

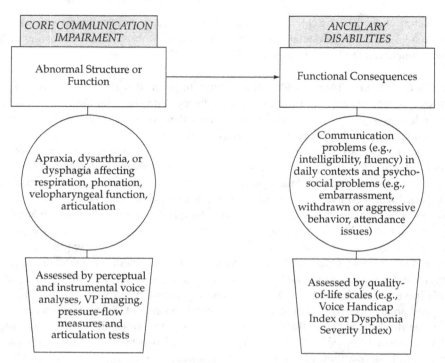

FIGURE 9.1   Assessment of motor speech disorders using the World Health Organization's classification of functioning, disability, and health (ICF).

Laryngeal and Alaryngeal Voice Disorders

There were major changes in the assessment and treatment of voice disorders in the last hundred years. The speech pathologist became involved in the processes of diagnosis and remediation that were previously the province of physicians and singing teachers. Recently, there has been increased research in the area of normal and disordered vocal physiology, and assessment and treatment are being changed further by the technological advances in microcomputers and electronics. Instruments are available for diagnosis and treatment that help to objectify behaviors that were previously unobservable and fleeting. It is an exciting time for clinicians who deal with voice disorders.

The proliferation of new instrumentation and research, however, should not obscure the fact that we have developed some very effective clinical procedures over the years that do not require equipment. Many authorities continue to believe that the listening skill and judgment of the well-trained clinician are the most important tools in a voice evaluation. Yet, measured vocal components help SLPs track areas of aberrance and therapeutic changes with precision—something welcomed by third-party payors and those of us concerned with evidence-based practice. Voice diagnosis combines the subjective and the objective as does all clinical work, and the clinician must be able to shift from the mental set of the scientist to that of the wine taster and back again. In this chapter, we will touch upon both subjective and objective aspects of vocal assessment.

Many adults and some children are referred to the speech pathologist by their physician for voice disorders resulting from medical difficulties or surgical intervention. The clinician also frequently comes in contact with children as the result of screening large numbers of youngsters in school settings or by teacher or parent referral. Prevalence figures for voice disorders among school-age children vary considerably in the literature, but probably hover around 6% (Duffy et al., 2004; McNamara & Perry, 1994). From our experience, it would appear that substantially less than 1% of school-age children are presently receiving voice therapy, and this is usually for chronic hoarseness. The prevalence of voice disorders among adults tends to be higher than in children, especially among certain vocally demanding professions like teaching (Yiu, 2002).

THE NATURE OF VOCAL DISTURBANCES

The imprecision of labels, which is the bane of voice study, begins with the term *voice* itself. Some definitions restrict the term to the generation of sound at the level of the larynx, while others include the influence of the vocal tract upon the generated tone, and still others broaden the definition to ultimately include aspects of tonal generation, resonation, articulation, and prosody. In this chapter, we will limit our discussion of voice to disorders affecting the laryngeal mechanism, including cancer of the larynx and its subsequent treatment. Disorders of resonance will be discussed in Chapter 11.

A framework to conceptualize voice and voice disturbance is shown in Figure 10.1. The auditory characteristics of pitch, loudness, and quality constitute one dimension of our paradigm. These are the primary perceptual attributes of the voice and relate generally to the fundamental frequency, amplitude, and complexity of the signal.

Pitch that is too high, too low, too invariant, or inappropriately variant for the speaker or the circumstances constitutes a voice disorder. The loudness of the speaking voice is usually judged according to the speaking circumstance, with the aberrant ranging from the total lack of voice (aphonia) to the inappropriately loud. For our purposes, the term *quality* refers to the perceived pleasantness, or appeal, of the voice. Although this perception is linked to both the phonatory and resonatory characteristics of the speaker, we will consider only the disturbance of phonation in this chapter. Many terms have been used to describe vocal quality, yet roughness or hoarseness and breathiness seem to be the two most widely accepted.

The physical systems that most directly influence the vocal production are the respiratory, phonatory, and resonatory-articulatory systems, but they are not the only systems that influence the voice; the endocrine and neural systems may also impact voice production.

The respiratory system provides the motive force for voice production, and ultimately the resultant airstream becomes the vibrator that embodies all of the characteristics that the ear eventually senses. The importance of the airstream to vocal production is not really the issue at this

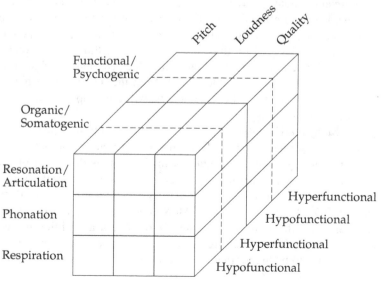

FIGURE 10.1 An organizational schema of voice disorders.

point, but there is some question as to the influence of the respiratory mechanism upon the various vocal characteristics and the serious reader is referred to companion articles on physically examining the abdominal wall and the diaphragm by Hixon and Hoit (1998, 1999). Suffice it to say, the respiratory mechanism must be capable of the following:

1. Providing an adequate amount of air so that the speaker can sustain speech with ease to allow for natural phrasing and prosodic factors
2. Providing adequate control of the flow of air so that the mechanism can, when necessary, either initiate or arrest the speech signal
3. Providing an airstream that is not so indebted to active muscle contraction that it encourages unnecessary muscle tension in the respiratory and phonatory mechanisms

Knowledge of the elements of laryngeal function is crucial in guiding the diagnostic process. To be an efficient sound source, the larynx must perform a valving action upon the flow of air that establishes alternate, regular pressure changes within the body of air. In order to do this, the vocal folds must be capable of (1) performing a wide range of valving actions, from completely open and unrestricted to closed and totally restricted; (2) valving completely along the length of the vocal folds; (3) closing and opening during phonation with just the right amount of energy to avoid extreme tension during the closing phase; (4) moving in a natural way that is free from superimposed and undue tension; and (5) making small, subtle, instantaneous adjustments, done continuously to alter the various vocal characteristics (these adjustments must allow for a variety of cyclic variations in the potential time of glottal opening and closing, from the long closing time of the glottal fry to the short closing time of the falsetto voice). The vocal folds must also be (1) of approximately equal size and shape so that they can move in synchrony with one another and (2) of appropriate size (length and mass) for the age and sex of the person.

The glottal tone is complex and rich in higher harmonics, but only through the resonant and damping effects of the vocal tract do the speech sounds achieve their identity. For the resonating chambers of the vocal tract to be efficient, they must be flexible in size, shape, texture, and relationship with one another.

The term *functional* should imply more than the simple absence of measurable organic deviation; it should imply that the diagnostician has found some active agent of etiology and that the agent is nonorganic. The term *functional* has unfortunately come to mean diagnosis by default.

Figure 10.1 identifies functional/psychogenic and organic/somatogenic as clinically meaningful categories. The term *functional* refers to those disorders where the learned, psychic, or maladaptive behavior has resulted in faulty vocal production, but not in physical alteration. If physical change has resulted from the functional cause, however, the proper designation is *psychogenic*. Similarly, if the original factor was physical or organic, then the term *organic* is justified; but if the physical difference results in behavioral change—that is, emotional response or faulty compensatory adjustments—the term *somatogenic* is appropriate.

The terms *hyperfunctioning* and *hypofunctioning* refer, respectively, to an excess or insufficiency of laryngeal tension and, as such, could apply to a wide variety of organic or functional disorders.

The term *voice disorders,* then, refers to abnormal pitch, loudness, or vocal quality according to sex, age, status, temporary physiological state, purpose of the speaker, and elements of the speaking circumstances. Vocal disorders may be primarily organic or functional and may be affected by any of the primary systems.

THE DIAGNOSTIC PROCESS

Before beginning our discussion of the diagnostic format, let us restate that this chapter will not cover the many and varied types of voice disorders; such information is available to the student in other sources (Boone, McFarlane, Von Berg, & Zraick, 2010; Rubin, Sataloff, & Korovin, 2006; Stemple & Glaze, 2009).

Our major focus will be on the actual planning, preparation, and execution of voice diagnoses. Diagnosis is intended to assess the parameters of the voice, determine the etiology and/or perpetuating factors, and outline a logical course of intervention, if warranted. Key components of the evaluative process include:

- Case history (including referral input, client interview, client's own impact ratings)
- Perceptual vocal assessment
- Acoustic analyses (low and/or high tech)
- Aerodynamic analysis (when available)
- Visual assessment
- Trial therapy probes

This process, then, addresses both aspects of the disorder per se as well as the impact of the disability as advocated by the World Health Organization (2002). This is shown in Figure 10.2.

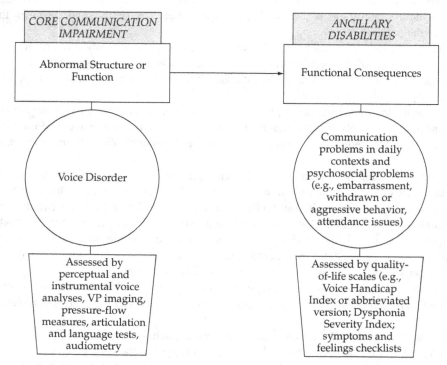

FIGURE 10.2 Assessment of voice using the World Health Organization's classification of functioning, disability, and health (ICF).

The Total Case History

The diagnostic process begins with a careful scrutiny of the original statement of the problem as provided by the referral source. Four perspectives guide our evaluation of this information: Who? What? When? and Why? This is followed by case history questionnaires and interviews, and also gathers patient impact ratings.

SIZING UP REFERRAL INFORMATION   It is important to know *who* presents the original complaint about the client's voice. We have found that the "best" source from a motivational standpoint is the client, but any individual who might have a significant impact upon the client may be a satisfactory referral source. If the client does not consider the voice to be a problem, treatment may not be in order or, if it is, this denial may necessitate counseling and educating as precursors to the actual voice treatment.

In the schools, it is often the classroom teacher who notices a vocal difference in a student and makes a referral to the SLP. Awareness training may be necessary in the early sessions here, too. It should be pointed out, however, that without prior training, such as listening experiences during inservice programs, classroom teachers are not particularly good at recognizing and referring students with voice disorders.

Next, consider *what* is described as the problem. When a description of the problems comes from the person with whom we will be working, we listen not only to the actual words spoken, but to the way in which they are presented. One of the best sources of information about the impact of the problem upon the individual is the way in which it is described. Case history questionnaires invariably ask for a description of the voice problem: when it started and what might have caused it.

In considering *when* the referral was made, three things are of concern. First, it is important to know when in the sequence of development of the problem the referral was made. Is this a long-standing problem that has only recently become serious, or is it a relatively new phenomenon that has been detected early? Second, what is this person's age and maturational level? Certain vocal changes are to be expected before puberty and would be considered normal, but a similar vocal quality at a later maturity level may be abnormal. Third, does this problem appear in cycles? For example, the client may suffer from this vocal change only during "hay fever" season. The time of year of the referral may provide some important diagnostic information.

Why was the referral made? The reason may vary from something as simple as an impending trip ("I just have to sound better than this by the first of August") to fears of serious medical problems. In evaluating the reasons for referral, it is important to keep in mind that contacting a speech clinician is often seen as psychologically safer than going to medical doctors or psychologists. This points up the importance of secondary referrals.

Sometimes the SLP refers the individual to other specialists for their input into the total assessment process; referrals work in both directions. Laryngologists often refer clients to SLPs for behavioral vocal intervention. Equally often, persons with voice problems seek the help of SLPs without first seeing a doctor. In most cases of phonatory voice disorders, some type of referral for medical or psychological evaluation will be necessary. We must remember that SLPs diagnose the voice and its characteristics, whereas medical doctors—particularly laryngologists—diagnose the vocal mechanism per se. It is not within the province of the SLP to diagnose nodules, inflammation, cancer, or the like; the SLP does assess the parameters of the voice that may or may not reflect such structural changes. Voice disorders may be caused by life-threatening situations such as carcinoma of the larynx or something as simple as vocal misuse. The importance of medical referral, then, is obvious. Structural changes such as ulcers, polyps, tumors, or nodules may be detected by the laryngologist through laryngeal examination (and confirmed by tissue biopsy). Auditory symptoms such as hoarseness or harshness of the voice and/or sensory complaints (e.g., laryngeal pain, lumps, and the like) should prompt the clinician to make the referral. Hoarseness lasting beyond 14 days, particularly in persons over the age of 40, should be referred on a suspicion of being a serious, life-threatening condition until proven otherwise. The need for a medical diagnosis cannot be underestimated because of the life/health implications for the client, the legal implications for the practicing clinician, and the requirement of third-party reimbursement agencies that services provided be "medically necessary."

It is widely accepted that the speech pathologist and the laryngologist should ideally cultivate a close working relationship when dealing with voice cases. Each professional can provide significant information to the other, and *voice treatment* that attempts to alter one or more parameters of the voice, such as pitch, should not begin without a laryngological examination. A *vocal hygiene* program, which does not alter the voice but teaches care of it, can begin with many clients prior to laryngoscopic examination. Thus, waiting for medical examination in cases of vocal abuse should not be used as a reason to postpone enrollment in an intervention program.

During an examination by a medical specialist, indirect laryngoscopy will be accomplished via a mirror. Direct laryngoscopy may be accomplished by use of a rigid or flexible endoscope. In cases of infants or preschool children, for whom such procedures are difficult, the laryngologist may use direct laryngoscopy under anesthesia. Videostroboscopy also is available in many laryngologists' offices and sophisticated voice centers. Videostroboscopy allows real-time observation of the condition and function of the vocal folds. This method will be discussed later in the chapter. The SLP will be interested in the findings of the laryngeal examinations for several reasons and may wish to personally view the folds to better understand the reported findings and diagnosis. Many SLPs perform videostroboscopy.

First, the examination can document any physical alteration to the vocal mechanism (e.g., nodules, polyps) that may account for vocal differences.

Second, the speech pathologist will want to have the extent of any vocal fold pathology documented as baseline information if voice therapy is indicated so that alterations in the client's voice over time, as the result of treatment, might be correlated with concomitant organic changes that show in future laryngological examinations. Forms containing drawings of the vocal apparatus have been recommended so that the physician can make notes indicating the size and location of abnormalities or the image may be stored in a computer file. Either way, this could become part of the client's record and be used for comparisons over time as evidence of intervention effectiveness.

A third reason the speech pathologist will be interested in the laryngeal examination is that surgical intervention may be recommended as the treatment of choice for a particular patient. A dialogue between the clinician and the doctor may be necessary to discuss this decision and to discuss recommendations regarding the appropriateness of follow-up voice therapy.

Finally, the absence of organic deviations on the laryngoscopic examination may suggest more functional bases for the client's disorder. Such knowledge would have direct implications for the direction of voice treatment and may also indicate that other referrals by the speech pathologist (e.g., to a psychologist) are in order.

A general medical evaluation or specific neurological or endocrinological examination may be indicated in certain cases. When dysfunction of the peripheral or central nervous system appears to be a possible contributing factor to the voice disorder, as in dysarthria (see Chapter 9), referral is indicated.

During a routine screening of all college students entering the teacher education and certification program, Susan came to our attention. Susan's voice was weak, and she had difficulty projecting it louder or trying to shout when requested to do so. On questioning, it was revealed that her voice tires easily throughout the day and a slight hoarseness is typical. This prompted us to inquire further—trying to unravel the mystery of Susan's voice problem and wondering about a possible endocrinological basis. Suspicions of a hyperactive thyroid gland became stronger when Susan complained of nervousness and irritability, generalized muscle weakness, and fatigue—making it difficult for her to complete her aerobics routine at the local gym (one day her legs trembled and were so weak she could not rise from a squat), excessive sweating, weight loss—which she was happy about even though she still ate lots of food, suffered from insomnia, and had irregular menstrual periods. Her once-radiant skin had turned sallow in recent months. Referral to a physician was made and hyperthyroidism (Grave's disease) was diagnosed.

CASE HISTORY QUESTIONNAIRE AND INTERVIEW   The SLP should directly interview the client and, in the case of a child, the parents, teachers, and others of significance should be consulted as well. Much information about daily use of the voice, possible phonotraumas (abuses), and functional impacts can be gathered from informants. There are many excellent sources for guidance in taking an adequate case history with an emphasis on voice disorders, and many of these sources provide forms for the clinician's use (Boone, McFarlane, Von Berg, & Zraick, 2010 ; Rubin, Sataloff, & Korovin, 2006). Table 10.1 lists sample case history questions that we routinely ask during a client interview. Table 10.2 may be used as a checklist on which clients may indicate any coexisting sensory symptoms (Pindzola, 1987). In the following section, we will elaborate on those case history topics most relevant to vocal diagnosis and

TABLE 10.1	Sample Questions to Ask in the Case History Intake

1. What are your voice concerns?
2. When did these voice issues begin?
3. Did this begin suddenly or develop slowly?
4. What conditions surrounded the onset of these vocal concerns (colds, illness, surgery, personal problems, etc.)?
5. When is your voice better? When is it worse?
6. Describe the daily use of your voice (typical weekday behaviors and job demands on the voice; typical weekend activities).
7. Are there specific situations when voice trauma occurs? (Inquire about the frequency of common misuses and abuses such as excessive crying, throat clearing, coughing, smoking, screaming, etc.).
8. Describe your general health (sinus problems; allergies; illnesses; injuries to head, neck or scrotum; endocrine disorders; heart disease; surgery; use of medications; fatiguability; smoking/drinking habits; etc.).
9. What medications do you take?
10. What has your doctor told you about your voice (or why has the doctor referred you)?

TABLE 10.2	Checklist of Sensory Symptoms

Mark (X) all symptoms associated with the voice problem.

_____ 1. Frequent throat clearing

_____ 2. Frequent coughing

_____ 3. Vocal fatigue that progresses with use of the voice

_____ 4. Irritation or pain in the voice box or throat

_____ 5. Strain, bulging, or tenderness of neck muscles

_____ 6. Swelling of veins and/or arteries in the neck

_____ 7. Feeling of a foreign substance or "lump" in throat

_____ 8. Ear irritation, tickling, or earache

_____ 9. Frequent sore throats

_____ 10. A tickling, soreness, or burning sensation in the throat

_____ 11. Scratchy or dry throat

_____ 12. Tension and/or tightness in the throat

_____ 13. A feeling that talking is an effort

_____ 14. Pain or difficulty swallowing

_____ 15. Pain or burning sensation at the base of the tongue

subsequent intervention, but it is helpful to realize that the information in both these tables opens the exploration into how the voice is impacting the client's quality of life.

Family Data. For a young client, information regarding the parental occupation, number of siblings, history of family adjustment, other voice problems within the family, and general health pattern of the family tells us a great deal about the young client's social and physical milieu. Generally, the following characteristics may be considered potentially remarkable and should be explored further: (1) too much or too little structure and organization to the home; (2) premium placed on verbal competition; (3) interparental friction; (4) unusual sibling competition; (5) history of voice disorders; (6) poor parental adjustment; (7) history of extended recurrent health problems; and (8) general level of concern for physical and health problems. For the adult client, we are interested in many of the same issues, particularly occupation, number of persons living in the home, and health problems or communication disorders among those living in the home.

> Barbara was a 32-year-old mother of twins. Both 4-year-old boys were described as rambunctious, and Barbara was the archetypical housewife. She also cared for her mother-in-law, who was hard of hearing, a bit senile, and lived in the same home. Barbara just could not understand why she had developed bilateral vocal nodules and why the doctor insisted on her enrolling in voice therapy. Clearly, family information of this type suggests etiological factors of vocal abuse and provides behavioral change as a direction for treatment.

Onset of the Problem. In many instances, the beginning of the voice problem will have great diagnostic significance. It is important to investigate not only the nature of the onset, but also the circumstances surrounding it. Physical or psychological trauma may have equally instant effects upon voice production. In some cases, extended questioning may be necessary because it is common for clients to repress uncomfortable incidents of the past. A sudden onset within hours suggests the high probability of a conversion vocal disorder or a neurological origin (such as stroke), whereas many other types of vocal disturbances develop gradually (mass and approximation lesions, degenerative disease, etc.).

Although the abrupt onset of a vocal disorder is traumatic and startling, most voice disorders are of insidious origin. Many people cannot pinpoint the exact date of the onset and tend to indicate when people first noticed or remarked about their voices. Since a gradual onset is not necessarily specific to organic or functional etiologies, the examiner must look to other data for final answers. Probably more important than the rate of development is information on coincident factors such as the client's general health and emotional state.

Course of Development. A careful description of the developmental stages of the voice disturbance may provide helpful diagnostic information. The course of the development of the voice disorder may be found to parallel a chronic medical problem, cumulating vocational stress, certain periods of physical maturation, changes in family relationships, or developing financial crises. We want to know how the problem has changed since its onset, and we want to know about any circumstances surrounding variability of the voice disturbance. For instance, were there changes in the voice disorder during its development that might be correlated with changes in personal habits (e.g., smoking, use of alcohol), work conditions (e.g., excessive noise, stress), or medical conditions (e.g., sinus, allergy)? The clinician will want to keep in mind that once a voice disorder has been firmly established, only a minimal amount of tension, misuse, or abuse will be necessary to perpetuate the problem.

Description of Daily Vocal Performance and Problem Variability. While the course-of-development questions seek a historical perspective, we need information on factors that influence the voice at the time of the evaluation. For instance, we might ask the client to describe his or her daily routine and relate it to talking. Does the problem become worse through the day? Does it become better as the day progresses? It is especially important in cases of childhood vocal pathology to obtain an accurate picture of the youngster's typical use of voice and instances of misuse or abuse.

Social Adjustment. Assessment of the personality characteristics of the individual may assist the diagnostician in interpreting other information. Formal personality testing is not within the jurisdiction of the speech pathologist, but each clinician is expected to be perceptive and sensitive to clues about the client's basic adjustment to life. Classification of voice characteristics with specific personality types has not provided overwhelming evidence of definite relationships; but the personality and the voice interact in a complex fashion, and this results in many symptomatic characteristics.

Vocation. We are interested in the vocation of our voice client for two reasons. First, we must determine if the occupation demands a great deal of talking and if that talking is under adverse conditions. Not all teachers develop "teacher's nodules," however, and the vocation must be judged in relation to the person. Several writers have postulated that there is a personality type that develops vocal nodules. We have found many of these people to be tense, energetic, high-strung, and verbally aggressive. Place this type of person in an occupational setting that demands a great deal of speaking under tension, and a bit of poor judgment in choosing adaptive procedures, and the chances of finding an individual with vocal nodules could be greatly enhanced.

A second factor in our evaluation of the vocation of an individual is to assess the possibility of changing aspects of the client's job routine or behavior at work if the vocation has a deleterious effect on the voice disorder.

We worked with a college professor who taught several large lecture classes to groups of over 150 students. His vocal abuse and misuse during these presentations had resulted in small nodules for which voice therapy was recommended. In an effort to be audible, dynamic, and authoritative, he had been speaking loudly, with a lower pitch, and excessive tension. We explored the possibility of his using a lavalier microphone in the large lecture rooms, and this effectively eliminated an abusive situation that was vocationally related.

Health. Realizing that the voice is influenced by many physiological systems, a complete medical history and examination are necessary in many instances. A history of the general health and physical development of the client should be obtained, along with information about specific illnesses, surgeries, and medications. The clinician should also obtain data concerning the general energy level and health-related habits such as smoking, drinking, and drug usage.

Patient Impact Ratings. The last part of the case history phase of assessment seeks to ascertain, from the client's perspective, the degree of impact the voice is having on the client's daily functioning. It is in vogue to refer to these as quality of life scales. Such topics evolved in the interview questioning (recall Table 10.2 and Figure 10.2 as regards daily performance, social adjustment, vocation) but now need to be objectified with scoreable tools that are normed, reliable, and valid. Instruments of this type can be used pre- and post-treatment to assess effectiveness and change in quality of life (Awan & Roy, 2009; Hakkesteegt et al., 2010). In this sense, quality of life scales and assessments are evaluative probes and reevaluations that monitor change and the impact of intervention. A list of quality of life and patient symptom assessment scales is presented in Table 10.3. A few are also highlighted here.

The Voice Handicap Index (VHI) and abbreviated versions of the VHI are now in common clinical use. The 30-question VHI (Jacobson et al., 1997) explores three patient domains using a 0–4 rating scale. In the physical domain, the client rates statements such as, "I feel as though I have to strain to produce voice." In the functional domain statements tap into daily impacts such as, "My voice makes it difficult for people to hear me." An example of a statement in the emotional domain is, "My voice problem upsets me." Seven- and 10-question abbreviated versions of the VHI exist in experimental form. The literature, however, suggests the 30-item VHI is statistically sound, and clinicians often administer the VHI in the initial diagnostic session and periodically thereafter to monitor treatment progress, both physically and behaviorally. A pediatric version of the Voice Handicap Index (P-VHI) exists as well, and will be mentioned in Chapter 11.

Although specific to unilateral vocal fold paralysis cases, a validated 36-item Voice Outcomes Survey is available (Gliklich, Glovsky, & Montgomery, 1999).

The Dysphonia Severity Index (DSI) is another handicap scale in popular use. The DSI features more of a focus on severity as a function of perceived vocal quality. It weighs a combination of actual acoustic measures: the highest vocal frequency (fundamental frequency expressed in Hertz), the lowest intensity (in dB), the maximum phonation time (MPT in seconds), and jitter (percentage derived from requisite equipment). Scored between +5 for a normal voice to −5 for a severely dysphonic voice, the more negative the client's index, the worse the vocal quality. The DSI is normed and valid according to Wuyts et al. (2000) and is highly correlated with the Voice Handicap Index.

TABLE 10.3	A List of Some Quality of Life and Symptom Impact Scales for Children and Adults

Iowa Patient's Voice Index (IPVI) (Karnell et al., 2007)
 A simple 3-item patient perception questionnaire developed by Verdolini and colleagues at the University of Iowa and studied for reliability by Karnell

Dysphonia Severity Index (DSI) (Wuyts et al., 2000)
 See text for description

Patient Questionnaire of Voice Performance (PQVP) (Carding & Horsley, 1992)
 Has patient self-rate aspects of his or her own vocal performance to yield an impact score (e.g., 12 = normal functioning, 60 = severe dysphonia); often used with nonorganic dysponic cases

Pediatric Voice Handicap Index (pVHI) (Zur et al., 2007)
 Assesses physical, functional, and emotional attributes

Pediatric Voice Outcomes Survey (pVOS) (Hartnick et al., 2003)
 Assesses physical, social, and school attributes in children ages 2–18

Pediatric Voice-Related Quality of Life (PVRQOL) (Boseley et al., 2006)
 Assesses physical and social-emotional attributes

Singing Voice Handicap Index (SCHI) (Jacobson et al., 2007)
 Subjective assessment useful with patients that sing

Voice Activity and Participation Profile (VAPP) (Ma & Yiu, 2001)
 Assesses perception of voice problem, activity limitation, and social participation restrictions at work and play in a 28-item questionnaire

Vocal Disability Coping Questionnaire (VDCQ) (Epstein et al., 2009)
 Assesses information-seeking, avoidance, and social support attributes

Voice Handicap Index (VHI) (Jacobson et al., 1997)
 Assesses physical, functional, and educational attributes in 30 questions

Voice Outcome Surgery (VOS) (Gliklich et al., 1999)
 Assesses functional, social, and work attributes; was designed for used in cases of unilateral vocal fold paralysis

Voice Performance Questionnaire
 Twelve multiple-choice questions, available online at http://www.entuk.org/clinical_outcomes/documents/PVQ

Voice-Related Quality of Life (V-RQOL) (Hogikyan et al., 1999)
 Assesses physical and social-emotional attributes in a 10-item questionnaire designed to be completed two weeks prior to the voice evaluation. The V-RQOL was developed at the University of Michigan Vocal Health Center and is available free online at http://www.entnet.org

Voice Symptom Scale (VoiSS) (Deary et al., 2003)
 Assesses the voice and patient reports of communication problems, throat infections, psychological distress, voice sound and variability problems, and phlegm

PERCEPTUAL, ACOUSTIC, AND AERODYNAMIC ASSESSMENT

The first step in voice analysis is simply listening to the client in an analytical manner. Obviously, this listening process is largely judgmental. Much of what we do in a routine voice assessment is perceptual and subjective. As such, rating scales, profiles, checklists, and assessment outlines are the order of the day. A checklist, such as the simple one shown in Table 10.4, may guide the clinician

TABLE 10.4	Checklist of Vocal Characteristics

Pitch

1	2	3	4	5	6	7							

Description						Severity					
—Too high	1	2	3	4	5	6	7
—Too low	1	2	3	4	5	6	7
—Invariant	1	2	3	4	5	6	7
—Pitch breaks	1	2	3	4	5	6	7
—Diplophonia	1	2	3	4	5	6	7
—Repetitive pattern	1	2	3	4	5	6	7

Loudness

1	2	3	4	5	6	7

Description						Severity					
—Excessive	1	2	3	4	5	6	7
—Inadequate	1	2	3	4	5	6	7
—Uncontrolled variation	1	2	3	4	5	6	7
—Repetitive pattern	1	2	3	4	5	6	7
—Invariant	1	2	3	4	5	6	7
—Tremulous	1	2	3	4	5	6	7

Quality

1	2	3	4	5	6	7

Description						Severity					
—Hoarseness	1	2	3	4	5	6	7
—Harshness	1	2	3	4	5	6	7
—Breathiness	1	2	3	4	5	6	7
—Hypernasal	1	2	3	4	5	6	7
—Hyponasal	1	2	3	4	5	6	7
—Other (describe)	1	2	3	4	5	6	7

Judgment of Vocal Tension

—Aphonia/whisper
—Breathy phonation
—Normal
—Hypertension
—Hypertension/intermittent phonation

Overall Judgment of Voice

1	2	3	4	5	6	7

Note: 1 = normal; 7 = severely disordered.

TABLE 10.5	An Annotated Listing of Some of the Available Rating Scales and Evaluation Materials

The Boone Voice Program for Adults (3rd ed.)
(Boone, 2000)
Both diagnosis and remediation procedures for vocal disorders are contained in this kit.

The Boone Voice Program for Children (2nd ed.)
(Boone, 1993)
Screening, evaluation, and referral instructions are included in a manual with this remediation kit. Also provided are the necessary forms and stimulus materials.

Systematic Assessment of Voice (SAV)
(Shipley, 1990)
This is a comprehensive inventory of tasks, strategies, and guidelines for assessing functional and organic voice problems in children and adults. It contains reproducible lists of words, phrases, sentences, passages for oral reading, case history forms, letters to parents, and so forth.

Voice Assessment Protocol for Children and Adults
(Pindzola, 1987)

This protocol directs and quantifies clinical observations of voice. The following vocal parameters are assessed: pitch, loudness, quality, breath features, and rate.

Voice Diagnostic Protocol
(Awan, 2001)
This manual compiles methods of low-cost vocal analyses including history-taking and perceptual analysis of vocal frequency, intensity, quality, examination of structures, evaluation of respiratory and phonatory control, and effects of excessive muscular tension. Each diagnostic procedure is explained and normative data and interpretations of results are provided. Includes a CD-ROM.

CAPE-V
See text for description.

GRBAS
See text for description.

---

in a cursory appraisal of the various characteristics of the voice. What is important to assess is not the overall voice, but a decomposition of the voice into its various attributes of pitch/frequency, loudness/intensity, quality, and myriad other features that vary with the rating scale used. Many voice assessment tools (rating scales, profiles, checklists, open-ended observation forms, and the like) are available; Table 10.5 lists some of the more commonly used resources. Yet it must be stated that the reliability, validity, and standardization norms of such tools are disappointing, if not lacking. Unfortunately, this is true of the two widely used scales, the GRBAS and the CAPE-V, which were developed to avoid such shortcomings (Biddle et al., 2002). We provide a brief word about each.

The GRBAS Scale was developed by the Japanese Society of Logopedics and Phoniatrics and was first described in English by Hirano (1981). GRBAS represents the parameters of grade, roughness, breathiness, asthenia, and strained quality. Each parameter is rated on a 4-point scale (0 = normal, 3 = extreme problem).

The Voice Special Interest Division 3 of ASHA developed a "more objective" rating scale called Consensus Auditory Perceptual Evaluation-Voice, or CAPE-V. In CAPE-V, the voice is assessed in sustained vowel production, sentence production, and conversational speech, describing how consistently the voice is produced and assigning a severity rating of consistent, mild, moderate, or severely deviated. This rating is done for each vocal attribute: roughness, breathiness, strain, pitch, loudness, and overall.

The research literature is robust in assessing reliability and validity of perceptual voice scales and quality of life scales. A case in point is the work by Karnell et al. (2007). The clinician-rated vocal attributes of GRBAS and CAPE-V perceptual scales were compared and both were found to be reliable, though CAPE-V was said to be more sensitive to small vocal differences.

However, these two scales showed less agreement with the patient-administered vocal attributes and quality of life impact scales of V-RQOL and IPVI (see Table 10.3).

Let us now turn our attention to a discussion of the vocal parameters and how they are routinely assessed. As in evaluating other communication disorders, the clinician must realize that the type of sample obtained affects how "ecologically valid" it is. For instance, in the case of a child with vocal nodules who is suspected of being a vocal abuser, it would be ideal to observe the youngster in a play situation with others, during school activities, and in the home environment. Most often, a variety of sampling activities is used in the evaluation, ranging from conversation, counting, coughing, singing the scale, and prolonging isolated speech sounds. The point here is that the clinician should be aware that a broad sampling of vocal performance is needed in order to make correct judgments on any parameter of the voice.

Five voice areas of pitch, loudness, quality, breath features, and rate/rhythm are routinely assessed in clients through a marriage of perceptual and simplistic acoustic analysis, as with a stopwatch and pitch pipe or piano keyboard. More sophisticated technological appraisals also are becoming routine in a variety of clinical settings. Let's review the five areas of vocal assessment from perceptual, acoustic, and aerodynamic vantage points.

FEATURE ASSESSMENT

PITCH Clinicians routinely evaluate various pitch characteristics of the client's voice. Pitch is a perceptual phenomenon that correlates with the valving rate of the vocal folds. Rightly or wrongly, clinicians interchange the terms *pitch* and *frequency* when talking about a client's voice. *Pitch determination* of the speaking fundamental frequency, also known as habitual pitch, can be accomplished with musical-matching methods using low tech—pitch pipe or keyboard—or by high-tech instrumental analysis, as shown in Table 10.6 . The client's speaking fundamental frequency can then be compared to normative data, based on age and sex. Table 10.7 shows average fundamental frequencies for a representative sample of ages, synthesized from the literature.

Pitch determination methods can also be used to locate a client's optimal pitch. *Optimal pitch* is a controversial concept that supposes each person has an optimal or natural pitch range at which he or she *should* be speaking. If we accept the premise of optimal performance, then, when optimal pitch does not match habitual pitch, habitual pitch may need to be raised or lowered in treatment. The determination of optimal pitch is by no means precise. In addition, it should be emphasized that optimal pitch is not a single note, but a range of notes where the vocal mechanism appears to function best with the least muscular tension. Various vegetative (natural, involuntary, and nonspeech sounds) and range singing techniques have been proposed for eliciting optimal pitches from clients; once elicited and recorded, the value of the optimal pitch can be determined musically or instrumentally. Table 10.8 summarizes some of the more commonly used methods for eliciting a client's optimal pitch. Later in the chapter, we will discuss how these techniques are useful as probes or facilitators of voicing abilities.

The normal voice is characterized by *pitch variability,* also known as *intonation* or *inflection*. The voice is abnormal when there is a lack of pitch variability or when pitch fluctuations are excessive. Dysarthrias may be characterized by monopitch where a limited range of notes are used monotonously. Monopitch and restricted pitch ranges are also associated with superior laryngeal nerve paralysis, additive lesions, and other disorders. Excessive pitch variability or prosodic excess may be heard in the dysarthrias, particularly spastic, ataxic, and hyperkinetic forms (Duffy, 2005). Dysarthria voice samples often exhibit frequency variations, especially on

TABLE 10.6 Some Available Software for Vocal Assessments

Computerized Speech Laboratory (CSL) (http://www.kayelemetrics.com/)
  This company's website contains purchasing information for this expensive, freestanding equipment; considered the gold standard for research and clinical analysis of voice; entire CSL includes popular components known as the VisiPitch and the Multi-Dimensional Voice Program

Multi-Speech (http://www.kayelemetrics.com/)
  This company's website contains purchasing information for this low-cost, Windows-based speech analysis system akin to the CSL; performs a variety of voice analyses

Praat: Doing Phonetics by Computer (http://www.fon.hum.uva.nl/praat)
  Allows for various free spectral, pitch and format analyses as well as for jitter and shimmer

Sona-Spech II (http://www.kayelemetrics.com/)
  This company's website contains purchasing information for this affordable alternative to the VisiPitch for measuring speech and vocal behaviors

Speech Analyzer (http://www.sil.org/computing/speechtools/speechanalyzer.htm)
  Downloadable analyzer for viewing sound files as a waveform, pitch plot, spectrum, or various F1 vs. F2 displays

Speech and Hearing Laboratory (http://www.speechandhearing.net/laboratory/tools.html)
  Site contains various software tools that are free and downloadable; site describes signal displays and acoustic analyses available

The Voice Diagnostic Protocol (Awan, 2001)
  Part of a commercially available assessment package; contains a CD ROM for the clinician's computer when a microphone is added

TABLE 10.7 Average Fundamental Frequencies and Nearest Musical Note for Selected Ages

Age	Sex	Mean Fundamental	Musical Note
1–2	either	445 Hz	A4
3	either	390 Hz	G4
6	either	320 Hz	E4
10	male	235 Hz	A3#
15	male	165 Hz	E3
20–29	male	120 Hz	B2
50–59	male	118 Hz	A2#
60–69	male	112 Hz	A2
80–89	male	146 Hz	D3
10	female	265 Hz	C4
15	female	220 Hz	A3
20–29	female	227 Hz	A3#
50–59	female	214 Hz	G3#
60–69	female	209 Hz	G3#
80–89	female	197 Hz	G3

TABLE 10.8 Some Techniques for Determining Optimal Pitch

Resonance-Swell Method
Have client hum at the same intensity up the scale, and note whether the voice becomes louder or swells in a given range of pitches. Client and/or clinician should listen for this swell in loudness.

Loud-Audible Sigh
Client should take a deep breath and produce /a/ as a loud sigh. Listen most carefully for the pitch at the onset of the sigh because one tends to lower the pitch during the sound. Optimal is said to be the onset tone.

Yawn-Sigh
The client should yawn and sigh audibly in a relaxed manner. Yawning opens the throat and minimizes the constriction around the larynx.

Vegetative Techniques
Listen to the natural, spontaneous laugh, cough, throat clearing, or grunt of the client. These vegetative forms of phonation may be representative of optimal pitch.

Inflection Methods
Have the client say "um hum" using a rising inflection with lips closed, as though he or she were spontaneously and sincerely agreeing with what was just said. In addition, the clinician could have the client say "hello" in a natural, spontaneous, and sincere way. An automatic affirmative utterance often approximates optimal pitch. A related method is to have the client say "hello" with rising inflection, as though asking a question. The slight inflection may reveal a more optimal voice.

Pushing or Pulling Techniques
The client should attempt to phonate /a/ of optimal quality while pushing down or pulling up on his or her chair. This method may be particularly useful for clients with disordered closure of the vocal folds.

Pitch Range Methods
The type of phonation may be do-re-mi or ah-ah-ah or one-two-three, and so on. The client phonates the entire vocal range from the lowest sound that can be produced to the highest, excluding falsetto. One-third of this range should represent optimal pitch. An alternate, and popular, method is to have the client phonate his or her entire vocal range from the lowest note to the highest, including falsetto. The total range is then divided by one-fourth to locate the optimal. For example, calculate the number of full-step notes in the client's range and then locate the note that is one-fourth of the way from the bottom.

sustained vowel productions. Hearing-impaired and deaf speakers also often utilize excessive pitch fluctuation.

Diplophonia refers to the presence of two or more simultaneous pitches or tones in the voice and may be caused by separate or unequal vibratory sources. Possible causes include a paralyzed vocal fold vibrating at a rate different from the healthy one, a vibration of a growth or lesion, simultaneous adduction of the ventricular folds and true folds, and even an innocuous saliva globule.

Pitch breaks most often occur in a person using an inappropriately low-pitched voice. Intermittently, the pitch will suddenly break upward toward a more optimal level. Any condition that adds to the mass or size of the vocal folds may alter their vibratory characteristics. Pitch breaks may be one symptom of additive lesions such as, but not limited to, nodules, polyps, and tumors.

To summarize our discussion of pitch, the clinician must observe the client, measure pitch features, and seek answers to the following questions: What is the client's habitual pitch (speaking fundamental frequency), and is this pitch appropriate for the person's age, sex, and body stature? What is an optimal level for the client to use? Is a normal amount of pitch variability present in the speaking voice, or is the voice monotoned or widely varying and sing-songed in pattern? Are pitch breaks present? Is diplophonia present?

LOUDNESS   Perceptual judgments of vocal loudness are common, but instrumentation is available for measuring intensity (e.g. sound level meter, CSL). Of interest during the assessment is whether the *loudness level* is appropriate for the speaking situation. In normal conversational speech, some three feet from the speaker, the average sound intensity is 65 dB (range 55–75 dB). Typical loudness levels may be abnormal in various pathologies. Adults with dysarthria may speak too softly (as in Parkinsonism) or with a booming voice (as in some spasticities and dystonias). Lack of vocal loudness is characteristic of paralyzed cords and psychogenic disorders. Vocal abuse cases often speak with excessive effort and loudness, at least in some situations; the end result, however, may be hypofunctional loudness.

The clinician should also note if the typical loudness level can be maintained comfortably, without trailing off, or whether there is a *degree of effort*. Listen for loudness that trails off at the end of a sentence, which may be typical in vocal fold paralysis, dysarthrias, or obstructive lesions. *Phonation breaks* or momentary skips of loudness are abnormal and may indicate difficulty maintaining vocal fold adduction and vibration.

A certain amount of *loudness variability* is normal and is reflected in the stress patterns of the language. In addition to critically listening to conversational speech, we often ask the client to read "with feeling" sentences such as the following:

Get out of here, get out of here!
I don't know, I said I don't know!
I need more money, Dad, I'm broke!
Where did she go? I can't find her.
Will you cut that out!

We have observed that lack of loudness variability may take two differing forms of monoloudness; excess and equal stress patterns are typical of many dysarthrias, whereas the monoloud but weak and "bland" voice is typically seen in affective disorders and some forms of dysarthria.

The clinician may wish to have the client demonstrate his or her *loudness range,* from soft to maximal levels. Whispering and shouting can be requested. One method is to ask the client to count, beginning softly and increasing loudness with higher and higher numbers. Restricted loudness range is often seen in clients with respiratory involvement, particularly the dysarthrias.

Loudness abuses is one example of phonotrauma that may be situation-oriented. For instance, conversational levels may be appropriate but frequent loud talking or screaming (as in lectures, sermons, cheerleading, playground activities, etc.) may be perpetuating a vocal disorder. Questions asked in the interview should probe the client's daily uses of the voice with the purpose of discovering situational abuses.

After appraising the client's voice, the clinician should then have answers to the following questions about loudness: Is the loudness level that is used appropriate for the speaking situation? Can the level be maintained comfortably without undue strain? Can the level be maintained throughout the entire utterance or does it begin to trail off? Are loudness breaks present? Is the loudness variable in order to reflect stress and emphasis patterns of English or is the client monoloud? Can loudness vary from minimal (whispered) to maximal (shouted) levels? What, if any, situations are frequently encountered in which loudness abuse occurs?

QUALITY   The descriptive terminology used with disorders of vocal quality reflects the perceptual nature of the judgments. It can be argued that the clinician's ear is the best tool for describing the quality of a voice—and many clinicians use just that. However, rather sophisticated equipment is also available to study, categorize, and "objectify" acoustical parameters of the voice. Technology is available to measure periodicity of vocal fold vibrations, changes in amplitude (shimmer, and this is proving to be an important, objective measure to ascertain), changes in frequency (jitter), and opening-closing characteristics. (The Computerized Speech Lab from Kay Elemetrics has many software options for voice measures.) Still, deciding whether a voice is breathy, harsh, or hoarse is done most efficiently by critical listening.

Vocal quality is affected by the manner of vocal fold vibration. Many terms of vocal quality appear in the literature including "breathy," "harsh," or "hoarse"; hoarseness is the most prevalent. Designations such as "strident" and "husky" are used less frequently. With the popularity of CAPE-V, standardized terms are often limited to roughness, breathiness, and strain.

The breathy voice is characterized by an audible escape of air through partially closed folds. The lack of firm adduction may be due to obstruction by a mass or lesion, a paralyzed cord, or muscular incompetence.

The voice displaying effort and force is the harsh voice. Harshness is usually perceived in a phonatory milieu of hard glottal attacks, low pitch, intensity problems, and overadduction of the vocal folds. Equivalent terms are "roughness" and "unpleasantness," although "strident," "coarse," "grating," "rasping," "rough," "metallic," and "guttural" have been used as synonyms for "harshness."

The hoarse voice incorporates the features of both breathiness and harshness. As such, turbulent air flow, rough/aperiodic vibrations, low pitch, and neck muscle strain may be evident. Hoarseness is a common symptom of many vocal pathologies and should be recognizable by all SLPs. In particular, the public school clinician should be familiar with the auditory symptoms of hoarseness as a warning sign of vocal abuse and related lesions in children. The clinician must make medical referrals as appropriate. In addition, the clinician must educate teachers through inservice programs to recognize voice disturbances in students so that teacher referrals to the SLP will be accomplished.

The perception of vocal quality also is affected by *glottal approximation*. The hard glottal attack refers to an abrupt impact or strong initiation of speech. Extra effort is used to start the vibrations of tightly adducted folds. Presumably, then, prior to phonation there is too much tension in laryngeal muscles. Conversely, soft attack is an abnormally weak glottal approximation. Breathiness usually precedes this phonation. The astute clinician is listening for symptoms of an inappropriate glottal approximation.

The measures of jitter (frequency perturbation) and shimmer (amplitude perturbation), typically on a sustained vowel, are becoming more commonplace because of jitter's and shimmer's utility in early detection of pathology, even when the laryngologist sees no obvious lesion or tissue change. Speech pathologists working in concert with laryngologists will be called upon to obtain measures of jitter and shimmer on their patients. The sound spectrogram has long been a favorite piece of equipment for the voice scientist and clinician. Isshiki, Yanigahara, and Morimoto (1966) proposed that narrowband analyses can provide measures of hoarseness. They described four types:

- Type 1 shows the slightest degree of hoarseness where the distinct harmonic component is mixed with the noise component, which is limited within the formant region of the vowels; vowels to use are /u, o, a, e, i/.
- Type 2 shows a slight noise component in the high frequency region (3000–5000 Hz). The noise components predominate over the harmonics, most noticeable for the vowels /e/ and /i/.
- Type 3 shows only noise in the second formant of /i/ and /e/; there is also a further intensification of noise above 3000 Hz.
- Type 4 is characterized by noise in the second formant of /e/, /i/, and /a/ and in the first formant of /a/, /o/, and /u/. In these formant regions, the harmonic components are hardly noticeable.

The clinician can use the typing system of Isshiki, Yanigahara, and Morimoto for baseline, objective documentation of a patient's hoarseness. Spectrographic reassessments and retyping could be used as a barometer of improvement through treatment.

Quality can also be affected by resonance imbalances; however, these problems will be discussed in Chapter 11.

BREATH   Breathing variables affect laryngeal function in general, and vocal loudness and rate of speech in particular. Several features of the respiratory system and breath management are typically assessed in a voice evaluation. In this section, an overview of the following assessment techniques is presented:

- Observation of breathing
- Vital capacity measures
- Attention to noises
- Words per breath
- Maximum phonation time (MPT)
- Maximum exhalation time (MET)
- S/Z ratio
- Mean flow rate (MFR)
- Phonation threshold pressure (PTP)
- Phonation quotient (PQ)
- Subglottal pressure measure

Any or all of these measures aid in the clinical decision process.

The clinician may first want to observe the *predominant region* used for breath support. The diaphragm is the principle muscle of inhalation and various thoracic muscles assist when needed in expanding the lung-thoracic unit. Diaphragmatic breathing involves descent of the diaphragm and expansion of the abdomen during inhalation. Although quite normal—and a preferred way of breathing for both song and speech—it is difficult if not impossible to observe in a clothed, seated client. Expansion of the chest, not the shoulders, in a slight heaving motion is more observable; this type of thoracic breathing is used by many people. Clavicular breathing, in contrast, is characterized by shoulder elevation, upper thoracic tension (in the area of the clavicle or collar bone), and neck muscle strain. Clavicular breathing is an inefficient method of lung expansion for inhalation, as it involves too much effort for too little breath. The clinician should try to observe the region predominately used for breathing by clients; many hyperfunctional voice cases employ this inefficient form of breathing.

The maximum amount of air that can be exhaled following maximal inhalation is called *vital capacity*. The relationship of vital capacity to speech production is somewhat a matter of conjecture at this point. Vital capacity is apparently related to several factors, such as body size, physical condition, and sex. There is little or no research to vindicate those who have worked to increase the vital capacity of their voice clients. On the other hand, it is logical to assume that an individual with an extremely small amount of available air would find it difficult to sustain phonation and might resort to increased laryngeal tension and forcing to maintain normal or near-normal phrasing. It is probably not so much the volume of air as it is the individual's ability to control the airflow.

Equipment, such as the spirometer, is necessary to measure vital capacity. Clinically, however, we have found that a vital capacity insufficient for normal speech purposes was so obvious from normal observation that further formal testing was not necessary. Vital capacity measurements may be of particular concern in cases of emphysema, later stages of Parkinson's disease, and cerebral palsy in children. Related to lung volume are indications of the client's tidal volume, inspiratory reserve volume, expiratory reserve volume, and air flow rates, which some authorities recommend measuring clinically (Boone, McFarlane, Von Berg, & Zraick, 2010.).

Inhalation for speech should be quick and quiet. The clinician should listen for *associated noises* such as gasps and vocalizations during inhalation as the client speaks. Rating scales may also prompt the clinician to judge their conspicuousness or severity. *Inhalatory stridor* refers to noticeable phonatory sounds during inhalation and may be common in cases of vocal fold paralysis and dysarthrias.

When respiratory support is inadequate for normal speech, clients may breathe more frequently. In addition, fewer words (or syllables) may be spoken per breath group. These two factors contribute to the perception of "choppy" speech. The clinician should assess *words per breath;* a patient who can only utter six or so words per air charge is displaying poor breath support. Occasionally, a patient may say an excessive number of words per breath group. Research as to what is excessive is, however, lacking. Perhaps upward of 12 or 13 words per breath group is typical of normal speakers. Increased speaking rates and loss of intelligibility may be the negative by-products of too many words per breath.

Of interest in a voice evaluation is the maximum duration that a client can sustain sound plus air. *Maximum phonation time* (MPT) is typically measured with a stopwatch as the client prolongs certain voiced phonemes, such as /a/ or /z/. This surprisingly simple assessment is quite sensitive to vocal dysfunction along the glottal edge and so it is a must in any voice evaluation. Speyer et al. (2010) have shown its reliability across various methods of assessment. A similar measure is that of *maximum exhalation time* (MET), where a voiceless phoneme such as /s/ is used. The clinician should provide several trials, instruct the client to use a deep breath, and record the longest sustained attempt. A general rule of thumb that is easy to remember and clinically useful is that elementary school-age children (6 to 10 years old) should be able to prolong /a/ for at least 9 seconds, regardless of sex; adult males average 25 to 35 seconds MPT; adult females average 15 to 25 seconds MPT; and 12 seconds for persons over age 65. Related to the measures of MPT and MET is the clinical procedure of computing the *S/Z ratio.* The S/Z ratio is a quick-screening device used to determine how much of a voice problem may be related to respiration control and how much may be the result of laryngeal problems. Clients who have laryngeal pathology will have less control of the air stream during the production of a prolonged /z/. Using a stopwatch, two trials are given for the prolongation of both the voiceless /s/ and the voiced /z/ phonemes. The best or longest /s/ and the longest /z/ are used in calculating the S/Z ratio. If the S/Z ratio is greater than 1.2 for a child or 1.4 for an adult, a laryngeal pathology, especially of the glottal edge, may exist (Boone, McFarlane, Von Berg, & Zraick, 2010). Gelfer and Pazera (2006) discuss various methods of elicitation and ratio calculation for optimal reliability. We wish to reiterate that the physical examination of the abdominal wall and diaphragm (Hixon & Hoit, 1998, 1999) is worth considering by the SLP, and straightforward assessment forms are provided by those researchers.

Aerodynamic tests can assess properties of phonation, including subglottal pressure, supraglottal pressure, glottal impedance, and the volume velocity of the air flow at the glottis. Hirano (1981) states that the values of these four parameters vary during the opening and closing maneuvers of the glottis and may be difficult to measure. For example, the determination of subglottal pressure necessitates an invasive approach (such as a tracheal puncture), and glottal resistance must be mathematically calculated since it cannot be measured directly. The measure of *mean flow rate* (MFR), however, is often done as an office procedure.

The MFR of a sustained vowel, such as /a/, spoken at a natural pitch and loudness level, has been used clinically to evaluate phonatory function. The patient sustains the vowel for a maximum period of time while wearing a mask fitted tightly to the face or using a mouthpiece with the nose clamped. The mask or mouthpiece is coupled to a spirometer, pneumotachograph, or hot-wire anemometer. The MFR is obtained by dividing the total volume of air used during phonation by the duration of phonation. Normal values of the MFR range from 40 to 200 ml/sec in adult males and females. The MFR is greater than normal in cases of recurrent laryngeal nerve paralysis. Values for MFR in cases of nodules, polyps, polypoid swelling (Reinke's edema), and neoplastic tumors also exceed the normal range but are not as marked as with recurrent laryngeal nerve paralysis. In contrast, MFR values are typically within normal limits for the conditions of laryngitis, contact granuloma, and spastic dysphonia. Therefore, MFR is diagnostically important and may be used to probe or reevaluate progress in treatment.

Another aerodynamic measure that may be calculated is that of *phonation quotient.* Hirano (1981) calculates the phonation quotient (PQ) by dividing the vital capacity (VC) by the maximum phonation time (MPT):

$$PQ = \frac{VC}{MPT}$$

He also reports that the phonation quotient has a high positive relationship to the MFR and therefore is a reasonable, clinical substitute for MFR when no equipment for air flow measurement is available. Normal values of the PQ in adults and children are typically between 120 to 190 ml/sec. High phonation quotients are associated with recurrent laryngeal nerve paralysis and additive lesions of the folds, such as nodules, polyps, polypoid swelling, and neoplasms.

Subglottal and phonation threshold pressure measures are also aerodynamic and may be ascertained with a special face mask to be less intrusive. Normal values of subglottal pressure during habitual phonation are typically 5 to 10 cm H_2O, but these values change with variations in vocal intensity and fundamental frequency. Pressure values are abnormally high in laryngeal carcinoma, recurrent nerve paralysis, laryngocele, and perhaps even in functional dysphonias. Phonation threshold pressure (PTP) is the amount of air pressure necessary to set the vocal folds in motion at the lowest intensity level. Often this is 2–3 H_2O pressure, though humidity and a host of other variables can affect PTP values. As reviewed by Yendle (2010), there is a need to standardize methods of measuring PTP as this is a sensitive measure of glottal edge dysfunction. Excess vocal fold mass, bowing during approximation, and paralysis of movement require higher amounts of PTP than do healthy larynges.

RATE AND RHYTHM   Although traditionally not part of vocal evaluations, the *rate* at which a client talks should be assessed as rate can affect or be affected by other variables of speech and the voice. Often excessive rates are related to poor breathing features and improper phrase groupings. The client may try to say too many words on one breath, giving the perception of an excessive rate of speech, as in Parkinsonism. The converse may also occur. Frequent air intakes may give the perception of choppiness—the client may only be able to say a few words, then breathe, then say a few more words, then breathe, and so forth. The result is not only a choppy *rhythm* but an overall slowness of speech owing to the increased pause time. Rate changes may also interfere with intelligibility, as is so typical of the dysarthrias.

Rate is typically expressed as words per minute or syllables per minute. It can be quite cumbersome to measure an entire speech sample for the determination of rate. Therefore, we offer the following efficient and clinically useful estimation method (tape-recording for later playback is recommended): Count the number of words in a 60-second sample of "connected" speech. If no connected 60-second samples are available on the tape recording, then count the number of words in whatever connected sample is available and mathematically calculate words per minute. For example, if a 20-second speech sample contains 50 words, then, on the average, the person is talking at 150 words per minute (60 seconds divided by 20 seconds = 3, and 3 times 50 words = 150 wpm). An alternative method, useful for determining rate of speech during reading, is to give the client a reading passage with prenumbered words. Allow the client to read aloud for 1 minute, as timed with a stopwatch, and note how many of the words were read.

Conversational speech rates for children and for adults were discussed in Chapter 7. At the present time, we do not know what constitutes a speech rate that is "too fast" or "too slow," and so the clinician's judgment of normalcy is important. Rate determinations may be most necessary with neurological voice disorders.

VISUAL ASSESSMENT

Technological advances have permitted us to view laryngeal function, and much of this technology is in clinical application: fiber-optic, video stroboscopy, and laryngographic techniques are proving useful in the assessment of neurologic dysfunction, vocal fold lesions, morphologic changes of the folds, and abnormal phonatory function. The serious reader should consult the work of Titze (1994) and Hirano (1981), who have done much to standardize the clinical examination of the voice. These equipment-based approaches require costly and specialized instrumentation, an experienced operator, cooperative patients, and the interpretation of complicated graphs and mathematical formulas (Dejonckere, 2000). The allure of greater understanding and objectivity is strong, and such equipment is becoming de rigueur in a well-equipped medical clinic. It is something welcomed by third-party payors and evidence-minded clinicians alike. We will mention endoscopic assessment.

Perhaps the best view of the larynx is provided by a rigid endoscope because the image may be magnified. When the image is well lit, the physician can diagnose disease and the SLP can document laryngeal function. When done repeatedly over time, the SLP can track changes in function as a result of treatment. Rigid endoscopy, however, assumes phonation on a sustained vowel (like "eeee"), not connected speech. Flexible endoscopy allows a view of the entire larynx (as well as the nasopharynx), and images during connected speech and singing are possible. The drawbacks include a small image, need for excellent light (halogen), or better yet, stroboscopic lighting (xenon strobe). Physicians often fail to detect laryngeal pathologies with flexible endoscopy, but SLPs find functional viewing during speech/singing useful. Regardless of method, structural observations by the SLP should include appraisal of the following attributes:

- Smoothness of glottal margins
- Color of laryngeal tissue
- Vocal fold mobility
- Observation of the mucosal wave
- Mucosal pliability versus stiffness
- Pattern of glottic closure
- Symmetry of movement
- Location and size of any mass
- Information about the open/closed quotients

INFORMAL ASSESSMENT PROBES

We have now explained both the perceptual-informal and the technological-formal methods of voice appraisal for a variety of situations; see Figure 10.3. We also like the process of diagnosis and treatment decision making outlined by Pannbacker (1999) specific to cases with vocal nodules. Clearly, most SLPs operate in work settings with limited instrumentation available. Over the years, then, clinicians have developed effective behavioral techniques for assessing, probing, treating, and reassessing laryngeal voice disorders. Indeed, the process of voice therapy is behavioral; that is, we as clinicians use strategies, techniques, devices, and even psychological "tricks" to change or alter a client's voice. Of course, this presupposes that the changes are somehow better for the client—the voice sounds better, less effort is expended in its production, further

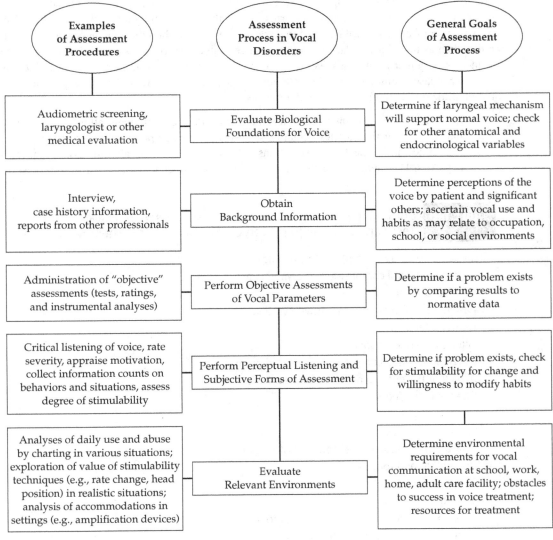

FIGURE 10.3 Critical assessment process in vocal disorders.

damage is not being inflicted on the vocal mechanism, and so forth. But just completing a voice evaluation, where deviant vocal parameters have been analyzed, in and of itself does not suggest how to proceed clinically. As clinicians, we want to know what we can do to make the client's voice "better." Here we enter the world of trial therapy—a necessary component of assessment—and the use of facilitating techniques to probe the client's potential to alter his or her voice for the better. Let us now highlight some of these probe techniques in hopes that clinicians will try out the client's ability to modify and improve parameters of the voice during the initial diagnostic evaluation. By doing so, the clinician will be able to accomplish two important things: a meaningful prognosis and a direction for intervention.

Patients with hypofunctional voice problems often show improved phonatory abilities by increasing glottal tension. The clinician should probe which maneuvers, if any, are successful in improving the voice. Do any of the so-called optimal pitch techniques help, such as grunting, pushing, pulling, throat clearing, or coughing (see Table 10.8)? An intentional hard glottal attack, even if accompanied by increased tension in the arms and trunk while pushing forcefully, may facilitate approximation of the vocal folds. Used this way, these may be thought of as hypertonic techniques rather than as techniques to achieve optimal pitch. Table 10.9 presents a useful sampling of techniques used by many clinicians over the years that may facilitate, or improve, voice production.

Two case examples may illustrate how the use of hypertonic probe techniques in the evaluation affected treatment recommendations.

Mrs. Hernandez was involved in a rather messy divorce settlement after 22 years of marriage. Over the past few months, she has experienced periodic losses of voice—sometimes during heated conversations but occasionally for an afternoon or an entire day. Mrs. Hernandez indicated that the voice was reduced to a whisper during these

---

TABLE 10.9   Some Circumlaryngeal Reposturing and Resonant Facilitating Techniques for the Improvement of Voice as Trial Therapy

To improve adduction and phonatory abilities:
    Gutzmann lateral compression of thyroid lamina
    Head turning or tilting
    Pushing or pulling concomitant with voicing
    Hard glottal attacks
To alter pitch and/or quality:
    Gutzmann frontal compression of thyroid prominence
    Any/all of the optimal pitch techniques (Table 10.7)
    Change in loudness
    Change in speech rate
    Soft glottal attacks
    Relaxation of musculature/reduction of tension
    Lip bubbles and tongue trilling
    Easy, resonant counting
    Singing, humming
    Slow, exagerrated nasal words (noon, moon)
    Alteration of respiratory patterns

episodes and was not hoarse as with laryngitis. The current episode of voice loss, and the reason she was seeing a speech-language pathologist, had lasted over a week. The clinician was not able to get Mrs. Hernandez to speak above a whisper in the evaluation; she showed no potential to talk, sing, or shout. The clinician was able to elicit, rather quickly, a cough and a throat-clearing maneuver that contained true phonated sound. A diagnosis of hysterical aphonia was made and, because of the rehabilitation potential displayed for phonation, treatment was recommended immediately. After three sessions of behavioral shaping, beginning with vegetative eliciting techniques, the client was speaking normally. Referral was then made for psychological support services.

Mrs. Osborne, age 42, presented with unilateral vocal fold paralysis subsequent to thyroid surgery. The laryngologist referred the patient for voice improvement therapy. Teflon injection was contraindicated, as it would further compromise the reduced glottal airway. The patient presented with stridor during physical exertion; the speaking voice was hoarse and of limited loudness. Hoarseness diminished and loudness improved when the speech-language pathologist exerted medial pressure against the thyroid lamina on the side of the paralyzed fold (a rendition of the Gutzmann medial compression technique). Other hypertonic facilitating techniques were helpful, as well, in improving Mrs. Osborne's voicing abilities. With medical management contraindicated, the clinician felt compensatory strategies involving increased muscular effort and glottal attack were appropriate and realistic. Treatment was recommended along these lines.

Vocal quality improvements can also be brought about by changes in the manner of speaking. Adjustments in the respiratory, phonatory, and articulatory processes impact on the overall perception of the voice. We provide one case example here.

Greg was a college student referred to us by the university infirmary. Greg had gone to see the doctor with general complaints of not feeling well, simply in an effort to get a medical excuse for missing a class exam for which he had not studied. The doctor could find nothing wrong with Greg but was concerned by his "gravel-sounding, hoarse voice." Indirect laryngoscopy revealed normal structures and referral was made to our speech clinic. Greg's voice was pitched abnormally low and the quality was indeed abnormal. The aberrant quality was the more conspicuous problem. He indicated that his voice always sounded like this and gave him no trouble other than fatigue after any day of heavy talking. Part of our evaluation session was spent with "trial and error" attempts to change Greg's voice. Some things we tried had no effect, others made him sound more harsh, and a few techniques seemed to bring out a "better" voice. In particular, raising Greg's pitch slightly decreased the harshness. The higher pitch, he assured us, felt comfortable. We hypothesized that Greg was using an inappropriately low and harsh voice, perhaps to project a more masculine image, and that the functional disorder would remediate quite well. Treatment was recommended to improve the harsh quality by raising pitch.

Prognosis

Prognosis has several aspects. First, there is the question of spontaneous remission of the presenting symptoms. Will this individual display an improvement in voice without intervening therapy? Second, how much improvement can be expected following the prescribed clinical program? That is, to what degree is the voice therapy, as projected, going to be effective? Third, how permanent are the gains shown in therapy going to be? Is the vocal improvement such that continuous therapy will be necessary to maintain optimal voice performance? (Medicare and most third-party reimbursement agencies will not fund "maintenance therapy.") Finally, would some other clinical procedure be of greater benefit to the client?

A variety of factors have potential prognostic value in voice cases. Some of the variables are directly observable and subject to quantification; others are much more subjective. The factors appear to fall into three broad categories: characteristics of the disorder, the person, and the environment. Those factors include:

1. ***Duration of the Problems.*** Generally disorders of long standing have greater resistance to clinical treatment.
2. ***Etiological Factors.*** Two factors are relevant here. First, is the cause of the problem identifiable? Second, is the cause of the problem alterable? And if so, is the type of necessary habilitating service available?
3. ***Degree of Secondary Psychological Components.*** Generally, the greater the degree of psychological disturbance, the poorer the prognosis.
4. ***Variability and General Flexibility of the Voice.*** Generally, the more the client is able to alter his or her vocal behavior, the better the prognosis. This underscores the importance of probing for vocal change with facilitating techniques during the initial session.
5. ***Auditory and Imitative Skills.*** The better the client is at hearing differences in quality, pitch, and loudness, coupled with the ability to imitate these differences, the more favorable the prognosis.
6. ***Impact or Degree of Disability.*** The greater the impact of the voice difference upon the individual, the better the chances for cooperation and motivation. Generally, too, if the family of the client is supportive, the outlook is more favorable. This relates to the World Health Organization's emphasis on impact (Figure 10.2).
7. ***Structural Integrity of the Vocal Mechanism.*** Clearly, the more the speech mechanism is disrupted anatomically or neurologically, the more limited the prognosis will be.

CONCLUSION TO VOCAL (LARYNGEAL) DISORDERS

This chapter has covered a great deal of information. But what are a reasonable number of measures important to track pre-, peri-, and post-treatment as evidence of progress and outcome? The ones we try to collect on each client include:

- Patient, family, and SLP ratings of the voice (e.g., features of pitch, loudness, quality, and so forth)
- Perceived sensory symptoms, including phonatory effort
- Average fundamental frequency during reading and monologue
- Frequency range utilized during reading and monologue
- Maximum phonation time (MPT of a vowel)
- Jitter (expressed as a percentage)
- Laryngeal appearance

Certainly more can be added to this list, but we feel comfortable that these are reasonable measures that can be reevaluated often to document change—or lack of it. Evidence of this type also satisfies our accountability to the client and to third-party payors.

The evaluation of voice disorders is a challenge to the speech pathologist. It requires the ability to deal with older adults as well as young children. The clinician must often work closely with medical personnel and other allied health workers, which necessitates knowing procedures and terminologies that are peripheral to speech-language pathology. The clinician must also remain abreast of current technological developments in electronics, surgery, and medical technology. Finally, the clinician must keep interpersonal clinical skills finely honed so that psychological aspects of vocal disorders can be detected and dealt with through treatment or referral.

ASSESSMENT OF THE LARYNGECTOMEE

We now turn to a discussion of the loss of voice due to laryngeal excision. Laryngeal excision is done primarily to preserve the life of the patient, most often because of the presence of cancer. However, the surgeon, in removing the malignant tumor and a healthy margin of tissue, is also conscious of the need to provide as great a chance for continued vocal function as is possible. Surgery may include excision of the total larynx, half of the larynx, one vocal fold and part of the other, removal of the anterior section of the thyroid cartilage and both vocal folds, or various other combinations. In cases of early detection, subtotal laryngectomies are becoming more routine, and the surgeon is often able to reconstruct a serviceable larynx and preserve voice. It is important that the SLP know exactly what procedures were undertaken, because the rehabilitation program will vary relative to the type of surgery and the condition of the remaining structures.

The assessment of a person who has undergone a total laryngectomy is inherently different from the initial assessment of persons with other communication disorders. We do not approach the initial session to solve the problem/no problem issue. When we get a referral to see a laryngectomee, we immediately know that the ability to speak has been lost—there is a problem and the diagnosis is obvious. We also know that some form of intervention will be necessary to reestablish a means of communication for the patient. What needs to be assessed is the current status of the patient (physically, psychologically, and the like), the potential for rehabilitation, and the direction (or directions) that the intervention program should take. Questions floating through the clinician's mind are likely to include: Is the patient psychologically ready to begin rehabilitation in earnest? What is the physical health of the patient like, both in general and as related to the laryngeal surgery? Are there cultural, educational, or intellectual limitations that may affect the short- and long-term courses of treatment? And, most important, for which avenues of communication does the patient show potential or preference (e.g., gestures, artificial devices, esophageal speech, tracheoesophageal speech)?

These days, patients who undergo total laryngectomy routinely have a primary tracheoesophageal fistula created for speech. The scope of this book does not allow for a discussion of all alaryngeal speech options and their dynamic assessments (e.g., artificial larynx, traditional esophageal speech) though Table 10.10 provides a summary of these. We will confine our discussion to an overview of the basic assessment process for all patients, then summarize what is done with a patient receiving a tracheoesophageal fistula.

The evaluation process involves the collection of background information, current status indicators, and trial therapy, among other things. The clinician's insights, judgments, and competencies with trial therapy techniques are crucial, as the evaluation session is truly the initial treatment session as well.

Once the patient is talking, it is important subjectively and objectively to appraise the quality of the speech. Research has provided us with yardsticks with which to measure the progress of our patients. Reevaluation materials are available for this purpose.

TABLE 10.10 Overview of Three Forms of Alaryngeal Speech Rehabilitation

Esophageal Speech

- Vibratory sound source is tissue in the upper esophageal segment (UES) and/or where the trachea joins the esophagus (P-E segment)
- Exhaled lung air cannot be delivered to this area; a different source of air must insufflate the segment
- Techniques for generating this air include injection and inhalation
- Injection uses articulators to increase air pressure, forces a ball of air through the muscle sphincter at the top of the P-E segment
- Inhalation involves decreasing air pressure in a rapidly expanding thorax (below that of room air pressure) so that air insufflates the esophagus
- Control of the egress of air is crucial for articulation intelligibility
- Length of utterance (number of syllables) per air charge is limited
- Speech frequency is low and quality is rough in traditional esophageal speech
- Main advantage: does not require purchase or maintenance of special equipment
- Main disadvantage: difficult and slow to learn

Artificial Larynx Speech

- Vibratory sound source is an external mechanism: either electronic (battery powered) or pneumatic (oral air to a rubber membrane)
- Placement of electrolarynx often on neck, chin or cheek but intraoral tubing available to deliver sound into mouth as done in pneumatic type
- Relies on resonance in the vocal tract and articulation of sound
- Device usually held by nondominant hands
- Speech quality often mechanical with strong volume
- Electrolarynx speech phrasing can be continuous and so training on pausing promotes intelligibility
- Main advantage: easy to learn and provides immediate speech
- Main disadvantages: requires use of one hand, is visually conspicuous, cost to purchase and to maintain (recharge battery)

Tracheoesophageal (TE) Speech

- Surgeon creates a puncture (fistula) in the wall separating trachea and esophagus. A one-way valve (prosthesis) is placed into the puncture site to allow exhaled lung air to pass into the esophagus. This air vibrates the PE segment for sound production
- The one-way valve allows lung air to pass into the esophageal segment without food and liquids leaking into the trachea
- Occlusion of one-way valve prosthesis with thumb or finger makes speech possible; often a prosthetic speaking valve is coupled to allow hands-free speech
- Use of lung air affords speech that is near-normal in breath support and phrasing
- Vibration of PE segment results in lower vocal frequency and rougher quality than in laryngeal speech
- Main advantages: lung air is used for speech and, apart from healing time, speech is instantaneous or easy to acquire
- Main disadvantages: additional surgical step is necessary for the puncture, some patients are not good candidates for TE speech, routine maintenance of all purchased devices necessary, and the danger of aspiration if liquids leak through a malfunctioning valve

THE COUNSELING PROCESS

The evaluation will seek to determine a patient's rehabilitation potential and to provide information necessary to shape the direction of treatment. But the evaluation process also has the goal of providing information, support, and emotional release for the patient and the patient's family. The clinician must wear many hats. In this section, let us explore the clinician's role in the preoperative visit, family and spouse counseling, arranging or assisting with the visit by another laryngectomee, and postoperative counseling of the patient.

The Preoperative Visit

Ideally, the surgeon requests that a preoperative visit be made by the SLP. When the physician informs the patient of the cancer, a thousand thoughts must surge through the patient's mind: Will I die? Will I be disfigured? Will my family be able to look at me? Will I talk again? Will I lose my job? Private thoughts such as these may happen so forcefully and quickly that the patient does not absorb much of what else the physician says. We often see patients with only a small understanding of the surgery and its many consequences for daily living. Explanations offered by the physician, then, can be supplemented at a later meeting by the speech pathologist. A preoperative visit is an ideal time to meet the patient, who can still talk, ask questions, express feelings and fears, and so forth. The clinician must be emotionally and professionally capable of dealing with the issues of this meeting. It can be a time when grown men cry, when women react with such anger as to order you out of their room, when denial is apparent, and/or when the patient needs desperately to hear some words of hope and optimism.

One goal of the first meeting, then, is to provide emotional release and support. The clinician must remember in the preoperative visit that the patient is facing a trauma unparalleled in his or her lifetime. The first confrontation is no social chat and may well demand all of the professional proficiency the clinician can muster. Occasionally, the clinician might find that the patient is not capable of dealing rationally with the topic immediately before surgery and, in these cases, it may be preferable to postpone detailed discussion until after recovery.

Another major goal of the first meeting is to provide some information about the operation and the implications for speech. After consultation with the physician, every attempt should be made to present a clear discussion of the anatomical changes. Charts and diagrams are helpful. We often give the patient some booklets or pamphlets, available from the International Association of Laryngectomees (IAL) of the American Cancer Society (contact the IAL for a list of available materials). The paperback *Voice Restoration for the Laryngectomized* (Sansing, 1997) also is a thoughtful gift to a patient.

We explain that many communication avenues exist. At this time, we decide on an appropriate short-term method (e.g., writing, gesturing, pointing to pictures), depending on literacy, vision, and manual dexterity abilities or limitations. We arrange for the hospital, family, speech services, social services, or other department or agency to make the necessary supplies available immediately after surgery (e.g., paper/pencil, wipe-off writing boards, picture communication boards, synthetic speech devices, and so forth). We may also introduce other methods that the patient may learn to use, such as esophageal speech and speech with an artificial larynx unless tracheoesophageal fistula is planned. The introduction must offer the optimism that he or she may actually speak again, but care must be taken not to overwhelm the patient with too many details at this point.

Family-Spouse Counseling

Providing adequate information to the family can have far-reaching clinical implications. The spouse and immediate family also must understand the anatomy of the operation. Often, clinicians stress what the laryngectomee will be unable to do; and although this information is important, it is also important to stress to the family what the patient will be able to do. We generally attempt to have a frank discussion with the spouse about the typical reactions of the family. If a problem can be identified before it develops, it may be easier to control. The tendency to dominate the silent mate (or parent) must be controlled, as must the inclinations to infantilize, overindulge, and pity. Often we have to warn the family not to shout at the patient—they may think that someone who cannot talk also does not hear well. Some families readily admit to a feeling of repulsion because of the physical changes; this can be easily conveyed to the patient. The silent mate is sometimes excluded from conversation and decision making in the family. The clinician must be sensitive to the fact that the spouse will have significant concerns. The fear of death, reduced income, new responsibilities, social changes, and alterations in the marital (and sexual) relationship may be topics for discussion. One of the primary purposes of the clinician's visit with the family members is to let them know that their feelings are understood. It is expected that the clinician will be warm, sincere, and insightful, but we resist the temptation to dictate any specific attitude beyond this because each patient will require a somewhat different approach. Some need to be dealt with gently, others straightforwardly and frankly. Find the level and type of interaction your patient and his or her family respond to best and use it.

Materials available from the IAL are useful in spouse-family counseling. Many different pamphlets can provide the family with information and inspiration. We also like to arrange a viewing of one or more videos; the patient should attend with the family. The IAL film list should be consulted for something appropriate. Family counseling, then, seeks to ensure that the family is emotionally and physically ready to assist in the rehabilitation program and care of their loved one.

Laryngectomee Visitation

It is ideal when the surgeon and/or the SLP can arrange for the patient to be visited by a laryngectomee either before or after the surgery. The laryngectomee visitor, by his or her sheer presence, offers the patient hope: Here is a person who survived cancer, survived the operation, learned to talk, perhaps returned to work, and generally has gotten back into life. The laryngectomee can offer to the patient sincere understanding of the emotional turmoil—he or she has been down that road—and may be the best paraprofessional to offer advice and empathy. The laryngectomee visitor is also a model of alaryngeal speech. The patient hears firsthand what practiced esophageal speech and/or artificial larynx speech sound like. Visitors are also great at explaining the importance of personal drive and daily practice.

Postoperative Counseling

If preoperative referrals were not made, the postoperative meetings will offer the opportunity for emotional release, support, and information sharing. All that we have described in the previous sessions needs to be accomplished now. If preoperative visits were done, then postoperatively the speech clinician is ready to move forward with the rehabilitation program, which involves a balance between treating and reassessing the patient's emotional, physical, and speech status.

The first few postoperative days may be the emotional low point for the patient. Frequent and brief visits may provide the support needed. The speech pathologist should also ensure that the patient has a means of communicating. Earlier we mentioned planning for written messages, picture communication boards, and the like. The clinician, with physician knowledge, may introduce artificial larynx devices for immediate speech if a primary tracheoesophageal fistula was not created for speech. The interested student is urged to consult any of the many excellent sources describing the available devices, their types, and how to begin training a patient in their use. We would like to suggest the classic book on artificial devices by Salmon and Goldstein (1978) and the edited text on alaryngeal speech by Salmon (1999).

BACKGROUND AND CURRENT STATUS INFORMATION

The evaluation of the newly laryngectomized patient truly began with the first preoperative meeting and has continued through all subsequent contacts. Where the patient is psychologically, physiologically, and intellectually is important to know, and these places keep changing. Dynamic assessments, rather than static evaluations, are the order of the day. Yet, as in traditional evaluations of a patient, we need to collect background as well as current status information. We begin by reading the patient's hospital chart with particular emphasis on the initial (admitting) medical report, the surgical report, the daily notes by the nursing staff, and the family history critique provided by the social worker.

In determining the potential for speech, a thorough case history is helpful with laryngectomized patients. Three facets are particularly crucial. It is important to know the extent of the surgery, the degree of involvement of related structures such as the tongue or pharynx, general health of the patient, and medical prognosis. The second critical area is the individual's vocation and interests. We find it most helpful to plan our clinical work about the patient's preferred activities. It is also important to know if the person will be able to continue in those vocations and hobbies that involve communication. A third variable related to the patient's potential for learning traditional esophageal speech is attitude and motivation. Some patients are depressed, discouraged, and unmotivated, while others evidence a high level of interest in recovering their communication abilities. This is a subjective judgment on the clinician's part, but it is one of those intangible variables that certainly relates to the potential of the patient to speak again.

Many texts have compiled lists of the necessary medical and background information helpful in planning a rehabilitive program and they offer case history forms. Table 10.11 lists questions that guide us in the thorough collection of information on a patient. In addition to shaping the treatment program, such information provides prognostic insights.

A necessary part of the evaluation concerns the current status of the patient's oral-motor abilities. Chapter 9 provided details on an oral examination; suffice it to say that we thoroughly evaluate the tongue, lip, and jaw mobility. Articulation may be affected if surgery involved the hyoid bone, which is an anatomical connection for many muscles of the tongue, mandible, and pharynx. In addition, it is not uncommon that surgical alterations were necessary to contain concomitant oral, lingual, or lymph node cancers. Some information about the previous articulation, speech, and language patterns of the patient is also helpful. For example, we have had poor

| TABLE 10.11 | Laryngectomee Case History Outline |

1. *Surgical Factors*
   Date of surgery
   Extent of surgery
   Postoperative complications
   Irradiation/other treatment procedures
2. *Physical-Mental Factors*
   General physical condition
   Upper respiratory health
   Status of oral structures
   Hearing acuity
   Other physical factors or conditions
   Cognitive-mental clarity
   Educational background

3. *Emotional Factors*
   Level of negative emotion/depression
   Level of motivation
   Degree of dependency on spouse/family
   Other personality traits or problems
4. *Social Factors*
   Home/family situation
   Occupational aspects
   Hobbies/pastimes
   Smoking and drinking habits
   Social network/sociability
   Family attitudes and acceptance

success with alaryngeal speech intelligibility in cases where, premorbidly, the patient was edentulous and seldom wore dentures.

An assessment of the patient's hearing acuity also is desirable. Since a high percentage of laryngectomees are above the age of 55, it is common to find a presbycusic hearing loss. A moderate-to-severe hearing loss may hinder the learning process and, of necessity, shape the direction of the rehabilitation program.

Mr. Wayne Johnson, a 61-year-old white male, was admitted with a 6-month history of hoarseness. Examination by otolaryngologist revealed a hard mass in the neck at the angle of the jaw (at the area of the middle one-third of the left anterior lymphatic chain), and dysplasia involving the left aryepiglottic fold, false fold, and true fold. Biopsy confirmed locations with the finding of squamous cell carcinoma. A left radical neck dissection and total laryngectomy were performed.

Background information, contained in the report from social services, included mention that Mr. Johnson was a salesman and lived in an affluent resort community on a lake and golf course. He and his wife golfed several times a week and enjoyed all water sports, including skiing.

The speech pathologist, after reading the medical chart, began to wonder about the quality of life for Mr. Johnson following laryngectomy. Being a salesman, communication and meeting the public are necessary parts of his job. Will he return to work? Will he experience a loss of earnings from lost commissions? (The public might not buy from an unusual-sounding person.) Will the company "urge" him to take early retirement? Could the company shift his duties from sales force to office work? To be sure, questions such as these were not only going through the mind of the speech pathologist but also of the patient and his wife. The clinician felt that an impending return to work would be a strong motivator for Mr. Johnson to speak. The clinician also had thoughts concerning his avocations and knew future counseling would have to deal with these issues. Mr. Johnson almost certainly would play golf again, but with a reduction in general strength, head-neck rotation abilities, and a less effective golf swing because of the radical neck dissection. The lake lifestyle posed particular dangers. Stoma breathers generally are advised to stay clear of water. Skiing is out for Mr. Johnson, as is swimming; riding in a motor boat carries a certain risk (accidents do happen). Will Mr. Johnson adjust to these restrictions? He could wade in the water and even try to snorkel with a special breathing device for laryngectomees, but clearly his lifestyle is in for a drastic change. Of prime importance, however, is the containment of cancer, his survival, and a return of the ability to communicate.

EARLY SPEECH ATTEMPTS WITH A TRACHEOESOPHAGEAL PROSTHESIS

The evaluation may proceed differently with patients planning to have a tracheoesophageal puncture (TEP), also known as tracheoesophageal fistulization.

In this procedure, the surgeon places a hole (puncture or fistula) in the membranous wall between the trachea and the esophagus, thus providing a route or connection between these two structures. A prosthesis placed in this opening will allow for pulmonary air to be routed into the top of the esophagus under certain conditions. Breathing is still done through the stoma. Aspiration of saliva, liquids, and foods is minimized by the one-way directionality of the prosthetic device. The conditions that allow for diverting exhaled air into the esophagus, rather than out the stoma, are digital occlusion of the prosthesis opening, located in the stoma, or the use of a valving device to reroute the airstream.

Upon muscular effort, air diverted into the esophagus will be compressed, and forced through the top of the closed esophagus, thereby setting the pharyngoesophageal segment into vibration. This segment is the sound source or pseudoglottis; articulation of the sound is accomplished in the usual manner in the upper vocal tract. In essence, tracheoesophageal speech (TE speech) is esophageal in nature, yet supported by the pulmonary system. Tracheoesophageal speech obviates the need to learn traditional esophageal speech via injection or inhalation methods and is, therefore, easily mastered. Furthermore, the use of lung air provides acoustic and perceptual advantages over traditional esophageal speech.

Hospitalization for healed laryngectomees who come back for only the TEP procedure is brief; some surgical procedures can even be done on an outpatient basis or as an office procedure. Primary punctures also can be done on newly laryngectomized patients. Bosone (1999) reports many surgeons prefer to do a total laryngectomy, pharyngeal constrictor myotomy, and TEP at the same time. Others prefer that the patient convalesce before puncture. Screening for candidacy, fitting of the device, and instructing in the care and use of the device often is done solely by the speech pathologist, sometimes in concert with the nurse and doctor. Fluent conversational speech typically is acquired rapidly. The SLP, then, has a brief but vital role to play in the rehabilitation of TEP patients.

The success of any method depends, in part, on the proper selection of candidates for that method. Patient selection criteria and contraindications for tracheoesophageal puncture were established early on by Singer and Blom (1980); see the following list. Fagan and Isaacs (2002), in their work in South Africa, suggest that eligibility screening need not focus on social class and literacy but merely on manual dexterity and cognitive function.

1. Motivation to undergo the procedure and sustained motivation to care for the prosthesis on a daily basis.
2. Absence of physical or mental limitations to the daily care and fitting (insertion) of the prosthesis. In particular, the patient should have adequate vision and eye-hand coordination to place the prosthetic device while in front of a mirror. Manual dexterity (e.g., absence of arthritis) is necessary for the handling of the prosthesis and all associated materials (particularly if a tracheostoma valve is also used).
3. Good general health. Weak, feeble persons do not do well with TEP; however, conditions such as chronic pulmonary disease, diabetes, and alcoholism do not necessarily rule out candidacy.
4. Concern for hygiene in cleansing of the device, in neck tissue care (adhesives used with the valve can be irritating to sensitive skin), and in touching/handling all materials.
5. Adequate stoma characteristics. In particular, the stoma must not be retracted behind the manubrium. Size of the opening should be a minimum of 1 cm across the axis, but for some procedures 2 cm are needed. An excessively large stoma can be corrected somewhat by tape.
6. Recovery from postsurgical radiation treatment, if any.
7. Absence of chronic tracheitis or ulceration.
8. Absence of a history of unplanned fistulas, pharyngoesophageal stricture (spasm), or flap reconstruction. The presence of any of these conditions, however, does not necessarily rule out TEP candidacy but suggests the need for a more detailed assessment. A barium esophagram may yield findings suggesting that dilation may be necessary to maintain an adequate opening for airflow and voice.

In this regard we need to explain that the primary reason for failure with tracheoesophageal speech is spasms of the pharyngoesophageal segment. Spasms make the vibration and production of sound difficult, if not impossible. The spasms usually can be relaxed by surgically cutting some of the muscle fibers in the pseudoglottis. The need for this surgical procedure, called a myotomy, can be predicted with a simple screening test. The speech pathologist, or surgeon, or both perform an air insufflation procedure, where air is introduced into the esophagus and the patient is asked to phonate. Good phonation, of course, indicates that the patient's pharyngoesophageal segment is capable of vibration, and therefore a myotomy would not be needed. Such a patient is considered an excellent candidate for TEP. As mentioned previously, some surgeons do a myotomy on all patients at the time of primary surgery, whether necessary or not. There is some evidence that this results in poorer speech in some patients (Bosone, 1999). A recent alternative to surgical relaxation of the pharyngeal constrictor muscles is the injection of Botox. Reports of Botox's effectiveness are beginning to appear in the literature (Bosone, 1999). It is always best to identify patients early who will benefit from middle and inferior constrictor myotomy. Henley and Souliere (2009) give a preoperative injection of Xylocaine to produce a partial blockage for speech to confirm that myotomy will benefit the patient. Getting a patient started in the use of tracheoesophageal speech is a complex issue. We will attempt to subdivide the tasks and provide an overview of each.

PROSTHESIS FITTING   The speech pathologist is often responsible for fitting the patient with a prosthesis of proper size. Brands differ in size, features, and design to optimize individual patient fit. The Blom-Singer Voice Prosthesis, Low Pressure Voice Prosthesis, and the Duckbill Voice Prosthesis are in frequent use and are available in various lengths of optimal fit.

Following typical TEP surgery, a catheter is left in place for 24 to 72 hours to prevent closure of the puncture site. After that, a prosthesis should be fitted and voice will be possible. The speech pathologist should recheck the patient in four to five weeks and refit the prosthesis, if necessary. Occasionally, after the edema subsides, a shorter prosthesis is more appropriate.

The process of fitting the prosthesis is as follows: Instruct the patient not to swallow. Remove the catheter that has been in place since the surgery. Insert a depth gauge or the fistula measurement probe through the stoma and into the puncture; feel it "pop" into place. Pull out slightly until the retention collar is firmly against the puncture opening and read the distance on the imprinted probe. This indicates the length of prosthesis needed.

Once the size of the needed prosthesis has been determined, insert one, applying double-faced tape on the flanges, if necessary (depending on design). Once in place, have the patient drink some water to make sure there is no leakage around or through the prosthesis. Demonstrate digital occlusion for the patient and instruct him or her to try to talk on exhalation while the stoma/prosthesis opening is occluded with the clinician's thumb or finger. If voice is not produced, assess the reason(s) why (see next section). If successful, continue talking practice. Later, allow the patient to do his or her own digital occlusion. Indwelling prostheses, those placed by the physician or SLP and which last in place about six months, are becoming quite popular. These eliminate some of the need for screening candidacy with regard to manual dexterity, personal hygiene, and especially the need daily to insert the device and secure it in place.

VOICE FAILURE ASSESSMENT   If the patient is unable to produce voice, the speech pathologist should try to determine whether the problem lies with the prosthetic device or with the patient.

Common problems of voice failure owing to patient factors include the following: (1) The patient may be using excessive finger pressure against the stoma. (2) The patient may be using inadequate expiratory pressure. A weak, feeble patient is a poor candidate for TE speech because of the energy necessary to overcome the air resistance of the plastic devices. Alternately, perhaps the patient simply needs to be instructed to use more effort and more air in speech attempts. Other devices (styles and brands) may be tried as well; each model differs in its air-flow resistance. An ultralow resistance model may work for the patient. (3) Salivary secretions may have accumulated, blocking the pharynx. In this case, the speech will sound "gurgly." Expectoration should solve the problem. (4) A most likely reason for the absence of voice is the presence of pharyngoesophageal spasm. Perhaps the air insufflation pretest was not done prior to TEP. At any rate, do the insufflation test to see if voice is possible with the prosthesis removed. A myotomy or Botox relaxing may be necessary to counteract the spasms.

Voice failure may be due to problems with the prosthetic device. These problems are often easily identified and rectified. In these cases, the patient would have voice without the prosthesis (with stoma digital occlusion or with the air insufflation test), but no voice with a faulty prosthesis in place. (1) The patient may be unable to produce voice because the prosthesis is inserted upside down. Remove and reinsert the prosthesis. (2) The valve slit may be stuck together on devices with a slit (duckbill) design. (3) Incorrect prosthesis length could be the reason for lack of voice. A device that is too long, particularly a device with a slit design that would be so impeded, may be touching the posterior wall of the esophagus. Refitting the patient with a shorter device and/or changing to a different design (nonslit, flap-door) is in order. A prosthesis that is too short would not have the tip residing in the lumen of the esophageal tube. A slit-designed tip would be impeded from passing its air into the esophagus. Try rotating the placement a bit. A longer prosthesis may be necessary. (4) Occlusion of the port may block air flow and hence voice. Clearing of saliva (or other matter) is in order.

If the patient has used TE speech for a period of time and begins to experience a change in the voice, or loss of it, troubleshooting to find and eliminate the cause is necessary. We recommend the work of Bosone (1999) and of Bunting (2004) for troubleshooting ideas. Telemedicine also is finding a place in the troubleshooting and assessment of swallowing, the stoma, and overall communication status in postlaryngectomy patients via cameras and remote technology (Ward et al., 2009).

TRACHEOSTOMA VALVE   Talking with the voice prosthesis requires digital occlusion (finger or thumb). This may be an unnecessary inconvenience. After a few weeks' experience with the voice prosthesis, the patient may be a candidate for using a tracheostoma valve (various styles and brands exist). More and more often, the patient is trained with a valve at the same time the prosthesis is introduced. The valve is fitted into the stomal opening; naturally, the patient still wears the voice prosthesis. Again, these are tasks that are within the purview of the SLP responsible for assessing and rehabilitating the laryngectomee.

TRACHEOSTOMA VALVE CONTRAINDICATIONS   The valve fits into a flexible circular housing which is attached to the skin area surrounding the stoma with nonirritating adhesive. When positioned over the stoma, the valve diaphragm remains in a fully open position during quiet breathing and routine physical activity. For speech, a slight increase in exhalation causes the valve diaphragm to close and divert air into the esophagus. The valve automatically reopens when exhalation decreases at the completion of an utterance.

A tracheostoma valve must be maintained by the patient; it is easily disassembled for cleaning. The diaphragm can be replaced by the patient without return to the manufacturer.

Four contraindications to using a valve seem to exist: (1) Patients with high phonatory pressure may blow the seal often; (2) a very recessed or irregular stoma may not accommodate the valve; (3) patients with excessive tracheal discharge may occlude or dangerously hinder the operation of the valve; and (4) inadequate pharyngoesophageal segments preclude usable speech, even with a valve.

VALVE FITTING   Select the diaphragm thickness that does not inadvertently close on the patient during routine physical exertion or heavier than usual exhalation. Conversely, do not select one too thick as to require excessive exhalation for the generation of voice. A practical method for fitting involves the "stair-step" test. Have the patient try a diaphragm sensitivity while going up and down some stairs. The speech pathologist and patient should carefully watch for valve closure as breathing deepens during this exertion. If the valve closes, remove it and try the next-thicker size. Repeat the stair-step test until the proper diaphragm size has been determined. Some patients may wish to purchase two diaphragms: one for general use and a thicker one for use while dancing, exercising, and the like.

Patients should be instructed not to sleep with the tracheostoma valve in place. In addition, patients may find it helpful to remove the valve from its housing when they feel an urge to cough or forcefully exhale. This prevents blowing the seal and the necessity of cleaning and reapplying the adhesive. Some models contain a spring action valve (rather than the usual butterfly valve) with a cough relief valve that is said to eliminate blowout from a cough or instance of high airway pressure production.

VOICE TREATMENT SESSIONS Treatment begins with prosthesis fitting, usually done by the speech pathologist, as described previously. Once fitted, demonstrate digital occlusion for the patient. Instruct the patient to try to talk (on exhalation) while the prosthesis opening is digitally occluded. If voice is not produced, assess reasons that it is not. If successful, continue talking practice. Later, allow the patient to do his or her own finger occlusion. It is simple, yet the coordination needs to be practiced.

Concomitant with speech practice, the patient should be trained in the placement of the prosthesis and the valve, if applicable. Instructions as to taping and/or gluing should be detailed for some types of devices, allowing for much supervised practice. Care and cleaning of the devices should be taught as well. Usually by the third session, the patient is independent in talking with the prosthesis and in its placement, adhesion, and daily care.

We would like to offer a few observations about these first few sessions. One aspect of treatment may involve the unlearning of esophageal speech techniques in the patient who spoke esophageally prior to TEP. The two forms of speech are incompatible. Patients using esophageal speech must break whatever habits they have developed and return to what amounts to their prelaryngectomy form of speaking with lung air. This is usually easily achieved; yet, patients may require the speech pathologist to guide and monitor their unlearning or deconditioning of the esophageal speech habit.

Train the patient to use the proper amount of finger pressure on the prosthesis opening at the stoma. There is a tendency to push too forcefully at first. Similarly, patients may need the speech pathologist's help in learning the minimal amount of expiratory pressure needed to drive the system. Some patients begin learning TE speech with a valve, using an excessive amount of air pressure. This can result in "blowing a seal" or loosening of the valve housing. If the housing develops a broken seal, it becomes difficult to close the valve and utilize the prosthesis for voice production. Instead, the air leak becomes audible and speech breakdown occurs. When this happens, the patient must manually hold the housing down while speaking, until there is an opportunity to reapply the housing. This is less of a problem with low-resistance prostheses. Regular prostheses have a higher resistance to opening and to air flowing through them. A greater air pressure buildup is required of the speaker, with the danger of straining the glued seal of the housing.

In addition to learning the minimal amount of pressure needed on which to speak, the patient must learn proper ways to adhere the device to prevent blowout. Applying the proper amount of glue is important, as is getting the taped collar onto the housing without wrinkles in it, and applying it to the neck evenly. This is highly individualistic and must be learned by each patient with the help of the speech pathologist and sheer practice.

ONGOING ASSESSMENTS: A DYNAMIC PROCESS

Assessing the proficiency of alaryngeal speech and refining that speech in treatment sessions are two intertwined processes. The direction that treatment should take is directly related to how well the patient is doing in the various components of speech. Ideally, the patient's status changes for the better on a daily or weekly basis, making frequent reassessments a necessity. Dynamic, ongoing assessments, then, suggest to the clinician (1) what to work on, (2) how much therapeutic time needs to be devoted to certain tasks, and (3) what tasks or steps in the program may be skipped or bypassed. This last item points out that reassessments serve as probes as to what the patient can already do without training, as well as measures of achievement.

TE speech is produced with exhaled lung air, but this does not mean that TE speech will be equivalent to normal, laryngeal speech. More air will be expended in TE speech because of the resistance of the prosthetic device and routing passage. Hence, duration of sustained phonation and number of words spoken per breath will be shorter than normal. Lung air will permit variety in pitch and loudness, but the pseudoglottis may tend to restrict it. The result of all this is that TE speech is generally superior to esophageal speech but inferior to normal speech on most measures.

A prime area of dynamic assessment is that of articulatory intelligibility. Tracheoesophageal speakers need to constantly monitor and improve articulation proficiency with voiced/voiceless cognates and phonemes that pose perceptual confusion. We mention "jip–chip–ship" as an example of potential difficulties.

Regarding specific data pertinent to the assessment of TE speech, we would like to mention the works of Robbins, Fisher, and Blom (1984) and Pindzola and Cain (1989). These studies show good agreement in their data. Pindzola and Cain compared TE speakers, esophageal speakers, and normal speakers on certain criteria, including the following points:

1. Speech rate differed among the three groups of speakers. Normal talkers averaged 170 wpm, TE speakers averaged 152 wpm, and esophageal speakers averaged 94 wpm.
2. The fundamental frequency of the TE speakers was slightly lower than expected of normal males of the same age. TE speech averaged 108 Hz. Esophageal speech was much lower, with an average of 84 Hz. Lung air offers advantages here, even though the pharyngoesophageal segment acts as the pseudoglottis in both forms of alaryngeal speech.
3. The range of fundamental frequency, or pitch variability, was equivalent among the three groups. This indicates that both TE and esophageal speakers can achieve use of intonation with the pseudoglottis.
4. The number of words spoken per breath, or per air charge, showed the expected pattern: Normal speakers averaged 12 words per breath, TE speakers averaged 8 words per breath, and esophageal speakers averaged 3.5 words per air charge.

We agree with Lewin (1999), who observes that many SLPs discharge TE patients prematurely—once they can manage the technical apparatus—since speech is usually immediate. However, further treatment is merited to perfect the patient's intonation, loudness variability and stress, fluency, intelligibility, and naturalness, as is the prevention of the development of extraneous behaviors during communication.

Table 10.12 presents items of speech proficiency that we like to address in treatment sessions. Ongoing evaluations are done such that measures and ratings are taken as soon as the laryngectomee is talking as well as periodically throughout treatments. These frequent reassessments tell us areas in need of attention, when improvements have plateaued, or are not expected, based on outcomes reported in the literature (Bellandese, Lerman, & Gilbert, 2001; Lewin, 1999; Pindzola & Cain, 1989; Robbins et al., 1984; Van Rossum et al., 2002).

Carpenter (1999) presents a useful rating form for assessing alaryngeal speech subskills. TE speech is rated on respiratory support, stoma seal, duration, quality, loudness, pitch, articulation, timing, prosody, and presence of audible or visible distractors. Carpenter also asserts that alaryngeal speech proficiency may be assessed along three straightforward parameters: intelligibility, naturalness, and distractors.

With regard to functional communication outcomes, existing voice or neurological instruments, rather than specific alaryngeal instruments, tend to be used. For example, Schuster et al. (2004) employed the Voice Handicap Index (VHI, discussed earlier in this chapter) with TE speakers and found it a useful individual barometer but not good at identifying "scores" typical of laryngectomees as a group.

TABLE 10.12	Alaryngeal Treatment Items and Outcome Assessment Parameters (Item Proficiency Rated on a 5-Point Scale)

- *Maximum Phonation Time (MPT):* Duration of a vowel held for 9 to 17 seconds
- *Fundamental Frequency (F0):* Should approximate F0 values of laryngeal speakers of similar age group; special attention if female laryngectomee; utilize "telephone test" for gender rating
- *Intonation (F0 Variance):* Achieved via changes in subneoglottic air pressure and flow rates; practice at word/sentence level; humming/singing scale or songs
- *Overal Intensity/Speech Loudness:* Adequate for communication; ability to increase when needed via changes in subneoglottic air pressure and flow rates (Caution: Increased loudness may lead to extraneous noises and poor speech quality.)
- *Stress/Loudness Variability:* Clarity of lexical stress (OBject vs. obJECT) and of contrastive stress (BEV loves Bob vs. Bev loves BOB)
- *Articulatory Precision:* Proficiency with voiced–voiceless contrasts; intelligibility of problematic phonemes such as plosives, fricatives and affricates especially when in initial position
- *Speech Rate:* Correlated with speech naturalness; measured either as syllable rate or as word rate; measured during both speaking (goal of 120 wpm) and reading (goal of 166 wpm); goal rates to approximate laryngeal values as close as feasible
- *Fluency:* Degree of momentary periods of aphonia, with goal of zero; aphonic blocks (akin to stuttering blocks) often due to unwanted oral injection of air or by swallowing just prior to TE speech attempt; disfluency can also be due to pharyngeal constrictor spasm
- *Extraneous Behaviors:* Prevention or minimalization of things such as stoma noise, air leakage, valve thumping, neck tension or unusual posturing, observable mucus, oral/stoma odors, and so forth

Carpenter (1999), on the other hand, has proposed a cursory form for an alaryngeal speaker to rate both his or her overall *effectiveness* and overall *satisfaction* in three communication settings. Basically the person rates whether they talk as "much" or as "well" as they "need" to and "want" to. The University of Washington Quality of Life (UM-QOL) scale has been used following total laryngectomy (Kazi et al., 2007). Lastly, the European Organization for Research and Treatment of Cancer Quality of Life Questionnaire-C30 (EORTC QLQ-C30) has been used in tandem with the head and neck module (EORTC QLQ-H&N35) in various follow-up studies involving laryngectomized persons (Boscolo-Rizzo et al., 2008; Hanna et al., 2004; Relic et al., 2001).

PROGNOSIS

At the end of the evaluation sessions, we should have obtained pertinent case history data, and we should have provided information to the patient and the family about the anatomical changes and potential communication methods. We should also have a good idea about the patient's current method of communication and potential for treatment. As a review of much of what we have said in this chapter, we offer the following list of prognostic indicators for success.

1. The patient should have competent anatomical structures for the method or methods of speech chosen. The pharyngoesophageal segment must be adequate for TE speech. The tendency for esophageal spasms (as pretested with air insufflation) must be addressed for success.

2. The severity, extent, and type of surgery seem not to be related to the acquisition of speech. Yet this assessment may be highly individualistic.

3. Patients should be of good general health. Feeble patients generally do not do well in learning TE speech, which requires energy to persist in the rehabilitation process.

4. While TE puncture can be done at any time, the date of the surgery relative to the enrollment in the speech rehabilitation program is important. The prognosis for proficient speech after waiting is affected by other habits that have developed and are difficult to break.

5. Patients with a positive attitude and motivation to practice often throughout the day tend to be the successful ones.

6. Those planning to return to work seem to have an extra ounce of motivation to master speech and to do so more quickly than those staying home or in an institution.

7. Patients who have family support at home, willing communication partners, and people willing to participate in the rehabilitation program and to help with daily practice generally do quite well.

8. Patients who are literate and willing to read and study materials about laryngectomy rehabilitation seem to make good progress. They make good use of workbooks, stimuli lists, and the like in daily practice.

To conclude, then, we have shown the multitude of complex issues involved in the assessment, counseling, prognosing, and reassessment of persons with laryngectomies. The focus was on the SLP's role with patients having the tracheoesophageal procedure.

11

Assessment of Resonance Imbalance

Disorders of voice, particularly disorders of vocal quality, may be due to defective transmission of sound through the vocal tract. Sound generation at the level of the larynx occurs normally, and so these are not laryngeal disorders discussed in Chapter 10. Problems of resonance may be classified as hyponasality, hypernasality, nasal emission, cul-de-sac resonance, or thin/effeminate resonance. The assessment of resonance imbalance will be the focus of this chapter.

CATEGORIES OF ABNORMAL RESONANCE

The *denasal* or *hyponasal* voice lacks the normal nasal resonance expected on /m/, /n/, and /ŋ/ in English. Often these articulatory distortions resemble /b/, /d/, and /g/, respectively. The vocalic elements may also take on the characteristics of talking with a head cold. Hyponasality usually results from some blockage or obstruction in the nasopharynx or nasal cavity. This obstruction may stem from congestion, nasal polyps, or various structural deformities. The speech of children with cochlear implants also may display inconsistent hyponasality on vocalic speech elements and the normally nasal consonants of /m/, /n/, and /ŋ/, making them sound denasal (Teoh & Chin, 2009).

Hypernasality is an excessive amount of nasal resonance during the production of vowels and vocalic elements. The nasal cavity is not adequately separated from the oral cavity during speech. Such velopharyngeal incompetence, or VPI, may stem from neuromuscular deficits or structural defects. Congenital clefts of the hard or soft palate are obvious examples of structural defects frequently leading to hypernasality, and we will discuss these conditions later in the chapter. Not only can hypernasality result from clefts of the hard or soft palate, but also from submucous clefts, velums with inadequate length, or pharyngeal dimensions that are too large. A neuromuscular deficit, such as a paralyzed or paretic velum, or dysfunction of the pharyngeal constrictor muscles may be attributed to trauma-induced dysarthria or disease-related dysarthria. Diseases such as myasthenia gravis, muscular dystrophy, and poliomyelitis often affect velopharyngeal functioning.

Hypernasality may be pronounced or only slightly apparent; in addition, it can be continuous or intermittent. In mild intermittent cases, the excess nasality on vowels may be most noticeable in the context of nasal consonants. This represents assimilation nasality and indicates a velum that can function but moves too slowly during connected speech.

Nasal emission is an audible escape of air through the nares during the production of pressure consonants, such as plosives, fricatives, and affricates. Implicated in this condition is an incompetent velopharyngeal mechanism. Nasal emission is different from the resonance imbalance of hypernasality, although the two problems may co-occur.

Cul-de-sac resonance typically occurs in the oropharynx, largely owing to posterior tongue retraction. This resonance imbalance is heard as a muffled and hollow-sounding voice with a pharyngeal focus. In addition, Peterson-Falzone (1982) states that cul-de-sac resonance can result from an anterior nasal obstruction and a posterior aperature (opening). Cul-de-sac resonance associated with tongue retraction often occurs on a functional basis, as well as in patients with deafness, flaccid and spastic dysarthria, athetoid cerebral palsy, or oral verbal apraxia (Boone et al., 2010; Prater & Swift, 1984). The degree of this nasality may be reduced in hearing impaired individuals with increases in speaking rates (Dwyer, Robb, & O'Beirne, 2009).

Thin vocal resonance, also known as an *effeminate voice quality,* seems related to an anterior tongue posture. The habitually high and excessively anterior tongue position is almost always due to functional, not organic, reasons. Prater and Swift (1984) explain:

> The voice sounds very weak and lacking in resonance, particularly for the back vowels . . . patients . . . articulate with a minimal oral opening and with little range of movement of the jaw. Because of . . . anterior tongue carriage and . . . restricted oral movement for articulation, the general impression . . . is that this type of speaker is using immature, baby-like, effeminate speech. Often, the speaker's vocal pitch is also elevated slightly, which aids in this perception of vocal immaturity and effeminacy. (p. 241)

CASE HISTORY AND GENERAL VOICE ASSESSMENT

The evaluation of a resonance disorder is often an outgrowth of a general voice evaluation; the clinician may not know beforehand the specific nature of a patient's problem. Consequently, the evaluation session proceeds along the lines described in Chapter 10. Suffice it to say that, first, a case history interview is done. Routine information is gathered, but particular questions need to be asked concerning the patient's description of the voice problem and known or suspected causes of the disorder. Oronasopharyngeal injuries, structural defects, and surgeries need to be thoroughly discussed. Second, the oral peripheral examination is crucial to the evaluation of resonance disorders; and, third, all parameters of the voice must be assessed.

Any of the assessment instruments mentioned in Chapter 10 would be appropriate to use. A Voice Assessment Protocol for Children and Adults (Pindzola, 1987) is useful in assessing a multitude of vocal parameters. It evaluates the resonance of the patient's voice on a severity continuum. The patient may be scored as exhibiting normal resonance balance, cul-de-sac resonance, hyponasality (slight or intermittent vs. moderate to severe), hypernasality on vocalic elements (slight, intermittent, or assimilative vs. moderate vs. severe), and nasal emission on pressure consonants (slight or intermittent vs. moderate to severe).

The popular, and reliable, Consensus Auditory-Perceptual Evaluation of Voice (CAPE-V), you will recall, is a measuring tool sponsored by ASHA's Special Interest Division 3, Voice and Voice Disorders. The article by Kempster et al. (2009) is a good source for the free instrument and also for documentation forms. CAPE-V rates six voice quality features: overall severity, roughness, breathiness, strain, pitch, and loudness. The astute reader will note that resonance is not among these attributes. The CAPE-V form includes two unlabeled scales allowing the SLP to

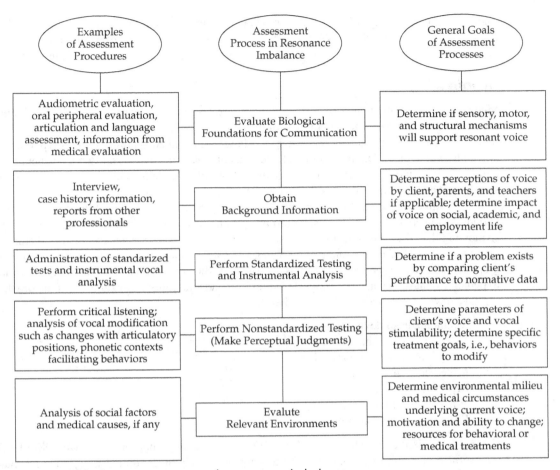

FIGURE 11.1 Critical assessment process in resonance imbalance.

document other salient perceptual features. It is here that the clinician can rate the type and degree of nasality (or any other vocal features desired).

Additionally, various commercially available treatment programs include an assessment instrument. An example pertinent to resonance is found within the *Hypernasality Modification Program: A Systematic Approach* by Ray and Baker (2002). This product includes a Resonance Evaluation to profile resonance in 16 structured phonetic contexts and purports being useful for ages 6 to adults. After a thorough, overall voice assessment, emphasis is given to the appraisal of the resonance imbalance. Specific techniques can be employed by the SLP. Figure 11.1 displays the process we recommend.

ASSESSMENT TECHNIQUES AND PROBES FOR RESONANCE IMBALANCE

In this section, we would like to discuss techniques requiring little or no instrumentation that the SLP can and should do to assess the various resonance imbalances. Before concluding the evaluation, we feel very strongly that the clinician should experiment, or probe, to see what improvements, or changes in general, can be effected in the patient's voice. Some writers have discussed this as *stimulability*. Wilson (1987) maintains that the ability of a patient to produce a clear voice upon stimulation means that voice treatment has a good chance of being successful.

Hyponasality

Since denasality is often due to obstruction in the nasal cavity, an examination of the nasal region is in order during the oral peripheral part of the assessment. Additionally, during the case history intake, the patient may indicate knowledge of having a deviated septum, nasal polyp, enlarged adenoids, and the like. On the other hand, the basis of a patient's hyponasality may be neuromuscular in origin and may reflect improper timing of velar movements. Case history questions should probe for trauma- or disease-related etiologies.

To evaluate a patient for hyponasal voice quality, SLPs rely on critical listening. While the patient is conversing or reading a standard paragraph, the clinician acutely listens for denasality shadowing the vowel portions of speech and, in particular, listens for the articulatory distortions or substitutions of b/m, d/n, and g/k. By using specially constructed phrases, sentences, or paragraphs that have a preponderance of nasal phonemes, the clinician has a heightened opportunity to perceive denasal resonance. Suggested stimuli include the following examples, some of which we have devised or borrowed from the literature:

> Mama made some lemon jam.
> I know a man on the moon.
> Many a man knew my meaning.
> Mike needs more milk.
> My mom makes money.
> When may we know your name?
> I'm naming one man among many.

Having the patient count aloud from 90 to 100 is contextually appropriate, as well. Word pairs are useful in detecting hyponasality: "bake"/"make," "rib"/"rim," "dine"/"nine," "mad"/"man," "wig"/"wing," "bag"/"bang." In hyponasality, nasal resonance would be lacking and so, for example, the "bake"/"make" pair would sound like "bake"/"bake."

Another clinical task that is helpful in revealing hyponasal speech is to have the patient read a list of words initiated with the /m/ phoneme. Bzoch (2004) suggests these 10 words: "meat," "moat," "mit," "moot," "mate," "mut," "met," "Mert," "mat," and "might." While the patient is reading, or repeating, each word from the list twice, the clinician alternately compresses and releases the patient's nostrils. In normal velopharyngeal function, the resonance becomes hypernasal when the nares are occluded, but no resonance change is heard in true hyponasality. Bzoch counts the number of words with no change in resonance and uses this figure as an index of hyponasality.

Operating on this same principle is the humming technique. The inability of a patient to hum or to hum clearly is suggestive of hyponasality (Prater & Swift, 1984).

> Carmen Perez has fluctuating hyponasality. The severity of her hyponasality changes on a daily basis, but there is a more noticeable fluctuation with the seasons. Carmen's ear, nose, and throat doctor observed nasal cavity characteristics typical of allergic inflammation: tissue coloration changes and hypertrophy of the nasal turbinates secondary to edema. The planned course of treatment involved use of prescribed antihistamines and the option of undergoing a lengthy allergen tolerance program.

Hypernasality

Judgments about resonance are truly judgments of a perceptual nature; a well-tuned clinical ear is essential—and adequate—for the SLP. Critical listening by the clinician while the patient converses and/or reads a passage can be supplemented by rating the severity of the hypernasality on a rating scale. Let us highlight a few others.

Classical methods rate the severity of hypernasality from mild to very severe. A typical perceptual system categorizes speech into five levels of nasal severity as follows:

- *Normal Nasality.* Speech has enough nasality to sound normal, but not so much as to call attention to it unless specifically listening for it.
- *Mild Nasality.* Nasality is apparent as the person speaks. It is somewhat greater than that of most speakers but would probably cause little or no distraction if not listening for it.
- *Moderately Nasal.* Nasality is obviously present and is moderately distracting to the listener.
- *Severely Nasal.* Nasality is prominent, is a highly distracting feature in the speech, and makes listening to the message difficult.
- *Very Severely Nasal.* Nasality is so distracting that it dominates all aspects of speech and makes hearing the message extremely difficult.

The Buffalo III Resonance Profile (Wilson, 1987) continues in wide use. It is a 12-item supplement to Wilson's more general Buffalo III Voice Profile and is used when a patient has been rated 2 or higher on the nasal or oral resonance items of that voice profile. The profile for resonance uses a 5-point rating scale where 1 is normal and 5 is very severe. Twelve parameters are then so rated: hypernasal resonance, hyponasal resonance, oral resonance, cul-de-sac resonance, nasal emission, facial grimaces, language level, articulation, speech intelligibility, speech acceptability, velopharyngeal competency, and overall resonance rating.

The SLP can use a "listening tube" to heighten the perception of a patient's hypernasality, thus facilitating its recognition. We have used a makeshift listening tube fashioned from the plastic headsets provided by the airlines for in-flight movies. Prater and Swift (1984) explain an alternate construction and the use of a listening tube:

> The listening tube consists of a glass or plastic olive-shaped tip that is attached to a 2- to 3-foot piece of rubber tubing. Before beginning hypernasality assessment procedures, the nasal olive should be inserted into the patient's nostril and the free end of the tubing should be inserted into the clinician's ear. With this device in place, even the slightest degrees of nasal emission or hypernasality can be easily detected in the patient's speech. (pp. 55–56)

A commercially available Oral and Nasal Listener is available from Super Duper Publishing (http://www.superduperinc.com).

The SLP may try a simple procedure sometimes known as the "nasal flutter test." Have the patient repeat in an alternate fashion the vowels /a/ and /i/ while the clinician alternately compresses and releases the patient's nostrils. It is presumed that if velopharyngeal closure is adequate, there will be no noticeable difference in vowel quality as the nostrils are pinched. Conversely, if the clinician hears an increase in the nasal resonance during the nose-occluded condition, velopharyngeal incompetence may be suspected. The resonance quality change has also been described as a flutterlike sound; hence, the name of the test procedure.

Bzoch (2004) recommends a similar nose-occluded–unoccluded test procedure using plosive-vowel-plosive syllables. Ten vowels are tested in a /b—t/ context: "beet," "bit," "bait," "bet," "bat," "bought," "boat," "boot," "but," "Bert." In a person with normal velopharyngeal closure, the nose-occluded and unoccluded conditions sound the same.

Articulation tests involve both consonants and vowels and so can be fair measures of velopharyngeal closure, nasal emission, and hypernasality. Consonant environments influence the amount of nasality perceived on vowels. From least influential to most influential are /z, v, d, g, f, s, t, k/. It would seem, therefore, that nasality on vowels should be studied in these consonantal environments.

The perception of hypernasality can be heightened by using context-controlled stimuli. Having the patient count aloud from 60 to 100 is an insightful, yet simple, assessment procedure. We offer the following summary of the counting task, which is a useful indicator of velopharyngeal incompetence and the symptoms of hypernasality, nasal emission, and hyponasality.

1. The 60 series of numbers may reveal velopharyngeal incompetence and nasal emission due to the frequent occurrence of the /s/ pressure phoneme.
2. The 70 series may reveal assimilative hypernasality owing to the embedded /n/ phoneme.
3. The 80 series should reveal normal or near-normal articulation and resonance.
4. The 90 series should sound normal when produced by a patient with hypernasality because of the frequent production of nasal consonants. The patient with hyponasality may display the articulatory substitution of d/n.

The SLP can test for sound confusions in cases of suspected velopharyngeal incompetence. Have the patient read or repeat word pairs, such as "bake"/"make," "rib"/"rim," "dine"/"nine," "mad"/"man," "wig"/"wing," "bag"/"bang." In a patient with VPI, both sounds are hypernasal, making the "bake"/"make" pair, for example, sound like "make"/"make."

Instrumentation is also available that purports to detect or measure hypernasality. We maintain that hypernasality is a perceptual phenomenon and must be assessed perceptually. Attempts to measure hypernasality "objectively" are really attempts to measure velopharyngeal function, oral and nasal airflows, and the like. Although these data certainly relate to judgments of hypernasality, they are not measures of hypernasality per se. We will discuss instrumentation used to measure aspects of velopharyngeal function later in this chapter when we discuss the cleft palate population.

Once the SLP has determined that the patient exhibits some degree of hypernasality, the evaluative session should turn to discovering what, if any, techniques and manipulations lessen the perception of nasality. Together, the patient and clinician should experiment to find "what works," and in doing so they are arriving at a prognosis for change and are mapping the direction of future treatment, if warranted.

The variability of the hypernasality as it relates to phonetic context should be explored. Does the perception of hypernasality diminish or worsen in sentences loaded with high vowels? with low vowels? with numerous nasal consonants? with many pressure consonants?

Does the degree of hypernasality improve when the patient speaks with "open-mouth articulation," where there is exaggerated mouth opening, and where speech sounds are enunciated with exaggerated movement? Air takes the path of least resistance, so by opening the anterior oral cavity wider, air will tend to flow outward rather than through the narrower, but opened, velopharyngeal port.

The SLP should also probe for possible improvements in hypernasality with changes in speaking rate, pitch, and loudness. These may be prime areas of manipulation in compensatory treatment programs. It is likely that perceived hypernasality is lessened at higher pitch and intensity levels. The role of muscular fatigue can also be explored by having the patient determine whether there are times during the day that nasality is better or worse.

At the beginning of the second grade, Belinda Johnston was noticed by the SLP during school-wide screenings. The child's voice was hypernasal and nasal emission occurred inconsistently on words starting with /s/, /f/, and /p/. Belinda was failed on this brief screening and the SLP followed up on the case. In a telephone conversation with the mother, the clinician learned that Belinda had a tonsillectomy and adenoidectomy during the previous Easter break because of frequent ear infections and sore throats. The mother stated that Belinda's voice has sounded "unusual" only since the surgery, but she was told by the doctor that it would improve with time. The first-grade teacher confirmed that Belinda's voice sounded normal the previous year. As six months had elapsed since the surgery, the SLP and mother agreed to initiate appropriate school system procedures for a formal speech evaluation and subsequent intervention. In the evaluation, hypernasality was confirmed and its severity rated, as was the consistency and severity of nasal emission. The oral peripheral examination revealed several indicators of submucous clefting. There was a midline notching of the uvula (slight bifidity), an anteriorly placed velar dimple, midline translucency of the palate, and a highly vaulted hard palate. Velar movement occurred symmetrically, but contact with the posterior pharyngeal wall could not be observed with certainty. Air came out the nose when the clinician used the modified tongue–anchor technique, and Belinda was unable to blow up a balloon.

The SLP wondered whether traditional adenoidectomy should have been done on this child—the oral exam revealed several factors that would contraindicate a routine removal (Finkelstein et al., 2002). (The adenoid's bulk compensated for the child's VPI.) The school SLP desired objective confirmation of the suspicions of VPI, available with sophisticated instrumentation, and expert opinions of the proper behavioral course of action, if any. Belinda was referred to the craniofacial team at a metropolitian hospital a hundred miles away.

The SLP at a rehabilitation hospital received Delondo Hayes as a transfer patient from an acute care facility. Mr. Hayes was a 22-year-old automobile crash victim who had sustained brain stem and spinal cord injuries. The clinician noted in the initial speech consult that Mr. Hayes was partially paralyzed and used a wheelchair. His conversational speech was slow, slurred, and excessively hypernasal. In the oral examination, the speech pathologist also noted absence of gag reflex and weak lingual muscles. The patient was diagnosed with the motor speech disorder of flaccid dysarthria. Early treatment efforts would be directed at oral muscle mobility and precision of articulation. Slow speech rates would be accepted—indeed, encouraged—as a means of achieving target articulatory placements, including velar gestures. The hypernasality would be monitored for four to six weeks of rehabilitation before considering further alternatives.

Nasal Emission

Since nasal emission and hypernasality can both be due to insuffient velopharyngeal closure, it makes sense that they often co-occur; yet, we must keep in mind that the two problems are separate entities.

The assessment of nasal emission involves looking and listening. The expulsion of air through the nostrils may be so obvious as to flare the nares of the speaker. In contrast, in an attempt to decrease the outward flow of air, the person may constrict the nares. The clinician, then, looks for facial (nasal) grimaces.

Critical listening is crucial for the SLP to accurately diagnose the presence of nasal emission. Sometimes the emitted air is obviously noisy; in fact, *nasal snort* is a descriptive term encountered in this body of literature. At other times, the nasal emission is barely audible or detectable only with special techniques, as we shall see.

A frequent way to assess the presence of nasal emission is by administering a single-word articulation test. Attention should be directed toward production of pressure plosives, fricatives, and affricates. The results of the articulation test should answer the following questions for the clinician:

1. Does the speaker misarticulate fricatives, plosives, and affricates that have been demonstrated to require high intraoral breath pressure?
2. Do the misarticulations involve audible nasal emission?
3. Are there evidences of facial grimacing during the production of these consonants?
4. Does occluding the nostrils (preventing an air leakage) result in normal production of them?
5. Regarding nasal emission, are voiced consonants less defective than their voiceless cognates? Typically, the required amount of oral air pressure is greater for voiceless phonemes.
6. Are single consonants less affected than blends?
7. Are consonants in the initial or final position in words articulated correctly more often than medial consonants are?
8. Does the patient use compensatory articulation patterns, such as glottal stop, pharyngeal stop, mid-dorsum palatal stop, pharyngeal fricative, posterior nasal fricative, and so forth?

In addition to, or in place of, a formal articulation test, the clinician may listen for nasal emission in specially designed words and sentences. Have the patient read or repeat stimuli loaded with pressure consonants, such as the following clinical favorites:

Pick the peas.
Pappa piped up.
Polish the shoes.
Bessie stayed all summer.
We'd better buy a bigger dog.
Follow Sally, Charley.
People, baby, paper, Bobby, puppy, bubble, pepper, B. B., piper, bye bye.

Likewise, the clinician can listen carefully as the patient counts aloud. The numbers between 60 and 79 are especially evocative of nasal emission.

The SLP can use simple items to enhance the detection and monitoring of nasal air emission. A small mirror held under the patient's nostril will fog as air escapes. We have used a dental mirror with its convenient handle or a small lipstick mirror. Fog on the mirror during the patient's attempts at prolonging fricatives, repeating VCV syllables containing pressure consonants (such as /ipi ipi ipi/, /upu upu upu/), or saying the pressure-loaded sentences previously listed is strongly suggestive of velopharyngeal incompetence. These same procedures may be done with wisps of cotton on a wooden tongue depressor held beneath the nose when a mirror is not available. We find the cotton's sensitivity less reliable, though.

The listening tube, described previously, is also useful for assessing nasal emission. An apparatus of clear plastic cylinder, styrofoam piston, and tubing with a nasal olive is available commercially as the See-Scape (from PRO-ED at http://www.proedinc.com). We would like to mention that all devices used to detect and visualize the nasal emission of air are useful in treatment as well as in assessment.

After determining that a patient has nasal emission, the clinician should probe for techniques that diminish air escape. If none is found, behavioral treatment may be contraindicated, and physical management necessary. Here are some techniques the SLP can try.

Have the patient use light articulatory contacts on pressure consonants—the plosives, fricatives, and affricates. A complementary technique that may diminish nasal emission is that of open-mouth articulation, as was suggested for hypernasality.

Perhaps having the patient extend the vowel portions of speech will lessen the emphasis placed on pressure consonant articulation and so improve nasal emission. The fluency-enhancing techniques that involve vowel/syllable prolongations, found in many stuttering approaches, may prove useful with some patients. Reduced rates of speech may also be useful, especially in patients who show velar movement potential but suffer from sluggish timing maneuvers.

Cul-de-sac Resonance

The hollow voice quality of this disorder is typically due to hyperfunction of the tongue. Speech is produced with the tongue posteriorly positioned in the oral cavity and oropharynx regions. The SLP should try to observe this posterior retraction when possible; having the patient phonate an open vowel, such as /a/, may facilitate viewing of the posterior tongue placement.

De facto diagnosis may come from probing for improvements in the cul-de-sac resonance. Experiment by having the patient read sentences or word lists loaded with phonemes that promote anterior tongue placement and inhibit lingual retraction. Prater and Swift (1984) suggest the following phonemes for developing clinical stimuli:

Tongue-tip: /t/, /d/, /s/, and /z/

Front vowels: /i/, /I/, and /e/

Front consonants: /w/, /hw/, /p/, /b/, /f/, /v/, /θ/, and /l/

It has been noted in the literature that hearing-impaired and deaf speakers often use too slow a rate of speech. The slow rate of speech seems attributable to altered syllable durations, which, in turn, adversely affects speech intelligibility and voice quality. Increasing the speaking rates of hearing-impaired persons may improve their perceived hypernasality or their cul-de-sac resonance and should be attempted by the SLP.

Thin Vocal Resonance

The thin, effeminate voice quality usually is related to anterior tongue carriage, and thus the oral resonance of vowels and consonants is affected. By moving the place of the primary articulatory constriction more forward in the oral cavity, energy loci are shifted to higher frequencies, and vocalic formats are likewise elevated. The perception of effeminacy may be increased by the patient's use of an elevated fundamental frequency and/or exaggerated use of the upper range for pitch inflections. Pitch, as well as quality, should be evaluated in these patients. To assess thin resonance, have the patient read sentences or word lists containing many back vowels and back consonants (such as /k/ and /g/). Note whether there is an improvement in resonance with this probe technique.

ASSESSMENT ASSOCIATED WITH CLEFT PALATE

In addition to the information presented on assessing hypernasality and nasal emission, we would like to elaborate on the diagnostic process used with patients who have clefts of the hard or soft palate or who have had repairs—either surgical or prosthedontic—to their structures. The dramatic improvement of surgical and other rehabilitative procedures for the individual with a cleft has been encouraging. We recommend the tutorial article on the nature, assessment, and treatment of velopharyngeal dysfunction by Dworkin, Marurick, and Krouse (2004). Students also may find the Web resources in Table 11.1 of interest. Though some individuals use terms carelessly and interchangeably, we wish to clarify that a velopharyngeal dysfunction is differentiated as follows:

1. *Velopharyngeal insufficiency*—refers to abnormal structures, and so speech treatment cannot alter the problem alone.
2. *Velopharyngeal incompetence*—refers to abnormal functions, and so speech treatment can play a key role in retraining mislearned speech behaviors.

In the diagnosis of communication problems associated with cleft palate, the SLP is typically a member of a team. The craniofacial team is a well-accepted clinical entity, and in many communities represents the ultimate in interdisciplinary cooperation between SLPs, audiologists, psychologists, surgeons, otolaryngologists, radiologists, prosthedontists, orthodontists,

---

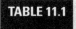**TABLE 11.1** Web Resources of Interest Concerning Cleft Lip, Cleft Palate, and Pharyngoplasty

http://www.widesmiles2.org

This is a detailed site with much usable information for the parent of a child with a cleft, including newborn feeding, emotional support with chat rooms, before and after surgical photos, and other helpful information. The SLP will benefit as well from viewing the general information and the explanations of primary and secondary surgeries. Pertinent also is material comparing and contrasting the three surgical options for velopharyngeal incompetence: pharyngeal flap, the double-reversing Z-plasty (Furlow), and the sphincter pharyngoplasty.

http://www.plasticsurgery.org/Patients_and_Consumers/Procedure/ Reconstructive_Procedures/Cleft_Lip_and_Palate

The website of the American Society of Plastic Surgeons provides simple illustrated explanations of surgeries for clefts of the lip and palate.

http://www.google.com

Do a video search for cleft palate speech to see and hear samples before and after surgery, including change following pharyngeal flap surgery.

http://www.ich.ucl.ac.uk

Search the Institute for Children's Health, located in the United Kingdom, for a variety of cleft-related information including speech appliances for pictures and information on speech bulbs and palatal lifts.

http://www.cleftline.org/publications/speech.htm

The Cleft Palate Foundation presents parents with information, factsheets, and publication resources.

TABLE 11.2	Areas Typically Appraised in Suspected Cases of Velopharyngeal Dysfunction (* denotes optional task or physician-directed)

Case History

Articulation and Intelligibility—formal tests, informal stimuli

Resonance—perceptual scales, listening tubes, various other devices

Intraoral Examination

Pressure-Flow Studies—nasometer, oral manometer

Endoscopy—with rigid or fiberoptic scopes

*Radiographic Studies—cephalometry (still, lateral x-rays), videofluoroscopy, cinefluorography, tomography (laminagraphy), and/or computerized tomography (CT) scanning

*Others—accelerometry, electromyography, ultrasound, MRI, electro-palatography

Stimulability Testing (Probes)

Impact/Quality of Life Scale

pedodontists, and educational personnel. The SLP is expected to inform the team members about the patient's communication abilities and disabilities, predict the effects of contemplated rehabilitative procedures, serve as the primary agent for change in the patient's speech-language skills, and stay in tune with how any communication difference or disorder may be impacting the person's daily life. As discussed by Boone et al. (2010), if there is tissue deficiency or velar weakness with reduced range of motion, behavioral therapy alone will not normalize the velopharyngeal anatomy and function. Realistic intervention, they say, must begin with a thorough evaluation, not only a perceptual speech and voice analysis but aerodynamic studies, acoustical analysis, and videoendoscopic studies to better judge the velopharyngeal mechanism. The speech pathologist should endeavor to evaluate, or have evaluated at an appropriate facility, many aspects of velopharyngeal functioning such as those outlined in Table 11.2. We also urge that the SLP keep in mind the framework of Figure 11.2 provided by the World Health Organization (2004) so that any impacts on daily life, education, and socialization are not overlooked.

Case History

The routine case history data may need to be augmented for the cleft palate patient. Knowledge of the type and extent of cleft, as well as a description of the surgical, prosthodontic, orthodontic, and other rehabilitative procedures performed would be helpful. Some statement of the patient's current medical status and plans for future intervention procedures will also help direct the evaluative process. If the clinician is not a formal member of a craniofacial team, copies of reports from other professionals who have dealt with the patient should be obtained.

Critical Listening, Intelligibility, and Articulation Testing

The initial interaction between clinician and young patient should occur as soon as possible when a cleft is detected. Prebabbling age is not too soon, so that parents can be advised of speech and language stimulation approaches. The goal is to foster a phonetic inventory that minimizes nasal substitutions and glottal stops and encourages use of oral consonants (Hardin-Jones, Chapman, & Scherer, 2006). Not only does this develop good articulation and prevent development of stubborn

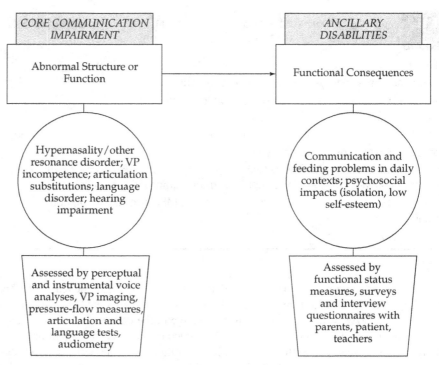

FIGURE 11.2 Assessment of speech associated with cleft palate and velopharyngeal incompetence using the World Health Organization's classification of functioning, disability, and health (ICF).

and inappropriate articulation, it also helps prepare the toddler for eventual imaging evaluation of the velopharyngeal mechanism. With a conversational patient, the SLP must apply critical listening skills to assess the individual's total communicative effectiveness. This involves systematically shifting perceptual sets from one aspect of the patient's speech to another. The SLP should listen for the presence of a resonance imbalance (such as hypernasality, hyponasality, nasal emission, or a combination) and rate its severity. The clinician also should listen to and rate the speech intelligibility. The serious reader is referred to Whitehill's (2002) critical review of intelligibility assessment in cleft speech. Next, the SLP should assess the general articulatory pattern. Is there an obvious preponderance of a particular type of error (such as glottal stops or pharyngeal fricatives)? Does the articulation appear to alter with differing communication situations, speech, or stress patterns? Next, listen to the language of the patient, particularly if he or she is a young child, and check for appropriate word choice, sentence complexity, and structure. The rate and rhythm of the patient's speech should be noted. Are there any other vocal quality differences (such as hoarseness)? Is there a facial grimace, constriction of the nares, or any other behavior that detracts from the individual's total communicative effectiveness?

After formulating a general impression of the patient's speech patterns, detailed phonology and articulation testing should be done. Standard articulation tests may be satisfactory for cleft palate individuals, but there are several considerations that may be best examined by "specialized" articulation tests and context-controlled stimuli. Certainly, all of the functional, perceptual, and sensory factors that affect the normal person could be active, but in cleft palate individuals there are added possibilities. Most important are the degree of velopharyngeal closure and the resultant airflow and intraoral pressure. The deviant geography of the oral cavity may contribute to this problem, which is complicated by the fact that the oral structure may well have undergone several architectural changes within the first few years of life. The SLP must keep in mind that this individual has been trying to produce standard sounds with a nonstandard structure, and under these conditions unique compensatory adjustments may have been made. The patient may have increased the airflow in order to build up adequate oral pressure, or minimized it to lessen nasal escape; in the latter case, we say that the patient is producing weak pressure consonants.

Many patients with velopharyngeal incompetency/insufficiency adopt compensatory articulations, including glottal stop substitutions, pharyngeal fricatives, velar fricatives, and aspirant productions of vowels and consonants; other, unusual compensations may also be used. Double articulations commonly do involve glottal or pharyngeal constriction simultaneously with valving at the lips or in the linguapalatal region. But other labial-lingual double articulations, or LLDAs as they are called, do exist. Gibbon and Crampin (2002) can be consulted in this regard.

Keep in mind that it is entirely possible for the compensatory habits that developed before the final surgical adjustments to persist after competence of the velopharyngeal mechanism is established and the patient can make the correct articulatory movements. Stimulability probes therefore are important in determining the patient's prognosis for change. Articulation errors may also be related to an existing or prior hearing loss.

In summary, the clinician analyzes speech samples, elicited productions and phonetic inventories for overall intelligibility and analysis of patterns, keeping in mind the main goal: to distinguish speech errors that may be due to faulty velopharyngeal or other structural deviations from speech errors that are compensatory or developmental. Trost-Cardamone and Bernthal (1993) provide a chart of guidelines for deciding on a direction for intervention based on these analyses.

Nasal Resonance

Resonatory voice disorders are frequently heard in individuals with clefts. The assessment process described earlier in this chapter, then, certainly applies to the diagnostic workup of a patient with a cleft palate. Any quality aberration is possible in persons with clefts of the palate, but high-probability disorders are hypernasality and nasal emission, since both are related to inadequate velopharyngeal closure. It is worth mentioning that the clinician should attempt to determine to what extent the resonance imbalance is related to functional factors such as tension, fatigue, and learning or to organic factors such as neurological dysfunction or the structural defect of the cleft itself. We would like to restate that listener evaluation of a speaking voice is the best way for the clinician to judge the resonance parameter, but instrumentation is available for related measures.

The Oral Peripheral Examination

Although velopharyngeal closure cannot be visualized in an oral examination, it is important to examine the orofacial region of patients who manifest resonation disorders. The examination is an initial step in determining the general relationships among all structures in the vocal tract. For instance, the clinician can get a gross picture of palatal shape, total and effective velar lengths, movement ability and symmetry of movement of the velum, and dimensions of the pharynx and can determine if any defects, such as fistulas of the palate, are present. If the SLP has any concerns regarding structure or function, the physician should be consulted.

Procedures for appraising the structure and function of the oral and peripheral regions are described in the literature (Dworkin & Culatta, 1996; St. Louis & Ruscello, 2000). General information on conducting an oral peripheral examination is provided in Chapter 9. We offer a few special comments here.

Perhaps the most important thing for the SLP to do with the naked eye when velopharyngeal incompetency/insufficiency is suspected is to determine the effective length of the velum and the location of the velar dimple. The effective velar length is that portion of the elevated velar tissue used in closure of the nasopharynx during phonation. The effected length can be estimated from intraoral inspection of the velar dimple during phonation relative to nasopharyngeal depth. The velar dimple on the oral surface of the velum is an indication of the point of maximum elevation on the nasal surface of the velum. It typically occurs at 80% of the total velar length. The more anteriorly the dimple is placed (say, at the 50% mark), the less the effective velar length, and the greater the degree of velopharyngeal incompetence.

Examination of the palate may reveal oronasal fistulas that are not always readily visible. What is the shape of the palatal vault? Is the coloration a healthy pink, or do there appear to be white or blue tinted regions? Is there a palatal translucency observed during the oral exam when, in a dark room, a flashlight is shined into a nostril? Upon palpation, does the bony substructure feel firm and have normal posterior edges? If there is a fistula, the degree to which it affects articulation or resonance should be explored.

When overt clefting is present, the type and extent can be appraised. Many hospital-based craniofacial teams have devised specialized oral examination forms that contain diagrams of the lips and palate on which to mark the patient's features. The use of an individualized diagram not only documents the extent of the cleft but also facilitates communication among the team professionals.

Special Assessment Procedures for Velopharyngeal Function

As previously indicated, the oral peripheral examination does not allow for definitive judgments of velopharyngeal adequacy to be made. In addition, an articulation test, whether published or informal, is but an indirect measure of the client's velopharyngeal function. Other techniques, many involving instrumentation, are available to directly or indirectly assess the velopharyngeal mechanism. We maintain that no single measure is adequate for appraisal of velopharyngeal function; and we also believe that articulation testing and resonance assessment *must* be part of any diagnostic process. Despite advances in so-called objective acoustic measures of hypernasality (e.g., 1/3 octave spectra analysis), perceptual judgement remains the primary means for accessing levels of nasality (Vogel et al., 2009). Let us describe some of the other assessment procedures that are available for routine and/or sophisticated diagnostic sessions.

The tongue-anchor technique (Fox & Johns, 1970) is still used to estimate static closure ability. The patient is required to maintain intraoral pressure by puffing up the cheeks. If this procedure is accomplished, the patient is asked to protrude the tongue and then puff up the cheeks (to prevent lingual valving). The clinician holds the patient's nostrils while this exercise is done to aid in impounding pressure. If no air escapes when the nostrils are released, it is assumed that velopharyngeal closure is adequate.

As previously mentioned, informal and subjective measures of velopharyngeal leakage can be obtained by observing fog on a mirror held beneath the patient's nose, by seeing wisps of cotton move when so placed, by using listening tubes of various design, and by critically listening to controlled stimuli spoken in nose-occluded–unoccluded conditions.

The oral manometer is an affordable piece of equipment helpful in discriminating between persons with good and poor velopharyngeal closure. The patient either blows or sucks as forcefully as possible into/from a mouthpiece. The exhalation task yields a positive pressure reading from the manometer guages, while the inhalation task gives a negative reading. A ratio is obtained by comparing pressures achieved in the nostrils-open and nostrils-occluded conditions. A normal ratio of 1.00 is suggestive of velopharyngeal closure adequacy, particularly if an open bleed valve was used to inhibit compensatory maneuvers, such as tongue-palate valving. Ratios less than 1.00 may be indicative of VPI, hypernasal speech, and reduced intelligibility in cleft palate patients; ratios less than 0.89 are particularly poor indicators.

Air pressure and airflow techniques are based on the fact that VPI results in a decrement of intraoral air pressure and an increase in airflow through the nose. Consequently, pressure and flow measurements can be part of the total diagnostic workup; they are often used for research purposes. Pressure transducers, such as strain gauge transducers, are used to measure air pressures while airflow meters are used to measure volume rates of airflow. Types of flow meters include warm-wire anemometers, pneumotachographs, and thermistors. The pneumotachograph is perhaps the most commonly used and requires the use of a face mask to collect the airflow and direct it through a sensing screen. Air pressure and flow instrumentation is expensive and complex. However, Realica, Smith, Glover, and Yu (2000) adopted a common U-tube manometer using a Y-connector to measure oral and nasal airflow as well as pressure quantitatively. This is a simple means of assessing velopharyngeal incompetence.

Other instruments measure oral and nasal sound pressures. A ratio formed between the two measures, expressed as a percentage, is referred to as *nasalence.* Nasalence is highly correlated with perceptual judgments of nasality. Kay Elemetrics (http://www.kayelemetrics.com) markets the Nasometer, a computer-based system that uses this method for clinical assessments while the patient speaks controlled phonetic syllables or words, but also for treatment feedback where the patient views the monitor. Use of a Nasometer is quite feasible with young children who are not bothered by the special headset and microphone. The SLP also may wish to repeat the measure over treatment sessions as the nasalence score can be an objective indicator of improvement or lack thereof. This can be an excellent, and quick, tool for reassessments that also satisfy third-party payors.

Direct visualization of the velopharyngeal closure mechanism is in order when articulation and nasal resonance have been determined to be abnormal. Direct visualization involves methods such as radiographic, ultrasonic, endoscopic, MRI, and electropalatography. The SLP may perform these with a medical team or, in some cases, have direct responsibility. Let us say a brief word about each. Radiographic methods involve low doses of radiation to visualize the structures, including soft tissues. The SLP should work closely with the radiologist in selecting the most appropriate radiographic method and conditions of study. Knowledge of the literature is important in selecting which speech and nonspeech tasks to have the patient perform.

Ultrasound offers a noninvasive means of visualizing lateral pharyngeal wall movement during speech. This technique involves placing an ultrasonic transducer against the neck. Soft tissues and air in the pharyngeal cavities transmit the pulse differently, thus creating an image on the display screen.

Direct visualization is easily accomplished through an invasive technique that uses viewing devices called endoscopes (or similar instrument name like nasopharyngoscope). Rigid forms of endoscopy useful in observing velopharyngeal closure are the oral panendoscope and the nasal endoscope. Flexible endoscopes use fiber-optic bundles. We again remind the reader that closure, or lack of it, is best viewed from above, and so the flexible fiberscope inserted through the nasal cavity is used quite often. Most, if not all, hospitals now have the necessary equipment and the SLP may perform the procedure. Cooperative patients can be examined while seated and performing speech and nonspeech tasks. Even young children tolerate well a flexible optic tube placed nasally (Hay et al., 2009).

The electropalatography (EPG) involves the orthodontist designing an artificial palate containing some 62 embedded electrodes. The acrylic is placed such that articulator contact during speech can be mapped in synchrony with the acoustic signal. The EPG allows study of articulator placements.

Magnetic resonance imaging (MRI) is proving to be an effective method of monitoring levator veli palatini muscle activity at rest and during speech (Ettema et al., 2002). The SLP may or may not have access to some of the instruments but should know that they are available. In this age of high technology, it can be expected that access to such equipment from universities, medical centers, and clinics will become easier and more widespread. More important, objective instrumental analysis done before and after medical, prosthedontic, and behavioral speech-language treatment are becoming *de rigeur* as outcomes evidence. We note, in particular, the use of pre- and postnasalance measures.

Auditory Acuity and Language Ability

The high incidence of auditory acuity problems among children with cleft palate has been well documented. For this reason, it is absolutely essential that every patient have a hearing examination. These examinations should include both air and bone conduction testing and should be a part of every speech diagnosis.

The SLP will wish to see the child or infant as soon as possible. Typically, in major hospitals, once an infant is born with an orofacial anomaly, the work of a multidisciplinary team is set into motion. The SLP, as part of the team, will work closely with the parents—through counseling and training—to prevent future communication problems. During this early contact the parents can be informed about the need for normal speech and language stimulation, what to expect from their child regarding speech and language production, and the need for frequent audiometric testing. Some speech clinicians use established language stimulation programs as a preventive measure with these children, especially since vocabulary expansion tends to develop slowly in these toddlers (Hardin-Jones, Chapman, & Scherer, 2006).

SELF-ESTEEM AND DAILY IMPACT

Children with clefts, nasal emission, and nasality issues often find in playgroups and in school that they are the brunt of teasing, ridicule, and social exclusion because they may look and sound different. Parents, teachers, SLPs, and other healthcare team members need to anticipate these reactions and take steps to minimize their psychosocial impacts on the child. Indeed, a goal of medical and speech-voice intervention is "to fix" the structures and functions to the extent possible so that other negative consequences do not occur. The framework of the World Health Organization (2002) that was depicted in Figure 11.2 is helpful to remember. Although assessing the quality of life following intervention is an emerging body of literature, we wish to mention some tools that show promise for SLPs as well as surgeons.

Boseley and Hartnick (2004) administered a Pediatric Voice Outcomes Survey (PVOS) to the parents of children (mean age 5 years) pre- and post-surgery for velopharyngeal incompetency. They specifically compared outcomes between sphincteroplasty and superiorly based pharyngeal flap and found the PVOS to be a valid tool for functional impact. The SLP might well use the PVOS to track daily-living changes and perceived functional adjustments as a function of speech treatment.

Chapter 10 presented other adult and pediatric scales that the SLP may wish to use to track surgical and/or speech resonance treatment outcomes with regard to daily impact and quality of life.

PROGNOSIS ASSOCIATED WITH RESONANCE IMBALANCE

Let us now return to our general discussion of resonance imbalance and list some of the prognostic indicators for the treatment of resonatory disorders. We freely admit that much is speculation or opinion or is simply based on assumptions of etiology. Research documenting clinical effectiveness is sorely needed.

1. Prater and Swift (1984) state that voice treatment for cul-de-sac resonance usually is not successful in patients with neurologic involvement of the articulators, which includes conditions such as oral apraxia, athetoid cerebral palsy, flaccid dysarthria, and spastic dysarthria. Patients with functional cul-de-sac resonance and, to a lesser extent, deaf speakers can benefit from intervention directed toward anterior positioning of the tongue.

2. Thin resonance, with its assumed functional etiology, is remediated easily only in patients motivated to change. Treatment efforts should be directed toward correcting tongue carriage. The clinician may benefit from knowledge of male-female communication differences when assisting a patient to reduce the effeminate aspects of speech. The emerging literature on communication treatment for transsexuals may be used as a resource.

3. Hyponasality, when due to some nasal obstruction, necessitates physical management. Speech treatment alone is not likely to be beneficial.

4. The patient's motivation to change is paramount in predicting the outcome of voice treatment.

5. A favorable prognosis for treatment is indicated if the clinician was able to elicit a better voice resonance from the patients during the assessment. This phase of activity may be termed the probe, stimulability, or trial therapy phase where various techniques are tried with the patient to assess potential for change. Indeed, it is on this basis that treatment should be prescribed.

There are several indications and contraindications to speech treatment for individuals with cleft palate. Kummer (2007) provides some practical auditory and visual probes and techniques for individuals with velopharyngeal dysfunction We will cite some treatment indicators here. Much of what is listed applies to cases of hypernasality and nasal emission in the absence of clefting.

1. Speech treatment is contraindicated for patients with clearly inadequate velopharyngeal closure; physical management is warranted. As discussed in this chapter, evidence of velopharyngeal inadequacy should come from a variety of sources, including articulation testing showing consistent hypernasality and nasal emission, observation of nasal grimacing, imaging evidence, oral examination findings of an anteriorly displaced velar dimple and/or excessive nasopharyngeal dimensions, and pressure-flow measures.

2. Since home programs are essential in most therapeutic approaches, motivated and cooperative patients and their parents are a requirement for enrollment in a speech intervention program.

3. Speech treatment is not warranted, or is low priority, when the patient needs language and communication improvement.

4. Patients with boderline velopharyngeal closure may not be good candidates for speech treatment and the risk of developing inappropriate articulatory and laryngeal compensation is real. Likewise, nasality treatment is contraindicated if the patient presents with hoarseness (though hygiene treatment directed at reduction of hoarseness may be in order).

5. Patients who demonstrated improvement during the assessment probes are good candidates for speech treatment. Especially favorable are reduced hypernasality when employing exaggerated, open-mouth articulation and a marked difference in velar activity when gagging and phonating.

6. Some patients with inadequate velopharyngeal closure cannot benefit from further physical management. The SLP may opt to provide compensatory treatment. The goal, then, is not normal-sounding speech, but the best speech of which the patient is capable. Tasks used in the assessment probes may be appropriate treatment techniques in that the perception of hypernasality is reduced by their use. These tasks include increased mouth opening, low and forward placement of the tongue, auditory training, exaggerated articulation movements, light and quick articulatory contacts, overall slowed rate of speech, and altered pitch and/or loudness levels.

CONCLUSION

Information has been presented in this chapter in agreement with the profession's preferred practice patterns for resonance and nasal airflow assessment by the SLP (ASHA, 2004). Specifically, the SLP:

1. Evaluates oral, nasal, and velopharyngeal function for speech production
2. Identifies and describes the individual's underlying strengths and weaknesses that affect communication performance
3. Explores any effects on the individual's activities and participation in everyday communication contexts
4. Identifies any contextual factors that serve as barriers to or facilitators of successful communication and participation.

The expected outcomes of our assessment may result in the following (ASHA, 2004):

1. Diagnosis of a speech disorder
2. Clinical descriptions of the current characteristics of a resonance or nasal airflow disorder (such as from perceptual, acoustic, articulatory, aerodynamic, and imaging measures)
3. Identification of any co-occurring communication disorders or differences (e.g., auditory, cognitive-linguistic, articulatory, phonatory)
4. Prognosis for change (with or without other intervention measures)
5. Recommendations for SLP intervention and other measures (e.g., surgical, prosthedontic, educational)
6. Referral for other assessments or services

The evaluation of disorders of resonance is a challenge to the SLP. The clinician must often work closely with medical personnel and other allied health workers, which necessitates knowing procedures and terminologies that are peripheral to speech-language pathology. The clinician also must remain abreast of current technological developments in electronics, surgery, and medical technology. Finally, the clinician must keep interpersonal clinical skills finely honed so that psychological aspects of vocal disorders can be detected and dealt with through treatment or referral.

12

Multicultural Issues in Assessment

At this point in this textbook, we have completed our overview of the general diagnostic process and how it applies to evaluating the most common areas of communication disorders. We hope that the reader can see the importance of evaluating the biological bases of communication, gathering case history/interview information, performing standardized and nonstandardized testing, and evaluating the client's communication environment in terms of demands, supports, and obstacles to remediation. This approach to assessment is broad based and may be perceived as too detailed and time consuming by clinicians accustomed to using mainly standardized tests in evaluating clients. However, one area in which such an approach is indispensable to the speech-language pathologist is in dealing with cultural differences in assessment. It has been well known for some time that standardized testing presents a serious threat to fair assessment of children from diverse language groups (Kamhi, Pollock, & Harris, 1996; Taylor & Payne, 1983; Vaughn-Cooke, 1983, 1986). As a result, children from diverse linguistic and cultural backgrounds tend to score lower on these measures, and these lower scores could result in a disproportionate number of minority children being placed in special education programs. Fagundes, Haynes, Haak, and Moran (1998) summarize some of the types of bias possible on standardized tests:

> The typical types of bias on standardized tests that can have a negative effect on culturally diverse children are *situational bias* (examination format is threatening to child), *directions bias* (directions for test can be misinterpreted by child), *value bias* (asking child to give moral/ethical judgments that may differ culturally from the examiners'), *linguistic bias* (presumption that the child is a standard English speaker), *format bias* (test procedures are inconsistent with child's cognitive style), *cultural misinterpretation* (negative interpretation of client behavior when it is culturally appropriate), and *stimulus bias* (test is highly object/picture-oriented when child is socially oriented). (p. 148)

Roseberry-McKibbin and O'Hanlon (2005) cite several questionnaire studies that indicate SLPs working in public school settings find gaps in their knowledge about unbiased methods of assessing students who speak a language other than English and are English language learners. They make a case for not using standardized tests but, instead, alternative assessment strategies.

The alternative process involves preassessment activities of taking a detailed language history, parent interview, teacher interview, and whether the student communicates effectively with linguistically and culturally similar peers. They recommend taking a language sample, using dynamic assessment and nonword repetition tasks (discussed later in this chapter). While our profession is aware of the importance of multicultural issues and has issued guidelines for bilingual assessment, most clinicians surveyed report that they have not been adequately trained in such practices (Caesar & Kohler, 2007). In fact, most clinicians surveyed report that they use English standardized tests more frequently than nonstandardized methods in assessment of bilingual students.

This chapter provides a brief overview of the critical importance of multicultural issues in the assessment of communication disorders.

POPULATION AND PROFESSIONAL TRENDS

If birthrates and immigration trends continue as predicted, the population of the United States will become increasingly diverse by the middle of the twenty-first century. Specifically, there will be significant increases in African American, Hispanic, and Asian groups and the population of citizens with white, European backgrounds will remain relatively stable or even decrease. By the year 2050, it is predicted that white Americans with European ancestry will no longer be the predominant segment of the population. In some states (e.g., Texas, California) where there are large groups of Hispanic and Asian citizens, this is already the case. This trend is not just a wild prediction or theory, but is based on data from the Bureau of Labor Statistics. Figure 12.1 shows the United States population by different cultural groups. The present edition of this text is being prepared prior to the availability of the 2010 United States Census, so we rely on the 2000 census figures. As we will discuss later in this chapter, these figures change dramatically if one examines specific regional or local areas. Evidence of the reality that the country is becoming more diverse is seen in initiatives begun by governmental agencies, school systems, universities, and the workplace. Not only is there increased cultural diversity in all of these settings, but all of these organizations are realizing the growing importance of considering bilingualism, appreciation of cultural differences, and the short-sightedness of an ethnocentric view. Learning language in a bilingual environment does not negatively affect first language learning in children with normal intelligence (Owens, 2005) or even children with Down syndrome (Bird, Cleave, Trudeau,

	Total Population	% of Population
White	211,460,626	75.1
African American	34,658,190	12.3
American Indian/Alaska Native	2,475,956	0.9
Asian	10,242,998	3.6
Native Hawaiian/Pacific Islander	398,835	0.1
Other	15,359,073	5.5
Two or more races	6,826,228	2.4
Hispanic or Latino	35,305,818	12.5
Total population	281,421,906	100.0

FIGURE 12.1 Population of the United States by race.
Source: 2000 Census.

Thordardottir, Sutton, & Thorpe, 2005). Speech-language pathologists are frequently called upon to assess children who come to the United States through international adoption. These children represent many different languages/cultures and arrive in the country as infants or toddlers. Although this kind of assessment is challenging, research has shown that assessing prelinguistic communication and vocabulary comprehension using measures such as the Communication and Symbolic Behavior Scales and the MacArthur-Bates Communicative development scales reliably predicted language outcomes at age 2 (Glennen, 2007). Research has shown that many children who are adopted from overseas ultimately perform well by school age. For example, Scott, Roberts, and Krakow (2008) found that a cohort of children adopted from China performed average or above on tests of oral and written language in the early elementary grades.

The American Speech-Language-Hearing Association (ASHA) has a long-standing position on consideration of multicultural issues in assessment of communication disorders (Battle et al., 1983). The position of ASHA on assessment (we will not discuss aspects of treatment) embodies several important points. First, ASHA emphasizes that no social dialect of English is a communication disorder, but a legitimate variety of English that is used by its speakers for communication and social solidarity. Dialects are inextricably woven into the history and fiber of a culture and cannot be separated from the culture as a whole. Thus, the SLP should not devalue dialects or enroll a person in treatment for dialectal variations as being a pathological form of communication. Second, the position paper indicates that while a person may be speaking a dialect of English, that certainly does not preclude that person from manifesting a clinically significant communication disorder that is not related to that dialect. For example, a speaker of African American English can have a fluency, voice, language, or phonological disorder unrelated to his or her dialect. Third, ASHA mandates that the speech-language pathologist must possess competencies to distinguish between communication disorders and dialectal differences and be familiar with procedures for culturally unbiased testing to make this determination. It is important to remember that the use of a dialect may change with geographical region, socioeconomic level, conversational partner, and age. For example, Craig and Washington (2004) studied 400 typically developing African American children in the Detroit area to determine if dialect changes occurred as children aged. It was found that there was a significant downward shift in dialect production by first grade. The researchers also found that students who made the shift by decreasing their use of dialect tended to have significantly higher scores on standardized tests of reading and vocabulary. They hypothesize that perhaps children who are more linguistically advanced are more sensitive to pragmatic aspects of language and thus reduce dialect production. Similarly, Thompson, Craig, and Washington (2004) sampled the use of African American English (AAE) in 50 third graders in three contexts: picture description, oral reading of a Standard American English (SAE) text, and writing. All children used AAE in describing pictures, but less AAE was shown in the literacy condition (reading). There was also more AAE used in picture description than in writing. More morphosyntactic features of AAE were used in writing compared to other conditions. The oral reading used more phonological features of AAE, and the picture description used more phonological and morphosyntactic features than other conditions. This study supports the idea that literacy activities may promote dialect shifting in young African American children.

The three points mentioned above carry several important implications for the speech-language pathologist. First, wherever the SLP is employed he or she will be part of a local and regional environment. This environment will be made up of many cultural groups, which will vary in their size depending on the region of the country. As a resident of this environment, the SLP is professionally bound to become familiar with all cultural groups and dialectal variations commonly encountered in clinical work. We are not indicating that every SLP needs to become an expert on *all* cultures or dialects, just the ones that he or she will be dealing with on a clinical level. The second implication is that the SLP must seek standardized test instruments that represent the cultural populations indigenous to his or her environment or develop local norms that *do* represent regional cultures. We will discuss this issue later in the present chapter. A third implication is that the SLP should become familiar with nonstandardized testing tasks that can help to distinguish between a disorder and a dialectal difference. We will address these procedures in a subsequent section.

CULTURAL DIFFERENCES IN PERCEPTIONS OF DISABILITY AND COMMUNICATION

A major implication of multicultural issues on assessment concerns the diverse belief systems of the various cultural groups regarding disabilities and communication. Some cultures believe that a handicapping condition is a situation that nothing can or should be done about, or that the help for this condition is spiritual rather than clinical (Cheng, 1989). If the clinician charges into the initial interview with a client and makes a host of recommendations without addressing cultural attitudes toward remediation, the suggestions may fall on unsympathetic ears. The clients may also be offended and not return for treatment. Rodriguez and Olswang (2003) provide a recent example. They used both questionnaires and interview methodologies to study 30 Mexican American and 30 Anglo American mothers of children between the ages of 7 and 8 with language impairment to determine their beliefs about child rearing, education, and language impairment. The Mexican American mothers attributed extrinsic factors (e.g., God's will, schools) as the cause of their child's language impairment while Anglo American mothers cited intrinsic factors (e.g., medical condition, family history, personality). The Mexican American mothers also held a more traditional and authoritarian view of the educational system in that their role in the child's education was less as compared to Anglo mothers. This may have implications for parent programs. Most authorities believe that it is important to incorporate both the culture of the family and mainstream culture into treatment and literacy programs. Hammer, Rodriguez, Lawrence, and Miccio (2007) surveyed mothers of bilingual Puerto Rican children and found that they felt it important to include both traditional and progressive beliefs in their interactions. The researchers recommend that in clinical programs we use the family's traditional beliefs as a framework, but it is also important to inform families about expectations of the school culture as well. In a study of Mexican immigrant mothers, interview data were gathered on maternal perceptions of their children's communication, emergent literacy, and speech/language treatment program. The researchers found that most mothers were aware that their children exhibited some delay in communication and felt that the cause of such difficulties related to medical problems or familial history. The mothers tended to focus more on speech intelligibility/expressive language than on emergent literacy skills. They also felt it would be helpful if professionals could speak Spanish and provide more information about treatment programs (Kummerer, Lopez-Reyna, & Hughes, 2007). Clearly, this highlights the critical nature of gathering data from families through ethnographic interviews, and it also focuses on the significance of promoting an awareness of the importance of emergent literacy.

There is a growing literature in communication disorders concerning multicultural issues, and it is the ethical responsibility of every student and clinician to become familiar with this body of work. We cannot serve our clients well unless we take this cultural information into account.

INTERVIEWING AND COUNSELING ISSUES

Although multicultural issues affect all aspects of any profession, there are some important factors to consider in interviewing that relate to our burgeoning multicultural society. First, as mentioned in Chapter 2, the clinical interview represents the meeting of two or more individuals who each bring with them unique experiences, perceptions, views, values, and characteristics. When two people meet in a professional setting, the nature of the clinical relationship itself is sometimes problematic. That is, some people simply have trouble coming to a clinical situation, even if they are dealing with a clinician from the same culture as their own. When client and clinician represent differing cultural or racial backgrounds, there is an additional potential obstacle to overcome. Some clients may not feel as comfortable when they must reveal certain information to a stranger, and this discomfort may be intensified when the clinician represents a different race or culture. The solution for this is clearly not to make certain that clients and clinicians are culturally homogeneous. Given the diverse nature of our society, this would be impossible from a scheduling standpoint and unwise from a philosophical one. The best way to deal with cultural diversity in clinical situations is to make certain that clinicians have a sensitivity for cultural differences and a knowledge of multicultural issues in assessment and treatment. The American Speech-Language-Hearing Association has mandated that every accredited training program in communication disorders infuse multicultural information into each area of academic preparation and clinical practicum. Hopefully, our students will have increased opportunity to deal with culturally different clients, parents, and children and develop their interpersonal skills with, and knowledge of, these groups.

A second important implication of multicultural influence on interviewing concerns the specific information that is exchanged. We have indicated that much of the information exchanged in a clinical interview is of a highly personal nature and possibly charged with considerable affect. Many cultures (e.g., Native Americans and certain Asian groups) find it difficult to share personal information with unfamiliar people. Thus, in the interview it may be extremely uncomfortable for them to reveal some types of data. The clinician must be sensitive to such cultural beliefs and not press the client to provide information too soon. In some cases it will be necessary to conduct multiple interviews and establish a strong relationship with the clients before they will give information or take advantage of clinician suggestions for treatment. This issue alone is a strong indictment of some rigid policies in which an evaluation is expected to be completed in an hour or two, or IEP goals must be written in limited time frames. We must learn that different cultures may require alterations in our methods if we are to serve them optimally.

An obvious multicultural influence on interviewing is the possibility of dealing with the many children and adults from bilingual backgrounds. In some cases, the clinician must be bilingual, and in others the interviewer must make use of interpreters. The use of an interpreter, however, is a very specialized operation and the clinician must be certain that the person has adequate knowledge and experience to perform this specialized task. In some areas of the country, there is an increased likelihood that the SLP will encounter a bilingual population, and he or she should reflect on how these clients will be served appropriately in assessment and treatment. It is not possible to provide adequate services to these populations without a knowledge of and sensitivity to multicultural issues. Lynch (1992) describes the ideal interpreter as someone who is (1) proficient in the language (including specific dialect) of the family as well as that of the interventionist, (2) trained and experienced in cross-cultural communication and the principles (and dynamics) of serving as an interpreter, (3) trained in the appropriate professional field relevant to the specific family–interventionist interaction, and (4) able to understand and appreciate the respective cultures of both parties and to convey the more subtle nuances of each with tact and sensitivity. Lynch (1992) cautions against the use of family members as interpreters because they rarely meet the above criteria and could inject significant bias and family difficulties into the clinical situation. Most authorities on the use of interpreters emphasize the importance of thorough preparation of the interpreter prior to the clinical encounter in terms of the goals and purposes of the evaluation, potentially sensitive clinical and family issues, the format of the interview, and any technical terms and paperwork to be used in the conference. It is helpful to introduce all people present and clarify the goals and purposes of the interview so the family will know what to expect. Diligent clinicians may take the time to learn several social phrases in the language of the family so that greetings, saying thank you, and leave-taking can be done in a manner comfortable to the clients. This demonstrates respect for the family and shows that the clinician is making an attempt to understand and appreciate cultural differences. During the interview it is customary for the clinician to address remarks and questions to the family, not the interpreter. Also, while listening to the family, it is appropriate to look at the person who is speaking, not just at the interpreter. In this situation it is clearly beneficial to avoid technical jargon and figurative language that not only is difficult to translate, but may be confusing to the clients. As the interview progresses, especially in the portion where information is provided to the clients, it is wise to periodically check the family's understanding of facts presented and any recommendations given by the clinician. Finally, most experts on the use of interpreters recommend a debriefing session in which the clinician and interpreter can discuss the information collected, any difficulties encountered in the conference, any problems with the interpreting process, and any subtle impressions gleaned by the interpreter that go beyond the literal translation of the client's utterances (e.g., anger, hostility, fear, etc.). Although such impressions are subjective on the part of the interpreter, they may represent important information about the family's acceptance of the problem, perceptions of the clinical situation, and possible compliance with a treatment program. Good interpreters are difficult to find and often "burn out" quickly because of the time commitment, being asked to appear with little advance notice, and sometimes not being adequately compensated for their work. As a result, the SLP must do everything possible to develop and cultivate mutually beneficial relationships with interpreters.

CULTURAL DIFFERENCES IN INCIDENCE AND PREVALENCE OF DISORDERS

In many areas of communication disorders, cultural differences in the occurrence of various disorders have been reported. For example, in the area of audiology, there are systematic differences in the occurrence of otitis media along racial lines, with the following occurrence from high to low: Native Americans, Hispanic, white, and African American. Also, African Americans have less hearing loss with aging as compared to white Americans. In clefts of the lip and palate there is also a difference in occurrence, with Native Americans and Asians having more clefts than African Americans.

Fluency Disorders from a Multicultural Perspective

Ours is an ethnically diverse society, and we are only beginning to appreciate how cultural values might affect the incidence, development, and ultimate treatment of communication disorders such as stuttering. Multicultural sensitivity on the part of the SLP is necessary. Early examinations of stuttering within cultures and across nations were motivated by theorists espousing environmental

TABLE 12.1 Cultural Variables and Stuttering

Gender/Sex

There is unequivocal evidence that more males than females stutter, regardless of the society or national origin.

Family and Societal Issues

Early research suggested that discipline, humiliation, and indulgence affect the occurrence of stuttering.

Parents of children who stutter display temperament and attitude differences (Yairi, 1997).

Persons who stutter, on the whole, though research is equivocal, show sensitive temperaments and inhibitions (as reviewed by Yasiri & Ambrose, 2005).

Living in a volatile society, such as Israel, may also affect stuttering (Amir & Ezrati-Vinacour, 2002).

Demographics

Equivocal research suggests that stuttering is more prevalent in urban, rather than rural areas (Brady & Hall, 1976). Yet, Dykes (1995) found that rural areas had a greater prevalence of stuttering (0.49%) than urban areas did (0.34%).

Bilingualism

It is generally accepted that bilingual children are more likely to stutter than monolingual speakers. Borsel et al. (2001) cites a prevalence rate of 2.8% among bilinguals versus nearly 1% in the general population. In contrast, Montes and Erickson (1990) found no significant differences in the occurrence of stuttered speech behaviors in English and Spanish bilingual children. They also noted that the types of disfluencies associated with second language learning are often misidentified as stuttering.

Race and Ethnicity

There is a long history of research comparing stuttering among different cultures, including among Eskimos and various tribes of native Americans; however, recent investigation are lacking. Also, little is known about stuttering in the Asian American community. Prevalence of stuttering among Puerto Ricans living in New York City was reported by Leavitt (1974) to be 0.84%, a value similar to that of whites; by comparison, the prevalence among Puerto Ricans living in San Juan was 1.5%. African American research is presented in separate tables.

---

etiologies of stuttering. Table 12.1 cites issues regarding culture and stuttering as presently understood. Table 12.2 summarizes differences in the nonstuttering disfluencies of African American and white children, adults, and aged persons, whereas Table 12.3 provides an overview of stuttering-like disfluencies among these same groups. The reader is cautioned that more current research is emerging. Borsel et al. (2001) state that stuttering is more prevalent among bilinguals than monolinguals, that stuttering can affect one or both languages, and that the two languages may be equally or differently affected.

Vocal and Resonance Disorders

The need for multicultural understanding pervades the SLP's work with patients exhibiting disorders of the voice, including those who have been laryngectomized, and disorders of resonance. Diagnosis of these areas was covered in Chapters 10 and 11, but some elaboration from a cultural perspective is warranted.

TABLE 12.2	Some Studies of Black and White Nonstuttering Speakers of Various Age Groups during Disfluencies

Children

- Preschool black and white children of low and of middle socioeconomic levels did not show different types of disfluency (Ratusnik, Kirilluk, & Ratusnik, 1979).
- Disfluencies of preschool black children did not differ between males and females; amounts of disfluencies, especially revisions, declined with age (3.5 through 5.5 years) (Anderson, 1976).
- No significant differences were found between disfluencies of black and white first-grade children; both groups exhibited 7–8% disfluency (Brutten & Miller, 1988).
- Black preschool children had more repetitions, prolongations, and revisions during narrative discourse than in conversational speech (Robinson & Davis, 1992).

Young and Aged Adults

- Black college football players displayed greater amounts of word and phrase repetitions than did white athletes (Robinson & Crowe, 1987).
- Black males and females, aged 61–91, had slower speech rates and greater disfluency rates (especially revisions and repetitions) than did white speakers (Walker et al., 1981).
- Black and white males, aged 65–85, of matched socioeconomic levels were compared; no significant fluency differences were found for race or socioecomomic level with regard to speaking rates, articulatory rates, or frequencies of interjections (approximately 4.75%), revisions (1.22%), and whole-word repetitions (0.83%) (Pindzola, 1990).

Cultural factors interact with both environmental surroundings and lifestyle choices. Environmental factors are thought to cause or perpetuate some voice disorders. Where one lives matters. Noise, air pollution, and relative humidity are factors that singularly or in combination may cause or maintain a particular disorder. There also is a growing awareness of the effects of lifestyle, including diet, smoking, rest/sleep, drug use, exercise, and alcohol consumption, on the functions of the larynx, upper airway, and the digestive tract (Shin & Bellenir, 1998).

Hoarseness is the predominant dysphonia in children up to age 18, with vocal nodules being the most frequent cause of hoarseness. Evidence suggests that African American youth from economically depressed inner cities exhibit more than twice the incidence of hoarseness as compared to white youngsters in other communities. Likewise, Hispanic American teenagers from Southern California have more than twice the incidence of dysphonia as white adolescents in the same or similar communities (Shin & Bellenir, 1998).

Others too have noted that the incidence of laryngeal pathologies in children seems to vary as a function of gender and ethnicity, and so the clinician will benefit from good skills for multicultural interaction. Dobres et al. (1990) examined medical charts in an admittedly modest-sized sample and discerned that Asian Americans have the greatest male-to-female incidence ratio (4.3:1), whites the second greatest (1.8:1), and African Americans the lowest (1.4:1). Of 30 laryngeal pathologies, it is worth noting that vocal nodules were more prevalent in white male children as compared to white females. Asian American gender differences were in the same direction, but the opposite pattern was seen among African American children, females showing a higher incidence.

Differential health-related conditions (smoking, drinking, nutritional factors) and environmental exposures no doubt affect the incidence of respiratory tract carcinomas in multicultural

TABLE 12.3	Some Studies Comparing Stuttering-Like Disfluencies among Blacks and Whites of Various Age Groups

Children

- Analysis of matriarchial families in Tennessee suggests more females stutter among blacks than among whites; male-to-female sex ratios were reported as 2.4:1 among blacks and 5:1 among whites (Goldman, 1967).
- Patriarchial black families had sex ratios of stuttering similar to sex ratios for whites (Goldman, 1967).
- The male-to-female ratio of stuttering prevalence in African Americans is similar to that of whites; both were 3.5:1 (Dykes, 1995).
- Black male nonstuttering children had closer relationships with their mothers and received more consistent discipline than did black male children who stuttered (Powell, 1967).
- The high prevalence of stuttering among Alabama school children (2.1% prevalence) was attributed to the large population of blacks in the schools (78% black, 22% white) (Gillespie & Cooper, 1973).
- African American male and female students have prevalence rates twice that of white males and females (Dykes, 1995).
- Proctor et al. (2001) examined over 3,400 preschoolers and found stuttering prevalence overall was 2.46% with no group differences among African Americans, European Americans, and other minorities.

Young and Aged Adults

- In a Chicago community college, the prevalence of stuttering was 2.7% for blacks and 0.8% for whites (Conrad, 1992).
- Among young adults, racial patterns of disfluency may exist: Whites tend to display overt repetitions and prolongations, while blacks tend to be more covert and severe. This may be a cultural response to conceal lack of verbal prowess among blacks (Leith & Mims, 1975).
- No known studies of aged adults exist beyond speculations posed by Manning and Monte (1981).

populations. According to the National Cancer Institute's data set (current up through 2006 and available at http://www.cancer.gov), the incidence of cancer of the larynx among U.S. minority groups is greatest among African Americans, followed by Hawaiians, Hispanics, Japanese, Chinese, Filipinos, and then Native Americans. By extension, the clinician should be cognizant of cultural differences when assessing and rehabilitating laryngectomized persons.

Shin and Bellenir (1998) cite similar uneven distributions from the oncology literature with regard to laryngeal carcinoma. The Surveillance, Epidemiology, and End Results Program of the National Cancer Institute, mentioned above, has gathered data for nearly 40 years from nine regions of the United States. Indications are that the African American population has laryngeal cancer at a rate 50% higher than whites. Hispanic Americans over the age of 65 present with an even higher incidence of laryngeal cancer, while Native Americans have a relatively low incidence. Shin and Bellenir believe that ethnic risk factors for laryngeal cancer include diet, lifestyle choices, cultural attitudes toward illness and health care providers, and differences in medical services.

Disorders of vocal resonance are distributed differently along multicultural lines, particularly in cases of cleft lip and palate. A cleft of the lip, palate, or both is one of the most common congenital abnormalities, with a prevalence ranging from under 1 in 1,000 births to over 2.69 in 1,000 births around the world. In the United States, approximately 45% of infant clefts are non-Caucasian. For minority groups in the United States, the highest incidence of cleft palate per 1,000 population is among Chinese/Chinese Americans (over 4.0), then Hawaiians and Japanese/Japanese Americans, followed by Native Americans, Latino Americans, and least African Americans (less than 0.8) (McLean et al., 2004; Meyerson, 1990; Vanderas, 1987). Vanderas also reviewed the incidence of different kinds of clefting (lip, palate, lip and palate), with most minority groups following the general population trend toward cleft lip with palate. A notable exception is that among African Americans a cleft palate only occurs more often.

LANGUAGE ASSESSMENT: THE MOST PROBLEMATIC AREA

Adult Language, Related Adult and Child Motor Speech Disorders, and Dysphagia

Neurological disease and accident can affect anyone, regardless of ethnicity. Public health demographics, however, show that neurological impairments affect individuals from the multicultural community to a disproportionate extent. Cerebrovascular accident is the leading cause of neurological impairment among African Americans, Hispanics, and certain Asian/Pacific Americans. Primary risk factors for CVA in these groups include hypertension (exacerbated by underutilization of healthcare services and high-cholesterol diets), arteriosclerosis (accentuated by diets high in fats and salt), sickle cell anemia (reduced red blood cells affects oxygen-carrying capacity, and sickle-shaped cells fail to pass through smallest blood vessels in the brain), and substance abuse (e.g., crack causes vasoconstriction that may lead to stroke). These sobering statistics make clear, then, that a speech-language pathologist specializing in neurogenic communication disorders can expect a diverse caseload. Patients from varied ethnic and cultural backgrounds may, in greater numbers, have aphasia, other adult language disorders, apraxias, and/or dysarthrias. The propensity toward neurological disease also may be reflected in the number of cases of adult and pediatric swallowing disorders.

In discussing neurogenic communication disorders in Hispanic Americans, Reyes (1995) notes that the case history must be expanded to include information regarding each of the patient's languages. Reyes recommends collecting the following additional case history information for optimal case planning and management:

1. Languages spoken in the home, community, and in school during childhood and premorbidly
2. Degree of speaking, reading, and writing proficiency in each language premorbidly
3. Frequency and type of code switching premorbidly (i.e., alternating use of two languages at the word, phrase, clause, or sentence level)
4. Language in which television, movies, radio, and newspapers were most often received premorbidly
5. Proficiency of significant others in each language (spouse, children, parents, siblings)
6. Attitudes of self and of significant family members toward bilingualism

Roberts (2001) also discussed aphasia assessment and treatment with bilingual and culturally diverse patients, stating that assessment is impacted along with recovery styles. She notes that tests may be culturally biased. Nonaphasic, nonwhite adults tend to score differently than nonaphasic whites on narrowly focused aphasia tests such as the Arizona Battery for

Communication Disorders and the Boston Naming Test (Armstrong et al., 1996; Roberts, 2000). Black versus white performance differences were also noted, though not as striking, in broader language tests such as the Boston Diagnostic Aphasia Examination (BDAE), the Western Aphasia Battery (WAB), and the Minnesota Tests for the Differential Diagnosis of Aphasia (MTDDA) (Molrine & Pierce, 2002). Ulatowska et al. (2001) compared interpretative abilities of African Americans with and without aphasia. They conclude that fable and proverb discourse tasks are valuable supplemental measures for characterizing communication competence in African American adults who have aphasia.

Paradis and Libben (1987) designed the Bilingual Aphasia Test (BAT). The BAT exists in over 60 languages and tests all language modalities. It also has a section that tests translation abilities between more than 100 pairs of languages. Additional information on the aspects of bilingual and multicultural aphasia is available from the National Aphasia Association (http://www.aphasia.org); in 2007 this organization formed a multicultural task force. ASHA (http://www.asha.org) also has special-interest groups devoted to neurogenic disorders (division 2) and to cultural and linguistic diversity (division 14). With regard to bilingual aphasia, we highly recommend the tutorial published in an ASHA journal by Lorenzen and Murrary (2008). Adults with strokes or other neurologic conditions often present with motor speech disorders as well. According to ASHA (2008), information on the prevalence of neurogenic communication disorders among adults in the United States includes the following points of interest.

1. Prevalence of Parkinson's disease in industrialized countries is 0.3% of the general population and over 1% of the population over age 60. People of all ethnicities are affected and men more so than women. Motor speech and voice are commonly affected within the communication realm.
2. Huntington's disease is rare, genetic and fatal. It affects only 5 in 100,000 people. Motor speech and cognition difficulties are typical.
3. Amyotrophic lateral sclerosis is a progressive, ultimately fatal motor disease affecting less than 3 in 100,000 people. Men are twice as likely as women to be affected. Oropharyngeal dysfunction is common along with voice quality dysphonia followed by loss of speaking ability. (A computerized alternative device is used by the world-renowned physicist, Stephen Hawking.)

The incidence of traumatic brain injury is high in both industrialized and nonindustrialized countries (Leon-Carrion et al., 2005). As covered in Chapter 9, TBIs are most common among youth and young adults because of work and play accidents. The pattern of TBI damage often includes motor speech, language, and cognitive deficits.

As reviewed earlier in this chapter, culturally diverse infants are more likely to be born prematurely, with low birth weight, and/or with medical complications stemming often from inadequate maternal diet and other culturally related environmental situations. The pediatric population is at high risk for neurological compromise; cerebral palsy is one such outcome common in diverse cultures and persons of low socioeconomic status. Pediatric feeding and swallowing difficulties are a common sequela in low-birth-weight babies and those with cerebral palsy. The Cerebral Palsy International Research Foundation (http://cpirf.org) follows the epidemiology of cerebral palsy throughout six countries (excluding the United States) and notes an increasing trend: In the 1970s, cerebral palsy occurred in 1.7 per 1,000 live births, whereas 2006 statistics report an incidence range of 2.12 to 2.45 per 1,000. Children with cerebral palsy may need the services of a speech-language pathologist for a host of issues including articulation and feeding. The SLP working in a pediatric dysphagia practice will need to adjust his or her interactions to those of the caregivers of these tiny patients. Feeding and swallowing issues eventually make their way to the school SLP who also will need skills with family and cultural issues (Davis-McFarland, 2008).

For more information on this, the interested reader is referred to the book *Communication Disorders in Multicultural Populations* (Battle, 2002) and in particular the section on neurogenic disorders in both adult and pediatric populations. Another excellent resource for speech-language pathologists is the book *Multicultural Neurogenics* (Wallace, 1997). Topics covered include cultural preferences in food (helpful in dysphagia practice), family involvement, time constraints, attitude toward authority, and suggestions on adapting assessment procedures. Neurological and swallowing impairments are discussed from the perspectives of African American, Indian, Hispanic, and Asian cultures.

Child Language/Phonology

Brown (1973) has noted that there are striking similarities in children's early language acquisition cross culturally. That is, children from a variety of cultures tend to develop the same types of early word combinations, presumably because these semantic relations rest on concepts developed in the sensorimotor period of cognitive development. While we may not find differences in word combinations across cultures, there may certainly be variations in prelinguistic and single-word development in various groups. Several recent studies of early language assessment in Hispanic children have been reported. Patterson (1998) studied 102 bilingual children with the Language Development Survey (LDS). Expressive vocabulary size increased with age, and there were gender differences in favor of the females. The article presents means, medians, and ranges of vocabulary size and potential screening guidelines. Thal, Jackson-Maldonado, and Acosta (2000) administered the Spanish-language version of the MacArthur Communicative Development Inventory to children aged 20 and 28 months. Results of the CDI were compared with language sample data on the children to determine the validity of the instrument. Results support the validity for assessing expressive vocabulary in children of these age groups using the scale. Another area that clinicians evaluate in early language cases is caretaker–child interaction. Cross-cultural studies of caretaker–child interaction have demonstrated cultural differences in interaction style, play, speech register, use of objects in joint referencing, parenting, family values/beliefs, and general opportunities for interaction (Bornstein, Tal, & Tamis-Lemonda, 1991a; Bornstein et al., 1991b; Fogel, Toda, & Kawai, 1988; Heath, 1983, 1989; Saville-Troike, 1986; Schieffelin, 1985; Watson-Gegeo & Gegeo, 1986). Anderson-Yockel and Haynes (1994) found differences in parental questioning behaviors during joint book reading between lower socioeconomic-level African American and white mother–toddler dyads. It is important for clinicians to realize that all cultural groups have differences and similarities to one another. For example, Mexican American mothers engage in joint book sharing with their children and use many strategies reported in mainstream populations during this type of activity. However, no cultural group is monolithic. Socioeconomic level, for instance, may be a variable that highlights performance differences even within the same cultural group. Rodriguez, Hines, and Montiel (2009) found that Mexican American mothers from both lower and middle socioeconomic levels showed many similarities to each other and mainstream populations. However, the lower SES group used less positive feedback and yes/no questions as compared to middle-class mothers.

These potential cultural differences in caregiver–child interaction must be taken into account as the clinician examines parents and children in clinical settings. Social interactions and selection of activities for joint referencing may be very different in the home environment, and we should not expect everyone to interact in the same way when using "mainstream" toys and objects provided in clinical settings. Clinicians must endeavor to learn more about child rearing and interaction in different cultures and should not impose ethnocentric views on the families we serve.

In older children, however, there have been significant differences reported in the development of grammatical morphemes, phonology, vocabulary, specific sentence types, and pragmatics (Dillard, 1972; Gutierrez-Clellen, 1996; Hester, 1996; Hyter & Westby, 1996; Mount-Weitz, 1996; Owens, 2005; Quinn, Goldstein, & Pena, 1996; Taylor, 1986a, 1986b; Williams & Wolfram, 1977; Wyatt, 1996). Especially when assessing school-age and adolescent students, it is of paramount importance that the SLP consider cultural differences. Stockman, Karasinski, and Guillory (2008) have shown that typically developing African American preschool children in Headstart programs initiate and respond to requests for conversational repairs in much the same manner as children speaking Standard English. While the frequency of occurrence of specific repair types differed somewhat, the categories of conversational repairs were consistent with those found in prior research on pragmatic development. The authors recommend that in assessment of conversational repairs clinicians should expect similar performance in children speaking African American and Standard English. It has been shown that school-age children speaking African American English evidence similar category types of cohesive devices as reported for children who speak Standard English (Horton-Ikard, 2009).

Gutierrez-Clellen (1999) outlines assessment implications for the public school SLP in assessment of literacy skills in bilingual children. The article views reading and spelling skills as reciprocal processes, and children with limited English proficiency may benefit from an integrated team approach to learning speaking, reading, and writing. There is even some evidence that children who are more able to shift between African American English and Standard American English in their written work tend to have higher reading achievement scores on standardized tests even when controlling for socioeconomic level. Interestingly, the ability to style shift in oral language tasks as measured by dialect density metrics was not as predictive as written language style shifting (Craig, Zhang, Hensel, & Quinn, 2009). Bilingual children learning English and Spanish in the preschool period tend to score within the typical developmental range as compared to monolingual children by the end of kindergarten. Research has shown that language growth in both English and Spanish is reasonably predictive of reading abilities in both languages (Hammer, Lawrence, & Miccio, 2007). Therefore, it is prudent to monitor language growth during later preschool years in both languages through regular evaluation of bilingual children.

Any intervention approach assumes adequate assessment. It is important that we test bilingual children across a variety of tasks that assess semantic performance and that both of the child's languages be used in the assessment (Pena, Bedore, & Rappazzo, 2003). Although we have not yet developed widely accepted specific procedures for evaluation of clients from a variety of cultures, most authorities suggest that multiple assessment measures should be used (Hamayan & Damico, 1991; Stockman, 1996; Vaughn-Cooke, 1983; Washington, 1996). The most promising avenues appear to be criterion-referenced testing, use of ethnographic techniques, and more nonstandardized as opposed to standardized procedures (Lidz & Pena, 1996; Robinson-Zanartu, 1996; Stockman, 1996). Anderson (1996) compared use of the SPELT-P and a nonstandardized description task designed by the investigator in evaluating the use of specific grammatical forms in Spanish-speaking children. The nonstandardized description task was more effective in evaluating the children's knowledge of the grammatical forms that were evaluated. The children performed significantly better on the nonstandardized task. Pena and Quinn (1997) studied differences in Puerto Rican and African American children's language performance on a familiar task (description) and on a task that was viewed as culturally less familiar (one-word labeling). They found that the familiar task for both groups was more sensitive to differentiating children with language disorder from those who were normally developing. Gutierrez-Clellen, Restrepo, Bedore, Pena, and Anderson (2000) discuss specific length and complexity measures for Spanish grammar to use in analysis of language samples. They provide clinical implications for assessment of Spanish-speaking children with differing levels of English proficiency. Some preliminary normative data are beginning to emerge for certain cultural groups on nonstandardized tasks. For instance, Craig and Washington (2002) studied 100 typically developing African American preschool and kindergarten children in order to provide performance data on the following measures: mean length of communication units, amount of complex syntactic productions, number of different words, responses to WH-questions, and understanding of passive/active sentences. More recently, Craig, Washington, and Thompson (2005) examined the same variables in African American children between first and fifth grade. The results of both studies provide preliminary reference information on these measures for African American children and are appropriate for use in culturally fair assessment.

Phonology, as an area of language, carries its own considerations of dialectal influences. African American English (AAE) has been sampled in isolated word contexts (Bleile & Wallach, 1992; Cole & Taylor, 1990; Haynes & Moran, 1989; Seymour & Seymour, 1981; Simmons, 1988; Washington & Craig, 1992) and in connected speech (Seymour, Green, & Huntley, 1991; Stockman, 1993; Stockman & Stephenson, 1981; Vaughn-Cooke, 1976; Wolfram, 1989). Most research has shown more similarities than differences between Standard English and AAE (Stockman, 1996). We know that AAE, like other dialects, changes with age and geographical region. Most differences in AAE are reported in medial and final word positions, and the initial word position shows the fewest alterations. Deletion of final consonants is one of the most frequently studied features of AAE. Moran (1993) has shown that when final consonants are deleted in AAE, the preceding vowel is systematically lengthened, which demonstrates knowledge of the deleted segment and not simply an "open syllable." Typically, there are only a few specific classes of phonological differences between Standard English and AAE reported in the literature (Williams & Wolfram, 1977; Wolfram, 1991, 1994). These differences mainly center on the /th/ and /r/ phonemes, final cluster reductions, and final consonant deletions. While there are many subtleties to be noted across word positions, canonical shapes, and word boundaries, it is clear the phonological differences are not numerous. More recent research has begun to focus on important areas such as phonological awareness. Thomas-Tate, Washington, and Edwards (2004) administered the Test of Phonological Awareness (TOPA) to 56 lower SES African American first graders. The performance of these children on the TOPA led the researchers to question whether the test results in lower scores for dialect speakers, since these children exhibited average scores on standardized tests of reading skills. Since there is a strong correlation between phonological awareness and reading, and there was not good agreement between TOPA scores and reading tests, the authors question whether dialect may have played a role in lower TOPA scores. It is important that tests of phonological awareness, which is just emerging as a significant area in our field, are developed with the goal of controlling any cultural bias. In many areas of assessment we can take some comfort that results of studies on English-speaking children are similar to those speaking other languages. For example, Goldstein, Fabiano, and Iglesias (2004) compared imitative and spontaneous productions of single words in 12 Spanish-speaking children with phonological disorders. In 62% of the cases, imitated and spontaneous productions were identical. The authors recommend that sampling in both modalities can add important information to an evaluation of phonology in Spanish-speaking children. In Hispanic/Latino children, several studies report useful information for the diagnostician. Two major Spanish dialects in the United States are Mexican American and Caribbean (Puerto Rican). Goldstein and Iglesias (1996) describe phonological patterns in terms of phonological processes. The children did not exhibit a percentage of occurrence of greater than 10% with the exception of consonant cluster reduction, which diminished at about the age of 4:6. The two most common processes were CCR and liquid simplification. The article provides a nice summary of phonological features of Puerto Rican dialect as well as a list of lexical items for use in assessment. Yavas and Goldstein (1998) provide information about common and uncommon phonological patterns across several languages and discusses the influence of one language upon another. In assessment the authors state: "The information gathered in a phonological assessment for bilingual children is similar to that collected for monolingual children; case history, oral-peripheral examination, hearing screening, language (e.g., syntax, semantics), voice, fluency and phonological patterns" (p. 49). In Chapter 5 of the present text, we discussed the importance of assessing narratives. We also indicated that narratives may vary with a person's cultural background (Gutierrez-Clellen & Quinn, 1993; Johnson, 1995; Miller, Gillam, & Pena, 2001). Proficiency in the oral production of language is important for development of literacy skills, especially in the case of children who are bilingual. This means that educators should monitor both English and Spanish oral language abilitites as well as literacy gains in both languages, especially in kindergarten and the early grades (Uccelli & Paez, 2007). Literacy programs that emphasize a rich variety of language uses have been advocated for bilingual students. Uccelli and Paez (2007) suggested not only vocabulary augmentation but work on constructing age-appropriate narratives in both languages, suspecting that generalization across languages may occur; however, this needs to be verified by further research.

We are now beginning to see research on sampling and elicitation of narratives in other cultures. For instance, Fiestas and Pena (2004) elicited two narratives using two different methods of sampling; a single picture and a wordless picture book. Narratives were also elicited in both languages (Spanish-English). For the book task, children produced narratives of equal complexity. There were more attempts and initiating events in Spanish, and more consequences in English. The single picture elicitation resulted in more variability. The authors feel that the wordless book task is a viable assessment method for bilingual children. In another study by Muñoz, Gillam, Peña, and Gulley-Faehnle (2003), 24 low SES Latino preschool children produced oral narratives in response to a wordless picture book. The narratives were analyzed for story structure (complete/incomplete episodes), productivity (total number of words, number of different words), sentence organization (number of utterances, C-unit length, percent of grammatically acceptable utterances). There were no differences in productivity measures between older (age 5) and younger (age 4) groups, but there were differences in sentence organization and story structure. This may suggest that the productivity measures that differentiate development in mainstream children may not be as sensitive in young Latino children. However, the authors felt that the sentence organization and story structure measures may be more valid for this population. Some studies of narratives show few differences between cultural groups. For example, Curenton and Justice (2004) studied 67 low-income children between the ages of 3 and 5 who were African American and Caucasian. They used a wordless picture book to generate a narrative, and they examined simple/complex elaborated noun phrases, adverbs, conjunctions, and mental/linguistic verbs (think, know, tell). There were no differences between the cultural groups, and there was a systematic increase in use of decontextualized language between ages 3 and 5. Use of decontextualized language is thought to be associated with academic success and literacy development.

It is important to consider sociocultural factors such as family structure, child play routines, urban versus rural, and length of residence in the country. There may also be cultural differences to be taken into account in gathering a speech sample. Ideally, phonological skills should be assessed in all of the child's languages. To do this, the SLP may have to rely on support personnel, interpreters, translators, bilingual speech pathology assistants, or family members. This is a very complicated process. It is beyond the scope of this chapter to outline all the possible linguistic variations produced by the various cultural groups in the United States (e.g., African American, Native American, Hispanic, Asian). The references cited above will provide a good beginning for the clinician in learning about cultural influences on language. It is the ethical responsibility of each SLP to at least become familiar with the dialects spoken in his or her geographical area. Dialectal differences *must* be considered in making judgments about the existence of a disorder, in selecting evaluation procedures, and in recommending treatment goals. Most cultural groups will exhibit differences in their language and communication that are attributable to bilingual or bidialectal influences on English. No other area of communication (e.g., voice, fluency) is affected as significantly as language. To make matters even more complicated, most language tests are designed using a Standard English model, and scoring procedures may mandate that deviation from this model should be counted as an "error." Therefore, the latter parts of the present chapter will focus on some assessment techniques that have been developed to minimize cultural bias in language evaluation.

In the area of standardized language testing, the importance of the population tested in the development of the instrument cannot be overemphasized. This is important not only to see how children from different cultures respond to the test stimuli, but the scores they make on the test contribute to the standardization sample or "norms" of the test. It is axiomatic in the psychometric literature that norms are not valid if the standardization sample differs significantly from the local population tested. Although many test instruments that are currently used have included children of different cultural groups in their norming samples, the percentage of these children may not be reflective of the proportion of such children in many local areas. For example, the general population of the United States is composed of approximately 12% African Americans; however, the concentration of this cultural group in many cities and states may be several times this proportion. As an illustration, let us look through the microscope at selected states in the country (Figure 12.2) and their percentage of cultural makeup mainly for African American and Hispanic residents (the "other" category includes Native American, Pacific Islander, and Asian individuals). It is clear from this table that many states have significantly more than the national average of African Americans, for example. If we turn to a more powerful lens and focus on cities in the United States (Figure 12.3), you can see that the percentages of the various cultures change drastically. The 2000 census statistics show that more than half of the United States population lives in the 39 largest metropolitan areas. It is questionable, at best, to use a test that had included only 9% African American children in its standardization sample if one is working in a community where over 60% of the children represent this cultural group. A second problem with the standardization samples in their reflection of cultural differences may surface in a lack of specific description of the groups in the norming sample. For instance, saying that 120 African American children were included in the norming sample does not provide any information on their socioeconomic level or whether or not they spoke African American English. If the children were not dialectal speakers, then their scores may have no relevance for evaluators who want to compensate for language bias on the test or to compare these scores to a population in the inner city where dialectal usage is a prominent feature. If a clinician uses a standardized test on dialect speakers and scores it differently from the procedure used with the normative sample, the norms

State	African American	Other Nonwhite	Hispanic
Alabama	26.0	1.2	1.7
Arkansas	15.7	1.5	3.2
Arizona	3.1	6.9	25.3
California	6.7	9.2	32.4
Colorado	3.8	3.3	17.1
Florida	14.6	2.1	16.8
Georgia	28.7	2.5	5.3
Hawaii	1.8	51.3	7.2
Illinois	15.1	3.6	12.3
Louisiana	32.5	1.8	2.4
Maryland	27.9	4.3	4.3
Michigan	14.2	2.4	3.3
Mississippi	36.3	1.1	1.4
Montana	0.3	6.8	2.0
New York	15.9	5.9	15.1
North Carolina	21.6	2.6	4.7
South Carolina	29.5	1.2	2.4
Texas	11.5	3.4	32.0
Wyoming	0.8	3.0	6.4

FIGURE 12.2   Selected states and their cultural makeup (percent).
Source: 2000 U.S. Census.

should not be used because the test was not scored the same way as it was during test development. There is some question, however, that scoring a test differently would even make a difference in some cases. For instance, Rhyner, Kelly, Brantley, and Krueger (1999) used the Bankson Language Screening Test 2 and the Structured Photographic Expressive Language Test-Preschool on 99 preschoolers who represented low-income SES. They state: "Presently, there are no standardized language screening tests that include normative data on African American children or children of any social class who do not speak the SAE dialect" (p. 50). In this study the children had very high failure rates, even with scoring modifications that took into account AAE dialect. Evidently, administration of standardized tests even with alternative scoring is not the ultimate solution to cultural bias in assessment. Recently, however, a new standardized testing procedure has been developed (Seymour, Roeper, DeVilliers, & DeVilliers, 2005). Preliminary studies have shown it to be valid and nonbiased for African American and Standard English children and that it can distinguish African American dialect speakers from African American children with language impairments. The test is called the *Diagnostic Evaluation of Language Variation* (DELV) and it has a screening test, a criterion-referenced edition, and a norm-referenced edition available. The norms are based on U.S. Census figures and are demographically adjusted for children ages 4 through 9. The test examines syntax, phonology, semantics, and pragmatics. Since phonological development in African American English and Mainstream American English have been shown to have different developmental trajectories, it is recommended that only features that share similar developmental patterns between the two language groups be used in diagnosis of language impairment. Pearson, Velleman, Bryant, and Charko (2009) provide a summary of developmental milestones for speakers of African American

City	African American	Other Nonwhite	Hispanic
Albuquerque	3.1	14.8	39.9
Atlanta	61.4	4.1	4.5
Baltimore	64.3	2.5	1.7
Boston	25.3	15.7	14.4
Charlotte	32.7	7.3	7.4
Chicago	36.8	17.3	26.0
Cleveland	51.0	5.2	7.3
Dallas	25.9	20.4	35.6
Denver	11.1	19.7	31.7
Detroit	81.6	3.8	5.0
El Paso	3.1	20.1	76.6
Fresno	8.4	36.2	39.9
Houston	25.3	22.2	37.4
Los Angeles	11.2	36.5	46.5
Memphis	61.4	3.2	3.0
Miami	22.3	6.2	65.8
New Orleans	67.3	3.4	3.1
New York	26.6	23.7	27.0
Philadelphia	43.2	9.6	8.5
San Francisco	7.8	37.7	14.1
Tucson	4.3	21.6	35.7
Washington, DC	60.0	6.8	7.9

FIGURE 12.3 Selected cities and their cultural makeup (percent).
Source: 2000 U.S. Census.

English who are learning Mainstream American English as a second dialect. They recommend using a nonbiased test such as the Dialect Sensitive Language Test (DSLT) and use features that develop similarly in AAE and MAE to differentiate children who are typically developing from those with language impairment.

The concept of *local norms* has been discussed for years in the psychometric literature (Adler, 1990; Evard & Sabers, 1979; Omark, 1981; Popham, 1981; Seymour, 1992). Owens (2004) states:

> Often the norming sample does not represent the population with which the speech-language pathologist is using the assessment procedure. In this situation, the norms are inappropriate and should not be used. This situation occurs most frequently with minority or rural children or with children from lower socioeconomic groups. In these cases, local norms should be prepared by following the norming procedure described in the test manual. Some tests, such as the Test of Language Development-Intermediate (TOLD-I) and the CELF, explain this process in detail. (p. 65)

Some formal tests such as the TACL-R have developed software that the practitioner can use in generating local normative data and CELF-3. The SALT computer program also has a module for the clinician to use in generating local norms for conversational and narrative samples. The use of local norms does not mean ignoring national norms in evaluating a client. It is useful, however, to obtain both national and local perspectives in order to discover test biases and the most discriminating types of norms for identifying disorder versus cultural difference in performance. Recently, clinical research has suggested that a variety of tools and standard score cutoff levels may be useful in differentiating language difference from disorder. For example, Oetting, Cleveland, and Cope (2008) found that use of a standardized subtest of language comprehension could identify only 56% of school-age children with language impairment using a cutoff of –1 SD, but when a cutoff of –0.5 SD was used the percentage of those correctly classified rose to 81%. Further, when a nonword repetition task was added to the classification scheme, the correct identification increased to 90% (see later section on processing tasks). This suggests that when judicious use of locally determined cutoffs instead of arbitrary global cutoffs such as 1.5 SD are coupled with other nonbiased measurements such as nonword repetition tasks, our ability to diagnose effectively is increased. Stockman's (2010) recent review of assessment in African American populations also suggests use of multiple tools and procedures for unbiased evaluation.

NONSTANDARDIZED APPROACHES IN MULTICULTURAL ASSESSMENT

There are a number of nonstandardized techniques that have been suggested in the recent literature for use in multicultural assessment. Stockman (2010, p. 34) states: "The evidence so far shows that young speakers of AAE pass through the same basic stages of early development as do young SAE speakers. They develop at the same pace as SAE peers matched in age, social class and regional location. . . . A range of traditional and nontraditional strategies exist for distinguishing differences due to normal language dialect variation and those due to language impairment. This array of resources has enabled clinicians to embrace the value of using multiple sources of information to make diagnostic judgments about any child, not just an AA child."

While research on these techniques has emphasized the African American population, the concept could be applied to children from any cultural background. Each of the techniques will be briefly described in the following sections.

Minimal Competency Core

Stockman (1996) discusses the concept of a minimal competency core (MCC) for use in multicultural assessment. When we compare dialects to Standard English, we know that there are far more similarities than differences between the dialect and the standard language. For instance, African American kindergarten-age children appear to use regular and irregular past tense marking, and whether they represent middle or lower SES, the types of past tense marking are quite different from patterns reported in children with specific language impairment (Pruitt & Oetting, 2009). Many grammatical, morphological, semantic, and phonological forms are used similarly by speakers of dialects and those who speak Standard English. As a result, Stockman indicates, there are specific types of knowledge and skill that all children should be able to demonstrate that do not vary because of cultural background. Thus, we can expect that even when comparing two dialects, there are structures that both groups will use in communication. In other words, there are things that every 3-year-old child should be able to produce, no matter which dialect he or she is speaking, and these items constitute the minimal competency core. The inability to produce any of the elements in this basic set of structures should correlate well with the existence of language impairment. The elements in the MCC span phonological, pragmatic, semantic, and morphological areas. In phonology, the 3-year-old child should be able to produce the following consonants in the initial position of words and syllables: m, n, p, b, t, d, k, g, f, s, h, w, j, l, and r. Stockman (2008) has provided further data on a larger sample of Headstart children producing word initial consonant clusters and 13 singleton phonemes that should be correctly articulated by speakers of both AAE and SAE. Over 80% of the children passed the minimal competence phonetic core, and the pass/fail decisions tended to be significantly related to clinical delay.

Pragmatically, a child should be able to produce comments, descriptions, ask questions, request objects/actions, answer questions, initiate conversational repairs, and produce changes in his or her own utterances in response to repair requests. Semantically, the child should be able to use cases such as existence, state, locative state, action, locative action, specification, possession, time, and negation. Finally, a 3-year-old child should have an MLU above 2.7 and some evidence of nondialectal morphemes such as the present progressive (-ing). In order to evaluate the MCC, Stockman recommends that a spontaneous language sample be gathered during play and the sample should be examined for presence or absence of MCC components. The assumption is that children showing absence of MCC components at age 3 are at risk for language impairment, since these elements should not be missing due to use of a dialect.

Schraeder, Quinn, Stockman, and Miller (1999) utilized a minimal competency core in what they called "authentic assessment" for screening preschool children and compared the results to those using the Structured Photographic Expressive Language Test-Primary (SPELT-P). The MCC approach involved a 50-utterance language sample and making judgments as to whether a child exhibited specific MCC core behaviors. The study found that the MCC approach was more accurate than the use of the standardized test in agreeing with results of a multidisciplinary team evaluation. The MCC procedure took approximately 30 minutes longer than the administration of the SPELT-P; however, the added accuracy is probably worth the effort.

Contrastive Analysis

Another nonstandardized method for use in multicultural assessment is contrastive analysis. Contrastive analysis is a method for separating clinically significant errors from expressive speech/language patterns that are consistent with a client's first dialect. Basically, there are four steps involved in contrastive analysis (McGregor, Williams, Hearst, & Johnson, 1997). First, the clinician must become familiar with the dialect spoken by the client. Information on dialects is available from a variety of sources, including tutorial articles and textbooks. The ASHA website (http://professional.asha.org) provides many resources on specific characteristics of a variety of dialects if the reader uses the ASHA search engine and types in *dialect* as the search criterion. If the clinician can find no resources on a specific dialect, perhaps local norms should be gathered to determine characteristics of dialects likely to be seen in prospective clients in a particular area. At any rate, the first step in contrastive analysis is to become familiar with features of the dialect. The second step in contrastive analysis is to collect data using language sampling. This sample is evaluated by the clinician to determine if "differences from Standard English" occur in the transcript. We specify "differences" because any deviation from the Standard language may be either a "true error" or a dialectal variation. It has always struck us as curious when some clinicians use the term "dialectal errors," because if it is dialectal, by definition it cannot be an "error." At any rate, using a knowledge of the features of a dialect, the clinician must distinguish differences that are due to the client's dialect from true errors that represent differences not accounted for by dialectal variation. Seymour, Bland-Stewart, and Green (1998) found that shared features (noncontrastive) between AAE and SAE differentiated children with language disorders more effectively than contrastive features (those features that differ between AAE and SAE). The noncontrastive features that appeared to be problematic for children with language disorders were prepositions, the present progressive (-ing) articles, conjunctions, complex sentences, and modals. All of these features should not vary significantly due to dialect, and thus when a child has errors in these features, the likelihood of a disorder is increased. Seymour et al. (1998) also indicated that not all contrastive features are equal and performance profiles may overlap in some cases, and that the population with language disorders is highly variable in terms of errors that occur.

Dynamic Assessment

Dynamic assessment (DA) has been suggested as a means to determine if a child has a clinically significant difficulty learning language (Laing & Kamhi, 2003). Gutierrez-Clellen and Pena (2001) advocate the use of dynamic assessment to differentiate between language disorder and language difference. The assumption is that during dynamic assessment, children with language differences will exhibit more modifiability and those with legitimate language difficulties will show less modifiability. Children who score low on standardized tests (static measures) may do so because of a language disorder or a cultural or dialectal difference.

The assumption behind dynamic assessment in dealing with cultural differences is that children who can learn language in a short period of mediated assessment with little clinician effort and high learner responsivity probably have normal learning abilities. On the other hand, children who show difficulty learning linguistic-based material in a short period of mediated assessment may show a weakness in their ability to learn language and may be more likely to exhibit a language disorder. This method of differentiating dialect from disorder is not particularly time efficient, due to the time needed for mediated assessment, but it is another data point to use in reducing cultural bias. Ukrainetz, Harpell, Walsh, and Coyle (2000) studied two groups of Native American (Arapahoe and Shoshone) children identified as "stronger" or "weaker" language learners through teacher report and examiner classroom observation. The children participated in a dynamic assessment procedure. The modifiability scores and differences between pre- and post-test performance were consistently greater in the "stronger" group, suggesting that the DA procedure can identify children with differing levels of language abilities. Dynamic assessment used for this purpose may or may not be ultimately validated as a discriminator of disorder from difference. Learning linguistic material in a short time with minimal exposure is part of the basis of "fast-mapping" tasks, which are another possibility the clinician might use to evaluate short-term learning abilities. African American children from different socioeconomic levels can perform differently on specific language tasks. For example, Horton-Ikard and Weismer (2007) found that African American toddlers representing middle and lower SES backgrounds performed differently on two standardized vocabulary tests. The lower SES children scored significantly lower on the vocabulary tests as compared to middle-class children. Interestingly, the two groups performed similarly in a fast-mapping task where the children were asked to learn novel word meanings. This again illustrates that we cannot lump all children from a specific group (e.g., African Americans) and assume that there is no intragroup variation with such variables as socioeconomic class. Also, it underscores the importance of looking for bias in standardized tests and using informal tasks to show true abilities.

Processing Tasks

Processing tasks have been studied in attempting to differentiate dialect from disorder and have several potential advantages (Laing & Kamhi, 2003). These tasks can use stimuli that do not depend on a child's prior exposure with language or unique cultural experiences. One of the first studies of processing tasks for this purpose was by Campbell, Dollaghan, Needleman, and Jamosky (1997). They studied "majority" and "minority" children and gave them a standardized language test, which they referred to as a "knowledge-based" measure. They also gave the children two processing tasks (Competing Language Processing Task-CLPT; Nonword Repetition Task-NRT). They found that the minority subjects scored significantly lower than the majority subjects on the knowledge-based test, but there were no significant differences on the two processing tasks. Can we use nonword repetition tasks on children younger than age 5? Roy and Chiat (2004) developed a nonword repetition task for preschool children to determine if younger children could perform it and to examine relationships between NRT performance and linguistic ability in normally developing children. They found that most of the participants could perform the task, that performance was sensitive to age, and that NRT significantly correlated with performance on a receptive vocabulary test.

Several other studies (Bishop et al., 1996; Dollaghan & Campbell, 1998; Washington & Craig, 2004; Weismer et al., 2000) have shown that the nonword repetition task can differentiate children with language disorder from those with normal language. This is presumably because the NRT may require children to engage in a type of metaphonological task. As we know, any task that requires "meta abilities" is difficult for children with language impairment because it involves a conscious manipulation of linguistic or phonetic segments. Rodekohr and Haynes (2001) also studied the CLPT and the NRT as compared to a standardized language test. They found that the two processing tasks differentiated normal language and language-impaired children, just as the standardized test did. The children whose normal language was AAE, however, scored significantly lower on the standardized language test than the children whose normal language was Standard English. The implication of these studies is that processing tasks represent a nonculturally biased method of screening for language disorder. The tasks take less than five minutes to administer and can be used as part of a diagnostic battery. These tests are *not* diagnostic in nature by themselves and should never be used for this purpose, only as another indicator as to whether a child has a language impairment when viewed with other information about the client.

CONCLUDING REMARKS

The information provided in this chapter is, at best, cursory. This is because research projects, convention presentations, scientific articles, and textbooks in the area of multicultural issues in helping professions have exploded in the past decade. Our goal here was to stimulate students and clinicians to consider the significance of multicultural issues in assessment. One can easily see that evaluating a client without considering cultural and dialectal variables is a fool's errand. We want you to go beyond what we have summarized here and make an ongoing effort to study in this area. McCabe and Bliss (2003) say it well:

> The most important caveat of all is taken from the Hippocratic oath: First do no harm. We hope to help you avoid mishandling cultural differences between you and your student or client. To ignore such differences or to exaggerate them both have negative consequences. . . . Value diversity and include it in clinical contexts. (p. ix)

13

The Diagnostic Report

Only one very important phase of the evaluation remains to be considered: the preparation of the diagnostic report. Put the clinical situation, the interview, testing methods, results, and impressions in writing as soon as possible. Never trust a memory. Commit it to paper while the facial characteristics and voice inflections can still be remembered. Make the report "alive" so that others can experience what occurred just by reading about it. The raw data are of limited value to the clinician or other workers until they are assembled in a clear, precise, and orderly fashion.

A *diagnostic report* is a written record that summarizes the relevant information a clinician obtained—and how he or she obtained it—in his or her professional interaction with a client. It serves the following functions: (1) It acts as a guide for further services to the client—providing a clear statement of how the person was functioning at a given point in time, so that the clinician can document change or lack of change. (2) It communicates the clinician's findings to other professional workers; it provides answers to a number of clinical questions, including: Does the person have a problem? Will treatment be helpful? Will referrals be necessary? (3) It serves as a document for research purposes.

The importance of the first function should be obvious: Intelligent clinical plans evolve naturally from carefully prepared reports. The second purpose of diagnostic reports is to answer questions about clients so that other professionals can plan and provide appropriate services. In addition to transmitting necessary information, a carefully prepared examination report will also tend to establish the credibility of the SLP in the eyes of other workers. To state it another way, a written document is an extension of the diagnostician, and even minor errors in spelling or grammar may cast doubt upon the accuracy and attention to detail with respect to substantive material. Although the clinician may be highly skilled in testing and interviewing, competence may be evaluated by the clinician's written communications. Clinical reports are the principal way in which a clinician relates to other professionals.

FORMAT

There are several ways to organize a diagnostic report and books devoted to clinical documentation (Burrus & Haynes, 2009; Cornett, 2006; Goldfarb & Serpanos, 2009; Hegde & Davis, 2009;

Murray, 2003; Pannbacker et al., 2001; Shipley & McAfee, 2009). Because reports may vary, depending on the intended reader, no single schema is appropriate for all circumstances; in many instances, the format will be dictated by the agency the clinician serves. There appear to be three broad categories of report formats as a function of work setting:

- *University training programs and traditional clinics.* Student clinicians learn to write comprehensive reports that are robust in detail. These reports tend to be lengthy. They also typically contain numerous subheadings with a summary conclusion (and diagnosis) at the end of the report once all findings have been presented. This format also remains in wide use in most for-profit clinical settings because of its thoroughness of information, even when written with brevity.
- *Medical setting.* Clinicians writing reports for health professionals use a concise, textual writing style, typically no more than one to three pages in length. Often the clinical summary and functional level appear as the initial paragraph, so that physicians and other health care professionals may read the gist of the patient's situation quickly. Another report style utilized in these work settings is a concise outline format, often patterned by an acronym. The outline allows the reader to locate easily routine types of information in a standard location. Alternately, there are standard report forms that may be required by the medical setting and reimbursement agency that offer a fill-in-the-blank approach with only abbreviated space for textual results. Often the forms combine an assessment summary with a plan of treatment for physician approval. Forms from the Centers for Medicare and Medicaid Services (CMS) of the U.S. Department of Health and Human Services are of this type. The interested reader may view CMS forms (such as CMD 700 and CMS 806A) online at http://www.cms.hhs.gov/home/medicare.asp.
- *Public schools.* Clinicians prepare federally mandated reports that reflect required components. The writing style tends to be concise, as preprinted school system forms are often utilized.

Regardless of the format employed, a diagnostic report should be organized for easy retrieval of information and prepared in a manner that reflects high professional standards. Here are criteria that the clinician should use to judge a diagnostic report: Is it accurate? Is it complete? Is it efficiently written (clearly and with an economy of words)? Was it prepared promptly?

Figure 13.1 provides a generic format—one that we have found quite effective in university and traditional clinics, and that we recommend to the beginning clinician. It contains several major sections, which can be written in longhand for later typing or which can be stored as a template in a word-processing program for ease of editing. Commercial software also is available that provides a range of predesigned report templates. (Two examples can be found at http://www.treatwrite.com/simply and http://www.clinicianmagician.com/program_features.) Keatley, Miller, and Johnson (1998) provide a good overview of system considerations. We join Swigert (2006) and urge that, when using time-saving technology, the clinician ensure the report is individualized as a picture of a particular client. A good report always is more than a citation of scores.

Routine Information

In this section, we present basic identifying information—the client's name, sex, address, date of birth, telephone number, parent's name where relevant, and of course the date of the examination; an undated report is of very little use. In addition to these routine data, we generally identify the

I. Routine information

Name: File no.:

Sex: Code:

Address: Date:

Birth date: Phone no.:

Parents: Age at Evaluation:

Evaluated by: Referred by:

II. Statement of the Problem   Address:

III. Historical Information

IV. Evaluation

V. Clinical Impressions

VI. Summary

VII. Recommendations (and Prognosis)

_____
                                    Clinician

_____
                                  Supervisor

FIGURE 13.1 Format for diagnostic report.

referral source (parent, teacher, physician) and the evaluator. If the client is a school-aged child, we note the name and location of his or her school and the names of the teacher and the principal. The keystone of this initial section of the report is meticulous attention to accuracy. In this day of third-party reimbursement, this first section often indicates the client's diagnostic code as well. Appendix E of this text lists International Classification of Diseases (ICD) codes frequently used by the SLP.

Statement of the Problem

In this section, we include a succinct statement of the presenting problem. What is the complaint and who is making it? Be sure to distinguish between the client's complaint and the problem stated by the referral source. In most instances, the reason for referral is stated in the client's (or parent's) own words—always indicated by quotation marks.

Historical Information

Before seeing a client for evaluation, many clinicians request that the individual fill out a brief case history form. Alternately, this information can be gathered in a face-to-face interview. Rather than present a generic example of a case history form, we refer the reader to the case history forms cited in preceding chapters. Different information needs to be collected with specific disorders.

Information obtained from referral letters, the case history, and the intake interview are included in this section of the diagnostic report. Material regarding the client's development (general and speech and language); medical, educational, and familial history; and estimates of psychosocial and behavioral adjustments are summarized. Only the most pertinent items are included in the diagnostic report. Because most of the historical information is obtained by questioning the client, a parent, or other informants, we suggest that the clinician briefly describe the interview situation—type of rapport established, the frankness and completeness of the respondent's answers, and any other pertinent observations.

Evaluation

The results of the various tests and examinations are delineated in this section. Before describing the assessment procedures and results, however, we include an opening statement that describes how the client approached the clinical setting and the tasks used to evaluate the communication abilities: Was the client apprehensive, bored, fatigued, cooperative? The name of each test, an explanation of what it does and how it was administered, and the results obtained should be included. Should the clinician include statements about communication skills that are within normal limits at the time of the evaluation? It is standard practice for a complete diagnostic report to mention, even if briefly, all aspects of a client's speech, hearing, and language performance so that subsequent assessments can utilize the information as baseline observations. The information is simply presented, not interpreted, in this section of the report.

Clinical Impressions

In this section, we summarize our impressions of the individual and the communication impairment. What type of speech or language problem does the client have? How severe is it? What caused it? What factors seem to be perpetuating it? What impact has it had on the client and the client's family? How much does it interfere with everyday functioning? What are the prospects for treatment? Although we can offer interpretations here, we must still be able to support our impressions with information obtained during the interview or testing. Speculations based on previous clinical experience, such as similarity between the client and other cases the diagnostician has examined, should be clearly labeled as such.

Summary

The summary should be a concise (not more than a short paragraph) statement abstracting the salient features of the whole report. What is the communication disorder? What are the primary features of the disorder? What is the probable cause of the disorder? What is the prognosis (and general estimate of the predicted time frame) for recovery?

Recommendations

This is perhaps the most crucial portion of the report. We must now translate our findings into appropriate suggestions or directions that will help the client solve communication and related problems. Do we recommend further speech and language evaluations? Is a medical referral necessary? Is treatment indicated? What direction should be taken? By whom, and when? The task, then, is to crystallize all the disparate interactions we have had with the individual, collate all the data, and then provide a flexible blueprint for further action. We must attempt to answer the question: What happens now—where do we go from here? Try to make the recommendations specific and brief. Suggestions for treatment or a more lengthy plan of therapy can be outlined in a letter or follow-up report. One final warning: Do not recommend *specific* evaluations or remediation procedures to workers in other professions. It is improper, for example, to recommend a client for electroencephalography to a neurologist, or for dental braces to an orthodontist; the speech clinician would be chagrined if a physician referred a child and recommended the administration of a specific test. Be sure that your referrals for additional assessment are based on sound evidence; it is expensive, time consuming, and stressful to the client to make recommendations for comprehensive medical or psychiatric evaluation without serious and compelling reasons:

> Early in the diagnostic session with 5-year-old Mark we suspected the possibility of brain injury. Mindful of the family's limited finances, we wanted to document carefully all signs of apparent cerebral dysfunction before making a referral for a complete pediatric neurological evaluation. Observation revealed a number of serious symptoms: difficulty with motor coordination; labile emotions; rapid and slurred speech; perseveration; and blanking out spells. The necessity for referral was then obvious.

Recommendations and prognosis statements should not be misleading or unrealistic. A clinician's awareness of evidence-based practice can guide him or her in such matters. Consider the example provided by Roth and Worthington (2005) for a 60-year-old male with moderate aphasia whose stroke had been 10 years earlier:

> Based on Mr. Hanks's high level of enthusiasm, the prognosis for improvement in therapy is good.

Why is this prognostic statement inappropriate? First, a client's degree of enthusiasm is not a reliable indicator of success. Second and important, the amount of time that has elapsed since the stroke would warrant a more guarded prognosis, since the aphasia literature is clear that recovery of function is time sensitive. Third, the improvement of "what" is not specific.

Clinicians in a medical setting may record their findings in a "problem-oriented" format (Kent & Chabon, 1980). Problem-oriented medical records (POMR) feature a carefully defined and documented list of problems, which encompass all the significant difficulties a patient is experiencing. The list includes the presenting complaint as well as those problems identified by the members of the treatment team. For example, a patient who suffered a CVA might have right hemiparesis and aphasia leading to problems with daily activities (e.g., feeding, dressing), locomotion, language, intelligibility, and the like. Ideally placed at the front of the patient's file, this list of problems generated by the multidisciplinary team points to areas needing further assessment and/or intervention. All available information about the person is then organized under the four headings shown in Figure 13.2. The four headings of information form the acronym SOAP. Daily chart documentations, as well as diagnostic reports, can be written by using the SOAP format. Progress notes need to be concise. The SOAP format is employed by most medical disciplines and is an excellent tool for guiding professionals, including the SLP, toward brevity. The SOAP format ensures that key information on the day's (or week's) session is recorded. All that is necessary is a brief statement on the patient's level of cooperation, motivation, or frustration (subjective), a citation of what tasks were attempted and at what levels of stimulation or cueing (objectives), levels of accuracy to which tasks were performed (assessments), and logical next steps in the rehabilitation program (plan).

SUBJECTIVE	OBJECTIVE	ASSESSMENT	PLAN
Interview and case history	Test results	Collation of subjective and objective information	Additional testing Treatment options

FIGURE 13.2   The SOAP format for medical reports.

In recent years, there has been a growing trend in healthcare toward the use of "functional outcome measures," in which the patient's behaviors are assessed categorically relative to levels of function. The Functional Communication Measures, a component of ASHA's Program Evaluation System, have a broad range of clinical applicability.

Another example is the Functional Independence Measure (FIM) (Research Foundation, 1990). The FIM rates patient dependence-independence on a seven-level scale; the ratings are made by a multidisciplinary team on various categories, such as communication, social cognition, locomotion, self-care, and the like. Some facilities have used FIM levels to aid in patient selection and discharge decisions, as well as to track progress over time. The brevity of the FIM has led some agencies to more in-depth descriptors, such as a Pathway record.

A Pathway format typically organizes patient information in columns representing phases or changes over time. Phase 1 entries critique the patient's status at the time of admission, often using FIM levels (1–7 ratings). A stroke Pathway might include items in medical/nursing, nutrition, swallowing, mobility, self-care, cognition, communication, and others completed by the team. Pathways tracking also includes discharge planning and community reentry skills. Detailed Pathways can be appended by specific healthcare professionals for each area, as would be the case for a communication assessment by an SLP.

Public school clinicians use specialized procedures and report formats with components mandated by law (i.e., PL 94-142, PL 99-457, and PL 105-17 IDEA-A). As part of the IDEA legislation, a school's Intervention Assistance Team (IAT), which includes a child's parents, may suspect that a child has a disability and so initiate testing. Testing is called a multifactored evaluation because it covers a wide range of skills (e.g., cognitive, language, academic, social-emotional, and visual-motor skills). The SLP is an important team member. Although there is no mandated format for the IAT evaluation report, four main sections are typical: (1) identifying information, (2) background information, (3) assessment results, and (4) intervention plans. When all multifactorial components are compiled, the assessment team meets with the parents to explain the results. Information about the child's learning strengths and weaknesses is discussed and, based on federal regulations, the child's eligibility for special education services is decided.

If the child qualifies and the parents accept, the team determines how best to meet the child's educational needs. An Individualized Education Plan (IEP) must be written specifying goals for the school year. The IEP process is where the SLP details the speech-language goals for the child and the best presentation method for addressing the goals (e.g., in the classroom, through consultation, individual or small group pullout services, and so forth). The IEP is a student-focused plan devised by the team.

The updated standards in IDEA-A require that IEPs include parent involvement, focus on the general curriculum (so an SLP *must* collaborate with classroom teachers), verify team members as "qualified providers," mention needed accommodations, require assessments, and require progress reports. According to Blosser and Neidecker (2002), federal regulations specify the following IEP contents:

- Demographic information and a description of the student's communication impairment
- Present levels of educational performance
- Annual goals and short-term objectives
- Amount of special education or related services
- Supplementary aids and services (accommodations, assistive devices)
- Extent of participation with students without disabilities
- Projected dates for initiation of services and the anticipated frequency and duration of the services
- Objective criteria and evaluation procedures for determining on at least an annual basis whether the short-term instructional objectives are being achieved

The IEP is a working document; the IEP team—including the parents—can make alterations or eliminate goals, as appropriate. Figure 13.3 displays a portion of an IEP prepared for a child with a phonological disorder. The ASHA website provides a template for writing IEP goals and objectives, based on those of the state of Illinois.

Student: <u>David Grabowski</u>　　　　Birthdate: <u>1/7/04</u>　　　　Address: <u>224 Orchard</u>
Parents: <u>Gerard and Julie</u>　　　　District/School: <u>Beaver Grove Schools</u>
Grade: <u>First</u>　　　　　　　　　　District of residency: <u>Marquette County</u>
IEP conference date: <u>9/12/10</u>　　Projected IEP review date: <u>9/10/11</u>

Eligibility Statement: (What decision/description requires this service?)
David has difficulty with frictional manner of articulation production resulting in several substitutional errors: th/s, th/z, s/sh, ts/ch, dz/dj.

Current Eductional Level: (Where is child currently functioning?)
David is enrolled in a developmental first-grade classroom.

Special Services		
Goals	Objectives	Service description
1. David will produce *s, z* correctly at the word and sentence level. 2. David will produce *sh* correctly at the word and sentence level. 3. Progress reports will be sent to parents and teacher twice a year.	1. David will discriminate target sounds from other sounds with 90% accuracy. 2. David will produce target sounds at the beginning, middle, and end of single words with 90% accuracy. 3. David will correctly produce target sounds within sentences with 80% success.	Speech therapy

Dates of Services		Time in Programs	Responsible Individuals
Start	End	Daily	Speech-language clinician
9/19/10	5/1/11	Within small-group 20-minute sessions 2 times a week. In regular classroom rest of school week.	Supplementary aides
			None

Evaluation Plan: (How is it planned to ascertain that goals have been reached?)
1. Goldman-Fristoe Test of Articulation
2. Pre- and post-therapy word list containing target sounds
3. Five-minute sample of spontaneous speech

IEP Committee Members:

Name	Position
Ellen Mattson	Teacher
Roy Brown, Jr.	Principal
Rebecca Clark	Speech-language clinician
Gerard and Julie Grabowski	Parents

FIGURE 13.3　Individualized educational program.

This can be accessed at http://www.health.state.nm.us/.../SLP_SAMPLEANNUALPRO-GRESSREPORT.pdf. The U.S. Department of Education has published model formats for the IEP, as well as other related notices. These forms describe the minimal content needed to comply with regulatory requirements. To download the IEP format models and related information, visit http://idea.ed.gov.

The SLP in the schools is also responsible for writing the Individualized Family Service Plan (IFSP). The assessment of infants and toddlers (birth to 3 years) presents special considerations in terms of record keeping and evaluation procedures. Clearly, the family as well as the child's health are targets of assessment and possible intervention. Public Law 99-457 requires a multidisciplinary team approach to assessment of this population, since no single agency or discipline can meet the diverse needs of infants, toddlers, and their families. After assessment, the team is required by law to generate an IFSP that has the following components:

1. A statement of the child's present levels of development (cognitive, speech-language, hearing, motor, self-help, social)
2. A statement of the family's strengths and needs related to enhancing the child's development
3. A statement of major outcomes expected to be achieved for the child and family
4. The criteria, procedures, and time lines for determining progress
5. The specific early intervention services necessary to meet the unique needs of the child and family, including the method, frequency, and intensity of services
6. The projected dates for the initiation of service and the projected duration
7. The name of the case manager
8. The procedures for transition from early intervention into the preschool

One can readily see that the format of the IFSP has clear implications for assessment. First, it mandates family assessment that forces the SLP to focus on the child's total environmental system. Second, it requires that judgments be made in a variety of areas that need multidisciplinary cooperation (e.g., cognitive, social, language, motor, hearing). Third, it requires the practitioner to recommend evaluation procedures to be used to determine progress. The clinician needs to be prepared to address the issues included in the IFSP when he or she participates in staff meetings with other professionals subsequent to his or her evaluations of these children.

IDEA and IDEA-A mandated that schools should plan for the transition of a student with disabilities from school to work or other postsecondary activities from age 14 onward. The assessment of students of this age must be comprehensive to prognose and plan for educational, vocational, and social eventualities. The Individual Transition Plan (ITP) is another report format, similar to the IEP, which school-based speech-language pathologists write. Blosser and Neidecker (2002) can be consulted for details.

We would like to close this discussion of component parts and styles of the report by suggesting that the clinician or the employing agency audit a sample number of diagnostic reports for format compliance. Patient care audits are part of the national health care monitoring system for quality assurance. Patient care audits may focus on the quality of care provided patients through a variety of channels, including thoroughness of evaluation and diagnosis, treatment procedures, and audits of patient outcomes. The first is pertinent to this chapter: Files can be retrospectively analyzed to see whether or not routine components are present in the diagnostic report. Before doing a patient care audit of "quality of reports," the clinician or agency must have specified minimal requirements beforehand—such things as inclusion of the client's date of birth; mention of referral source, chart number, and date of evaluation; and performance of a hearing test, oral peripheral examination, and the like. Presetting some desired level of compliance is also necessary (e.g., "At least 90% of the audited reports will have . . ."). We recommend patient care audits, even if self-administered, as a good spot check of compliance with professional standards of information collection and reporting. When deficiencies are found, the clinician can target specific areas for needed improvement and/or can adjust clinical procedures and expectations.

Before leaving this discussion on formats, we wish to remind the reader that, after the initial diagnostic assessment, there are numerous opportunities to reevaluate the client. Indeed, this is the premise of this book that is reflected in its title. Subsequent formal evaluations, informal evaluations, probes, and progress documentation are necessary. The various formats we have presented are easily adapted to these purposes. Sample annual reevaluation and progress report formats can be viewed at http://www.health.state.nm.us/.../SLP_SAMPLEANNUALPRO-GRESSREPORT.pdf.

CONFIDENTIALITY

In our view, confidentiality is basic to any helping profession. All reports and records should be kept secure so that no harm or embarrassment comes to the persons we serve. The privacy and security of documentation must be maintained in compliance with the regulations of the Health Insurance Portability and Accountability Act (HIPAA). When a diagnostic report is released, we prefer to mail it to a specific person rather than to the agency itself. Before releasing any information about a client, however, we must secure the client's permission in writing; most speech and hearing centers have permission forms, which are completed prior to or during the diagnostic session.

Because clients and parents have a legal right (Public Law 93-380, Family Educational Rights and Privacy Act of 1974, known as FERPA) to read any report containing information about them, we often find it useful to send them a copy of the diagnostic findings. Before mailing the report, however, we always review our findings and recommendations with them. By going over the report with the clients or parents, we can be sure that they understand its contents.

Of interest is that Watson and Thompson (1983) researched parental perceptions of both diagnostic reports and conferences that followed the diagnostic session. Ninety percent of parents indicated understanding the clinical results as presented in a face-to-face conference. Likewise, 89% of the parents stated they understood the conclusions of the written report. Although these figures are high, they suggest that as clinicians there is room to improve our professional oral and written communication skills.

STYLE

In the interest of brevity, we shall simply enumerate several principles of style that we have found useful.

1. Make your presentation straightforward and objective, using a topical outline. Use simple, brief, but complete sentences. It is often helpful to write for a specific reader; picture the reader in your mind—the classroom teacher, physician, speech clinician—and then simply tell the story of what you observed and recommend regarding a particular client. When in doubt about a reader's level of understanding, it is better to err on the side of simplicity.

2. Use an impersonal style. Some clinicians use the first person when writing diagnostic reports, but in our view it is preferable to keep the "I" out of it; a reference to "the clinician" or "the examiner" is more in keeping with professional reports. We prefer to individualize the client described in the report, not the writer. Furthermore, we believe that not only does an impersonal style help to minimize the writer's verbal idiosyncracies, but it also tends to encourage objectivity.

3. Edit the report carefully to make certain that spelling and use of tenses, grammar, and punctuation are accurate. Errors, even trivial ones, undermine the confidence of the reader in the diagnostician. Remember, competence is judged to a great extent by the precision of your reporting.

4. Watch your semantics. Be wary of overused or nebulous words such as "nice," "hopefully," "good," and the like. Avoid pet expressions or stereotyped ways of phrasing information. One clinician used the phrase "in terms of" 13 times in a two-page diagnostic report. Another laced his reports with currently popular words like "input," "interface," and "scenario." Some writers use the word "feel" inappropriately in statements like "The clinician felt the client understood the diagnostic task"; we believe (not feel!) that the word should be reserved for discussing emotions or tactile sensations. Use abbreviations sparingly. Avoid superlatives unless they are clearly indicated.

5. Avoid preparing an "Aunt Fanny" report—a bland written statement that could represent anyone or is so filled with qualifications ("perhaps," "apparently," "tends to") that it reveals nothing—nothing, that is, except a timid diagnostician.

6. Make the report "tight." Do not leave gaps or ambiguity where it is possible to read between the lines. If findings in certain areas are unremarkable, always state this explicitly. Do not leave the reader to guess whether you have investigated all possible aspects.

7. A diagnostic report is no place to display your learning or to parade a large vocabulary. Pedantic reports are misunderstood or unread.

8. Stay close to the data until you wish to draw the observations together and make some interpretations. For example, tell the reader which sounds were in error instead of simply stating that the child sounds infantile.

9. The very essence of good style is the willingness to take the time and energy to write and rewrite the report until it communicates what the clinician did and what the clinician found in the diagnostic session.

THE WRITING PROCESS

Many students have difficulty writing reports. Most of them have found the task onerous, and a few are threatened and overwhelmed by the prospect of summarizing all that has been done. It has been our experience, however, that rather than have a writing deficiency, most of these students have a writing bias—they do not think they can do it. There are, of course, no quick and simple solutions; but we offer the following suggestions that have proven helpful to more than one beginning report writer.

Write on a daily basis. Each night—before retiring, for example—sit down and write a descriptive paragraph concerning something that happened to you that day. At the end of the week, review the writing you have done; edit, revise, ask yourself what you meant by each word or phrase. The best way to learn to write, in our opinion, is to write.

Get the message out and revise it later. It is especially important in writing reports to begin as soon as possible while the material is still fresh in your mind. A common error that some beginning writers make is to attempt to produce perfect writing in the initial draft. It does not matter how it looks at this point; you can always edit or have someone help you edit. When you meet barriers or mental blocks, do not linger; jump over them and go on with the rest of the report. When you come back later, you will find that your mind has filled in the blank spots.

It is helpful to have someone read and comment on the initial draft of your report. Although it is difficult to submit one's prose for dissection, ask the reader to be frank and honest in his or her editing. So many times, a phrase that seems clear to the writer who conceived it is vague or obscure to an objective reader.

FOLLOW-UP

The clinician's responsibilities do not end when the diagnostic report is finished and filed. A complete evaluation includes one final important task: a careful follow-up. It is the examiner's professional obligation to determine that the diagnostic activities and recommendations are translated into action; it is useless, perhaps even harmful, to identify and describe problems unless the individual is seen for further testing or treatment as soon as possible. When the diagnostician is also the clinician, the follow-up can be handled directly and with a minimum of paperwork. In an agency such as ours, however (a university speech and hearing clinic), we regularly refer clients to other workers for further assessment or treatment. We use the following questions as guidelines in implementing a follow-up program:

1. Did the intended readers receive the report? The best of secretaries occasionally misfiles a document, so we generally call the referral source within a week after the diagnostic to determine if the report has arrived.

2. Does the reader understand the contents of the report? What questions did it raise, if any, about the client? We always log these phone calls in the client's folder.

3. What is the disposition of the client? Is the client being seen for further testing? Is the client on a waiting list or being seen for treatment?

4. How is the client responding to treatment? We call the local worker, usually on a monthly basis, to assess how the client is doing in treatment relative to our recommendations. Not only does this convey our interest and assistance, it also helps the diagnostic team evaluate the efficacy of its work.

SUMMARY

According to ASHA (2004), comprehensive assessment must be sensitive to cultural and linguistic diversity and also address the World Health Organization's *International Classification of Functioning, Disability and Health* (2002). This framework has guided much of the information presented in this book. Likewise, this book has shared ASHA's view on the clinical process of assessment: that it may be static (using procedures designed to describe current levels of functioning) and/or dynamic (using hypothesis-testing procedures to identify potentially successful intervention procedures). The comprehensive diagnostic—and report writing—processes presented in this chapter, and indeed this book, echo the following aspects cited by ASHA as necessary and important.

- Collect and summarize the relevant case history, including medical status, education, vocation, and socioeconomic, cultural, and linguistic backgrounds.
- Review the client's auditory, visual, motor, and cognitive status.
- Interview the client and the family.

- Measure with standardized and nonstandardized methods the specific aspects of speech, spoken and nonspoken language, cognitive-communication, and swallowing function.
- Analyze associated medical, behavioral, environmental, educational, vocational, social, and emotional factors.
- Identify the potential for effective intervention strategies and compensations.
- Select assessment instruments with consideration for documented ecological validity.
- Follow up services to monitor communication and swallowing status and ensure appropriate intervention and support for individuals with identified speech, language, cognitive-communication and/or swallowing disorders.

Report writing in the profession takes many and varied forms but succinct, accurate, clear, and grammatically correct documentation is a necessity and reflects well on the SLP. Preferred practice patterns of documentation as presented in this chapter and summarized by ASHA (2004) follow:

- Documentation includes pertinent background information, results and interpretation, prognosis, and recommendations indicating the need for further assessment, follow-up, or referral. When intervention is recommended, information is provided concerning the frequency, estimated duration, and type of service (e.g., individual, group, home program) required.
- Documentation addresses the type and severity of the communication or related disorder or difference, associated conditions (e.g., medical or educational diagnoses) and impact on activity and participation (e.g., educational, vocational, social).
- Documentation includes summaries of previous services in accordance with all relevant legal and agency guidelines.
- Results of the assessment are reported to the individual and family/caregivers, as appropriate and with written consent.
- The privacy and security of documentation are maintained in compliance with HIPAA, FERPA, and other state and federal laws.

APPENDIX A

Early Child Language Assessment Interview Protocol

GENERAL INFORMATION
PERTINENT HISTORY

- Referral source:
- Parent's statement of the problem:
- History of prior assessments:
- History of prior treatments:
- Parental treatment attempts:
- Daycare/Preschool status:
- Number and relationships of people living at home:

BIOLOGICAL PREREQUISITES FOR COMMUNICATION DEVELOPMENT
BIRTH AND GENERAL HEALTH

- Pregnancy:
- Birth:
- History of child illnesses:
- Present state of child's health:

AUDITORY STATUS

- History of frequent colds:
- History of earaches and ear infections:
- Parent's estimation of hearing acuity:

NEUROLOGICAL STATUS

- Concussions/Unconsciousness:
- Seizures:
- Has the child been seen by a neurologist? For what condition?
- Does the child evidence any motor difficulties?

GENERAL DEVELOPMENT

- Concern about self-help skills?
- Concern about fine and gross motor development?
- Concern about social development?
- Concern about communication development?

SOCIAL PREREQUISITES FOR COMMUNICATION DEVELOPMENT

- Approximate time spent in social interaction on typical day:
- Who are the persons the child frequently interacts with?
- What are the activities associated with social interactions?
- Does the child exhibit any antisocial or socially inappropriate behaviors (avoiding interactions, consistent playing alone?)
- Does the child exhibit any self-stimulating behaviors (e.g., rocking, flapping arms, etc.)?
- Does the child maintain eye contact?
- Does the child regulate your behavior nonverbally through gestures or physical manipulation?
- Does the child use objects or repeat actions to get your attention?
- Does the child vocalize during his or her social interactions?
- Does the child joint reference with the caretaker?
- Describe the child's typical day in detail:

COGNITIVE PREREQUISITES TO COMMUNICATION DEVELOPMENT

Does the child exhibit play routines and behavior which would indicate the following attainments (specify example activity):

- Object permanence:
- Means–end:
- Immediate imitation:
- Functional use of objects:
- Deferred imitation:
- Symbolic play with own body:
- Symbolic play with objects:
- Symbolic play with surrogate objects:
- Distal pointing:
- Combining more than one object at a time in play:
- What are the child's most frequent play activities?

COMMUNICATION DEVELOPMENT

- Does the child exhibit phonetically consistent forms?
- Parent estimation of the number of single words used expressively?
- Parent estimation of MLU?
- Reports of presyntactic devices?
- Parent's report of semantic relation types?
- Parent estimate of language comprehension?
- Parent estimate of child's intelligibility?

APPENDIX B

Coding Sheet for Early Multiword Analysis

Child   *Post Stage I*

Utterance	Semantic Relation	Function	Initiation	Element
Pushing car	Action + Object	Regulate action	Child Initiated	-ing
Push it	Action + Object	Regulate action	Child Initiated	
Car going	Instrument + Action	Label/comment	Child Initiated	-ing
More car	Recurrence + X	Regulate action	Child Initiated	
Car all gone?	X + Disappearance	Questioning	Child Initiated	
Juice up there	Entity + Locative	Elicited imitation	Adult Initiated	
Gimme juice	Action + Object	Regulating action	Child Initiated	
That truck	Nomination + X	Answering	Adult Initiated	
Ball	Personal/Social	Label/comment	Child Initiated	
Me ball	Possessor + Possession	Protest	Child Initiated	
No	Personal/Social	Protest	Child Initiated	
Mommy throw	Agent + Action	Regulating action	Child Initiated	
Throw it	Action + Object	Regulating action	Child Initiated	
Go there	Action + Locative	Answering	Adult Initiated	
Horsie	General Nominal	Answering	Adult Initiated	
Big horsie	Attribute + Entity	Spontaneous imitation	Child Initiated	
Me riding	Agent + Action	Label/comment	Child Initiated	-ing
More ride	Recurrence + X	Questioning	Child Initiated	
Please	Personal/Social	Regulating action	Child Initiated	
Put on table	Action + Locative	Regulating action	Child Initiated	on

APPENDIX C

Summary Sheet for Early Multiword Analysis

Child: _____ Age: _____ Birth Date: _____ Sample Date: _____

Context of Sample (Include people and objects present):

Length of Sample in Time:

Activities Performed during Sample:

Mean Length of Utterance (Column 1 of Coding Sheet):

Total Number of Child Utterances (Column 1 of Coding Sheet):

Longest Utterance in Morphemes (Column 1 of Coding Sheet):

Number of Single-Word Responses (Column 1 of Coding Sheet):

Semantic Relations Evident in Sample (Column 2 of Coding Sheet):

Functions Evident in Sample (Column 3 of Coding Sheet):

Percentages of Child- and Adult-Initiated Utterances (Column 4 of Coding Sheet):

Post Stage I Elements Noted (Column 5 of Coding Sheet):

Semantic Relations Missing from Sample:

Functions Missing from Sample:

APPENDIX D

Data Consolidation in Limited Language Evaluations

IDENTIFYING INFORMATION

Name: Address:
Telephone: Parents:
Date of Evaluation: Date of Birth: Age:

DATA OBTAINED IN EVALUATION

case history
reports from professionals
hearing screening
oral peripheral
behavioral observation of caretaker—
    child
behavioral observation of clinician—
    child
parental checklist (lexicon)
adaptive behavior scale
general developmental battery
spontaneous communication sample

nonstandardized tasks
cognitive scale
comprehension test
language battery
other

ANALYSES PERFORMED ON DATA

MLU
distributional analysis
early multiword analysis (semantic
    relations/functions)
communicative gesture analysis
cognitive analysis of play
vocalization analysis
phonetic inventory
phonological analysis
caretaker—child interaction analysis
scoring of standardized measurements
analysis of social behavior (e.g., turn-taking,
    joint referencing)
scoring of nonstandardized procedures
other

AREAS OF STRENGTH (+) AND CONCERN (−)

Biological

Hearing _____
Neurological _____
Medical _____
Anatomical _____

Cognitive

Play level _____
SM substage _____
Symbolic play _____

Social

Reciprocity _____
Play partner _____

Adaptive Behavior

Self-help _____
Gross motor _____
Fine motor _____
Social _____

Communicative Intent

Imperatives _____
Declaratives _____
Level _____
Rate _____

Single Words

Number _____
Variety _____
Functions _____

Early Multiword Combinations	**Phonology**	**Caretaker Strategies**
Variety _____	Phonetic inv. _____	Joint referencing _____
Productivity _____	Processes _____	Model _____
MLU _____		

RECOMMENDATIONS

Referrals: Further Testing by SLP: Prognosis:

Treatment Directions:

APPENDIX E

Diagnostic and Procedural Codes

The *International Classification of Diseases, Ninth Revision, Clinical Modification (ICD-9-CM)* is based on the World Health Organization's index for classifying diseases numerically. The system has become the standard for maintaining health statistics. Importantly, diagnostic and inpatient procedural codes also are used for reimbursements by third parties, including Medicare. Inclusion of the ICD Code—and other types of codes—have become an important feature of the diagnostic report. ASHA's web site (http://www.asha.org) is an excellent source for coding information, and it is useful for staying abreast of coding changes that affect speech-language pathologists. An example of this is White's (2009) overview of voice, resonance, and cerebrovascular disease code expansions. Also through ASHA is McCarthy's (2006) 66-page tutorial on billing, coding, and calculating fees that is an excellent primer for the novice to this vast subject.

Codes covering various diagnoses within communication disorders have been summarized elsewhere (ASHA's web site mentioned above; Blosser & Neidecker, 2002; Buck, 2010). The rubric of ICD-9-CM codes designates the first 3 digits for the diagnostic category. Following the decimal, a fourth and even fifth digit may be necessary to further specify the disorder. For example, 315.3 denotes Developmental Speech or Language. The later is further delineated as:

315.31 Expressive language disorder

315.32 Mixed receptive-expressive language disorder

315.34 Speech and language developmental delay due to hearing loss

315.39 Other (developmental articulation disorder, dyslalia, phonological disorder)

All 5 digits, when available in a coding reference book, should be used or the claim may be denied. Another ICD-9-CM example is provided for the voice and resonance disorders code of 784.4:

784.40 Voice and resonance disorders, unspecified

784.41 Aphonia, loss of voice

784.42 Dysphonia, hoarseness

784.43 Hypernasality

784.44 Hyponasality

784.49 Other voice and resonance disorders

These examples have shown some commonly used *diagnostic codes* in speech-language pathology.

In addition to serving as diagnostic codes, ICD-9-CM codes also exist to describe *inpatient hospital procedures,* and speech-language pathologists in such work settings mark them on the superbill for the coding/billing personnel. Very typically the SLP works in a setting that sees outpatients, and so the SLP should code *outpatient procedures* using a different system for procedures while retaining the diagnostic code. Current Procedural Terminology, or CPT, codes describe procedures that "are done" with the client. CPT codes are necessary for reimbursement. Some examples of diagnostic procedural codes for billing include the following:

> 92506 Evaluation of speech, language, voice, communication, and/or auditory processing
>
> 92520 Laryngeal function study (aerodynamic testing, acoustic testing)
>
> 92597 Evaluation for use and/or fitting of voice device
>
> 92607 Evaluation for prescription of speech-generating AAC device
>
> 92610 Evaluation of oral and pharyngeal swallowing function

These are just a few of the many CPT codes useful to describe the diagnostic efforts. There are many other CPT codes for treatment procedures; however, a discussion of these is beyond the scope of this book.

CPT codes may be supplemented by the Healthcare Common Procedural Coding System (HCPCS), Level I and/or Level II. Although some procedures are coded in this system, the HCPCS often covers devices and supplies. Table E.1 provides an overview of the three types of codes described in this appendix. When submitting claims to third-party payors, it is necessary to include both a diagnostic code as well as a procedure code (whichever code type is appropriate), as it is the medical diagnosis that justifies why evaluative and/or treatment procedures were performed. Coding is an extensive and necessary component of practice in the communication disorders. The SLP is advised to read available resources, such as those cited at the beginning of this appendix, as well as to seek guidance from a coding specialist when beginning to file claims for reimbursement.

TABLE E.1   Coding Systems for SLPs at a Glance

	ICD-9-CM	CPT	HCPCS (Level I)
Purpose	Reporting diagnosis, disorders, symptoms	Reporting procedures (evaluation or treatment)	Reporting supplies and equipment; some procedures
Code Type	Three digits followed by decimal and, when possible, two more digits for greater specification (e.g., 784.51 Dysarthria) Include additional alphanumeric V-Code to report other factors esp. if in comprehensive rehabilitation (such as OT and PT) (e.g., V 573)	Five digits (e.g., 92610 Evaluation of oral and pharyngeal swallowing function)	Alphanumeric (e.g., audiology screening)
Oversight	U.S. Department of Health and Human Services	American Medical Association	Centers for Medicare and Medicaid

REFERENCES

Aase, D., Hovre, C., Krause, K., Schelfhout, S., Smith, J., and Carpenter, L. (2000). *Contextual Test of Articulation.* Eau Claire, WI: Thinking Publications.

Adamovich, B. (1998). "Outcomes Measurement in Cognitive Communication Disorders: Traumatic Brain Injury." In *Measuring Outcomes in Speech-Language Pathology,* ed. C. Frattali (New York: Thieme).

Adamovich, B., and Henderson, J. (1992). *Scales of Cognition Ability for Traumatic Brain Injury (SCATBI).* Chicago: Riverside Publishing.

Adams, M. (1977). "A Clinical Strategy for Differentiating the Normally Nonfluent Child and the Incipient Stutterer." *Journal of Fluency Disorders* 2:141–148.

Adler, S. (1990). "Multicultural Clients: Implications for the SLP." *Language, Speech and Hearing Services in Schools* 21:135–139.

ADVANCE (2010). "Landmark Study Suggests Verbal Apraxia Symptoms Are Part of Larger Syndrome." *ADVANCE for Speech-Language Pathologists & Audiologists* 20(1):20.

Allen, D., Bliss, L., and Timmons, J. (1981). "Language Evaluation: Science or Art?" *Journal of Speech and Hearing Disorders* 46:66–68.

Als, H., Lester, B., Tronick, E., and Brazelton, T. (1982). "Toward a Research Instrument for the Assessment of Preterm Infants' Behavior (APIB)." In *Theory and Research in Behavioral Pediatrics,* Vol. 1, eds. H. Fitzgeralt, B. Lester, and M. Yogman (New York: Plenum Press).

Ambrose, N., and Yairi, E. (1994). "The Development of Awareness of Stuttering in Preschool Children." *Journal of Fluency Disorders* 19:229–245.

Ambrose, N., and Yairi, E. (1999). "Normative Disfluency Data for Early Childhood Stuttering." *Journal of Speech, Language, and Hearing Research* 42:895–909.

American Heritage Dictionary (1985). Boston, MA: Houghton Mifflin.

American Speech-Language-Hearing Association (1995). *Directory of Speech-Language Pathology Assessment Instruments.* Rockville, MD.

American Speech-Language-Hearing Association (2004). "Preferred Practice Patterns for the Profession of Speech-Language Pathology." Available at http://www.asha.org/members/deskref-journals/deskref/default

American Speech-Language-Hearing Association (2005). "Evidence-Based Practice in Communication Disorders" [position statement]. Available at http://www.asha.org/members/deskref-journals/deskref/default

Amerman, J., Daniloff, R., and Moll, K. (1970). "Lip and Jaw Coarticulation for the Phoneme /æ/." *Journal of Speech and Hearing Research* 13:148–161.

Amir, O., and Ezrati-Vinacour, R. (2002). "Stuttering in a Volatile Society—Israel." Newsletter for the ASHA special interest division 14: *Perspectives on Communication Disorders and Sciences in Culturally and Linguistically Diverse Populations* 8(2):13–14.

Ammons, R., and Johnson, W. (1944). "Studies in the Psychology of Stuttering." *Journal of Speech Disorders* 9:39–49.

Anastasi, A. (1976). *Psychological Testing.* New York: Macmillan.

Anastasi, A. (1997). *Psychological Testing,* 7th ed. Upper Saddle River, NJ: Prentice Hall.

Anderson, B. (1976). "An Analysis of the Relationship of Age and Sex to Type and Frequency of Disfluencies in Lower Socioeconomic Preschool Black Children." *Dissertation Abstracts International* 7:75–81.

Anderson, R. (1996). "Assessing the Grammar of Spanish-Speaking Children: A Comparison of Two Procedures." *Language, Speech and Hearing Services in Schools* 27:333–344.

Anderson-Yockel, J., and Haynes, W. (1994). "Joint Book Reading Strategies in Working Class African American and White Mother-Toddler Dyads." *Journal of Speech and Hearing Research* 37:583–593.

Andersson, L. (2005). "Determining the Adequacy of Tests of Children's Language." *Communication Disorders Quarterly* 26(4):207–225.

Andrews, G., and Cutler, J. (1974). "Stuttering Therapy: The Relation between Changes in Symptom Level and Attitudes." *Journal of Speech and Hearing Disorders* 39:312–319.

Andrews, N., and Fey, M. (1986). "Analysis of the Speech of Phonologically Impaired Children in Two Sampling

Conditions." *Language, Speech and Hearing Services in Schools* 17:187–198.

Apel, K. (1999). "An Introduction to Assessment and Intervention with Older Students with Language-Learning Impairments: Bridges from Research to Clinical Practice." *Language, Speech and Hearing Services in Schools* 30: 228–230.

Apel, K., and Swank, L. (1999). "Second Chances: Improving Decoding Skills in the Older Student." *Language, Speech and Hearing Services in Schools* 30:231–242.

Applebee, A. (1978). *The Child's Concept of a Story: Ages 2 to 17.* Chicago: University of Chicago Press.

Aram, D., and Nation, J. (1980). "Preschool Language Disorders and Subsequent Language and Academic Difficulties." *Journal of Communication Disorders* 13:159–170.

Armstrong, L., Borthwick, S. E., Bayles, K. A., and Tomoeda, C. K. (1996). "Use of the Arizona Battery for Communication Disorders of Dementia in the UK." *European Journal of Disorders of Communication* 31:171–180.

Arndt, J., and Healey, E. C. (2001). "Concomitant Disorders in School-Age Children Who Stutter." *Language, Speech and Hearing Services in Schools* 32:68–78.

Arvedson, J. C. (1993). "Oral-Motor and Feeding Assessment." In *Pediatric Swallowing and Feeding,* eds. J. C. Arvedson and L. Brodsky (San Diego, CA: Singular Publishing).

Arvedson, J. (2009). *Evaluation of Pediatric Feeding and Swallowing* (DVD and manual). Washington, DC: ASHA.

Arvedson, J. C., and Brodsky, L. (2002). *Pediatric Swallowing and Feeding Assessment and Management.* San Diego, CA: Thomson Delmar.

ASHA (2004). *ASHA Supplement,* No. 222, 7:73–87.

ASHA (2007). "Childhood Apraxia of Speech Ad Hoc Committee on Apraxia of Speech in Children." Accessed from http://www.asha.org/docs/html/TR2007—00278.html

ASHA (2008). "Incidence and Prevalence of Speech, Voice and Language Disorders in Adults in the United States." Accessed from http://www.asha.org/research/reports/speech_voice_language.htm, 41(2):195–198.

ASHA Forum (2009). "Cluttering Information and Issues," a January 2009 forum conducted by ASHA. The archived discussion is available to ASHA members at the password-protected ASHA.com site.

Atkins, C., and Cartwright, L. (1982). "An Investigation of the Effectiveness of Three Language Elicitation Procedures on Headstart Children." *Language, Speech and Hearing Services in Schools* 13:33–36.

Awan, S. N. (2001). *The Voice Diagnostic Protocol: A Practical Guide to the Diagnosis of Voice Disorders.* Austin, TX: Pro-Ed.

Awan, S., and Roy, N. (2009). "Outcome Measures in Voice Disorders: Application of an Acoustic Index of Dysphonia Severity." *Journal of Speech, Language, Hearing Research* 52:482–499.

Bailey, D., and Simeonsson, R. (1988). *Family Assessment in Early Intervention.* Columbus, OH: Merrill.

Bain, B., and Olswang, L. (1995). "Examining Readiness for Learning Two Word Utterances by Children with Specific Expressive Language Impairment: Dynamic Assessment Validation." *American Journal of Speech-Language Pathology* 4:81–91.

Balason, D., and Dollaghan, C. (2002). "Grammatical Morpheme Production in 4-Year-Old Children." *Journal of Speech, Language, and Hearing Research* 45: 961–969.

Ball, E. (1993). "Assessing Phoneme Awareness." *Language, Speech and Hearing Services in Schools* 24:130–139.

Ball, M., & Gibbon, F. (2001). *Vowel Disorders.* Woburn, MA: Butterworth Heineman.

Baltaxe, C., and Simmons, J. (1975). "Language in Childhood Psychosis: A Review." *Journal of Speech and Hearing Disorders* 40:439–458.

Bankson, N., and Bernthal, J. (1990). *Bankson-Bernthal Test of Phonology.* Austin, TX: Pro-Ed.

Bariley, R., and Staskowski, M. (2009) *Dysarthria Intervention in Schools Team Development and Treatment Strategies.* Washinton, DC: ASHA.

Barlow, J. (2001a). "Recent Advances in Phonological Theory and Treatment." *Language, Speech and Hearing Services in Schools* 32:225–228.

Barlow, J. (2001b). "Case Study: Optimality Theory and the Assessment and Treatment of Phonological Disorders." *Language, Speech and Hearing Services in Schools* 32:242–256.

Barlow, J. (2002). "Recent Advances in Phonological Theory and Treatment: Part II." *Language, Speech and Hearing Services in Schools* 33:4–8.

Barnes, E., Roberts, J., Long, S., Martin, G., Berni, M., Mandulak, K., and Sideris, J. (2009). "Phonological Accuracy and Intelligibility in Connected Speech of Boys with Fragile X Syndrome or Down Syndrome." *Journal of Speech, Language and Hearing Research* 52:1048–1061.

Barrie-Blackley, S., Musselwhite, C., and Rogister, S. (1978). *Clinical Oral Language Sampling*. Danville, IL: Interstate.

Bartko, J. (1976). "On Various Intraclass Correlation Reliability Coefficients." *Psychological Bulletin* 83(5):762–765.

Bashir, A., Kuban, K., Kleinman, S., and Scavuzzo, A. (1983). "Issues in Language Disorders: Considerations of Cause, Maintenance and Change." In *ASHA Report No. 12*, eds. J. Miller, D. Yoder, and R. Shiefelbusch (Rockville, MD: American Speech-Hearing-Language Association.)

Bates, E. (1976). *Language in Context*. New York: Academic Press.

Bates, E. (1979). *The Emergence of Symbols: Cognition and Communication in Infancy*. New York: Academic Press.

Bates, E., Bretherton, I., and Snyder, L. (1988). *From First Words to Grammar*. Cambridge, MA: Cambridge University Press.

Battle, D., et al. (1983). "Position Paper—Social Dialects." *Journal of the American Speech-Language-Hearing Association* 25:23–24.

Battle, D. (2002). *Communication Disorders in Multicultural Populations*, 3rd ed. Boston, MA: Butterworth-Heinemann.

Battle, J. (1992). *Culture-Free and Self-Esteem Inventories*, 2nd ed. Austin, TX: Pro-Ed.

Bayles, K. A. (1984). "Language and Dementia." In *Language Disorders in Adults: Recent Advances*, ed. A. L. Holland (San Diego, CA: College-Hill).

Bayles, K. A., and Kaszniak, A. W. (1987). *Communication and Cognition in Normal Aging and Dementia*. San Diego, CA: College-Hill.

Bayles, K. A., and Tomoeda, C. K. (1993). *The Arizona Battery for Communication Disorders of Dementia*. Tucson, AZ: Canyonlands Publishing.

Bayles, K. A., and Tomoeda, C. K. (1994). *The Functional Linguistic Communication Inventory*. Tucson, AZ: Canyonlands Publishing.

Bayles, K. A., and Tomoeda, C. K. (2007). *Communication Disorders of Dementia*. San Diego, CA: Plural Publishing.

Beach, T. (2002). *Oral Motor Toolbox*. Austin, TX: Pro-Ed.

Beard, R. (1969). *An Outline of Piaget's Developmental Psychology for Students and Teachers*. New York: Basic Books.

Bedrosian, J. (1985). "An Approach to Developing Conversational Competence." In *School Discourse Problems*, eds. D. Ripich and F. Spinelli (San Diego, CA: College-Hill Press).

Bellandese, M. H., Lerman, J. W., and Gilbert, H. R. (2001). "An Acoustic Analysis of Excellent Female Esophageal, Tracheoesophageal, and Laryngeal Speakers." *Journal of Speech, Language and Hearing Research* 44:1315–1320.

Benedict, H. (1975). "Early Lexical Development: Comprehension and Production." *Journal of Child Language* 6:183–200.

Benson, J. E., and Lefton-Greif, M. A. (1994). "Videofluoroscopy of Swallowing in Pediatric Patients: A Component of the Total Feeding Evaluation." In *Disorders of Feeding and Swallowing in Infants and Children: Pathophysiology, Diagnosis, and Treatment*, eds. D. N. Tuchman and R. S. Walter (San Diego, CA: Singular Publishing).

Benton, A. L., and Hamsher, K. (1989). *Multilingual Aphasia Examination*. Palo Alto, CA: Psychological Corporation.

Bernhardt, B., and Holdgrafer, G. (2001a). "Beyond the Basics I: The Need for Strategic Sampling for In-depth Phonological Analysis." *Language, Speech and Hearing Services in Schools* 32:18–27.

Bernhardt, B., and Holdgrafer, G. (2001b). "Beyond the Basics II: Supplemental Sampling for In-depth Phonological Analysis." *Language, Speech and Hearing Services in Schools* 32:28–37.

Bernhardt, B., and Stoel-Gammon, C. (1994). "Nonlinear Phonology: Introduction and Clinical Applications." *Journal of Speech and Hearing Research* 37:123–143.

Bernthal, J., and Bankson, N. (1988). *Articulation and Phonological Disorders*. Needham Heights, MA: Allyn & Bacon.

Bernthal, J., Bankson, N., and Flipsen, P. (2009). *Articulation and Phonological Disorders*, 6th ed. Boston, MA: Allyn & Bacon.

Beukelman, D., and Mirenda, P. (1992). *Augmentative and Alternative Communication*. Baltimore, MD: Paul H. Brookes.

Beukelman, D., and Mirenda, P. (1998). *Augmentative and Alternative Communication: Management of Severe Communication Disorders in Children and Adults*. Baltimore, MD: Paul H. Brookes.

Beving, B., and Eblen, R. (1973). "Same and Different Concepts and Children's Performance on Speech Sound Discrimination." *Journal of Speech and Hearing Research* 16:513–517.

Biddle, A., Watson, L., Hooper, C., Lohr, K., and Sutton, S. (2002). "Criteria for Determining Disability in Speech-Language Disorders." From *Agency for Healthcare Research and Quality Evidence Report No. 52*, Department of Health and Human Services. Accessed October 20, 2006 at http://www.ncbi.nlm.nih.gov/books/bv.fcgi?rid=hstal1.chapter.76986

Bird, E. K., Cleave, P., Trudeau, N., Thordardottir, E., Sutton, A., and Thorpe, A. (2005). "The Language Abilities of Bilingual Children with Down Syndrome." *American Journal of Speech-Language Pathology* 14:187–199.

Bird, J., Bishop, D., and Freeman, N. (1995). "Phonological Awareness and Literacy Development in Children with Expressive Phonological Impairments." *Journal of Speech and Hearing Research* 38:446–462.

Bishop, D., North, T., and Donlan, C. (1996). "Nonword Repetition as a Behavioral Marker for Inherited Language Impairment: Evidence from a Twin Study." *Journal of Child Psychology and Psychiatry* 36:1–13.

Blache, S. (1978). *The Acquisition of Distinctive Features*. Baltimore, MD: University Park Press.

Blagden, C., and McConnell, N. (1983). *Interpersonal Language Skills Assessment*. Moline, IL: Linguisystems.

Blakely, R. W. (2001). "Treatment of Developmental Apraxia of Speech." In *Current Therapy Communication Disorders: Dysarthria and Apraxia*, ed. W. H. Perkins (New York: Thieme-Stratton).

Bleile, K., and Wallach, H. (1992). "A Sociolinguistic Investigation of the Speech of African American Preschoolers." *American Journal of Speech-Language Pathology* 1:54–61.

Blodgett, E., and Cooper, E. (1987). *Analysis of the Language of Learning: The Practical Test of Metalinguistics*. Moline, IL: Linguisystems.

Blood, G., Blood, I., Kreiger, J., and O'Connor, S. (2009). "Double Jeopardy for Children Who stutter: Race and Coexisting Disorders." *Communication Disorders Quarterly* 30(3):131–141.

Blood, G., and Conture, E. (1998). "Outcomes Measurement Issues in Fluency Disorders." In *Measuring Outcomes in Speech-Language Pathology*, ed. C. Frattali (New York: Thieme).

Bloodstein, O., and Ratner, N. (2008). *A Handbook on Stuttering*, 6th ed. Clifton Park, NY: Delmar.

Bloom, L. (1970). *Language Development: Form and Function in Emerging Grammars*. Cambridge, MA: MIT Press.

Bloom, L. (1973). *One Word at a Time: The Use of Single Word Utterances Before Syntax*. The Hague: Mouton.

Bloom, L., and Lahey, M. (1978). *Language Development and Language Disorders*. New York: Wiley.

Bloom, L., Lightbrown, P., and Hood, L. (1975). "Structure and Variation in Child Language." *Monographs of the Society for Research in Child Development* 40:1–41.

Blosser, J. L., and Neidecker, E. A. (2002). *School Programs in Speech-Language Pathology: Organization and Service Delivery*. Boston, MA: Allyn & Bacon.

Bondy, A., and Frost, L. (1998). "The Picture Exchange Communication System." *Seminars in Speech and Language* 19:373–389.

Boone, D. (1993). *The Boone Voice Program for Children*, 2nd ed. Austin, TX: Pro-Ed.

Boone, D. (2000). *The Boone Voice Program for Adults*, 3rd ed. Austin, TX: Pro-Ed.

Boone, D., McFarlane, S. C., Von Berg, S., and Zraich, R. (2010). *The Voice and Voice Therapy*, 8th ed. Boston, MA: Allyn & Bacon.

Bopp, K., Brown, K., and Mirenda, P. (2004). "Speech-Language Pathologists' Roles in the Delivery of Positive Behavior Support for Individuals with Developmental Disabilities." *American Journal of Speech-Language Pathology* 13:5–19.

Bopp, K., Mirenda, P., & Zumbo, B. (2009). "Behavior Predictors of Language Development over 2 Years in

Children with Autism Spectrum Disorders." *Journal of Speech, Language and Hearing Research* 52:1106–1120.

Bornstein, M., Tal, J., and Tamis-Lemonda, C. (1991a). "Parenting in Cross-Cultural Perspective: The United States, France and Japan." In *Cultural Approaches to Parenting,* ed. M. Bornstein (Hillsdale, NJ: Lawrence Erlbaum Associates).

Bornstein, M., Tamis-Lemonda, C., Pecheux, M., and Rahn, C. (1991b). "Mother and Infant Activity and Interaction in France and the United States: A Comparative Study." *International Journal of Behavioral Development* 14:21–43.

Borsel, J. A., Maes, E., & Foulon, S. (2001). "Stuttering and Bilingualism: A Review." *Journal of Fluency Disorders* 26:179–205.

Boscolo-Rizzo, P., Maronato, F., Marchiori. C., Gava, A., and Mosto, M. C. (2008). "Long-term Quality of Life After Total Laryngectomy and Postoperative Radiotherapy versus Concurrent Chemoradiotherapy for Laryngeal Preservation." *Laryngoscope* 118:300–306.

Boseley, M., Cunningham, M., Volk, M., and Hartnick, C. (2006). "Validity of the Pediatric Voice-Related Quality-of-Life Survey." *Archives of Otolaryngology, Head and Neck Surgery*, 132(7):717–720.

Boseley, M. E., and Hartnick, C. J. (2004). "Assessing the Outcome of Surgery to Correct Velopharyngeal Insufficiency with Pediatric Outcomes Surgery." *International Journal of Pediatric Otorhinolaryngology* 68(11):1429–1433.

Bosma-Smit, A., and Hand, L. (1996). *SmitHand Articulation and Phonology Evaluation (SHAPE).* Los Angeles: Western Psychological Services.

Bosone, Z. (1999). "Tracheoesophageal Speech: Treatment Considerations Before and After Surgery." In *Alaryngeal Speech Rehabilitation,* 2nd ed., ed. S. Salmon (Austin, TX: Pro-Ed).

Bothe, A. K. (2004). *Evidence-Based Treatment of Stuttering.* Mahwah, NJ: Erlbaum.

Boudreau, D. (2005). "Use of a Parent Questionnaire in Emergent and Early Literacy Assessment of Preschool Children." *Language, Speech and Hearing Services in Schools* 36:33–47.

Boudreau, D., and Hedberg, N. (1999) "A Comparison of Early Literacy Skills in Children with Specific Language Impairment and Their Typically Developing Peers." *American Journal of Speech-Language Pathology* 8:249–260.

Bowerman, M. (1973). "Structural Relationships in Children's Utterances: Syntactic or Semantic?" In *Cognitive Development and the Acquisition of Language,* ed. T. Moore (New York: Academic Press).

Bowerman, M. (1974). "Development of Concepts Underlying Language." In *Language Perspectives: Acquisition, Retardation, and Intervention,* eds. R. Schiefelbusch and L. Lloyd (Baltimore, MD: University Park Press).

Bowman, S., Parsons, C., and Morris, D. (1984). "Inconsistency of Phonological Errors in Developmental Verbal Dyspraxic Children as a Factor of Linguistic Task and Performance Load." *Australian Journal of Human Communication Disorders* 10:109–120.

Brackenbury, T., and Pye, C. (2005). "Semantic Deficits in Children with Language Impairments: Issues for Clinical Assessment." *Language, Speech and Hearing Services in Schools* 36:5–16.

Brady, N., Marquis, J., Fleming, K., and McLean, L. (2004). "Prelinguistic Predictors of Language Growth in Children with Developmental Disabilities." *Journal of Speech, Language and Hearing Research* 47:663–677.

Brady, W. A., and Hall, D. E. (1976). "The Prevalence of Stuttering among School-Age Children." *Language, Speech and Hearing Services in Schools* 7:75–81.

Braine, M. (1963). "The Ontogeny of English Phrase Structure: The First Phrase." *Language* 39:1–14.

Braine, M. (1976). "Children's First Word Combinations." *Monographs of the Society for Research in Child Development* 41:1–104.

Bransford, J., and Nitsch, K. (1978). "Coming to Understand Things We Could Not Previously Understand." In *Speech and Language in the Laboratory, School and Clinic,* eds. J. Kavanagh and W. Strange (Cambridge, MA: MIT Press).

Brazelton, T. (1984). *Neonatal Behavior Assessment Scale.* Philadelphia: Lippincott.

Bricker, D., Squires, J., and Mounts, L. (1995). *Ages and Stages Questionnaire (ASQ): A Parent-Completed, Child Monitoring System.* Baltimore, MD: Paul H. Brookes.

Brinton, B., and Fujiki, M. (1984). "Development of Topic Manipulation Skills in Discourse." *Journal of Speech and Hearing Research* 27:350–358.

Brinton, B., and Fujiki, M. (1989). *Conversational Management with Language-Impaired Children.* Rockville, MD: Aspen.

Bronfenbrenner, U. (1979). *The Ecology of Human Development.* Cambridge, MA: Harvard University Press.

Brown, L., Sherbenou, R., and Johnson, S. (2010). *Test of Nonverbal Intelligence–Fourth Edition* (TONI-4). Austin, TX: Pro-Ed.

Brown, R. (1973). *A First Language: The Early Stages.* Cambridge, MA: Harvard University Press.

Brown, R., and Fraser, C. (1963). "The Acquisition of Syntax." In *Verbal Behavior and Learning: Problems and Processes,* eds. C. Cofer and B. Musgrave (New York: McGraw-Hill).

Brunson, K., and Haynes, W. (1991). "Profiling Teacher/Child Classroom Communication: Reliability of an Alternating Time Sampling Procedure." *Child Language Teaching and Therapy* 7(2):192–212.

Brutten, E., and Dunham, S. (1989). "The Communication Attitude Test: A Normative Study of Grade School Children." *Journal of Fluency Disorders* 14:371–377.

Brutten, E. J., and Miller, R. (1988). "The Disfluencies of Normally Fluent Black First Graders." *Journal of Fluency Disorders* 13:291–299.

Brutten, E., and Shoemaker, D. (1974). *The Southern Illinois Behavior Check List.* Carbondale: Southern Illinois University.

Bryan, K. L. (1995). *The Right-Hemisphere Language Battery,* 2nd ed. London: Whurr Publishers.

Buck, C. (2010). *2010 ICD-9-CM, Volumes 1 & 2.* Maryland Heights, MO: Sanders Elsevier.

Bunting, G. (2004). "Voice Following Laryngeal Cancer Surgery: Troubleshooting Common Problems After Tracheoesophageal Voice Restoration." *Otolaryngologic Clinics of North America* 37(3):597–612.

Burrus, A., and Haynes, W. (2009). *Professional Communication in Speech-Language Pathology.* San Diego, CA: Plural.

Bzoch, K. (2004). *Communicative Disorders Related to Cleft Lip and Palate,* 5th ed. Austin, TX: Pro-Ed.

Cabell, S., Justice, L., Zucker, T., and Kilday, C. (2009). "Validity of Teacher Report for Assessing the Emergent Literacy Skills of At-Risk Preschoolers." *Language, Speech and Hearing Services in Schools* 40:161–173.

Caesar, L., & Kohler, P. (2007). "The State of School-Based Bilingual Assessment: Actual Practice versus Recommended Guidelines." *Language, Speech and Hearing Services in Schools* 38:190–200.

Calandrella, A., and Wilcox, M. (2000). "Predicting Language Outcomes for Young Prelinguistic Children with Developmental Delay." *Journal of Speech, Language and Hearing Research* 43:1061–1071.

Camarata, S., and Schwartz, L. (1985). "Production of Object Words and Action Words: Evidence for a Relationship between Phonology and Semantics." *Journal of Speech and Hearing Research* 28:323–330.

Campbell, J., and Shriberg, L. (1982). "Associations among Pragmatic Functions, Linguistic Stress and Natural Phonological Processes in Speech Delayed Children." *Journal of Speech and Hearing Research* 25:547–553.

Campbell, T., Dollaghan, C., Needleman, H., and Janosky, J. (1997). "Reducing Bias in Language Assessment: Processing Dependent Measures." *Journal of Speech, Language and Hearing Research* 40:519–525.

Canning, B., and Rose, M. (1974). "Clinical Measurements of the Speed of Tongue and Lip Movements in British Children with Normal Speech." *British Journal of Disorders of Communication* 9:45–50.

Caplan, D., and Bub, D. (1990). "Psycholinguistic Assessment of Aphasia." Miniseminar presented at the Annual Convention of the American Speech-Language-Hearing Association, Seattle, WA.

Capone, N. (2007). Tapping toddlers' evolving semantic representation via gesture. *Journal of Speech, Language and Hearing Research* 50:732–745.

Capone, N., & McGregor, K. (2004). "Gesture Development: A Review for Clinical and Research Practices." *Journal of Speech, Language and Hearing Research* 47:173–186.

Carding, P., and Horsley, I. A. (1992). An evaluation study of voice therapy in non-organic dysphonia." *International Journal of Language and Communication Disorders* 27(2):137–158.

Carpenter, M. (1999). "Treatment Decisions in Alaryngeal Speech." In *Alaryngeal Speech Rehabilitation,* 2nd ed., ed. S. Salmon (Austin, TX: Pro-Ed).

Carrow-Woolfolk, E. (1985). *Test for Auditory Comprehension of Language-Revised.* Allen, TX: DLM Teaching Resources.

Case, J. L. (1996). *Clinical Management of Voice Disorders,* 3rd ed. Austin, TX: Pro-Ed.

Case-Smith, J. (1988). "An Efficacy Study of Occupational Therapy with High-Risk Neonates." *The American Journal of Occupational Therapy* 42:499–506.

Catts, H. (1993). "The Relationship between Speech-Language Impairments and Reading Disabilities." *Journal of Speech and Hearing Research* 36:948–958.

Catts, H. (1997). "The Early Identification of Language-Based Reading Disabilities." *Language, Speech and Hearing Services in Schools* 28:86–89.

Catts, H., et al. (2001). "Estimating the Risk of Future Reading Difficulties in Kindergarten Children: A Research Based Model and Its Clinical Implications." *Language, Speech and Hearing Services in Schools* 32:38–50.

Cazden, C. (1970). "The Neglected Situation of Child Language Research and Education." In *Language and Poverty: Perspectives on a Theme,* ed. F. Williams (Chicago, IL: Rand-McNally).

Chabon, S., Udolf, L., and Egolf, D. (1982). "The Temporal Reliability of Brown's Mean Length of Utterance Measure with Post Stage V Children." *Journal of Speech and Hearing Research* 25:124–128.

Chafe, W. (1970). *Meaning and the Structure of Language.* Chicago, IL: University of Chicago Press.

Channell, R. (2003). "Automated Developmental Sentence Scoring using Computerized Profiling Software." *American Journal of Speech-Language Pathology* 12:369–375.

Chapey, R. (2001). " Cognitive Stimulation: Stimulation of Recognition/Comprehension, Memory, and Convergent, Divergent and Evaluative Thinking." In *Language Intervention Strategies in Aphasia and Related Neurogenic Communication Disorders,* 4th ed., ed. R. Chapey (Philadelphia, PA: Lippincott Williams and Wilkins).

Chapman, R. (1978). "Comprehension Strategies in Children." In *Speech and Language in the Laboratory, School and Clinic,* eds. J. Kavanagh and W. Strange (Cambridge, MA: MIT Press).

Chapman, R. (1981). "Exploring Children's Communicative Intents." In *Assessing Language Production in Children: Experimental Procedures,* ed. J. Miller (Baltimore: University Park Press).

Chappel, G., and Johnson, G. (1976). "Evaluation of Cognitive Behavior in Young Nonverbal Children." *Language, Speech and Hearing Services in Schools* 7:17–27.

Cheng, L., (1989). "Service Delivery to Asian/Pacific LEP Children: A Cross-Cultural Framework." *Topics in Language Disorders* 9:1–14.

Cherney, L. R., Pannelli, J. J., and Cantiere, C. A. (1994). "Clinical Evaluation of Dysphagia in Adults." In *Clinical Management of Dysphagia in Adults and Children,* 2nd ed., ed. L. R. Cherney (Gaithersburg, MD: Aspen Publishers).

Chiat, S., & Roy, P. (2007). "The Preschool Repetition Test: An Evaluation of Performance in Typically Developing and Clinically Referred Children." *Journal of Speech, Language and Hearing Research* 50:429–443.

Chomsky, N. (1957). *Syntactic Structures.* The Hague: Mouton.

Chomsky, N., and Halle, M. (1968). *The Sound Pattern of English.* New York: Harper and Row.

Clark, D. (1989). "Neonates and Infants At Risk for Hearing and Speech-Language Disorders." *Topics in Language Disorders* 10(1):1–12.

Clune, C., Paolella, J., and Foley, J. (1979). "Free Play Behavior of Atypical Children: An Approach to Assessment." *Journal of Autism and Developmental Disorders* 9:61–72.

Code, C., Heer, M., and Schofield, M. (1989). *The Computerized Boston.* Palo Alto, CA: Psychological Corporation.

Coggins, T., and Carpenter, R. (1978). "Categories for Coding Prespeech Intentional Communication." Unpublished manuscript, University of Washington, Seattle.

Cole, E., and St. Clair-Stokes, J. (1984). "Caregiver-Child Interactive Behavior: A Videotape Analysis Procedure." *Volta Review* 86: 200–217.

Cole, P., and Taylor, O. (1990). "Performance of Working-Class African American Children on Three Tests of Articulation." *Language, Speech and Hearing Services in Schools* 21:171–176.

Coleman, D., Cook, A., and Meyers, L. (1980). "Assessing Non-Oral Clients for Assistive Communication Devices." *Journal of Speech and Hearing Disorders* 45:515–527.

Coleman, R. F., Michel, J., and Lynn, P. (1987). "Use and Misuse of Instrumental Analysis in Clinical Voice Practice." Paper presented at annual convention of the American Speech-Language-Hearing Association, New Orleans, LA.

Compton, A. (1970). "Generative Studies of Children's Phonological Disorders." *Journal of Speech and Hearing Disorders* 35:315–339.

Compton, A. (1976). "Generative Studies of Children's Phonological Disorders." In *Normal and Deficient Child Language,* eds. D. Morehead and A. Morehead (Baltimore, MD: University Park Press).

Compton, A., and Hutton, S. (1978). *Compton-Hutton Phonological Assessment.* San Francisco, CA: Carousel House.

Compton, C. (1996). *A Guide to 100 Tests for Special Education.* Upper Saddle River, NJ: Globe Fearon Educational.

Conrad, C. (1992). "Fluency in Multicultural Populations." In *Communication Disorders in Multicultural Populations,* eds. L. Cole and V. Deal (Rockville, MD: ASHA).

Conti-Ramsden, G. & Durkin, K. (2008). "Language and Independence in Adolescents with and without a History of Specific Language Impairment (SLI)." *Journal of Speech, Language and Hearing Research* 51:70–83.

Conture, E. (2001). *Stuttering: Its Nature, Diagnosis and Treatment.* Needham Heights, MA: Allyn & Bacon.

Conture, E., and Curlee, R. (2008). *Stuttering and Related Disorders of Fluency,* 3rd ed. New York: Thieme.

Cooper, E. B., and Cooper, C. (2003). *Personalized Fluency Control Therapy for Adolescents and Adults.* Austin, TX: Pro-Ed.

Cooper, E. B., and Cooper, C. (2004). *Personalized Fluency Control Therapy for Children.* Austin, TX: Pro-Ed.

Cornett, B. S. (2006 Sept. 5). "Clinical Documentation in Speech-Language Pathology Essential Information for Successful Practice." *The ASHA Leader* 11(12):8–9, 24–25.

Cosby, M., and Ruder, K. (1983). "Symbolic Play and Early Language Development in Normal and Mentally Retarded Children." *Journal of Speech and Hearing Research* 25:404–411.

Costello, J., and Onstine, J. (1976). "The Modification of Multiple Articulation Errors Based on Distinctive Feature Theory." *Journal of Speech and Hearing Disorders* 41:199–215.

Cowley, M. (1980). *The View from 80.* New York: Viking.

Craig, H., and Evans, J. (1993). "Pragmatics and SLI: Within-Group Variations in Discourse Behaviors." *Journal of Speech and Hearing Research* 36:777–789.

Craig, H., and Washington, J. (2002). "Oral Language Expectations for African American Preschoolers and Kindergartners." *American Journal of Speech-Language Pathology* 11:59–70.

Craig, H., and Washington, J. (2004). "Grade-Related Changes in the Production of African American English." *Journal of Speech, Language and Hearing Research* 47:450–463.

Craig, H., Washington, J., and Thompson, C. (2005). "Oral Language Expectations for African American Children in Grades 1 through 5." *American Journal of Speech-Language Pathology* 14:119–130.

Craig, H., Zhang, L., Hensel, S., and Quinn, E. (2009). "African American English Speaking Students: An Examination of the Relationship between Dialect Shifting and Reading Outcomes." *Journal of Speech, Language and Hearing Research* 52:839–855.

Crais, E. (1995). "Expanding the Repertoire of Tools and Techniques for Assessing the Communication Skills of Infants and Toddlers." *American Journal of Speech-Language Pathology* 4:47–59.

Crais, E., Douglas, D., and Campbell, C. (2004). "The Intersection of the Development of Gestures and Intentionality." *Journal of Speech, Language and Hearing Research* 47:678–694.

Crais, E., and Roberts, J. (1991). "Decision Making in Assessment and Early Intervention Planning." *Language, Speech and Hearing Services in Schools* 22:19–30.

Crais, E., Watson, L., and Baranek, G. (2009). "Use of Gesture Development in Profiling Children's Prelinguistic Communication Skills." *American Journal of Speech-Language Pathology* 18:95–108.

Crary, M. A. (1988). "A Multifaceted Perspective on Developmental Apraxia of Speech." Paper presented to the convention of the Speech and Hearing Association of Alabama, Orange Beach, AL.

Crary, M., Haak, N. J., and Malinsky, A. (1989). "Preliminary Psychometric Evaluation of an Acute Aphasia Screening Protocol." *Aphasiology* 3:611–618.

Crystal, D., Fletcher, P., and Garman, M. (1976). *The Grammatical Analysis of Language Disability: A Procedure for Assessment and Remediation.* London: Edward Arnold.

Cunningham, R., Farrow, V., Davies, C., and Lincoln, N. (1995). "Reliability of the Assessment of Communicative Effectiveness in Severe Aphasia." *European Journal of Disorders of Communication* 30:1–16.

Curcio, F. (1978). "Sensorimotor Functioning and Communication in Mute Autistic Children." *Journal of Autism and Childhood Schizophrenia* 8:281–292.

Curenton, S., and Justice, L. (2004). "African American and Caucasian Preschoolers' Use of Decontextualized Language: Literate Language Features in Oral Narratives." *Language, Speech and Hearing Services in Schools* 35:240–253.

Dabul, B. (2000). *Apraxia Battery for Adults.* Austin, TX: Pro-Ed.

Dale, P. (1980). "Is Early Pragmatic Development Measureable?" *Journal of Child Language* 7:1–12.

Daly, D. A. (1986). "The Clutterer." In *The Atypical Stutterer: Principles and Practices of Rehabilitation,* ed. K. O. St. Louis (Orlando, FL: Academic Press).

Damico, J. (1980). "Clinical Discourse Analysis." Miniseminar presented at the convention of the American Speech-Language-Hearing Association, Detroit, MI.

Damico, J. (1985). "Clinical Discourse Analysis: A Functional Approach to Language Assessment." In *Communication Skills and Classroom Success: Assessment of Language-Learning Disabled Students,* ed. C. Simon (San Diego, CA: College-Hill).

Damico, J., and Oller, J. (1980). "Pragmatic Versus Morphological/Syntactic Criteria for Language Referrals." *Language, Speech and Hearing Services in Schools* 11:85–94.

Daniloff, R., and Moll, K. (1968). "Coarticulation of Lip Rounding." *Journal of Speech and Hearing Research* 11:707–721.

Davies, A. E., Kidd, D., Stone, S. P., and MacMahaon, J. (1995). "Pharyngeal Sensation and Gag Reflex in Healthy Subjects." *Lancet* 345:487–488.

Davis, B., and MacNeilage, P. (1990). "Acquisition of Correct Vowel Production: A Quantitative Case Study." *Journal of Speech and Hearing Research* 33(1):16–27.

Davis-McFarland, E. (2008). "Family and Cultural Issues in a School Swallowing and Feeding Program." *Language, Speech and Hearing Services in Schools* 33(2):199–213.

Deary, I., Webb, A., MacKenzie, K., Wilson, J., and Carding, P. (2004). "Short, Self-Report Symptom Scales: Psychometric Characteristics of the Voice Handicap Index-10 and the Vocal Performance Questionnaire." *Otolaryngology—Head and Neck Surgery* 131(3):232–235.

Deary, I. J., Wilson, J. A., Carding, P. N., and Mackenzie, L. (2003). "VoiSS—A Patient-Derived Voice System Scale." *Journal of Psychosomatic Research* 54(5):483–489.

Dejonckere, P. H. (2000). "Perceptual and Laboratory Assessment of Dysphonia." *Otolaryngology Clinics of North America* 33:731–750.

Dietrich, S., and Roaman, M. (2001). "Physiologic Arousal and Predictions of Anxiety by People Who Stutter." *Journal of Fluency Disorders* 26:207–225.

Dillard, J. (1972). *Black English.* New York: Random House.

Dinnsen, D. (1984). "Methods of Empirical Issues in Analyzing Functional Misarticulation." *Phonological Theory and the Misarticulating Child,* ASHA Monographs 22:5–17.

Dinnsen, D. (1985). "A Re-Examination of Phonological Neutralization." *Journal of Linguistics* 21:265–279.

Dinnsen, D., and O'Connor, K. (2001). "Implicationally Related Error Patterns and the Selection of Treatment Targets." *Language, Speech and Hearing Services in Schools* 32:257–270.

Dobres, R., Lee, L., Stemple, J. C., Kummer, A. W., and Kretschmer, L. W. (1990). "Description of Laryngeal Pathologies in Children Evaluated by Otolaryngologists." *Journal of Speech and Hearing Disorders* 55:526–532.

Dodd, B., Hua, Z., Crosbie, S., Holm, A., & Ozanne, A. (2006). *Diagnostic Evaluation of Articulation and Phonology (DEAP).* San Antonio, TX: Harcourt Assessment.

Dollaghan, C., and Campbell, T. (1998). "Nonword Repetition and Child Language Impairment." *Journal of Speech, Language and Hearing Research* 41:1136–1146.

Donaldson, M. (1978). *Children's Minds.* London: Fontana.

Dore, J. (1975). "Holophrases, Speech Acts and Language Universals." *Journal of Child Language* 2:21–40.

Dore, J., et al. (1976). "Transitional Phenomena in Early Language Acquisition." *Journal of Child Language* 3:13–28.

Drummond, S. S. (1993). *Dysarthria Examination Battery (DEB).* San Antonio: Communication Skill Builders.

Drumwright, A. (1971). *The Denver Articulation Examination.* Denver, CO: Ladoca Project and Publishing Foundation.

Dubois, E., and Bernthal, J. (1978). "A Comparison of Three Methods for Obtaining Articulatory Responses." *Journal of Speech and Hearing Disorders* 43:295–305.

Duchan, J., and Weitzner-Lin, B. (1987). "Nurturant-Naturalistic Intervention for Language Impaired Children: Implications for Planning Lessons and Tracking Progress." *Journal of the American Speech and Hearing Association* 29(7):45–49.

Duffy, J. R. (2005). *Motor Speech Disorders: Substrates, Differential Diagnosis, and Management,* 2nd ed. St. Louis, MO: Elsevier Mosby.

Duffy, M. C., Proctor, A., and Yairi, E. (2004). "Prevalence of Voice Disorders in African American and European American Preschoolers." *Journal of Voice* 18(3):348–353.

Dunst, C. (1980). *A Clinical and Educational Manual for Use with the Uzigiris and Hunt Scales of Infant Psychological Development.* Baltimore, MD: University Park Press.

Dworkin, J. P., and Culatta, R. A. (1996). *Dworkin-Culatta Oral Mechanism Examination and Treatment System.* Nicholasville, KY: Edgewood Press.

Dworkin, J., Marurick, M., and Krouse, J. (2004). "Velopharyngeal Dysfunction: Speech Characteristics, Variable Etiologies, Evaluation Techniques, and Differential Treatments." *Language, Speech and Hearing Services in Schools* 35(4):333–352.

Dwyer, C., Robb, M., and O'Beirne, G. (2009). The influence of speaking rate on nasality in the speech of hearing-impaired individuals. *Journal of Speech, Language, and Hearing Research* 56:1321–1333.

Dykes, R. L. (1995). "Prevalence of Stuttering among African-American School-Age Children in the South: A Survey of Speech-Language Pathologists' Caseloads." Unpublished master's thesis, Auburn University, AL.

Dyson, A. (1988). "Phonetic Inventories of 2- and 3-Year-Old Children." *Journal of Speech and Hearing Disorders* 53(1):89–93.

Dyson, A., and Robinson, T. (1987). "The Effect of Phonological Analysis Procedure on the Selection of Potential Remediation Targets." *Language, Speech and Hearing Services in Schools* 18:364–377.

Edmonds, P., and Haynes, W. (1988). "Topic Manipulation and Conversational Participation as a Function of Familiarity in School-Age Language-Impaired and Normal Language Peers." *Journal of Communication Disorders* 21:209–228.

Edmonson, W. (1969). *The Laradon Articulation Scale.* Denver, CO: Laradon Hall.

Edmonston, N., and Thane, N. (1992). "Children's Use of Comprehension Strategies in Response to Relational Words: Implications for Assessment." *American Journal of Speech-Language Pathology* 1:30–35.

Edwards, M. (1992). "In Support of Phonological Processes." *Language, Speech and Hearing Services in Schools* 23:233–240.

Ehlers, P., and Cirrin, F. (1983). "Topic Relevancy Abilities of Language-Impaired Children." Paper presented at the annual convention of the American Speech-Language-Hearing Association, Cincinnati, OH.

Ehren, B. (1993). "Eligibility, Evaluation and the Realities of Role Definition in the Schools." *American Journal of Speech Language Pathology* 2(1):20–23.

Ehren, B., Montgomery, J., Rudebush, J., and Whitmire, K. (2009). "Responsiveness to Intervention: New Roles for Speech-Language Pathologists." American Speech-Language-Hearing Association. Retrieved from http://www.asha.org/members/slp/schools/prof-consult/NewRolesSLP.htm

Eisenberg, A., and Smith, R. (1971). *Nonverbal Communication.* New York: Bobbs-Merrill.

Eisenberg, S. (2005). "When Conversation Is Not Enough: Assessing Infinitival Complements Through Elicitation." *American Journal of Speech-Language Pathology* 14:92–106.

Eisenberg, S., Fersko, T., and Lundgren, C. (2001). "The Use of MLU for Identifying Language Impairment in Preschool Children: A Review." *American Journal of Speech-Language Pathology* 10:323–342.

Eisenberg, S., Ukrainetz, T., Hsu, J., Kaderavek, J., Justice, L., & Gillam, R. (2008). "Noun Phrase Elaboration in Children's Spoken Stories." *Language, Speech and Hearing Services in Schools* 39:145–157.

Eisenson, J. (2008). *Examining for Aphasia,* 4th ed. Austin, TX: Pro-Ed.

Elbert, M. (1992). "Consideration of Error Types: A Response to Fey." *Language, Speech and Hearing Services in Schools* 23:241–246.

Elbert, M., and Gierut, J. (1986). *Handbook of Clinical Phonology: Approaches to Assessment and Treatment,* San Diego, CA: College-Hill.

Ellis-Weismer, S., Tomblin, J., Zhang, X., Buckwalter, P., Chynoweth, J., and Jones, M. (2000). "Nonword Repetition Performance in School-Age Children with and without Language Impairment." *Journal of Speech, Language and Hearing Research* 43:865–878.

Emerick, L. (1984). *Speaking for Ourselves: Self-Portraits of the Speech or Hearing Handicapped,* Danville, IL: Interstate.

Enderby, P., and Palmer, R. (2008). "The Standardized Assessment of Dysarthria Is Possible." In *Clinical Dysarthria,* ed. W. R. Berry (Austin, TX: Pro-Ed).

Enderby, P., Wood, V., and Wade, D., (2006). *Frenchay Aphasia Screening Test* (2nd ed.). Hoboken, NJ: Wiley.

Engler, L., Hannah, E., and Longhurst, T. (1973). "Linguistic Analysis of Speech Samples: A Practical Guide for Clinicians." *Journal of Speech and Hearing Disorders* 38:192–204.

Erickson, R. (1969). "Assessing Communication Attitudes among Stutterers." *Journal of Speech and Hearing Research* 12:711–724.

Epstein, R., Hiran, S. P., Stygall, J., and Newman, S. P. (2009). "How Do Individuals Cope with Voice Disorders? Introducing Voice Disability Coping Questionnaire." *Journal of Voice* 23(2):209–217.

Estes, K., Evans, J., and Else-Quest, N. (2007). "Differences in the Nonword Repetition Performance of Children with and without Specific Language Impairment: A Meta-Analysis." *Journal of Speech, Language and Hearing Research* 50:177–195.

Ettema, S. L., Kuehn, D. P., Perlman, A. L., and Alperin, N. (2002). "Magnetic Resonance Imaging of the Levator Veli Palatini Muscle During Speech." *The Cleft Palate-Craniofacial Journal* 39:130–144.

Evans, J., and Craig, H. (1992). "Language Sample Collection and Analysis: Interview Compared to Free-play Assessment Contexts." *Journal of Speech and Hearing Research* 35:343–353.

Evard, B., and Sabers, D. (1979). "Speech and Language Testing with Distinct Ethnic-Racial Groups: A Survey for Improving Test Validity." *Journal of Speech and Hearing Disorders* 44:271–281.

Ezrati-Vinacou, R., and Levin, I. (2004). "The Relationship between Anxiety and Stuttering: A Multidimensional Approach." *Journal of Fluency Disorders* 29(2):135–148.

Fagan, J., and Isaacs, S. (2002). "Tracheoesophageal Speech in a Developing World Community." *Archives of Otolaryngology—Head and Neck Surgery* 128:50–53.

Fagundes, D., Haynes, W., Haak, N., and Moran, M. (1998). "Task Variability Effects on the Language Test Performance of Southern Lower Socioeconomic Class African-American and Caucasian Five-Year-Olds." *Language, Speech and Hearing Services in Schools* 29:148–157.

Faircloth, M., and Faircloth, S. (1970). "An Analysis of the Articulatory Behavior of a Speech-Defective Child in Connected Speech and Isolated Word Responses." *Journal of Speech and Hearing Disorders* 35:51–61.

Farquhar, M. (1961). "Prognostic Value of Imitative and Auditory Discrimination Tests." *Journal of Speech and Hearing Disorders* 26:342–347.

Featherstone, H. (1980). *A Difference in the Family: Life with a Disabled Child.* New York: Basic Books.

Felsenfeld, S., Broen, P., and McGue, M. (1994). "A 28-Year Follow-Up of Adults with a History of Moderate Phonological Disorder: Educational and Occupational Results." *Journal of Speech and Hearing Research* 37:1341–1353.

Fenson, L., Marchman, V., Thal, D., Dale, P., Reznick, J., and Bates, E. (2006). *MacArthur-Bates Communicative Development Inventories.* Baltimore: Paul H. Brookes.

Fey, M. (1986). *Language Intervention with Young Children.* San Diego, CA: College-Hill.

Fey, M. (1992). "Articulation and Phonology: Inextricable Constructs in Speech Pathology." *Language, Speech and Hearing Services in Schools* 23:225–232.

Fey, M., and Leonard, L. (1983). "Pragmatic Skills of Children with Specific Language Impairment." In *Pragmatic Assessment and Intervention Issues in Language,* eds. T. Gallagher and C. Prutting (San Diego, CA: College-Hill).

Fiestas, C., and Pena, E. (2004). "Narrative Discourse in Bilingual Children: Language and Task Effects." *Language, Speech and Hearing Services in Schools* 35:155–168.

Fillmore, C. (1968). "The Case for Case." In *Universals in Linguistic Theory,* eds. E. Bach and R. Harms (New York: Holt, Rinehart, and Winston).

Finkelstein, Y., Wexler, D. B., Nachmani, A., and Ophir, D. (2002). "Endoscopic Partial Adenoidectomy for Children with Submucous Cleft." *The Cleft Palate-Craniofacial Journal* 39:479–486.

Finn, P. (1998). "Recovery Without Treatment: A Review of Conceptual and Methodological Considerations Across Disciplines." In *Treatment Efficacy for Stuttering: A Search for Empirical Bases,* eds. A. Cordes and R. Ingham (San Diego: Singular).

Fisher, H., and Logemann, J. (1971). *The Fisher-Logemann Test of Articulation Competence.* Boston, MA: Houghton-Mifflin.

Fleming, S., and Waver, A. (1987). "Index of Dysphagia: A Tool for Identifying Deglutition Problems." *Dysphagia* 1:206–208.

Fletcher, S. (1972). "Time-by-Count Measurement of Diadochokinetic Syllable Rate." *Journal of Speech and Hearing Research* 15:763–770.

Flipsen, P., Hammer, J., and Yost, K. (2005). "Measuring Severity of Involvement in Speech Delay: Segmental and Whole-Word Measures." *American Journal of Speech-Language Pathology* 14:298–312.

Fluharty, N. (2000). *Fluharty Preschool Speech and Language Screening Test-Second Edition.* Austin, TX: Pro-Ed.

Fogel, A., Toda, S., and Kawai, M. (1988). "Mother-Infant Face-to-Face Interaction in Japan and the United States: A Laboratory Comparison Using 3-Month-Old Infants." *Developmental Psychology* 24:398–406.

Folger, J., and Chapman, R. (1978). "A Pragmatic Analysis of Spontaneous Imitations." *Journal of Child Language* 5:25–38.

Folstein, M. F., Folstein, S. E., and McHugh, P. R. (1975). "Mini-Mental State: A Practical Method for Grading the Cognitive State of Patients for the Clinician." *Journal of Psychiatric Research* 12:189–198.

Foster, W., & Miller, M. (2007). "Development of the Literacy Achievement Gap: A Longitudinal Study of Kindergarten Through Third Grade." *Language, Speech and Hearing Services in Schools* 38:173–181.

Fox, D., and Johns, D. (1970). "Predicting Velopharyngeal Closure with a Modified Tongue-Anchor Technique." *Journal of Speech and Hearing Disorders* 35:248–251.

Frattali, C. (1998). "Measuring Modality-Specific Behaviors, Functional Abilities, and Quality of Life." In *Measuring Outcomes in Speech-Language Pathology,* ed. C. Frattali (New York: Thieme).

Frattali, C., Thompson, C. K., Holland, A., Wohl, C. B., and Ferketig, M. M. (1997). *ASHA Functional Assessment of Communication Skills for Adults.* Rockville, MD: American Speech-Language-Hearing Association.

Freed, D. B. (2000). *Motor Speech Disorders: Diagnosis and Treatment.* San Diego: Singular.

Fristoe, M., and Goldman, R. (1968). "Comparisons of Traditional and Condensed Articulation Tests Examining the Same Number of Sounds." *Journal of Speech and Hearing Research* 11:583–589.

Fuchs, D., Fuchs, L., Dailey, A., and Power, M. (1985). "The Effect of Examiner's Personal Familiarity and Professional Expertise on Handicapped Children's Test Performance." *Journal of Educational Research* 78:3–14.

Fudala, J., and Reynolds, W. (1993). *Arizona Articulation Proficiency Scale—2nd Edition.* Los Angeles: Western Psychological Services.

Fujiki, M., and Brinton, B. (1983). "Sampling Reliability in Elicited Imitation." *Journal of Speech and Hearing Disorders* 48:85–89.

Fujiki, M., Brinton, B., and Todd, C. (1996). "Social Skills of Children with Specific Language Impairment." *Language, Speech and Hearing Services in Schools* 27:195–202.

Fujiki, M., et al. (2001). "Social Behaviors of Children with Language Impairment on the Playground: A Pilot Study." *Language, Speech and Hearing Services in Schools* 32:101–113.

Furey, J., and Watkins, R. (2002). "Accuracy of Online Language Sampling: A Focus on Verbs." *American Journal of Speech-Language Pathology* 11:434–439.

Furuno, S., O'Reilly, K., Inatsuka, T., Husaka, C., Allmon, T., and Zeisloft-Falby, B. (1994). *The Hawaii Early Learning Profile.* Palo Alto, CA: VORT.

Gallagher, T. (1983). "Preassessment: A Procedure for Accomodating Language Use Variability." In *Pragmatic Assessment and Intervention Issues in Language,* eds. T. Gallagher and C. Prutting (San Diego, CA: College-Hill).

Garber, N. (1986). "A Phonological Analysis Classification for Use with Traditional Articulation Tests." *Language, Speech and Hearing Services in Schools* 17(4):253–261.

Garn-Nunn, P. (1986). "Phonological Processes and Conventional Articulation Tests: Considerations for Analysis." *Language, Speech and Hearing Services in Schools* 17(4):244–252.

Garn-Nunn, P., and Martin, V. (1992). "Using Conventional Articulation Tests with Highly Unintelligible Children: Identification and Programming Concerns." *Language, Speech and Hearing Services in Schools* 23:52–60.

Garrett, K., and Lasker, J. (2007). *The Oceanside, CA Multimodal Communication Screening Test for Persons with Aphasia* (MCST-A). Available online in multiple parts, http://aac.unl.edu/screen/screen.html; http://aac.unl.edu/screen/pictures.pdf; http://aac.unl.edu/screen/score.pdf

Garrett, K., and Moran, M. (1992). "A Comparison of Phonological Severity Measures." *Language, Speech and Hearing Services in Schools* 23:48–51.

Garvey, C. (1977a). "The Contingent Query: A Dependent Act in Conversation." In *Interaction, Conversation, and the Development of Language,* Vol. 5, eds. M. Lewis and L. Rosenblum (New York: Wiley).

Garvey, C. (1977b). "Play with Language and Speech." In *Child Discourse,* eds. S. Ervin-Tripp and C. Mitchell-Kernan (New York: Academic Press).

Gazella, J., and Stockman, I. (2003). "Children's Story Retelling under Different Modality and Task Conditions: Implications for Standardizing Language Sampling Procedures." *American Journal of Speech-Language Pathology* 12:61–72.

Geetha, Y. V., Pratibha, K., Ashok, R., and Ravingra, S. (2000). "Classification of Childhood Disfluencies Using Neural Networks." *Journal of Fluency Disorders* 25:99–117.

Gelfer, M. and Pazera, J. (2006). "Maximum Duration of Sustained /s/ and /z/ and the s/z Ratio with Controlled Intensity." *Journal of Voice* 20(3):369–379.

German, D. J. (1990). *The Test of Adolescent and Adult Word-Finding.* Austin, TX: Pro-Ed.

Gibbon, F. E., and Crampin, L. (2002). "Labial-Lingual Double Articulations in Speakers with Cleft Palate." *The Cleft Palate-Craniofacial Journal* 39:40–49.

Gierut, J. (2007). "Phonological Complexity and Language Learnability." *American Journal of Speech-Language Pathology* 16:6–17.

Gierut, J., Elbert, M., and Dinnsen, D. (1987). "A Functional Analysis of Phonological Knowledge and Generalization Learning in Misarticulating Children." *Journal of Speech and Hearing Research* 30(4):462–479.

Gilbertson, M., and Bramlett, R. (1998). "Phonological Awareness Screening to Identify At-Risk Readers: Implications for Practitioners." *Language, Speech and Hearing Services in Schools* 29:109–116.

Gillam, R., and Pearson, N. (2004). "Test of Narrative Language." Austin, TX: Pro-Ed.

Gillam, S., Fargo, J., and Robertson, K. (2009). "Comprehension of Expository Text: Insights Gained from Think-Aloud Data." *American Journal of Speech-Language Pathology* 18:82–94.

Gillespie, S. K., and Cooper, E. B. (1973). "Prevalence of Speech Problems in Junior and Senior High School." *Journal of Speech and Hearing Research* 16:739–743.

Ginsburg, H., and Opper, S. (1969). *Piaget's Theory of Intellectual Development: An Introduction.* Englewood Cliffs, NJ: Prentice-Hall.

Glaspey, A., & Stoel-Gammon, C. (2005). "Dynamic Assessment in Phonological Disorders." *Topics in Language Disorders* 25:220–230.

Glennen, S. (2007). "Predicting Language Outcomes for Internationally Adopted Children." *Journal of Speech, Language and Hearing Research* 50:529–548.

Gliklich, R. E., Glovsky, R. M., and Montgomary, W. W. (1999). "Validation of a Voice Outcome Survey for Unilateral Vocal Cord Paralysis." *Otolaryngology, Head & Neck Surgery* 120(2):153–158.

Goffman, E. (1963). *Stigma: Notes on the Management of Spoiled Identity.* Englewood Cliffs, NJ: Prentice Hall.

Goldfarb, R., and Serpanos, C. (2009). *Professional Writing in Speech-Language Pathology and Audiology.* San Diego: Plural.

Goldman, R. (1967). "Cultural Influences on the Sex Ratio in the Incidence of Stuttering." *American Anthropologist* 69:78–81.

Goldman, R., and Fristoe, M. (2000). *Goldman-Fristoe Test of Articulation-2.* Circle Pines, MN: American Guidance Service.

Goldstein, B., Fabiano, L., and Iglesias, A. (2004). "Spontaneous and Imitated Productions in Spanish-Speaking Children with Phonological Disorders." *Language, Speech and Hearing Services in Schools* 35:5–15.

Goldstein, B., and Iglesias, A. (1996). "Phonological Patterns in Normally Developing Spanish-speaking 3- and 4-Year-Olds of Puerto Rican Descent." *Language, Speech and Hearing Services in Schools* 27:82–90.

Goodglass, H., Gleason, J. B., Bernholtz, N. D., and Hyde, M. R. (1972). "Some Linguistic Structures in the Speech of a Broca's Aphasic." *Cortex* 8:191–212.

Goodglass, H., Kaplan, E., and Barresi, N. (2000). *The Assessment of Aphasia and Related Disorders.* Hagerstown, MD: Lippincott Williams & Wilkins.

Gordon, P., and Luper, H. (1992). "The Early Identification of Beginning Stuttering, I: Protocols." *American Journal of Speech-Language Pathology* 1:43–53.

Gordon-Brannan, M., and Hodson, B. (2000). "Intelligibility/Severity Measurements of Prekindergarten Children's Speech." *American Journal of Speech-Language Pathology* 9:141–150.

Gowie, C., and Powers, J. (1979). "Relations among Cognitive, Semantic and Syntactic Variables in Children's Comprehension of the Minimal Distance Principle: A Two-Year Developmental Study." *Journal of Psycholinguistic Research* 8: 29–41.

Graham, S., and Harris, K. (1999). "Assessment and Intervention in Overcoming Writing Difficulties: An Illustration from the Self-Regulated Strategy Development Model." *Language, Speech and Hearing Services in Schools* 30:255–264.

Gray, S., et al. (1999). "The Diagnostic Accuracy of Four Vocabulary Tests Administered to Preschool-Age Children." *Language, Speech and Hearing Services in Schools* 30:196–206.

Greenslade, K., Plante, E. & Vance, R. (2009). "The Diagnostic Accuracy and Construct Validity of the Structured Photographic Expressive Language Test–Preschool: Second Edition." *Language, Speech and Hearing Services in Schools* 40:150–160.

Gregory, H., Campbell, J., Gregory, C., and Hill, D. (2002). *Stuttering Therapy Rationale and Procedures.* Boston, MA: Pearson.

Grice, H. (1975). "Logic and Conversation." In *Studies in Syntax, Semantics and Speech Acts,* vol. 3, eds. P. Cole and J. Morgan (New York: Academic Press).

Groher, M. (1984). *Dysphagia: Diagnosis and Management.* Boston, MA: Butterworths.

Groher, M., and Crary, M. (2010). *Dysphagia Clinical Management in Adults and Children.* Maryland Heights, MO: Mosby Elsevier.

Grunwell, P. (1985). *Phonological Assessment of Child Speech (PACS).* San Diego, CA: NFER-Nelson; Windsor, UK: College-Hill Press.

Grunwell, P. (1988). *Clinical Phonology.* Baltimore, MD: Williams and Wilkins.

Guitar, B. (2006). *Stuttering: An Integrated Approach to Its Nature and Treatment.* Philadelphis, PA: Lippincott Williams & Wilkins.

Guitar, B., and Grims, S. (1977). "Developing a Scale to Assess Communication Attitudes in Children Who Stutter." Paper presented at the convention of the American Speech-Language-Hearing Association, Atlanta, GA.

Guitar, B., and McCauley, R. (2009). *Treatment of Stuttering: Established and Emerging Intervention.* Philadelphia, PA: Lippincott Williams & Wilkins.

Gummersall, D., and Strong, C. (1999). "Assessment of Complex Sentence Production in a Narrative Context." *Language, Speech and Hearing Services in Schools* 30:152–164.

Gurland, B. J., Copeland, J., Sharpe, L., and Kelleher, M. (1976). "The Geriatric Mental Status Interview (GMS)." *International Journal of Aging and Human Development* 7:303–311.

Gutierrez-Clellen, V. (1996). "Language Diversity: Implications for Assessment." In *Assessment of*

Communication and Language, eds. K. Cole, P. Dale, and D. Thal (Baltimore, MD: Brookes).

Gutierrez-Clellen, V. (1999). "Mediating Literacy Skills in Spanish-Speaking Children with Special Needs." *Language, Speech and Hearing Services in Schools* 30:285–292.

Gutierrez-Clellen, V., and Pena, E. (2001). "Dynamic Assessment of Diverse Children: A Tutorial." *Language, Speech and Hearing Services in Schools* 32:212–224.

Gutierrez-Clellen, V., and Quinn, R. (1993). "Assessing Narratives in Diverse Cultural/Linguistic Populations: Clinical Implications." *Language, Speech and Hearing Services in Schools* 24:2–9.

Gutierrez-Clellen, V., Restrepo, M., Bedore, L., Pena, E., and Anderson, R. (2000). "Language Sample Analysis in Spanish-Speaking Children: Methodological Considerations." *Language, Speech and Hearing Services in Schools* 31:88–98.

Hakkesteegt, M., Brocaar, M., and Wieringa, M. (2010). "The Application of the Dysphonia Severity Index and the Voice Handicap Index in Evaluating Effects of Voice Therapy and Phonosurgery." *Journal of Voice* 24(2):199–206.

Hall, K. M. (1992). "Overview of Functional Assessment Scales in Brain Injury Rehabilitation." *NeuroRehabilitation* 2:98–113.

Hall, N. (2004). "Lexical Development and Retrieval in Treating Children Who Stutter." *Language, Speech and Hearing Services in Schools* 35:57–69.

Hall, P. K., Hardy, J. C., and LaVelle, W. E. (1990). "A Child with Signs of Developmental Apraxia of Speech with Whom a Palatal Lift Prosthesis Was Used to Manage Palatal Dysfunction." *Journal of Speech and Hearing Disorders* 55:454–460.

Hall, P., and Tomblin, J. (1978). "A Follow-Up Study of Children with Articulation and Language Disorders." *Journal of Speech and Hearing Disorders* 43:227–241.

Halliday, M. (1975). *Learning How to Mean: Explorations in the Development of Language.* New York: Elsevier.

Halliday, M., and Hasan, R. (1976). *Cohesion in English.* London: Longman.

Hallowell, B., and Chapey, R. (2001). "Delivering Language Intervention Services to Adults with Neurogenic Communication Disorders." In *Language Intervention Strategies in Aphasia and Related*

Neurogenic Communication Disorders, 4th ed., ed. R. Chapey (Philadelphia, PA: Lippincott Williams and Wilkins).

Halper, A., Cherney, L. R., and Burns, M. S. (1996). *Rehabilitation Institute of Chicago Clinical Management of Right Hemisphere Dysfunction,* 2nd ed. Gaithersburg, MD: Aspen Publications.

Hamayan, E., and Damico, J. (1991). *Limiting Bias in the Assessment of Bilingual Students.* Austin, TX: Pro-Ed.

Hammer, C., Lawrence, F., & Miccio, A. (2007). "Bilingual Children's Language Abilities and Early Reading Outcomes in Head Start and Kindergarten." *Language, Speech and Hearing Services in Schools* 38:237–248.

Hammer, C., Rodriguez, B., Lawrence, F., & Miccio, A. (2007). "Puerto Rican Mothers' Beliefs and Home Literacy Practices." *Language, Speech and Hearing Services in Schools* 38:216–224.

Hanna, E., Sherman, A., Cash, D., Adams, F., Vural, E., Fan, C. Y., and Suen, J. (2004). "Quality of Life for Patients Following Total Laryngectomy vs. Chemoradiation for Laryngeal Preservation." *Archives of Otolaryngology—Head & Neck* Surgery 130(7):875–879.

Hardin-Jones, M., Chapman, K., and Scherer, N. (2006, June 13). "Early Intervention in Children with Cleft Palate." *The ASHA Leader* 11:8–9, 32.

Harris, G. (1985). "Considerations in Assessing English Language Performance of Native American Children." *Topics in Language Disorders* 5:42–52.

Harrison, L., & McLeod, S. (2010). "Risk and Protective Factors Associated with Speech and Language Impairment in a Nationally Representative Sample of 4- to 5-Year-Old Children." *Journal of Speech, Language and Hearing Research* 53:508–529.

Hartnick, C. J., Volk, M., and Cunningham, M. (2003). "Establishing Normal Voice-Related Quality of Life Scores with the Pediatric Population." *Archives of Otolaryngology, Head and Neck Surgery* 29(10):1090–1093.

Haskill, A., and Tyler, A. (2007). "A Comparison of Linguistic Profiles in Subgroups of Children with Specific Language Impairment." *American Journal of Speech-Language Pathology* 16:209–221.

Hay, I., Oates, J., Giannini, A., Berkowiz, R., and Rotenberg, B. (2009). "Pain Perception of Children Undergoing

Nasendoscopy for Investigation of Voice and Resonance Disorders." *Journal of Voice* 23(3):380–388.

Hayden, D., and Square, P. (1999). *Verbal Motor Production Assessment for Children.* San Antonio, TX: Psychological Corporation.

Haynes, W., Haynes, M., and Jackson, J. (1982). "The Effects of Phonetic Context and Linguistic Complexity on /s/ Misarticulation in Children." *Journal of Communication Disorders* 15:287–297.

Haynes, W., and Hood, S. (1978). "Disfluency Changes in Children as a Function of the Systematic Modification of Linguistic Complexity." *Journal of Communication Disorders* 11:79–93.

Haynes, W., and McCallion, M. (1981). "Language Comprehension Testing: The Influence of Cognitive Tempo and Three Modes of Test Administration." *Language, Speech and Hearing Services in Schools* 12:74–81.

Haynes, W., and Moran, M. (1989). "A Cross-Sectional Developmental Study of Final Consonant Production in Southern Black Children from Preschool through Third Grade." *Language, Speech and Hearing Services in Schools* 20:400–406.

Haynes, W., Moran, M., and Pindzola, R. (2011). *Communication Disorders in Educational and Medical Settings An Introduction for Speech-Language Pathologists, Teachers, and Allied Health Professionals,* Boston, MA: Jones & Bartlett Learning.

Haynes, W., and Oratio, A. (1978). "A Study of Clients' Perceptions of Therapeutic Effectiveness." *Journal of Speech and Hearing Disorders* 43:21–33.

Haynes, W., Purcell, E., and Haynes, M. (1979). "A Pragmatic Aspect of Language Sampling." *Language, Speech and Hearing Services in Schools* 10:104–110.

Healey, E. C., Scott, L., and Susan, M. (2004). "Clinical Application of a Multidimensional Approach for the Assessment and Treatment of Stuttering." *Contemporary Issues in Communication Disorders* 31:40–48.

Healy, T., and Madison, C. (1987). "Articulation Error Migration: A Comparison of Single-Word and Connected Speech Samples." *Journal of Communication Disorders* 20:129–136.

Heath, S. (1983). *Ways with Words.* Cambridge, UK: Cambridge University Press.

Heath, S. (1989). "The Learner as a Cultural Member." In *The Teachability of Language,* eds. M. Rice and R. Schiefelbusch (Baltimore, MD: Brookes).

Hebbeler, K., and Rooney, R. (2009). "Accountability for Services for Young Children with Disabilities and the Assessment of Meaningful Outcomes: The Role of the Speech-Language Pathologist." *Language Speech and Hearing Services in Schools* 40:446–456.

Hegde, M. (1987). *Clinical Research in Communication Disorders.* Boston, MA: Little, Brown.

Hegde, M. (2006). *Treatment Protocols for Stuttering.* San Diego, CA: Plural.

Hegde, M. N., and Davis, D. (2009). *Clinical Methods and Practicum in Speech-Language Pathology.* Clifton Park, NY: Delmar.

Heilbrun, C. (1998). *The Last Gift of Time: Life Beyond Sixty.* New York: Random House.

Heilmann, J., Miller, J., & Nockerts, A. (2010). "Using Language Sample Databases." *Language, Speech and Hearing Services in Schools* 41:84–95.

Heilmann, J., Miller, J., Nockerts, A., & Dunaway, C. (2010). "Properties of the Narrative Scoring Scheme Using Narrative Retells in Young School-Age Children." *American Journal of Speech-Language Pathology* 19:154–166.

Heilmann, J., Weismer, S., Evans, J., and Hollar, C. (2005). "Utility of the MacArthur-Bates Communicative Development Inventory in Identifying Language Abilities of Late-Talking and Typically Developing Toddlers." *American Journal of Speech-Language Pathology* 14:40–51.

Helm-Estabrooks, N. (1993). *Aphasia Diagnostic Profiles.* Chicago: Riverside.

Helm-Estabrooks, N., Ramsberger, G., Morgan, A. R., and Nicholas, M. (1989). *Boston Assessment of Severe Aphasia.* Austin, TX: Pro-Ed.

Henley, J., and Souliere, C. (2009). "Tracheoesophageal Speech Failure in the Laryngectomee: The Role of Constrictor Myotomy." *The Laryngoscope* 96(9):1016–1020.

Hester, E. (1996). "Narratives of Young African American Children." In *Communication Development and Disorders in African American Children,* eds. A. Kamhi, K. Pollock, and J. Harris (Baltimore, MD: Brookes).

Hickman, L. (1997). *The Apraxia Profile*. Boston: Pearson.

Hirano, M. (1981). *Clinical Examination of Voice*. Vienna, Austria: Springer-Verlag.

Hixon, T. J., and Hoit, J. D. (1998). "Physical Examination of the Diaphragm by the Speech-Language Pathologist." *American Journal of Speech-Language Pathology* 7:37–45.

Hixon, T. J., and Hoit, J. D. (1999). "Physical Examination of the Abdominal Wall by the Speech-Language Pathologist." *American Journal of Speech-Language Pathology* 8:335–345.

Hodson, B. (1985). *Computer Analysis of Phonological Processes*. PhonoComp, Box 46, Stonington, IL 62567.

Hodson, B. (1986). *The Assessment of Phonological Processes—Revised*. Austin, TX: Pro-Ed.

Hodson, B. (2003). *Computerized Analysis of Phonological Patterns (HCAPP)*. Wichita, KS: PhonoComp Software.

Hodson, B. (2004). *Hodson Assessment of Phonological Patterns-3*. Austin, TX: Pro-Ed.

Hodson, B., and Paden, E. (1991). *Targeting Intelligible Speech: A Phonological Approach to Remediation*, 2nd ed. Austin, TX: Pro-Ed.

Hoffman, P., Schuckers, G., and Ratusnik, D. (1977). "Contextual-Coarticulatory Inconsistencies of /s/ Misarticulation." *Journal of Speech and Hearing Research* 20:631–643.

Hogikyan, N. D., and Sethurama, G. (1999). "Validation of an Instrument to Measure Voice-Related Quality of Life (V-RQOL)." *Journal of Voice* 13:557–569.

Holland, A. (1975). "Language Therapy for Children: Some Thoughts on Context and Content." *Journal of Speech and Hearing Disorders* 40:514–523.

Holland, A., Frattali, C., and Fromm, D. (1999). *Communication Activities of Daily Living*, 2nd ed. Austin, TX: Pro-Ed.

Holland, A., and Thompson, C. (1998). "Outcomes Measures in Aphasia." In *Measuring Outcomes in Speech-Language Pathology*, ed. C. Frattali (New York: Thieme).

Horton-Ikard, R. (2009). "Cohesive Adequacy in the Narrative Samples of School-Age Children Who Use African-American English." *Language, Speech and Hearing Services in Schools* 40:393–402.

Horton-Ikard, R., & Weismer, S. (2007). "A Preliminary Examination of Vocabulary and Word Learning in African American Toddlers from Middle and Low Socioeconomic Status Homes." *American Journal of Speech-Language Pathology* 16:381–392.

Howe, C. (1976). "The Meanings of Two-Word Utterances in the Speech of Young Children." *Journal of Child Language* 3:29–47.

Huang, R., Hopkins, J., and Nippold, M. (1997). "Satisfaction with Standardized Language Testing: A Survey of Speech-Language Pathologists." *Language, Speech and Hearing Services in Schools* 28:12–23.

Hubbell, R. (1981). *Children's Language Disorders: An Integrated Approach*. Englewood Cliffs, NJ: Prentice Hall.

Hubbell, R. (1988). *A Handbook of English Grammar and Language Sampling*. Englewood Cliffs, NJ: Prentice Hall.

Hughes, D., Fey, M., and Long, S. (1992). "Developmental Sentence Scoring: Still Useful after All These Years." *Topics in Language Disorders* 12:1–12.

Hutchinson, T. (1996). "What to Look for in the Technical Manual: Twenty Questions for Users." *Language, Speech and Hearing Services in Schools* 27:109–121.

Hux, K., Morris-Friehe, M., and Sanger, D. (1993). "Language Sampling Practices: A Survey of Nine States." *Language, Speech and Hearing Services in Schools* 24:84–91.

Hymes, D. (1971). "Competence and Performance in Linguistic Theory." In *Language Acquisition: Models and Methods,* eds. R. Huxley and E. Ingram (New York: Academic Press).

Hyter, Y. (2007). Understanding children who have been affected by maltreatment and prenatal alcohol exposure. *Language, Speech and Hearing Services in Schools*, 38:93–98.

Hyter, Y., and Westby, C. (1996). "Using Oral Narratives to Assess Communicative Competence." In *Communication Development and Disorders in African American Children,* eds. A. Kamhi, K. Pollock, and J. Harris (Baltimore, MD: Brookes).

Ichord, R. N. (1994). "Neurology of Deglutition." In *Disorders of Feeding and Swallowing in Infants and Children: Pathophysiology, Diagnosis, and Treatment,* eds. D. N. Tuchman and R. S. Walter (San Diego, CA: Singular Publishing).

Impara, J., and Plake, B. (eds.) (1998). *Thirteenth Mental Measurements Yearbook.* Lincoln, NE: Buros Institute of Mental Measurements.

Ingham, J. (2003). "Evidence-Based Treatment of Stuttering: I. Definition and Application." *Journal of Fluency Disorders* 28:197–207.

Ingham, R. (2005). "Clinicians Deserve Better: Observations on a Clinical Forum Titled 'What Child Language Research May Contribute to the Understanding and Treatment of Stuttering (2004).'" *Language, Speech and Hearing Services in Schools* 36(2):152–155.

Ingram, D. (1976). *Phonological Disability in Children.* New York: Elsiever.

Ingram, D. (1981). *Procedures for the Phonological Analysis of Children's Language.* Baltimore, MD: University Park Press.

Ingram, D., and Ingram, K. (2001). "A Whole Word Approach to Phonological Analysis and Intervention." *Language, Speech and Hearing Services in Schools* 32:271–283.

Ingram, K., and Ingram, D. (2002). "Commentary on 'Evaluating Articulation and Phonological Disorders When the Clock Is Running.'" *American Journal of Speech-Language Pathology* 11:257–258.

Irwin, J., and Wong, P. (1983). *Phonological Development in Children 18 to 72 Months.* Carbondale: Southern Illinois University Press.

Isshiki, N., Yanigahara, N., and Morimoto, H. (1966). "Approach to the Objective Diagnosis of Hoarseness." *Folia Phoniatrica* 18:393–400.

Jackson, S., Pretti-Frontczak, K., Harjusola-Webb, S., Grisham-Brown, J., and Romani, J. (2009). "Response to Intervention: Implications for Early Childhood Professionals." *Language, Speech and Hearing Services in Schools* 40:424–434.

Jacobson, B., Cohen, S., Stewart, M., Ossoff, R., Garrett, C. G., Attia, A., Noordzij, J. P., and Cleveland, T. (2007, June). "Creation and Validation of the Singing Voice Handicap Index." *Annals of Otology, Rhinology & Laryngology.*

Jacobson, B., Johnson, A., Grywalski, C., Silbergleit, A., Jacobson, B., and Benniger, S. (1997). "The Voice Handicap Index (VHI): Development and Validation." *American Journal of Speech-Language Pathology* 6(3):66–70.

Jelm, J. M. (1990). *Oral-Motor/Feeding Rating Scale.* Tucson, AZ: Therapy Skill Builders.

Jelm, J. M. (2001). *Verbal Dyspraxia Profile.* DeKalb, IL: Janelle.

Johns, V., and Haynes, W. (2002). "Dynamic Assessment and Predicting Children's Benefit from Narrative Training." Paper presented at the convention of the American Speech-Language-Hearing Association, Atlanta, GA.

Johnson, C. (1995). "Expanding Norms for Narration." *Language, Speech and Hearing Services in Schools* 26:326–341.

Johnson, C., et al. (1999). "Fourteen-Year Follow-Up of Children with and Without Speech/ Language Impairments: Speech/Language Stability and Outcomes." *Journal of Speech, Language, and Hearing Research* 42:744–760.

Johnson, C., Beitchman, J., and Brownlie, E. (2010). "Twenty-Year Follow-Up of Children with and Without Speech-Language Impairments: Family, Educational, Occupational, and Quality of Life Outcomes." *American Journal of Speech-Language Pathology* 19:51–65.

Johnson, C., Weston, A., and Bain, B. (2004). "An Objective and Time-Efficient Method for Determining Severity of Childhood Speech Delay." *American Journal of Speech-Language Pathology* 13:55–65.

Johnson, J., Whinney, B., and Pederson, O. (1980). "Single-Word versus Connected Speech Articulation Testing." *Language, Speech and Hearing Services in Schools* 11:175–179.

Johnston, J. (1982). "Narrative: A New Look at Communication Problems in Older Language-Disordered Children." *Language, Speech and Hearing Services in Schools* 13:144–155.

Johnston, J. (2001). "An Alternate MLU Calculation: Magnitude and Variability of Effects." *Journal of Speech, Language, and Hearing Research* 44:156–164.

Johnston, J. (2006) *Thinking about Child Language: Research to Practice.* Eau Claire, WI: Thinking Publications.

Johnston, J., Miller, J., Curtiss, S., and Tallal, P. (1993). "Conversations with Children Who Are Language Impaired: Asking Questions." *Journal of Speech and Hearing Research* 36: 973–978.

Jokel, R., De Nil, L. and Sharpe, K. (2007). "Speech Disfluencies in Adults with Neurogenic Stuttering Associated with Stroke and Traumatic Brain Injury." *Journal of Medical Speech-Language Pathology* 15(3):243–262.

Justice, L. (2006). "Evidence-Based Practice Response to Intervention and the Prevention of Reading Difficulties." *Language, Speech and Hearing Services in Schools* 37:284–297.

Justice, L., Bowles, R., Kaderavek, J., Ukrainetz, T., Eisenberg, S., and Gillam, R. (2006). "The Index of Narrative Microstructure: A Clinical Tool for Analyzing School-Age Children's Narrative Performances." *American Journal of Speech-Language Pathology* 15:177–191.

Justice, L. and Ezell, H. (2004). "Print Referencing: An Emergent Literacy Enhancement Strategy and Its Clinical Applications." *Language, Speech and Hearing Services in Schools* 35:185–193.

Justice, L., Invernizzi, M., and Meier, J. (2002). "Designing and Implementing an Early Literacy Screening Protocol: Suggestions for the Speech-Language Pathologist." *Language, Speech and Hearing Services in Schools* 33:84–101.

Justice, L., and Kaderavek, J. (2004). "Embedded-Explicit Emergent Literacy Intervention I: Background and Description of Approach." *Language, Speech and Hearing Services in Schools* 35:201–211.

Kaderavek, J., and Justice, L. (2004). "Embedded-Explicit Emergent Literacy Intervention II: Goal Selection and Implementation in the Early Childhood Classroom." *Language, Speech and Hearing Services in Schools* 35:212–228.

Kaderavek, J., and Sulzby, E. (1998). "Parent–Child Joint Book Reading: An Observational Protocol for Young Children." *American Journal of Speech-Language Pathology* 7:33–47.

Kaderavek, J., and Sulzby, E. (2000). "Narrative Production by Children with and Without Specific Language Impairment: Oral Narratives and Emergent Readings." *Journal of Speech, Language and Hearing Research* 43:34–49.

Kadushin, A. (1972). "The Social Work Interview." New York: Columbia University Press.

Kahn, J. (1984). "Cognitive Training and Initial Use of Referential Speech." *Topics in Language Disorders* 5:14–18.

Kahn, L., and James, S. (1980). "A Method for Assessing the Use of Grammatical Structures in Language-Disordered Children." *Language, Speech and Hearing Services in Schools* 11:188–197.

Kahn, L., and Lewis, N. (2002). *Kahn-Lewis Phonological Analysis-2.* Circle Pines, MN: American Guidance Service.

Kamhi, A. (2004). "A Meme's Eye View of Speech-Language Pathology." *Language, Speech and Hearing Services in Schools* 35:105–111.

Kamhi, A., and Johnston, J. (1982). "Towards an Understanding of Retarded Children's Linguistic Deficiencies." *Journal of Speech and Hearing Research* 25:435–445.

Kamhi, A., Pollock, K., and Harris, J. (1996). *Communication Development and Disorders in African-American Children.* Baltimore, MD: Paul H. Brookes.

Kaplan, E., Goodglass, H., and Weintraub, S. (1983). *Boston Naming Test,* 2nd ed. Philadelphia, PA: Lea and Febiger.

Kaplan, N., and Dreyer, D. (1974). "The Effect of Self-Awareness Training on Student Speech Pathologist–Client Relationships." *Journal of Communication Disorders* 7:329–342.

Karnell, M., Melton, S., Childes, J., Coleman, T., Dailey, S., and Hoffman, H. (2007). "Reliability of Clinician-Based (GRBAS and CAPE-V) and Patient-Based (V-RQOL and IPVI) Documentation of Voice Disorders." *Journal of Voice* 21(5):576–590.

Katz, R. C. (2001). "Computer Applications in Aphasia Treatment." In *Language Intervention Strategies in Aphasia and Related Neurogenic Communication Disorders,* 4th ed., ed. R. Chapey (Philadelphia, PA: Lippincott Williams and Wilkins).

Kaufman, N. (1995). *Kaufman Speech Praxis Test for Children (KSPT).* Austin, TX: Pro-Ed.

Kay, J., Lesser, R., and Coltheart, M. (1997). *Psycholinguistic Assessments of Language Processing in Aphasia.* Hove, UK: Psychology Press.

Kazi, R., De Cordova, J., Kanagalingam, J., Venkitaraman, R., Nutting, C. M., Clarke, P., Rhys-Evans, P., and Harrington, K. J. (2007). "Quality of Life following Total Laryngectomy: Assessment Using the UW-QOL Scale." *Journal for Oto-Rhino-Laryngology, Head and Neck Surgery* 69(2):100–106.

Keatley, M. A., Miller, T. I., and Johnson, A. F. (1998). "Designing Automated Outcomes Management Systems." In *Measuring Outcomes in Speech-Language Pathology,* ed. C. M. Frattali (New York: Thieme).

Keenan, E., and Schieffelin, B. (1976). "Topic as a Discourse Notion: A Study of Topic in the Conversations of Children and Adults." In *Subject and Topic,* ed. C. Li (New York: Academic Press).

Keenan, J., and Brassell, E. (1974). "A Study of Factors Related to Prognosis for Individual Aphasic Patients." *Journal of Speech and Hearing Disorders* 39:257–269.

Keenan, J., and Brassell, E. (1975). *Aphasia Language Performance Scales.* Murfreesboro, TN: Pinnacle Press.

Kempster, G., Gerrott, B., Verdolini Abbott, K., Barkmeier-Kraemen, J., and Hillman, R. (2009). *American Journal of Speech-Language Pathology* 18:124–132.

Kenney, K., & Prather, E. (1984). "Coarticulation as Assessment in Meaningful Language." Tucson, AZ: Communication Skill Builders.

Kenny, D., Koheil, R., Greenberg, J., Reid, D., Milner, M., Roman, R., and Judd, P. (1989). "Development of a Multidisciplinary Feeding Profile for Children Who are Dependent Feeders." *Dysphagia* 4:16–28.

Kent, L., and Chabon, S. (1980). "Problem-Oriented Records in a University Speech and Hearing Clinic." *Journal of the American Speech and Hearing Association* 22:151–158.

Kent, R. (1982). "Contextual Facilitation of Correct Sound Production." *Language, Speech and Hearing Services in Schools* 13:66–76.

Kent, R., and Minifie, F. (1977). "Coarticulation in Recent Speech Production Models." *Journal of Phonetics* 5:115–133.

Kent, R., Miolo, G., and Bloedel, S. (1994). "The Intelligibility of Children's Speech: A Review of Evaluation Procedures." *American Journal of Speech-Language Pathology* 3:81–95.

Kent, R. D., Vorperian, H. K., and Duffy, J. R. (1999). "Reliability of the Multi-Dimensional Voice Program for the Analysis of Voice Samples of Subjects with Dysarthria." *American Journal of Speech-Language Pathology* 8:129–136.

Kertesz, A. (2006). *Western Aphasia Battery—Revised.* New York: Psych Corp.

King, R., Jones, C., and Lasky, E. (1982). "In Retrospect: A Fifteen-Year Follow-Up Report of Speech-Language Disorders in Children." *Language, Speech and Hearing Services in Schools* 13:24–32.

Kirk, C. (2008). "Substitution Errors in the Production of Word-Initial and Word-Final Consonant Clusters." *Journal of Speech, Language and Hearing Research* 51:35–48.

Kirk, C., & Gillon, G. (2007). "Longitudinal Effects of Phonological Awareness Intervention on Morphological Awareness in Children with Speech Impairment." *Language, Speech and Hearing Services in Schools* 38:342–352.

Kirk, S., and Kirk, W. (1971). *Psycholinguisic Learning Disabilities.* Urbana: University of Illinois Press.

Kirkwood, T. (2000). *Time of Our Lives: The Science of Human Aging.* Oxford: Oxford University Press.

Klecan-Aker, J., and Hedrick, D. (1985). "A Study of the Syntactic Language Skills of Normal School-Age Children." *Language, Speech and Hearing Services in Schools* 16:187–198.

Klee, T., Pearce, K., and Carson, D. (2000). "Improving the Positive Predictive Value of Screening for Developmental Language Disorder." *Journal of Speech, Language and Hearing Research* 43:821–833.

Klein, H. (1984). "Procedure for Maximizing Phonological Information from Single-Word Responses." *Language, Speech and Hearing Services in Schools* 15:267–274.

Klein, H., & Liu-Shea, M. (2009). "Between Word Simplification Patterns in the Continuous Speech of Children with Speech Sound Disorders." *Language, Speech and Hearing Services in Schools* 40:17–30.

Klein, M., and Briggs, M. (1987). "Facilitating Mother–Infant Communicative Interactions in Mothers of High-Risk Infants." *Journal of Childhood Communication Disorders* 10(2):95–106.

Klinger, L., and Dawson, G. (1992). "Facilitating Early Social and Communicative Development in Children with Autism." In Causes and Effects in Communication and Language Intervention, eds. S. Warren and J. Reichle (Baltimore: Brookes).

Koutsoftas, A., Harmon, M., & Gray, S. (2009). "The Effect of Tier 2 Intervention for Phonemic Awareness in a Response-to-Intervention Model in Low-Income Preschool Classrooms." *Language, Speech and Hearing Services in Schools* 40:116–130.

Kramer, P. (1977). "Young Children's Free Responses to Anomalous Commands." *Journal of Experimental Child Psychology* 24:219–234.

Kratcoski, A. (1998). "Guidelines for Using Portfolios in Assessment and Evaluation." *Language, Speech, and Hearing Services in Schools* 29:3–10.

Kummer, A. (2005). "Ankyloglossia: To Clip or Not to Clip: That's the Question." *The ASHA Leader* 10(17):6–7,30.

Kummer, A. (2007). *Cleft Palate and Craniofacial Anomalies: Effects on Speech and Resonance,* 2nd ed. New York: Thomson Delmar Learning.

Kummerer, S., Lopez-Reyna, N., & Hughes, M. (2007). "Mexican Immigrant Mothers' Perceptions of Their Children's Communicative Disabilities, Emergent Literacy Development and Speech-Language Therapy Program." *American Journal of Speech-Language Pathology* 16:271–282.

Kwiatkowski, J., and Shriberg, L. (1992). "Intelligibility Assessment in Developmental Phonological Disorders: Accuracy of Caregiver Gloss." *Journal of Speech and Hearing Research* 35:1095–1104.

Labov, W. (1970). "The Logic on Nonstandard English." In *Language and Poverty: Perspectives on a Theme,* ed. F. Williams (Chicago: Rand-McNally).

Lahey, M. (1988). *Language Disorders and Language Development.* New York: Macmillan.

Lahey, M., and Edwards, J. (1995). "Specific Language Impairment: Preliminary Investigation of Factors Associated with Family History and with Patterns of Language Performance." *Journal of Speech and Hearing Research* 38:643–657.

Laing, S., and Kamhi, A. (2003). "Alternative Assessment of Language and Literacy in Culturally and Linguistically Diverse Populations." *Language, Speech and Hearing Services in Schools* 34:44–55.

LaParo, K., Justice, L., Skibbe, L., and Pianta, R. (2004). "Relations Among Maternal, Child and Demographic Factors and the Persistence of Preschool Language Impairment." *American Journal of Speech-Language Pathology* 13:291–303.

LaPointe, L. (2005). *Aphasia and Related Neurogenic Language Disorders,* 3rd ed. New York: Thieme.

LaPointe, L., and Horner, J. (1998). *Reading Comprehension Battery for Aphasia (RCBA-2).* Austin, TX: Pro-Ed.

Larrivee, L., and Catts, H. (1999). "Early Reading Achievement in Children with Expressive Phonological Disorders." *American Journal of Speech-Language Pathology* 8:118–128.

Larson, V., and McKinley, N. (1995). "Language Disorders in Older Students." Eau Claire, WI: Thinking Publications.

Lawrence, C. (1992). "Assessing the Use of Age-Equivalent Scores in Clinical Management." *Language, Speech and Hearing Services in Schools* 23:6–8.

Least-Heat-Moon, W. (1982). *Blue Highways: A Journey into America.* Boston, MA: Atlantic—Little, Brown.

Leavitt, R. R. (1974). *The Puerto Ricans: Cultural Change and Language Deviance.* Tucson: University of Arizona Press.

Lee, L. (1974). *Developmental Sentence Analysis.* Evanston, IL: Northwestern University Press.

Lee, L., Koenigsknecht, R., and Mulhern, S. (1975). *Interactive Language Development Teaching.* Evanston, IL: Northwestern University Press.

Lefton-Greif, M. A. (1994). "Diagnosis and Management of Pediatric Feeding and Swallowing Disorders: Role of the Speech-Language Pathologist." In *Disorders of Feeding and Swallowing in Infants and Children: Pathophysiology, Diagnosis, and Treatment,* eds. D. N. Tuchman and R. S. Walter (San Diego, CA: Singular Publishing).

Leith, W., and Mims, H. (1975). "Cultural Influences in the Development and Treatment of Stuttering: A Preliminary Report." *Journal of Speech and Hearing Disorders* 40:459–466.

Leon-Carrion, J., Domingue-Morales, M., Martin, M., and Murillo-Cabezaz, F. (2005). "Epideminology of Traumatic Brain Injury and Subarachnoid Hemorrhage." *Pituitary* 8(3):197–202.

Leonard, L. (1971). "A Preliminary View of Information Theory and Articulatory Omissions." *Journal of Speech and Hearing Disorders* 36: 511–517.

Leonard, L. (1975). "On Differentiating Syntactic and Semantic Features in Emerging Grammars: Evidence from Empty Form Usage." *Journal of Psycholinguistic Research* 4:357–364.

Leonard, L. (1976). *Meaning in Child Language: Issues in the Study of Early Semantic Development.* New York: Grune and Stratton.

Leonard, L. (2009). "Is Expressive Language Disorder an Accurate Diagnostic Category?" *American Journal of Speech-Language Pathology* 18:115–123.

Leonard, L., Prutting, C., Perozzi, C., and Berkley, R. (1978). "Nonstandardized Approaches to the Assessment of Language Behaviors." *Journal of the American Speech and Hearing Association,* May:371–379.

Leonard, L., Steckol, K., and Panther, K. (1983). "Returning Meaning to Semantic Relations: Some Clinical Applications." *Journal of Speech and Hearing Disorders* 48:25–35.

Leonard, L., Weismer, S., Miller, C., Francis, D., Tomblin, J., and Kail, R. (2007). "Speed of Processing, Working Memory and Language Impairment in Children." *Journal of Speech, Language and Hearing Research* 50:408–428.

Levin, H. S., O'Donnell, V. M., and Grossman, R. G. (1979). "The Galveston Orientation and Amnesia Test: A Practical Scale to Assess Cognition after Head Injury." *Journal of Nervous System and Mental Disorders* 167:675–684.

Lewin, J. (1999). "Tracheoesophageal Communication: Beyond Traditional Speech Treatment." In *Alaryngeal Speech Rehabilitation,* 2nd ed., ed. S. Salmon (Austin, TX: Pro-Ed).

Lewis, B., and Freebairn, L. (1992). "Residual Effects of Preschool Phonology Disorders in Grade School, Adolescence and Adulthood." *Journal of Speech and Hearing Research* 35:819–831.

Lewis, B., Freebairn, L., Hansen, A., Miscimarra, L., Iyengar, S., & Taylor, H. (2007). "Speech and Language Skills of Parents of Children with Speech Sound Disorders." *American Journal of Speech-Language Pathology* 16:108–118.

Lidz, C. (1991). *A Practitioner's Guide to Dynamic Assessment.* New York: Guilford Press.

Lidz, C., and Pena, E. (1996). "Dynamic Assessment: The Model, Its Relevance as a Nonbiased Approach and Its Application to Latino American Preschool Children." *Language, Speech and Hearing Services in Schools* 27:367–372.

Lifter, K., Edwards, G., Avery, D., Anderson, S., and Sulzer-Azaroff, B. (1988). "Developmental Assessment of Children's Play: Implications for Intervention." Paper presented at the convention of the American Speech-Language-Hearing Association, Boston, MA.

Liles, B. (1985). "Cohesion in the Narratives of Normal and Language-Disordered Children." *Journal of Speech and Hearing Research* 28:123–133.

Liles, B. (1993). "Narrative Discourse in Children with Language Disorders and Children with Normal Language: A Critical Review of the Literature." *Journal of Speech and Hearing Research* 36:868–882.

Lippke, S., Dickey, S., Selmar, J., and Soder, A. (1997). *Photo Articulation Test,* 3rd ed. Danville, IL: Interstate Printers and Publishers.

Loban, W. (1976). *Language Development: Kindergarten through Grade Twelve.* Research Report No. 18. Urbana, IL: National Councils of Teachers of English.

Locke, J. (1980). "The Inference of Speech Perception in the Phonologically Disordered Child. Part I: A Rationale, Some Criteria, the Conventional Tests." *Journal of Speech and Hearing Disorders* 45:431–444.

Locke, J. (1983). "Clinical Phonology: The Explanation and Treatment of Speech Sound Disorders." *Journal of Speech and Hearing Disorders* 48:339–341.

Logemann, J. (1998). *Evaluation and Treatment of Swallowing Disorders.* Austin: Pro-Ed.

Logemann, J. (1998). "Efficacy, Outcomes, and Cost Effectiveness in Dysphagia." In *Measuring Outcomes in Speech-Language Pathology,* ed. C. Frattali (New York: Thieme).

Logemann, J. A., Veis, S., and Colangelo, L. (1999). "A Screening Procedure for Oropharyngeal Dysphagia." *Dysphagia* 14:44–51.

Long, S., and Channell, R. (2001). "Accuracy of Four Language Analysis Procedures Performed Automatically." *American Journal of Speech-Language Pathology,* 10:180–188.

Long, S., and Fey, M. (1993). *Computerized Profiling.* San Antonio, TX: The Psychological Corporation.

Long, S., Fey, M., and Channell, R. (2002). *Computerized Profiling,* Version 9.4.1, http://www.computerizedprofiling.org.

Longhurst, T., and File, J. (1977). "A Comparison of Developmental Sentence Scores for HeadStart Children in Four Conditions." *Language, Speech and Hearing Services in Schools* 8:54–64.

Longhurst, T., and Grubb, S. (1974). "A Comparison of Language Samples Collected in Four Situations."

Language, Speech and Hearing Services in Schools 5:71–78.

Longhurst, T., and Schrandt, T. (1973). "Linguistic Analysis of Children's Speech: A Comparison of Four Procedures." *Journal of Speech and Hearing Disorders* 38:240–249.

Longstreth, D. (1986). "The BELZ Dysphagia Scale." Paper presented at the annual convention of the American Speech-Language-Hearing Association, Detroit, MI.

Lorenzen, B., and Murrary, L. (2008) "Bilingual Aphasia: A Theoretical and Clinical Review." *American Journal of Speech-Language Pathology* 17:299–317.

Louko, L., and Edwards, M. (2001). "Collecting and Transcribing Speech Samples: Enhancing Phonological Analysis." *Topics in Language Disorders* 21:4.

Love, R. J. (2000). *Childhood Motor Speech Disorders Disability,* 2nd ed. Needham Heights, MA: Allyn & Bacon.

Lowe, R. (1986). *Assessment Link between Phonology and Articulation.* Moline, IL: Linguisystems.

Lucas, E. (1980). *Semantic and Pragmatic Language Disorders.* Rockville, MD: Aspen.

Ludlow, C. (1983). "Identification and Assessment of Aphasic Patients for Language Intervention." In *Contemporary Issues in Language Intervention,* eds. J. Miller, D. Yoder, and R. Schiefelbusch (Rockville, MD: American Speech-Language-Hearing Association).

Lund, N., and Duchan, J. (1988). *Assessing Children's Language in Naturalistic Contexts.* Englewood Cliffs, NJ: Prentice Hall.

Lund, N., and Duchan, J. (1993). *Assessing Children's Language in Naturalistic Contexts.* Englewood Cliffs, NJ: Prentice Hall.

Luterman, D. (1979). *Counseling Parents of Hearing-Impaired Children.* Boston, MA: Little, Brown.

Lutz, K. C., and Mallard, A. R. (1986). "Disfluencies and Rate of Speech in Young Adult Nonstutterers." *Journal of Fluency Disorders* 11:307–316.

Luyster, R., Qiu, S., Lopez, K., & Lord, C. (2007). "Predicting Outcomes of Children Referred for Autism Using the MacArthur-Bates Communicative Development Inventory." *Journal of Speech, Language and Hearing Research* 50:667–681.

Lynch, E. (1992). "Developing Cross-Cultural Competence." In *Developing Cross-Cultural Competence,* eds. E. Lynch and M. Hanson (Baltimore, MD: Brookes).

Ma, E., and Yiu, E. (2001). "Voice Activity and Participation Profile: Assessing the Impact of Voice Disorders on Daily Activities." *Journal of Speech, Language and Hearing Research* 44(3):511–524.

MacDonald, J., and Carroll, J. (1992). "A Social Partnership Model for Assessing Early Communication Development: An Intervention Model for Preconversational Children." *Language, Speech and Hearing Services in Schools* 23:113–124.

Manning, W. (2010). *Clinical Decision Making in Fluency Disorders.* Clifton Park, NY: Delmar.

Manning, W. H., and Monte, K. L. (1981). "Fluency Breaks in Older Speakers: Implications for a Model of Stuttering Throughout the Life Cycle." *Journal of Fluency Disorders* 6:35–48.

Mansson, H. (2000). "Childhood Stuttering: Incidence and Development." *Journal of Fluency Disorders* 25:47–57.

Marks, I. M. (1987). *Fears, Phobias and Rituals.* New York: Oxford University Press.

Martino, R., Pron, G., and Diamant, N. (2000). "Screening for Oropharyngeal Dysphagia in Stroke: Insufficient Evidence for Guidelines." *Dysphagia* 15:19–30.

Masterson, J. (1999). "Technological Applications for Speech and Language Assessments." *Seminars in Speech and Language* 20.

Masterson, J., & Bernhardt, B. (2001). *CAPES: Computerized Articulation and Phonology Evaluation System (Version 1.0.1).* San Antonio, TX: Psychological Corporation.

Masterson, J., Bernhardt, B., and Hofheinz, M. (2005). "A Comparison of Single Words and Conversational Speech in Phonological Evaluation." *American Journal of Speech-Language Pathology* 14:229–241.

Masterson, J., and Crede, L. (1999). "Learning to Spell: Implications for Assessment and Intervention." *Language, Speech and Hearing Services in Schools* 30:243–254.

Mattis, S. (1976). "Mental Status Examination for Organic Mental Syndrome in the Elderly Patient." In *Geriatric Psychiatry,* eds. R. Bellack and B. Karasu (New York: Grune and Stratton).

Maxwell, E., and Rockman, B. (1984). "Procedures for Linguistic Analysis of Misarticulated Speech." *Phonological Theory and the Misarticulating Child,* ASHA Monographs 22:69e.

Maxwell, S., and Wallach, G. (1984). "The Language-Learning Disabilities Connection: Symptoms of Early Language Disability Change over Time." In *Language Learning Disabilities in School-Age Children,* eds. G. Wallach and K. Butler (Baltimore, MD: Williams and Wilkins).

Mazza, P., Schuckers, G., and Daniloff, R. (1979). "Contextual-Coarticulatory Inconsistency of /∫/ Misarticulation." *Journal of Phonetics* 7:57–69.

McCabe, A., and Bliss, L. (2003). *Patterns of Narrative Discourse: A Multicultural Life Span Approach.* Boston, MA: Allyn & Bacon.

McCabe, A., Bliss, L., Barra, G., & Bennett, M. (2008). "Comparison of Personal versus Fictional Narratives of Children with Language Impairment." *American Journal of Speech-Language Pathology* 17:194–206.

McCarthy, J. (2006). "Billing, Coding, & Calculating Fees: Finding Solutions." Accessed online at http://www. asha.org/uploadFiles/practice/reimbursement/coding/billingcodes2006.pdf

McCathren, R., Warren, S., and Yoder, P. (1996). "Prelinguistic Predictors of Later Language Development." In *Assessment of Communication and Language,* eds. K. Cole, P. Dale, and D. Thal (Baltimore, MD: Brookes).

McCauley, R. (1996). "Familiar Strangers: Criterion Referenced Measures in Communication Disorders." *Language, Speech and Hearing Services in Schools* 27:122–131.

McCauley, R., and Skenes, L. (1987). "Contrastive Stress, Phonetic Context and Misarticulation of /r/ in Young Speakers." *Journal of Speech and Hearing Research* 30(1):114–121.

McCauley, R., and Strand, E. (2008). "A Review of Standardized Tests of Nonverbal Oral and Speech Motor Performance in Children." *American Journal of Speech-Language Pathology* 17:81–91.

McCauley, R., Strand, E., Lof, G., and Schooling, T. (2009). "Evidence-Based Systematic Review: Effects of Nonspeech Oral Motor Exercises on Speech." *American Journal of Speech-Language Pathology* 18:343–360.

McCauley, R., and Swisher, L. (1984a). "Psychometric Review of Language and Articulation Tests for Preschool Children." *Journal of Speech and Hearing Disorders* 49:34–42.

McCauley, R., and Swisher, L. (1984b). "Use and Misuse of Norm-Referenced Tests in Clinical Assessment: A Hypothetical Case." *Journal of Speech and Hearing Disorders* 49:338–348.

McClean, M. (1973). "Forward Coarticulation of Velar Movement at Marked Junctural Boundaries." *Journal of Speech and Hearing Research* 16:236–246.

McCollum, J., and Stayton, V. (1985). "Social Interaction Assessment/Intervention." *Journal of the Division for Early Childhood* 9:125–135.

McCullough, G. H., Wertz, R. T., Rosenbek, R. C., and Dinneen, C. (1999). "Clinicians' Preferences and Practices in Conducting Clinical/Bedside and Videofluoroscopic Swallowing Examinations in an Adult, Neurogenic Population." *American Journal of Speech Language Pathology* 8:149–163.

McDonald, E. (1964). *Articulation Testing and Treatment.* Pittsburgh, PA: Stanwix House.

McEachern, D., and Haynes, W. (2004). "Gesture-Speech Combinations as a Transition to Multiword Utterances." *American Journal of Speech-Language Pathology* 13:227–236.

McFadden, T. (1996). "Creating Language Impairments in Typically Achieving Children: The Pitfalls of 'Normal' Normative Sampling." *Language Speech and Hearing Services in Schools,* 27:3–9.

McGinty, A., & Justice, L. (2009). "Predictors of Print Knowledge in Children with Specific Language Impairment: Experimental and Developmental Factors." *Journal of Speech, Language and Hearing Research* 52:81–97.

McGregor, K., and Schwartz, R. (1992). "Converging Evidence for Underlying Phonological Representation in a Child Who Misarticulates." *Journal of Speech and Hearing Research* 35:596–603.

McGregor, K., Williams, D., Hearst, S., and Johnson, A. (1997). "The Use of Contrastive Analysis in Distinguishing Difference from Disorder: A Tutorial." *American Journal of Speech-Language Pathology* 6:45–56.

McLean, J., and Snyder-Mclean, L. (1978). *A Transactional Approach to Early Language Training.* Columbus, OH: Merrill.

McLeod, S., Hand, L., Rosenthal, J., and Hayes, B. (1994). "The Effect of Sampling Condition on Children's Productions of Consonant Clusters." *Journal of Speech and Hearing Research* 37:868–882.

McLeod, S., Van Doorn, J., and Reed, V. (2001). "Normal Acquisition of Consonant Clusters." *American Journal of Speech-Language Pathology* 10:99–110.

McNamara, A. P., and Perry, C. K. (1994). "Vocal Abuse Prevention Practices: A National Survey of School-Based Speech-Language Pathologists." *Language, Speech and Hearing Services in Schools* 25:105–111.

McNeil, M., and Prescott, T. (1978). *Revised Token Test.* Austin, TX: Pro-Ed.

McNeil, M. R., Robin, D. A., & Schmidt, R. A. (2008). "Apraxia of Speech: Definition, Differentiation, and Treatment." In *Clinical Management of Sensorimotor Speech Disorders,* 2nd ed., ed. M. R. McNeil (New York: Thieme).

McNeill, D. (1970). *The Acquisition of Language: The Study of Developmental Psycholinguistics.* New York: Harper & Row.

McReynolds, L., & Engmann, D. (1975). *Distinctive Feature Analysis of Misarticulations.* Baltimore: University Park Press.

McReynolds, L., and Huston, K. (1971). "A Distinctive Feature Analysis of Children's Misarticulation." *Journal of Speech and Hearing Disorders* 36:155–166.

Merrell, A., and Plante, E. (1997). "Norm Referenced Test Interpretation in the Diagnostic Process." *Language, Speech and Hearing Services in Schools* 28:50–58.

Merritt, D., and Liles, B. (1989). "Narrative Analysis: Clinical Applications of Story Generation and Story Retelling." *Journal of Speech and Hearing Disorders* 54:438–447.

Messick, S. (1975). "The Standard Problem: Meaning and Values in Measurement and Evaluation." *American Psychologist* 30:955–966.

Messick, S. (1980). "Test Validity and the Ethics of Assessment." *American Psychologist* 35:1012–1027.

Messner, A. H., and Lalakea, M. L. (2002). "The Effect of Ankyloglossia on Speech in Children." *Otolaryngology, Head and Neck Surgery* 127:539–545.

Meyerson, M. D. (1990). "Cultural Considerations in the Treatment of Latinos with Craniofacial Malformations." *Cleft Palate Journal* 27(3):279–288.

Miccio, A., Elbert, M., and Forrest, K. (1999). "The Relationship Between Stimulability and Phonological Acquisition in Children with Normally Developing and Disordered Phonologies." *American Journal of Speech-Language Pathology* 8:347–363.

Miles, S., Chapman, R., and Sindberg, H. (2006). "Sampling Context Affects MLU in the Language of Adolescents with Down Syndrome." *Journal of Speech, Language and Hearing Research* 49:325–337.

Millen, K., and Prutting, C. (1979). "Consistencies across Three Language Comprehension Tests for Specific Grammatical Features." *Language, Speech and Hearing Services in Schools* 10:162–170.

Miller, J. (1981). *Assessing Language Production in Children: Experimental Procedures.* Baltimore, MD: University Park Press.

Miller, J. (2002). *Systematic Analysis of Language Transcripts, Version 7.0.* Language Analysis Laboratory, University of Wisconsin–Madison.

Miller, J., and Chapman, R. (1981). "The Relation between Age and Mean Length of Utterance in Morphemes." *Journal of Speech and Hearing Research* 24:154–161.

Miller, J., and Chapman, R. (1995). *SALT: Systematic Analysis of Language Transcripts.* Madison: Language Analysis Laboratory, University of Wisconsin.

Miller, J., and Chapman, R. (2008). *Systematic Analysis of Language Transcripts (version 8-Computer Software).* Madison, WI: University of Wisconsin–Madison, Waisman Center, Language Analysis Laboratory.

Miller, J., and Paul, R. (1995). *The Clinical Assessment of Language Comprehension.* Baltimore, MD: Brookes.

Miller, L., Gillam, R., and Pena, E. (2001). *Dynamic Assessment and Intervention: Improving Children's Narrative Abilities.* Austin, TX: Pro-Ed.

Mimura, M., Kato, M., Sano, Y., Kojima, T., Naesar, M., and Kashima, H. (1998). "Prospective and Retrospective Studies of Recovery in Aphasia: Changes in Cerebral Blood Flow and Language Function." *Brain* 121:2083–2094.

Moll, K., and Daniloff, R. (1971). "Investigation of the Timing of Velar Movements during Speech." *Journal of the Acoustical Society of America* 50:678–684.

Molrine, C. J., and Pierce, R. S. (2002). "Black and White Adults' Expressive Language Performance on Three Tests of Aphasia." *American Journal of Speech-Language Pathology* 11:139–150.

Montes, J., and Erickson, J. G. (1990). "Bilingual Stuttering: Exploring a Diagnostic Dilemma." *Ethnotes* 1:14–15.

Montgomery, J., & Evans, J. (2009). "Complex Sentence Comprehension and Working Memory in Children with Specific Language Impairment." *Journal of Speech, Language and Hearing Research* 52:269–288.

Montgomery, J., Magimairaj, B., & Finney, M. (2010). "Working Memory and Specific Language Impairment: An Update on the Relation and Perspectives on Assessment and Treatment." *American Journal of Speech-Language Pathology* 19:78–94.

Moore-Brown, B., & Montgomery, J. (2006). "SLPs and RTI: Your Response Will Make the Difference." Paper presented at the Convention of the American Speech-Language-Hearing Association, Miami, FL.

Moran, M. (1993). "Final Consonant Deletion in African American Children Speaking Black English: A Closer Look." *Language, Speech and Hearing Services in Schools* 24:161–166.

Morehead, D., and Morehead, A. (1974). "From Signal to Sign." In *Language Perspectives—Acquisition, Retardation and Intervention* (Baltimore, MD: University Park Press).

Morris, N., and Crump, W. (1982). "Syntactic and Vocabulary Development in the Written Language of Learning Disabled and Non-Disabled Students at Four Age Levels." *Learning Disability Quarterly* 5:163–172.

Morris, S. (2009). "Test-Retest Reliability of Independent Measures of Phonology in the Assessment of Toddlers' Speech." *Language, Speech and Hearing Services in Schools* 40:46–52.

Morris, S. (2010). "Clinical Application of the Mean Babbling Level and Syllable Structure Level." *Language, Speech and Hearing Services in Schools* 41:223–230.

Morrison, J., & Shriberg, L. (1992). "Articulation Testing versus Conversational Speech Sampling." *Journal of Speech and Hearing Research* 35:259–273.

Morrison, M. (1998). *Let Evening Come: Reflections on Aging.* New York: Random House.

Mount-Weitz, J. (1996). "Vocabulary Development and Disorders in African American Children." In *Communication Development and Disorders in African American Children,* eds. A. Kamhi, K. Pollock, and J. Harris (Baltimore, MD: Brookes).

Mulac, A., Prutting, C., and Tomlinson, C. (1978). "Testing for a Specific Syntactic Structure." *Journal of Communication Disorders* 11: 335–347.

Muma, J. (1973a). "Language Assessment: The Co-Occurring and Restricted Structure Procedure." *Acta Symbolica* 4:12–29.

Muma, J. (1973b). "Language Assessment: Some Underlying Assumptions." *Journal of the American Speech and Hearing Association* 15: 331–338.

Muma, J. (1975). "The Communication Game: Dump and Play." *Journal of Speech and Hearing Disorders* 40:296–309.

Muma, J. (1978). *Language Handbook: Concepts, Assessment, Intervention.* Englewood Cliffs, NJ: Prentice Hall.

Muma, J. (1981). *Language Primer.* Lubbock, TX: Natural Child Publisher.

Muma, J. (1983). "Speech Language Pathology: Emerging Clinical Expertise in Language." In *Pragmatic Assessment and Intervention Issues in Language,* eds. T. Gallagher and C. Prutting (San Diego, CA: College-Hill Press).

Muma, J. (1984). "Semel and Wiig's CELF: Construct Validity?" *Journal of Speech and Hearing Disorders* 49:101–104.

Muma, J. (1985). "No News Is Bad News: A Response to McCauley and Swisher." *Journal of Speech and Hearing Disorders* 50:290–293.

Muma, J. (1986). *Language Acquisition: A Functionalistic Perspective.* Austin, TX: Pro-Ed.

Muma, J. (1998). *Effective Speech-Language Pathology: A Cognitive Socialization Approach.* Mahwah, NJ: Erlbaum.

Muma, J. (2002). "Construct Validity: The Essence of Language Assessment." Unpublished manuscript.

Muma, J., Lubinski, R., and Pierce, S. (1982). "A New Era in Language Assessment: Data or Evidence." In *Speech and Language,* Vol. 7, ed. N. Lass (New York: Academic Press).

Munoz, M., Gillam, R., Pena, E., and Gulley-Faehnle, A. (2003). "Measures of Language Development in

Fictional Narratives of Latino Children." *Language, Speech and Hearing Services in Schools* 34:332–342.

Murray, D., Ruble, L., Willis, H., & Molloy, C. (2009). "Parent and Teacher Report of Social Skills in Children with Autism Spectrum Disorders." *Language, Speech and Hearing Services in Schools* 40:109–115.

Murray, J. (2003, Oct. 21). "Responding to the Dysphagia Consult: A Report-Writing Primer." *The ASHA Leader* 8(19):4–5, 24–25.

Musselwhite, C., and Barrie-Blackley, S. (1980). "Three Variations of the Imperative Format of Language Sample Elicitation." *Language, Speech and Hearing Services in Schools* 11:56–67.

Myers, F. (1996). "Cluttering a Matter of Perspective." *Journal of Fluency Disorders* 21:175–186.

Myers, F., and St. Louis, K. (1996). *Cluttering: A Clinical Perspective.* San Diego, CA: Singular.

Myers, P. S. (2001). "Communication Disorders Associated with Right Hemisphere Damage." In *Language Intervention Strategies in Aphasia and Related Neurogenic Communication Disorders* (4th ed.), ed. R. Chapey (Philadelphia, PA: Lippincott Williams and Wilkins).

National Association of State Directors of Special Education (2005). http://www.nasdse.org

National Cancer Institute (1985). *Cancer Rates and Risks,* 3rd ed. Washington, DC: National Institutes of Health.

Nelson, K. (1973). "Structure and Strategy in Learning to Talk." *Monographs of the Society for Research in Child Development* 38:11–56.

Nelson, K. (1974). "Concept, Word and Sentence: Interrelations in Acquisition and Development." *Psychological Review* 81:267–285.

Nelson, N. (1998). *Childhood Language Disorders in Context,* 2nd ed. Boston: Allyn & Bacon.

Nelson, N. (2010). *Language and Literacy Disorders: Infancy Through Adolescence.* Boston: Allyn & Bacon.

Newhoff, M., and Leonard, L. (1983). "Diagnosis of Developmental Language Disorders." In *Diagnosis in Speech-Language Pathology,* eds. I. Meitus and B. Weinberg (Baltimore, MD: University Park Press).

Newman, R., and McGregor, K. (2006). "Teachers and Laypersons Discern Quality Differences between

Narratives Produced by Children with or without SLI." *Journal of Speech, Language and Hearing Research* 49:1022–1036.

Nicholas, J., & Geers, A. (2008). "Expected Test Scores for Preschoolers with a Cochlear Implant Who Use Spoken Language." *American Journal of Speech-Language Pathology* 17:121–138.

Nippold, M. (1988). "Figurative Language." In *Later Language Development: Ages Nine through Nineteen,* ed. M. Nippold (Austin, TX: Pro-Ed).

Nippold, M. (1993). "Developmental Markers in Adolescent Language: Syntax, Semantics and Pragmatics." *Language, Speech and Hearing Services in Schools* 24:21–28.

Nippold, M. (2009). "School-Age Children Talk about Chess: Does Knowledge Drive Syntactic Complexity?" *Journal of Speech, Language and Hearing Research* 52:856–871.

Nippold, M., Mansfield, T., Billow, J., & Tomblin, J. (2008). "Expository Discourse in Adolescents with Language Impairments: Examining Syntactic Development." *American Journal of Speech-Language Pathology* 17:356–366.

Nippold, M., Mansfield, T., Billow, J., & Tomblin, J. (2009). "Syntactic Development in Adolescents with a History of Language Impairments: A Follow-Up Investigation." *American Journal of Speech-Language Pathology* 18:241–251.

Nippold, M., Schwarz, I., and Undlin, R. (1992). "Use and Understanding of Adverbial Conjuncts: A Developmental Study of Adolescents and Young Adults." *Journal of Speech and Hearing Research* 35:108–118.

Norris, J. (1995). "Expanding Language Norms for School-Age Children and Adolescents: Is It Pragmatic?" *Language, Speech and Hearing Services in Schools* 26:342–352.

O'Brian, S., and Packman, A. (2004). "Self-Rating of Stuttering Severity as a Clinical Tool." *American Journal of Speech-Language Pathology* 13:219–226.

Oetting, J., Cleveland, L., & Cope, R. (2008). "Empirically Derived Combinations of Tools and Clinical Cutoffs: An Illustrative Case with a Sample of Culturally/Linguistically Diverse Children." *Language Speech and Hearing Services in Schools* 39:44–53.

Oller, K., et al. (1972). "Five Studies in Abnormal Phonology." Unpublished paper, University of Washington.

Olswang, L., Bain, B., Rosendahl, P., Oblak, S., and Smith, A. (1986). "Language Learning: Moving from a Context-Dependent to Independent State." *Child Language Teaching and Therapy* 2:180–210.

Olswang, L., and Carpenter, R. (1978). "Elicitor Effects on the Language Obtained from Young Language-Impaired Children." *Journal of Speech and Hearing Disorders* 43:76–86.

Olswang, L., Rodriguez, B., and Timler, G. (1998). "Recommending Intervention for Toddlers with Specific Language Learning Difficulties: We May Not Have All the Answers, But We Know a Lot." *American Journal of Speech-Language Pathology* 7:23–32.

Olswang, L., Stoel-Gammon, C., Coggins, T., and Carpenter, R. (1987). *Assessing Prelinguistic and Early Linguistic Behaviors in Developmentally Young Children.* Seattle: University of Washington Press.

Olswang, L., Svensson, L., Coggins, T., Beilinson, J., and Donaldson, A. (2006). "Reliability Issues and Solutions for Coding Social Communication Performance in Classroom Settings." *Journal of Speech, Language and Hearing Research* 49:1058–1071.

Omark, A. (1981). *Communication Assessment of the Bilingual, Bicultural Child: Issues and Guidelines.* Baltimore, MD: Pro-Ed.

O'Neill, D. (2007). "The Language Use Inventory for Young Children: A Parent-Report Measure of Pragmatic Language Development for 18–47-Month-Old Children." *Journal of Speech, Language and Hearing Research* 50:214–228.

Onslow, M. (1996). *Behavioral Management of Stuttering.* San Diego: Singular.

Opitz, V. (1982). "Pragmatic Analysis of the Communicative Behavior of an Autistic Child." *Journal of Speech and Hearing Disorders* 47:99–108.

Oratio, A. (1977). *Supervision in Speech Pathology: A Handbook for Supervisors and Clinicians.* Baltimore, MD: University Park Press.

Owens, R. (2004). *Language Disorders: A Functional Approach to Assessment and Intervention,* 4th ed. Boston: Allyn & Bacon.

Owens, R. (2005). *Language Development: An Introduction.* Needham Heights, MA: Allyn and Bacon.

Paden, E., and Moss, S. (1985). "Comparison of Three Phonological Analysis Procedures." *Language, Speech and Hearing Services in Schools* 16(2):103–109.

Palisano, R., Rosenbaum, P. L., Walter, S., Russell, D., Woods, E., and Galuppi, B. (1997). Development and reliability of a system to classify gross motor function in children with cerebral palsy. *Developmental Medicine and Child Neurology* 39:214–223.

Panagos, J., Quine, H., and Klich, P. (1979). "Syntactic and Phonological Influences in Children's Articulations." *Journal of Speech and Hearing Research* 22:841–848.

Pannbacker, M. (1999) "Treatment of Vocal Nodules: Options and Outcomes." *American Journal of Speech-Language Pathology* 8:209–217.

Pannbacker, M., Middleton, G., Vekovius, G., and Sanders, K. (2001). *Report Writing for Speech-Language Pathologists and Audiologists.* Austin, TX: Pro-Ed.

Paradis, M., and Libben, G. (1987). *The Assessment of Bilingual Aphasia.* Hillsdale, NJ: Lawrence Erlbaum Associates.

Patterson, J. (1998). "Expressive Vocabulary Development and Word Combinations of Spanish-English Bilingual Toddlers." *American Journal of Speech-Language Pathology* 7:46–56.

Paul, D., Frattali, C., Holland, A., Thompson, C., Caperton, C., and Slater, S. (1999). *Quality of Communication Life Scale (ASHA QCL).* Rockville, MD: American Speech-Language-Hearing Association.

Paul, R. (2001). *Language Disorders from Infancy through Adolescence: Assessment and Intervention.* St. Louis, MO: Mosby.

Paul, R. (2007). *Language Disorders from Infancy through Adolescence: Assessment and Intervention,* 3rd ed. St. Louis, MO: Mosby.

Paul, R., and Alforde, S. (1993). "Grammatical Morpheme Acquisition in 4-Year-Olds with Normal, Impaired and Late Developing Language." *Journal of Speech and Hearing Research* 36:1271–1275.

Paul, R., and Jennings, P. (1992). "Phonological Behavior in Toddlers with Slow Expressive Language Development." *Journal of Speech and Hearing Research* 35:99–107.

Paul, R., and Shriberg, L. (1982). "Association between Phonology and Syntax in Speech-Delayed Children." *Journal of Speech and Hearing Research* 25:536–546.

Pearson, B., Velleman, S., Bryant, T., & Charko, T. (2009). "Phonological Milestones for African American English-Speaking Children Learning Mainstream American English as a Second Dialect." *Language, Speech and Hearing Services in Schools* 40:229–244.

Peets, K. (2009). "The Effects of Context on the Classroom Discourse Skills of Children with Language Impairment." *Language, Speech and Hearing Services in Schools* 40:5–16.

Pena, E. (1996). "Dynamic Assessment: The Model and Its Language Applications." In *Assessment of Communication and Language,* eds. P. Cole, P. Dale, and D. Thal (Baltimore, MD: Brookes).

Pena, E., Bedore, L., and Rappazzo, C. (2003). "Comparison of Spanish, English and Bilingual Children's Performance Across Semantic Tasks." *Language, Speech and Hearing Services in Schools* 34:5–16.

Pena, E., Gillam, R., Malek, M., Ruiz-Felter, R., Resendiz, M., Fiestas, C., and Sabel, T. (2006). "Dynamic Assessment of School-Age Children's Narrative Ability: An Experimental Investigation of Classification Accuracy." *Journal of Speech, Language and Hearing Research* 49:1037–1057.

Pena, E., and Quinn, R. (1997). "Task Familiarity: Effects on the Test Performance of Puerto Rican and African American Children." *Language, Speech and Hearing Services in Schools* 28:323–332.

Pena, E., Quinn, R., & Iglesias, A. (1992). "The Application of Dynamic Assessment to Language Assessment: A Non-Biased Procedure." *Journal of Special Education* 26:269–280.

Perlin, W. S., and Boner, M. M. (1994). "Clinical Assessment of Feeding and Swallowing in Infants and Children." In *Clinical Management of Dysphagia in Adults and Children,* ed. L. R. Cherney (Gaithersburg, MD: Aspen Publications).

Peters, T. J., and Guitar, B. (1991). *Stuttering: An Integrated Approach to Its Nature and Treatment.* Baltimore, MD: Williams and Wilkins.

Peterson, R., Pennington, B., Shriberg, L., & Boada, R. (2009). "What Influences Literacy Outcome in Children with Speech Sound Disorder?" *Journal of Speech, Language and Hearing Research* 52:1175–1188.

Peterson-Falzone, S. (1982). "Resonance Disorders in Structural Defects." In *Speech, Language and Hearing,* vol. 2, *Pathologies of Speech and Language,* eds. N. Lass, L. McReynolds, J. Northern, and D. Yoder (Philadelphia, PA: W. B. Saunders).

Pigott, T., Barry, J., Hughes, B., Eastin, D., Titus, P., Stensil, H., Metcalf, K., and Porter, B. (1985). *Speech-Ease Screening Inventory (K-1).* Austin, TX: Pro-Ed.

Pimental, P. A., and Kingsbury, N. A. (2004). *Mini Inventory of Right Brain Injury.* Austin, TX: Pro-Ed.

Pindzola, R. H. (1988). *Stuttering Intervention Program: Age 3 to Grade 3.* Austin, TX: Pro-Ed.

Pindzola, R. H. (1990). "Disfluency Characteristics of Aged, Normal-Speaking Black and White Males." *Journal of Fluency Disorders* 15:235–243.

Pindzola, R. H. (2000). *A Voice Assessment Protocol for Children and Adults.* Austin, TX: Pro-Ed.

Pindzola, R. H., and Cain, B. H. (1989). "Duration and Frequency Characteristics of Tracheoesophageal Speech." *Annals of Otology, Rhinology, and Laryngology* 98(12):960–964.

Pindzola, R. H., Jenkins, M., and Lokken, K. (1989). "Speaking Rates of Young Children." *Language, Speech and Hearing Services in Schools* 20:133–138.

Pindzola, R. H., and White, D. (1986). "A Protocol for Differentiating the Incipient Stutterer." *Language, Speech and Hearing Services in Schools* 17:2–15.

Plante, E. (1996). "Observing and Interpreting Behaviors: An Introduction to the Clinical Forum." *Language, Speech and Hearing Services in Schools* 27:99–101.

Plante, E., and Vance, R. (1994). "Selection of Preschool Language Tests: A Data-Based Approach." *Language, Speech and Hearing Services in Schools* 25:15–24.

Plante, E., and Vance, R. (1995). "Diagnostic Accuracy of Two Tests of Preschool Language." *American Journal of Speech-Language Pathology* 4:70–76.

Pollack, E., and Rees, N. (1972). "Disorders of Articulation: Some Clinical Applications of Distinctive Feature Theory." *Journal of Speech and Hearing Disorders* 37:451–461.

Polmanteer, K., and Turbiville, V. (2000). "Family-Responsive Individualized Family Service Plans for Speech-Language Pathologists." *Language, Speech and Hearing Services in Schools* 31:4–14.

Poole, E. (1934). "Genetic Development of Articulation of Consonant Sounds in Speech." *Elementary English Review* 11:159–161.

Popham, J. (1981). *Modern Educational Measurement.* Englewood Cliffs, NJ: Prentice Hall.

Porch, B. (1981). *Porch Index of Communicative Ability.* Austin, TX: Pro-Ed.

Powell, H. (1967). "Child-Rearing Practices Reported for Young Male Negro Stutterers and Nonstutterers in Two South Carolina School Districts." *Dissertation Abstracts International* 28, no. 3A:1149–1150.

Powell, L., and Courtice, K. (1983). *Alzheimer's Disease.* Reading, MA: Addison-Wesley.

Powell, T. (1995). "A Clinical Screening Procedure for Assessing Consonant Cluster Production." *American Journal of Speech Language Pathology* 4:59–65.

Powell, T. (2008a). "An Integrated Evaluation of Nonspeech Oral Motor Treatments." *Language, Speech and Hearing Services in Schools* 39:422–427.

Powell, T. (2008b). "The Use of Nonspeech Oral Motor Treatments for Developmental Speech Sound Production Disorders: Interventions and Interactions." *Language, Speech and Hearing Services in Schools* 39:374–379.

Powers, M. (1971). "Functional Disorders of Articulation: Symptomatology and Etiology." In *Handbook of Speech Pathology and Audiology,* ed. L. Travis (Englewood Cliffs, NJ: Prentice Hall).

Prater, R. J., and Swift, R. W. (1984). *Manual of Voice Therapy.* Boston, MA: Little, Brown.

Prathanee, B. (1998). "Oral Diadochokinetic rate in adults." *Journal of the Medical Association of Thailand* 81(10):784–788.

Prather, E., Hedrick, D., and Kern, C. (1975). "Articulation Development in Children Aged 2 to 4 Years." *Journal of Speech and Hearing Disorders* 40:179–191.

Prelock, P., Beatson, J., Bitner, B., Broder, C., and Ducker, A. (2003). "Interdisciplinary Assessment of Young Children with Autism Spectrum Disorder." *Language, Speech and Hearing Services in Schools* 34:194–202.

Preston, J., and Edwards, M. (2007). "Phonological Processing Skills of Adolescents with Residual Speech Sound Errors." *Language, Speech and Hearing Services in Schools* 38:297–308.

Preston, J., and Edwards, M. (2010). "Phonological Awareness and Types of Sound Errors in Preschoolers with Speech Sound Disorders." *Journal of Speech, Language and Hearing Research* 53:44–60.

Price, L., Hendricks, S., and Cook, C. (2010). "Incorporating Computer-Aided Language Sample Analysis into Clinical Practice." *Language, Speech and Hearing Services in Schools* 41:206–222.

Prizant, B., and Wetherby, A. (1988). "Providing Services to Children with Autism (ages 0 to 2 years) and Their Families." *Topics in Language Disorders* 9(1):1–23.

Proctor, A. (1989). "Stages of Normal Noncry Vocal Development in Infancy: A Protocol for Assessment." *Topics in Language Disorders* 10:26–42.

Proctor, A., Duffy, M. C., Patterson, A., and Yairi, E. (2001). "Stuttering in African-American and European-American Preschoolers." *The ASHA Report* 6(15):141.

Pruitt, S., and Oetting, J. (2009). "Past Tense Marking by African American English Speaking Children Reared in Poverty." *Journal of Speech, Language and Hearing Research* 52:2–15.

Prutting, C., and Kirchner, D. (1987). "A Clinical Appraisal of the Pragmatic Aspects of Language." *Journal of Speech and Hearing Disorders* 52:105–119.

Puntil-Sheltman, J. (2002). "Medically Fragile Patients." *The ASHA Leader* (18):14–15.

Puranik, C., Lombardino, L., and Altmann, L. (2008). "Assessing the Microstructure of Written Language Using a Retelling Paradigm." *American Journal of Speech-Language Pathology* 17:107–120.

Quinn, R., Goldstein, B., and Pena, E. (1996). "Cultural/Linguistic Variation in the United States and its Implications for Assessment and Intervention in Speech-Language Pathology: An Introduction." *Language, Speech and Hearing Services in Schools* 27:345–346.

Quirk, R., and Greenbaum, S. (1975). *A Concise Grammar of Contemporary English.* New York: Harcourt Brace Jovanovich.

Rabidoux, P., and Macdonald, J. (2000). "An Interactive Taxonomy of Mothers and Children During Storybook Interactions." *American Journal of Speech-Language Pathology* 9:331–344.

Rafaat, S., Rvachew, S., and Russell, R. (1995). "Reliability of Clinician Judgments of Severity of Phonological

Impairment." *American Journal of Speech Language Pathology* 4:39–46.

Ratner, N. R. (2004). "Caregiver–Child Interactions and Their Impact on Children's Fluency Implications for Treatment." *Language, Speech and Hearing Services in Schools* 35:46–56.

Ratusnik, D. L., Kirilluk, E., and Ratusnik, C. M. (1979). "Relationship among Race, Social Status, and Sex of Preschoolers' Normal Disfluencies: A Cross-Cultural Investigation." *Language, Speech, and Hearing Services in Schools* 10:171–177.

Ray, B., and Baker, B. (2002). *Hypernasality Modification Program: A Systematic Approach.* Austin, TX: Pro-Ed.

Raymer, A. M., and Rothi, L. (2001). "Cognitive Approaches to Impairments of Word Comprehension and Production." In *Language Intervention Strategies in Aphasia and Related Neurogenic Communication Disorders,* 4th ed., ed. R. Chapey (Philadelphia, PA: Lippincott Williams and Wilkins).

Realica, R. M., Smith, M. K., Glover, A. L., and Yu, J. C. (2000). "A Simplified Pneumotachometer for the Quantitative Assessment of Velopharyngeal Incompetence." *Annals of Plastic Surgery* 44(2):163–166.

Rees, N., and Shulman, M. (1978). "I Don't Understand What You Mean by Comprehension." *Journal of Speech and Hearing Disorders* 43:208–219.

Reisberg, B., Ferris, S. H., and Crook, T. (1982). "Signs, Symptoms, and Course of Age-Associated Cognitive Decline." In *Aging,* Vol. 19, *Alzheimer's Disease: A Report of Progress,* eds. S. Corkin, K. L. Davis, J. H. Growdon, E. Usdin, and R. L. Wurtman (New York: Raven Press).

Relic, A., Mazemja, P., Arens, C., Koller, M., and Ganz, H. (2001). "Investigation Quality of Life and Coping Resources after Laryngectomy." *European Archives of Oto-Rhino-Laryngology* 258(10):514–517.

Rescorla, L. (1989). "The Language Development Survey: A Screening Tool for Delayed Language in Toddlers." *Journal of Speech and Hearing Disorders* 54:587–599.

Rescorla, L. (2002). "Language and Reading Outcomes to Age 9 in Late Talking Toddlers." *Journal of Speech, Language and Hearing Research* 45:360–371.

Rescorla, L. (2009). "Age 17 Language and Reading Outcomes in Late-Talking Toddlers: Support for a Dimensional Perspective on Language Delay." *Journal of Speech, Language and Hearing Ressearch* 52:16–30.

Rescorla, L., and Alley, A. (2001). "Validation of the Language Development Survey (LDS): A Parent Report Tool for Identifying Language Delay in Toddlers." *Journal of Speech, Language and Hearing Research* 44:434–445.

Rescorla, L., Alley, A., and Christine, J. (2001). "Word Frequencies in Toddlers' Lexicons." *Journal of Speech, Language and Hearing Research* 44:598–609.

Rescorla, L., and Goossens, M. (1992). "Symbolic Play Development in Toddlers with Expressive Specific Language Impairment (SLI-E)." *Journal of Speech and Hearing Research* 35:1290–1302.

Rescorla, L., Ratner, N., Jusczyk, P., and Jusczyk, A. (2005). "Concurrent Validity of the Language Development Survey: Associations with the MacArthur-Bates Communicative Development Inventories—Words and Sentences." *American Journal of Speech-Language Pathology* 14:156–163.

Rescorla, L., Ross, G., and McClure, S. (2007). "Language Delay and Behavioral/Emotional Problems in Toddlers: Findings from Two Developmental Clinics." *Journal of Speech, Language and Hearing Research* 50:1063–1078.

Research Foundation (1990). *Functional Independence Measure, Version 3.1,* from the Uniform Data Set for Medical Rehabilitation, Department of Rehabilitation Medicine, State University of New York at Buffalo.

Retherford, K. (2000). *Guide to Analysis of Language Transcripts.* Eau Claire, WI: Thinking Publications.

Reyes, B. (1995). "Considerations in the Assessment and Treatment of Neurogenic Communication Disorders in Bilingual Adults." In *Bilingual Speech-Language Pathology: A Hispanic Focus,* ed. H. Kayser (San Diego, CA: Singular Publishing).

Reynolds, C., & Horton, A. (2007). *Test of Verbal Comprehension and Fluency.* Austin, TX: Pro-Ed.

Rhyner, P., Kelly, D., Brantley, A., and Krueger, D. (1999). "Screening Low-Income African American Children Using the BLT-2S and the SPELT-P." *American Journal of Speech-Language Pathology,* 8:44–52.

Rice, M., Sell, M., and Hadley, P. (1990). "The Social Interactive Coding System (SICS): An On-Line, Clinically Relevant Descriptive Tool." *Language, Speech and Hearing Services in Schools* 21:2–14.

Rice, M., Smolik, F., Perpich, D., Thompson, T., Rytting, N., and Blossom, M. (2010). "Mean Length of Utterance Levels in 6-Month Intervals for Children 3 to 9 Years with and without Language Impairments." *Journal of Speech, Language and Hearing Research* 53:333–349.

Riley, G. (1981). *Stuttering Prediction Instrument for Young Children.* Austin, TX: Pro-Ed.

Riley, G. (2009). *The Stuttering Severity Instrument*, 4th ed. East Moline, IL: Linguasystems.

Ritterman, S., and Freeman, N. (1974). "Distinctive Phonetic Features as Relevant and Irrelevant Stimulus Dimensions in Speech Sound Discrimination Learning." *Journal of Speech and Hearing Research* 17:417–425.

Robbins, J., Fisher, H., and Blom, E. (1984). "A Comparative Acoustic Study of Normal, Esophageal, and Tracheoesophageal Speech Production." *Journal of Speech and Hearing Disorders* 49:202–210.

Roberts, J., Martin, G., Moskowitz, L., Harris, A., Foreman, J., and Nelson, L. (2007). "Discourse Skills of Boys with Fragile X Syndrome in Comparison to Boys with Down Syndrome." *Journal of Speech, Language and Hearing Research* 50:475–492.

Roberts, P. M. (2000). "Written Picture Name Agreement in French-English Bilinguals." Unpublished manuscript cited in *Language Intervention Strategies in Aphasia and Related Neurogenic Communication Disorders,* 4th ed., ed. R. Chapey (Philadelphia, PA: Lippincott Williams and Wilkins).

Roberts, P. M. (2001). "Aphasia Assessment and Treatment for Bilingual and Culturally Diverse Patients." In *Language Intervention Strategies in Aphasia and Related Neurogenic Communication Disorders,* 4th ed., ed. R. Chapey (Philadelphia, PA: Lippincott Williams and Wilkins).

Robertson, C., and Salter, W. (1997). *The Phonological Awareness Test.* East Moline, IL: Linguisystems.

Robinson, T. L., and Crowe, T. A. (1987). "A Comparative Study of Speech Disfluencies in Nonstuttering Black and White College Athletes." *Journal of Fluency Disorders* 12:147–156.

Robinson, T. L., and Davis, J. G. (1992). "Speech Fluency Skills in African American Preschoolers during Narrative Discourse." Paper presented at the annual convention of the American Speech-Language-Hearing Association, San Antonio, TX.

Robinson-Zanartu, C. (1996). "Serving Native American Children and Families: Considering Cultural Variables." *Language, Speech and Hearing Services in Schools* 27:373–384.

Rodekohr, R., and Haynes, W. (2001). "Differentiating Dialect from Disorder: A Comparison of Two Processing Tasks and a Standardized Language Test." *Journal of Communication Disorders* 34:255–272.

Rodriguez, B., Hines, R., and Montiel, M. (2009). "Mexican American Mothers of Low and Middle Socioeconomic Status: Communication Behaviors and Interactive Strategies During Shared Book Reading." *Language, Speech and Hearing Services in Schools* 40:271–282.

Rodriguez, B., and Olswang, L. (2003). "Mexican-American and Anglo-American Mothers' Beliefs and Values about Child Rearing, Education, and Language Impairment." *American Journal of Speech-Language Pathology* 12:452–462.

Rogers, B., Arvedson, J., Buck, G., Smart, P., and Msall, M. (1994). "Characteristics of Dysphagia in Children with Cerebral Palsy." *Dysphagia* 9:69–73.

Rogers, S. (1977). "Characteristics of the Cognitive Development of Profoundly Retarded Children." *Child Development* 48:837–843.

Roseberry-McKibbin, C., and O'Hanlon, L. (2005). "Nonbiased Assessment of English Language Learners: A Tutorial." *Communication Disorders Quarterly* 26(3):178–185.

Rosenbek, J., LaPointe, L., and Wertz, T. (1989). *Aphasia: A Clinical Approach.* Boston, MA: College-Hill.

Ross-Swain, D., and Fogle, P. (1996). *Ross Information Processing Assessment-Geriatric.* Austin, TX: Pro-Ed.

Ross-Swain, D., and Kipping, P. (2003). *SAFE: Swallowing Ability and Function Evaluation.* Austin, TX: Pro-Ed.

Roth, F. P., and Worthington, C. K. (2005). *Treatment Resource Manual for Speech-Language Pathology.* Clifton Park, NY: Delmar.

Roy, P., and Chiat, S. (2004). "A Prosodically Controlled Word and Nonword Repetition Task for 2 to 4 Year Olds: Evidence from Typically Developing Children." *Journal of Speech, Language and Hearing Research* 47:223–234.

Rubin, J., Sataloff, R. T., and Korovin, G. (2006). *Diagnosis and Treatment of Voice Disorders,* 3rd ed. San Diego, CA: Plural.

Ruder, K., and Bunce, B. (1981). "Articulation Therapy Using Distinctive Feature Analysis to Structure the Training Program: Two Case Studies." *Journal of Speech and Hearing Disorders* 46:59–65.

Rustad, R. A., DeGroot, T. L., Jungkunz, M. L., Freeberg, K. S., Borowick, L. G., and Wanttie, A. M. (1993). *The Cognitive Assessment of Minnesota.* Tucson, AZ: Therapy Skill Builders.

Rutter, M. (1978). "Diagnosis and Definition of Childhood Autism." *Journal of Autism and Childhood Schizophrenia* 8:139–169.

Rvachew, S. (2007). "Phonological Processing and Reading in Children with Speech Sound Disorders." *American Journal of Speech-Language Pathology* 16:260–270.

Rvachew, S., & Bernhardt, B. (2010). "Clinical Implications of Dynamic Systems Theory for Phonological Development." *American Journal of Speech-Language Pathology* 19:34–50.

Rvachew, S., Chiang, P., & Evans, N. (2007). "Characteristics of Speech Errors Produced by Children with and without Delayed Phonological Awareness Skills." *Language, Speech and Hearing Services in Schools* 38:60–71.

Ryan, B. (1974). *Programmed Therapy for Stuttering in Children and Adults.* Springfield, IL: Charles C Thomas.

Sabers, D. (1996). "By Their Tests We Will Know Them." *Language, Speech and Hearing Services in Schools* 27:102–121.

Sachs, J., and Devin, J. (1976). "Young Children's Use of Age Appropriate Speech Styles in Social Interaction and Role Playing." *Journal of Child Language* 3:81–98.

Sackett, D., Straus, S., Richardson, W., Rosenberg, W., and Haynes, R. (2000). *Evidence-Based Medicine: How to Practice and Teach EBM*, 2nd ed. Edinburgh, UK: Churchill Livingstone.

Salmon, S. J. (1999). *Alaryngeal Speech Rehabilitation,* 2nd ed. Austin, TX: Pro-Ed.

Salmon, S. J., and Goldstein, L. P. (1978). *The Artificial Larynx Handbook.* New York: Grune and Stratton.

Salvia, J., and Ysseldyke, J. (1981). *Assessment in Special and Remedial Education.* Boston, MA: Houghton-Mifflin.

Salvia, J., and Ysseldyke, J. (1995). *Assessment,* 7th ed. Boston, MA: Houghton-Mifflin.

Salvia, J., and Ysseldyke, J. (2004). *Assessment: In Special and Inclusive Education,* 9th ed. Boston: Houghton Mifflin.

Sander, E. (1972). "When Are Speech Sounds Learned?" *Journal of Speech and Hearing Disorders* 44:363–372.

Sansing, J. (1997). *Voice Restoration for the Laryngectomized.* Mentor, OH: Luminaud.

Sarno, M. T. (1969). *Functional Communication Profile.* New York: Institute of Rehabilitation Medicine.

Satcher, D. (1986). "Research Needs for Minority Populations." In *Concerns for Minority Groups in Communication Disorders,* eds. F. H. Bess, B. S. Clark, and H. R. Mitchell (Rockville, MD: ASHA Reports 16).

Saville-Troike, M. (1986). "Anthropological Considerations in the Study of Communication." In *Communication Disorders in Culturally Diverse Populations,* ed. O. Taylor (San Diego, CA: College Hill Press).

Schieffelin, B. (1985). "The Acquisition of Kaluli." In *The Cross-Linguistic Study of Linguistic Acquisition,* Vol. 1., ed. D. Slobin (Hillsdale, NJ: Lawrence Erlbaum Associates).

Schindler, J. S., and Kelly, J. H. (2002). "Swallowing Disorders in the Elderly." *The Laryngoscope* 112:589–602.

Schissel, R., and James, L. (1979). "A Comparison of Children's Performance on Two Tests of Articulation." *Journal of Speech and Hearing Disorders* 44:363–372.

Schlesinger, I. (1974). "Relational Concepts Underlying Language." In *Language Perspectives—Acquisition, Retardation and Intervention,* eds. R. Schiefelbusch and L. Lloyd (Baltimore: University Park Press).

Schlosser, R., & Wendt, O. (2008). "Effects of Augmentative and Alternative Communication Intervention on Speech Production in Children with Autism: A Systematic Review." *American Journal of Speech-Language Pathology* 17:212–230.

Schmauch, V., Panagos, J., and Klich, P. (1978). "Syntax Influences the Accuracy of Consonant Production in Language-Disordered Children." *Journal of Communication Disorders* 11:315–323.

Schmitt, L., Howard, B., and Schmitt, J. (1983). "Conversation Speech Sampling in the Assessment of Articulatory Proficiency." *Language, Speech and Hearing Services in Schools* 14:210–214.

Schraeder, T., Quinn, M., Stockman, I., and Miller, J. (1999). "Authentic Assessment as an Approach to Preschool Speech-Language Screening." *American Journal of Speech-Language Pathology* 8:195–200.

Schuele, C., and Boudreau, D. (2008). "Phonological Awareness Intervention: Beyond the Basics." *Language, Speech and Hearing Services in Schools* 39:3–20.

Schuell, H. (1973). *The Minnesota Test for Differential Diagnosis of Aphasia.* Minneapolis: University of Minnesota Press.

Schuster, M., Lohscheller, J., Hoope, U., Kummer, P., Eyshhobt, U., and Rosanowski, F. (2004). "Voice Handicap of Laryngectomees with Tracheosophageal Speech." *Folia Phoniatrica* 56(1):62–67.

Schwartz, A., and Goldman, R. (1974). "Variables Influencing Performance on Speech Sound Discrimination Tests." *Journal of Speech and Hearing Research* 17:25–32.

Schwartz, R. (1983). "Diagnosis of Speech Sound Disorders in Children." In *Diagnosis in Speech-Language Pathology,* eds. B. Weinberg and I. Meitus (Baltimore, MD: University Park Press).

Schwartz, R. (1992). "Clinical Applications of Recent Advances in Phonological Theory." *Language, Speech and Hearing Services in Schools* 23:269–276.

Scott, C. (1988). "Spoken and Written Syntax." In *Later Language Development: Ages Nine through Nineteen,* ed. M. Nippold (Austin, TX: Pro-Ed).

Scott, C., and Stokes, S. (1995). "Measures of Syntax in School-Age Children and Adolescents." *Language, Speech and Hearing Services in Schools* 26:309–319.

Scott, K., Roberts, J., and Krakow, R. (2008). "Oral and Written Language Development of Children Adopted from China." *American Journal of Speech-Language Pathology* 17:150–160.

Secord, W., and Donohue, J. (2002). *Clinical Assessment of Articulation and Phonology.* Greenville, SC: Super Duper Publications.

Secord, W., and Shine, R. (1997). *Secord Contextual Articulation Tests (S-CAT).* Sedona, AZ: Red Rock Educational Publications.

Seymour, H. (1992). "The Invisible Children: A Reply to Lahey's Perspective." *Journal of Speech and Hearing Research* 15:640–641.

Seymour, H., Bland-Stewart, L., and Green, L. (1998). "Differences Versus Deficit in Child African-American English." *Language, Speech and Hearing Services in Schools* 29:96–108.

Seymour, H., Green, L., and Huntley, R. (1991). "Phonological Patterns in the Conversational Speech of African American Children." Paper presented at the national convention of the American Speech-Language-Hearing Association, Atlanta, GA.

Seymour, H., Roeper, T., DeVilliers, J., and DeVilliers, P. (2005). "Treating Child Language Disorders: Lessons from African-American English." Paper presented at the convention of the American Speech-Language-Hearing Association, Atlanta, GA.

Seymour, H., and Seymour, C. (1981). "Black English and Standard American English Contrasts in Consonantal Development for Four- and Five-Year-Old Children." *Journal of Speech and Hearing Disorders* 46:276–280.

Shadden, B. (1988). *Communication Behavior and Aging: A Sourcebook for Clinicians.* Baltimore, MD: Williams and Wilkins.

Sharf, D. (1972). "Some Relationships between Measures of Early Language Development." *Journal of Speech and Hearing Disorders* 37:64–74.

Sheehy, G. (1996). *New Passages: Mapping Your Life across Time.* New York: Random House.

Shelton, R., Johnson, A., Ruscello, D., and Arndt, W. (1978). "Assessment of Parent-Administered Listening Training for Preschool Children with Articulation Deficits." *Journal of Speech and Hearing Disorders* 43:242–254.

Shelton, R., and McReynolds, L. (1979). "Functional Articulation Disorders: Preliminaries to Treatment." In *Speech and Language: Advances in Basic Research and Practice* (Vol. II), ed. N. Lass (New York: Academic Press).

Shigemori, Y. (1977). "Some Tests Related to the Air Usage during Phonation: Clinical Investigations." *Otologia* 23:138–166.

Shin, L. M., and Bellenir, K. (1998). *Health Reference Series,* Vol. 37. Detroit, MI: Omnigraphics, Inc.

Shine, R. (1980). "Direct Management of the Beginning Stutterer." *Seminars in Speech, Language and Hearing* 1(4):339–350.

Shine, R. E. (1988). *Systematic Fluency Training for Children*. Austin, TX: Pro-Ed.

Shipley, K. G. (1990). *Systematic Assessment of Voice (SAV)*. Oceanside, CA: Academic Communication Associates.

Shipley, K. G., and McAfee, J. G. (2009). *Assessment in Speech-Language Pathology: A Resource Manual*. Clifton Park, NY: Delmar.

Shorr, D. (1983). "Grammatical Comprehension Assessment: The Picture Avoidance Strategy." *Journal of Speech and Hearing Disorders* 48:89–92.

Shriberg, L. (1986). *Programs to Examine Phonetic and Phonologic Evaluation Records (PEPPER)*. University of Wisconsin, 1025 West Johnson St., Madison, WI 53706.

Shriberg, L. (1993). "Four New Speech and Prosody Voice Measures for Genetics Research and Other Studies in Developmental Phonological Disorders." *Journal of Speech and Hearing Research* 36:105–140.

Shriberg, L., and Kwiatkowski, J. (1977). "Phonological Programming for Unintelligible Children in Early-Childhood Projects." Paper presented to the convention of the American Speech and Hearing Association, Chicago, IL.

Shriberg, L., and Kwiatkowski, J. (1980). *Natural Process Analysis*. New York: John Wiley.

Shriberg, L., and Kwiatkowski, J. (1982a). "Phonological Disorders, I: A Diagnostic Classification System." *Journal of Speech and Hearing Disorders* 47:226–241.

Shriberg, L., and Kwiatkowski, J. (1982b). "Phonological Disorders, III: A Procedure for Assessing Severity of Involvement." *Journal of Speech and Hearing Disorders* 47:256–270.

Shriberg, L., and Kwiatkowski, J. (1988). "A Follow-Up Study of Children with Phonologic Disorders of Unknown Origin." *Journal of Speech and Hearing Disorders* 53:144–155.

Shriberg, L., and Kwiatkowski, J. (1994a). "Developmental Phonological Disorders, I: A Clinical Profile." *Journal of Speech and Hearing Research* 17:1100–1126.

Shriberg, L., Kwiatkowski, J., and Gruber, F. (1994b). "Developmental Phonological Disorders, II: Short-Term Speech Sound Normalization." *Journal of Speech and Hearing Research* 37:1127–1150.

Shriberg, L., Gruber, F., and Kwiatkowski, J. (1994c). "Developmental Phonological Disorders, III: Long-Term Speech Sound Normalization." *Journal of Speech and Hearing Research* 37:1151–1177.

Shriberg, L., Lohmeier, H., Campbell, T., Dollaghan, C., Green, J., & Moore, C. (2009). "A Nonword Repetition Task for Speakers with Misarticulations: The Syllable Repetition Task (SRT)." *Journal of Speech, Language and Hearing Research* 52:1189–1212.

Shulman, B. (1986). *Test of Pragmatic Skills, Revised*. Tucson, AZ: Communication Skill Builders.

Shumak, I. (1955). "A Speech Situation Rating Sheet for Stutterers." In *Stuttering in Children and Adults*, ed. W. Johnson (Mineapolis: University of Minnesota Press).

Shumway, S., and Wetherby, A. (2009). "Communicative Acts of Children with Autism Spectrum Disorders in the Second Year of Life." *Journal of Speech, Language and Hearing Research* 52:1139–1156.

Siegel, G. (1975). "The Use of Language Tests." *Language, Speech and Hearing Services in Schools* 6:211–217.

Sigelman, C. (1982). "Evaluating Alternative Techniques of Questioning Mentally Retarded Persons." *American Journal of Mental Deficiency* 86:511–518.

Silverman, F. (1984). *Speech Language Pathology and Audiology*. Columbus, OH: Merrill.

Silverman, F. (1995). *Communication for the Speechless*. Needham Heights, MA: Allyn & Bacon.

Silverman, S., and Ratner, N. B. (2002). "Measuring Lexical Diversity in Children Who Stutter: Application of *VOCD*." *Journal of Fluency Disorders* 27:289–304.

Simmons, J. (1988). "Fluharty Preschool and Language Screening Test: Analysis of Construct Validity." *Journal of Speech and Hearing Disorders* 53:168–174.

Simms-Hill, S., and Haynes, W. (1992). "Language Performance in Low-Achieving Elementary School Students." *Language, Speech and Hearing Services in Schools* 23:169–175.

Simon, C. (1987). "Out of the Broom Closet and into the Classroom: The Emerging SLP." *Journal of Childhood Communication Disorders* 11:41–66.

Simon, C. (1989). *Classroom Communication Screening Procedure for Early Adolescents (CCSPEA)*. Tempe, AZ: Communi-Cog Publications.

Singer, B., and Bashir, A. (1999). "What Are Executive Functions and Self-Regulation and What Do They Have to Do with Language-Learning Disorders?" *Language, Speech and Hearing Services in Schools* 30:265–273.

Singer, M., and Blom, E. (1980). "An Endoscopic Technique for Restoration of Voice after Laryngectomy." Paper presented at the annual meeting of the American Laryngologic Association, Palm Beach, FL.

Singh, S. (1976). *Distinctive Features: Theory and Validation*. Baltimore, MD: University Park Press.

Skahan, S., Watson, M., and Lof, G. (2007). "Speech-Language Pathologists' Assessment Practices for Children with Suspected Speech Sound Disorders: Results of a National Survey." *American Journal of Speech-Language Pathology* 16:246–259.

Skarakis-Doyle, E., Campbell, W., and Dempsey, L. (2009). "Identification of Children with Language Impairment: Investigating the Classification Accuracy of the MacArthur-Bates Communicative Development Inventories, Level III." *American Journal of Speech-Language Pathology* 18:277–288.

Skarakis-Doyle, E., and Dempsey, L. (2008). "The Detection and Monitoring of Comprehension Errors by Preschool Children with and without Language Impairment." *Journal of Speech, Language and Hearing Research* 51:1227–1243.

Skarakis-Doyle, E., Dempsey, L., and Lee, C. (2008). "Identifying Language Comprehension Impairment in Preschool Children." *Language, Speech and Hearing Services in Schools* 39:54–65.

Sklar, M. (1983). *Sklar Aphasia Scale*. Los Angeles: Western Psychological Services.

Smit, A. (1986). "Ages of Speech Sound Acquisition: Comparisons and Critiques of Several Normative Studies." *Language, Speech and Hearing Services in Schools* 17:175–186.

Smit, A. (1993a). "Phonologic Error Distributions in the Iowa Nebraska Articulation Norms Project: Consonant Singletons." *Journal of Speech and Hearing Research* 36:533–547.

Smit, A. (1993b). "Phonologic Error Distributions in the Iowa Nebraska Articulation Norms Project: Word

Initial Consonant Clusters." *Journal of Speech and Hearing Research* 36:931–947.

Smit, A., Hand, L., Frellinger, J., Bernthal, J., and Bird, A. (1990). "The Iowa Articulation Norms Project and Its Nebraska Replication." *Journal of Speech and Hearing Disorders* 55:779–798.

Smith, N. (1973). *The Acquisition of Phonology*. Cambridge, UK: Cambridge University Press.

Smith, V., Mirenda, P., and Zaidman-Zait, A. (2007). "Predictors of Expressive Vocabulary Growth in Children with Autism." *Journal of Speech, Language and Hearing Research* 50:149–160.

Snow, C. (1977). "The Development of Conversation between Mothers and Babies." *Journal of Child Language* 4:1–22.

Snyder, L. (1978). "Communicative and Cognitive Disabilities in the Sensorimotor Period." *Merrill Palmer Quarterly* 24:161–180.

Snyder, L. (1981). "Assessing Communicative Abilities in the Sensorimotor Period: Content and Context." *Topics in Language Disorders* 1:31–46.

Snyder-McLean, L., McLean, J., and Etter, R. (1988). "Clinical Assessment of Sensorimotor Knowledge in Nonverbal, Severely Retarded Clients." *Topics in Language Disorders* 8:1–22.

Sonies, B. C., Weiffenbach, J., Atkinson, J. C., Brahim, J., Macynski, A., and Fox, P. C. (1987). "Clinical Examination of Motor and Sensory Functions of the Adult Oral Cavity." *Dysphagia* 1:4.

Sparks, S. (1989). "Assessment and Intervention with At-Risk Infants and Toddlers: Guidelines for the Speech-Language Pathologist." *Topics in Language Disorders* 10(1):43–56.

Sparrow, S., Balla, D., and Cicchetti, D. (1984). *Vineland Adaptive Behavior Scales*. Circle Pines, MN: American Guidance Service.

Spaulding, T., Plante, E., and Farinella, K. (2006). "Eligibility Criteria for Language Impairment: Is the Low End of Normal Always Appropriate?" *Language, Speech and Hearing Services in Schools* 37:61–72.

Speyer, R., Bogaardt, H., Passos, V. L., Boodenburg, N., Zumach, A., Heijnen, M., Baijens, L., Fleskens, S., and Brunings, J. (2010). "Maximum Phonation Time: Variability and Reliability." *Journal of Voice* 24(3):281–284.

Square, P., and Weidner, W. E. (1981). *Differential Diagnosis of Developmental Apraxia.* Paper presented to the convention of the Speech and Hearing Association of Alabama, Birmingham, AL.

St. Louis, K., and Ruscello, D. (2000). *The Oral Speech Mechanism Examination,* 3rd ed. Austin, TX: Pro-Ed.

Staab, C. (1983). "Language Functions Elicited by Meaningful Activities: A New Dimension in Language Programs." *Language, Speech and Hearing Services in Schools* 14:164–170.

Stampe, D. (1969). "A Dissertation on Natural Phonology." Unpublished dissertation, University of Chicago.

Stark, R., Bernstein, L., and Demorest, M. (1993). "Vocal Communication in the First 18 Months of Life." *Journal of Speech and Hearing Research* 36:548–558.

Starkweather, C. W., and Givens-Ackerman, J. (1997). *Stuttering.* Austin, TX: Pro-Ed.

Starkweather, C. W., Gottwald, S. R., and Halfond, M. M. (1990). *Stuttering Prevention: A Clinical Method.* Englewood Cliffs, NJ: Prentice Hall.

Steckol, K., and Leonard, L. (1981). "Sensorimotor Development and the Use of Prelinguistic Performatives." *Journal of Speech and Hearing Research* 24:262–268.

Stemple, J. (1996). *Clinical Voice Pathology: Theory and Management.* Columbus, OH: Charles E. Merrill.

Stemple, J. C., and Glaze, L. E. (2009). *Clinical Voice Pathology: Theory and Management*, 4th ed. San Diego, CA: Plural.

Stiegler, L. (2007). "Discovering Communicative Competencies in a Nonspeaking Child with Autism." *Language, Speech and Hearing Services in Schools* 38:400–413.

Stockman, I. (1993). "Variable Word Initial and Medial Consonant Relationships in Children's Speech Sound Articulation." *Perceptual and Motor Skills* 76:675–689.

Stockman, I. (1996). "The Promises and Pitfalls of Language Sample Analysis as an Assessment Tool for Linguistic Minority Children." *Language, Speech and Hearing Services in Schools* 27:355–366.

Stockman, I. (2008). "Toward Validation of a Minimal Competence Phonetic Core for African American Children." *Journal of Speech, Language and Hearing Research* 51:1244–1262.

Stockman, I. (2010). "A Review of Developmental and Applied Language Research on African American Children: From a Deficit to Difference Perspective on Dialect Differences." *Language, Speech and Hearing Services in Schools* 41:23–38.

Stockman, I., Karasinski, L., and Guillory, B. (2008). "The Use of Conversational Repairs by African American Preschoolers." *Language, Speech and Hearing Services in Schools* 39:461–474.

Stockman, I., and Stephenson, L. (1981). "Children's Articulation of Medial Consonant Clusters: Implications for Syllabification." *Language and Speech* 24:185–204.

Stoel-Gammon, C. (1987). "Phonological Skills in 2-Year-Olds." *Language, Speech and Hearing Services in Schools* 18:323–329.

Stoel-Gammon, C. (1996). "Phonological Assessment Using a Hierarchial Framework." In *Assessment of Communication and Language,* vol. 6, eds. K. Cole, P. Dale, and D. Thal (Baltimore, MD: Paul H. Brookes).

Stoel-Gammon, C., and Dunn, C. (1985). *Normal and Disordered Phonology in Children.* Baltimore, MD: University Park Press.

Stokes, S., and Klee, T. (2009). "The Diagnostic Accuracy of a New Test of Early Nonword Repetition for Differentiating Late Talking and Typically Developing Children." *Journal of Speech, Language and Hearing Research* 52:872–882.

Stover, S., and Haynes, W. (1989). "Topic Manipulation and Cohesive Adequacy in Conversations of Normal Adults between the Ages of 30 and 90." *Clinical Linguistics and Phonetics* 3:137–149.

Straight, H. (1980). "Auditory versus Articulatory Phonological Processes and Their Development in Children." In *Child Phonology: Perception,* vol. 2, eds. G. Yeni-Komshian, C. Kavanagh, and C. Ferguson (New York: Academic Press).

Strandberg, T., and Griffith, J. (1969). "A Study of the Effects of Training in Visual Literacy on Verbal Language Behavior." *Journal of Communication Disorders* 2:252–263.

Strominger, A., and Bashir, A. (1977). "A Nine-Year Follow-Up of Language-Delayed Children." Paper presented at the convention of the American Speech-Language-Hearing Association, Chicago, IL.

Sturner, R., Heller, J., Funk, S., and Layton, T. (1993). "The Fluharty Preschool Speech and Language Screening Test: A Population-Based Validation Study Using Sample-Independent Decision Rules." *Journal of Speech and Hearing Research* 36:738–745.

Swanson, L., Fey, M., Mills, C., and Hood, L. (2005). "Use of Narrative-Based Language Intervention with Children Who Have Specific Language Impairment." *American Journal of Speech-Language Pathology* 14:131–143.

Swigert, N. (2006). "Clinical Documentation, Coding, and Billing." In B. Cornett, ed., "Professional Practice in Context: The Regulatory Environment." *Seminars in Speech and Language* 27(2):101–118.

Swigert, N. (2009). "Hot Topics in Dysphagia." *The ASHA Leader*, May 26:10–13.

Syder, D., Body, E., Parker, M., and Boddy, M. (1993). *Sheffield Screening Test for Acquired Language Disorders*. Windsor: NFER-Nelson.

Tager-Flusberg, H., Rogers, S., Cooper, J., Landa, R., Lord, C., Paul, R., Rice, M., Stoel-Gammon, C., Wetherby, A., and Yoder, P. (2009). "Defining Spoken Language Benchmarks and Selecting Measures of Expressive Language Development for Young Children with Autism Spectrum Disorders." *Journal of Speech, Language and Hearing Research* 52:643–652.

Tanner, D., and Cuthbert, V. (1999). *Quick Assessment for Aphasia*. Oceanside, CA: Academic Communication Association.

Tanner, D. D. (2001). "The Brave New World of the Cyber Speech and Hearing Clinic." *The ASHA Leader* 6:6–7.

Taylor, O. (1986a). *Nature of Communication Disorders in Culturally and Linguistically Diverse Populations*. San Diego, CA: College-Hill.

Taylor, O. (1986b). *Treatment of Communication Disorders in Culturally and Linguistically Diverse Populations*. San Diego, CA: College-Hill.

Taylor, O., and Payne, K. (1983). "Culturally Valid Testing: A Proactive Approach." *Topics in Language Disorders* 3:8–20.

Templin, M. (1957). *Certain Language Skills in Children: Their Development and Interrelationships*. Institute of Child Welfare, Monograph 26, Minneapolis: University of Minnesota Press.

Templin, M., and Darley, F. (1969). *The Templin-Darley Tests of Articulation*. Iowa City: University of Iowa, Bureau of Educational Research and Service.

Teoh, A. P., and Chin, S. B. (2009). "Transcribing the Speech of Children with Cochlear Implants: Clinical Application of Narrow Phonetic Transcriptions." *American Journal of Speech-Language Pathology* 18:388–401.

Terkel, S. (1980). *American Dreams: Lost and Found*. New York: Pantheon.

Terkel, S. (1986). *Hard Times: An Oral History of the Great Depression*. New York: Random House.

Terkel, S. (1993). *Race: How Blacks and Whites Think and Feel About the American Obsession*. Anchor Press.

Terkel, S. (2001). *Will the Circle Be Unbroken? Reflections on Death, Rebirth and Hunger for a Faith*. New Press.

Thal, D., DesJardin, J., and Eisenberg, L. (2007). "Validity of the MacArthur-Bates Communicative Development Inventories for Measuring Language Abilities in Children with Cochlear Implants." *American Journal of Speech-Language Pathology* 16:54–64.

Thal, D., Jackson-Maldonado, D., and Acosta, D. (2000). "Validity of a Parent-Report Measure of Vocabulary and Grammar for Spanish-Speaking Toddlers." *Journal of Speech, Language and Hearing Research* 43:1087–1100.

Thal, D., and Tobias, S. (1992). "Communicative Gestures in Children with Delayed Onset of Oral Expressive Vocabulary." *Journal of Speech and Hearing Research* 35:1281–1289.

Thomas, J., and Keith, R. *Looking Forward . . . The Speech and Swallowing Guidebook for People with Cancer of the Larynx or Tongue*, 4th ed. New York: Thieme.

Thomas-Tate, S., Washington, J., and Edwards, J. (2004). "Standardized Assessment of Phonological Awareness Skills in Low-Income African American First Graders." *American Journal of Speech-Language Pathology* 13:182–190.

Thompkins, C. A. (1995). *Right Hemisphere Communication Disorders: Theory and Management*. San Diego, CA: Singular Publishing.

Thompkins, C., and Lehman, M. (1998). "Outcomes Measurement in Cognitive Communication Disorders: Right Hemisphere Brain Damage." In *Measuring Outcomes in Speech-Language Pathology*, ed. C. Frattali (New York: Thieme).

Thompson, C., Craig, H., and Washington, J. (2004). "Variable Production of African American English across Oracy and Literacy Contexts." *Language, Speech and Hearing Services in Schools* 35:269–282.

Titze, I. (1994). *Principles of Voice Production.* Englewood Cliffs, NJ: Prentice Hall.

Toffler, A. (1981). *The Third Wave.* New York: Bantam Books.

Torgesen, J., and Bryant, B. (1994). *Test of Phonological Awareness.* Austin, TX. Pro-Ed.

Tough, J. (1977). *The Development of Meaning.* New York: Halsted Press.

Trost-Cardamone, J. E., and Bernthal, J. E. (1993). "Articulation Assessment Procedures and Treatment Decisions." In *Cleft Palate: Interdisciplinary Issues and Treatments,* eds. K. T. Moller and C. D. Starr (Austin, TX: Pro-Ed).

Tyack, D., and Gottsleben, R. (1974). *Language Sampling, Analysis and Training: A Handbook for Teachers and Clinicians.* Palo Alto, CA: Consulting Psychologists Press.

Uccelli, P., and Paez, M. (2007). "Narrative and Vocabulary Development of Bilingual Children from Kindergarten to First Grade: Developmental Changes and Associations among English and Spanish Skills." *Language, Speech and Hearing Services in Schools* 38:225–236.

Ukrainetz, T. (2006). "The Implications of RTI and EBP for SLPs: Commentary on L. M. Justice." *Language, Speech and Hearing Services in Schools* 37:298–303.

Ukrainetz, T., & Gillam, R. (2009). "The Expressive Elaboration of Imaginative Narratives by Children with Specific Language Impairment." *Journal of Speech, Language and Hearing Research* 52:883–898.

Ukrainetz, T., Harpell, S., Walsh, C., and Coyle, C. (2000). "A Preliminary Investigation of Dynamic Assessment with Native American Kindergartners." *Language, Speech and Hearing Services in Schools* 31:142–154.

Ulatowska, H., Wertz, R., Chapman, S., Keebler, M., Olness, G. S., Parsons, S., Miller, T., and Auther, L. (2001). "Interpretation of Fables and Proverbs by African Americans with and Without Aphasia." *American Journal of Speech-Language Pathology* 10:40–50.

Uzigiris, I., and Hunt, J. (1975). *Assessment in Infancy.* Urbana: University of Illinois Press.

Van Borsel, J., Maes, E., and Foulon, S. (2001). "Stuttering and Bilingualism: A Review." *Journal of Fluency Disorders* 26:179–205.

Van Riper, C., and Emerick, L. (1984). *Speech Correction: An Introduction to Speech Pathology and Audiology,* Englewood Cliffs, NJ: Prentice Hall.

Van Riper, C., and Irwin, J. (1958). *Voice and Articulation.* Englewood Cliffs, NJ: Prentice Hall.

Van Rossum, M. A., deKrom, G. Nootebom, S. G., and Queno, H. (2002). "Pitch Accent in Alaryngeal Speech." *Journal of Speech, Language, Hearing Research* 45:1119–1133.

Vanderas, A. P. (1987). "Incidence of Cleft Lip, Cleft Palate, and Cleft Lip and Palate Among Races: A Review." *Cleft Palate Journal* 24:216–225.

Vandiver, A. P. (1987). "Incidence of Cleft Lip, Cleft Palate, and Cleft Lip and Palate Among Races: A Review." *Cleft Palate Journal* 24:216–225.

Vanryckeghem, M., Hylebos, C., Brutten, G., and Peleman, M. (2001). "The Relationship Between Communication Attitude and Emotion of Children Who Stutter." *Journal of Fluency Disorders* 26:1–15.

Van Zaalen-op't Hof, Y., Wijnen, F., and De Jonckere, P. H. (2009). "Differentiating Diagnostic Characteristics between Cluttering and Stuttering—Part One," *Journal of Fluency Disorders* 24(3):137–154.

Vaughn-Cooke, F. (1976). "The Implementation of a Phonological Change: The Case for Resyllabification in Black English." *Dissertation Abstracts International* 38:234A.

Vaughn-Cook, F. (1983). "Improving Language Assessment in Minority Children." *Journal of the American Speech-Language-Hearing Association* 25:29–34.

Vaughn-Cook, F. (1986). "The Challenge of Assessing the Language of Nonmainstream Speakers." In *Treatment of Communication Disorders in Culturally and Linguistically Diverse Populations,* ed. O. Taylor (San Diego, CA: College Hill Press).

Velleman, S., and Vihman, M. (2002). "Whole-Word Phonology and Templates: Trap, Bootstrap, or Some of Each?" *Language, Speech and Hearing Services in Schools* 33:9–23.

Vogel, A., Ibrahim, H., Reilly, S., and Kilpatrick, N. (2009). A comparative study of two acoustic measures of hypernasality. *Journal of Speech, Language, and Hearing Research,* 52: 1640–1651.

Vygotsky, L. (1978). *Mind in Society: The Development of Higher Psychological Processes.* Cambridge, MA: Harvard University Press.

Wade, K., and Haynes, W. (1989). "Dynamic Assessment of Spontaneous Language and Cue Responses in Adult-Directed and Child-Directed Play: A Statistical and

Descriptive Analysis." *Child Language Teaching and Therapy* 5:157–173.

Wagner, R., Togersen, J., and Rashotte, C. (1999). *Comprehensive Test of Phonological Processing.* Austin, TX: Pro-Ed.

Walker, V. G., Hardiman, C. J., Hedrick, D. L., and Holbrook, A. (1981). "Speech and Language Characteristics of an Aging Population." In *Speech and Language: Advances in Basic Research and Practice,* ed. N. Lass (New York: Academic Press).

Wallace, G. (1997). *Multicultural Neurogenics.* Austin, TX: Pro-Ed.

Wallace, G. L. (1993). "Adult Neurogenic Disorders." In *Communication Disorders in Multicultural Populations,* ed. D. E. Battle (Boston, MA: Andover Medical Publishers).

Wallach, G., and Miller, L. (1988). *Language Intervention and Academic Success.* Boston, MA: College-Hill Press.

Ward, E., Crombie, J., Trickey, M., Hill, A., Theodoros, D., and Russell, T. (2009). "Assessment of Communication and Swallowing Post-Laryngectomy: A Telerehabilitation Trial." *Journal of Telemedicine and Telecare* 15:232–237.

Washington, J. (1996). "Issues in Assessing the Language Abilities of African American Children." In *Communication Development and Disorders in African American Children,* eds. A. Kamhi, K. Pollock, and J. Harris (Baltimore, MD: Brookes).

Washington, J., and Craig, H. (1992). "Articulation Test Performances of Low Income, African American Preschoolers with Communication Impairments." *Language, Speech and Hearing Services in Schools* 23:203–207.

Washington, J., and Craig, H. (2004). "A Language Screening Protocol for Use with Young African American Children in Urban Settings." *American Journal of Speech-Language Pathology* 13:329–340.

Watson, B. U., and Thompson, R. W. (1983). "Parent's Perception of Diagnostic Reports and Conferences." *Language Speech and Hearing Services in Schools* 14:114–120.

Watson, L. (1977). "Conversational Participation by Language-Deficient and Normal Children." Paper presented to the Convention of the American Speech and Hearing Association, Chicago, IL.

Watson-Gegeo, K., and Gegeo, D. (1986). "Calling Out and Repeating Routines in Kwara'ae Children's Language Socialization." In *Language and Socialization Across Cultures,* eds. B. Schieffelin and E. Ochs (Cambridge, UK: Cambridge University Press).

Webb, J., and Duckett, B. (1990). *The Rules Phonological Analysis.* Vero Beach, FL: The Speech Bin.

Weiner, F. (1979). *Phonological Process Analysis.* Baltimore, MD: University Park Press.

Weiner, F., and Ostrowski, A. (1979). "Effects of Listener Uncertainty on Articulatory Inconsistency." *Journal of Speech and Hearing Disorders* 44:487–493.

Weismer, S., Branch, J., and Miller, J. (1994). "A Prospective Longitudinal Study of Language Development in Late Talkers." *Journal of Speech and Hearing Research* 37:852–867.

Weismer, S., Tomblin, J., Zhang, X., Buckwalter, P., Chynoweth, J., and Jones, M. (2000). "Nonword Repetition Performance in School-Age Children with and Without Language Impairment." *Journal of Speech, Language and Hearing Research* 43:865–878.

Weiss, A. (2004). "Why We Should Consider Pragmatics When Planning Treatment for Children Who Stutter." *Language, Speech and Hearing Services in Schools* 35:34–45.

Weiss, A., Leonard, L., Rowan, L., and Chapman, K. (1983). "Linguistic and Nonlinguistic Features of Style in Normal and Language-Impaired Children." *Journal of Speech and Hearing Disorders* 48:154–163.

Weisz, J., and Zigler, E. (1979). "Cognitive Development in Retarded and Nonretarded Persons: Piagetian Tests of the Similar Sequence Hypothesis." *Psychological Bulletin* 86:831–851.

Wellman, B., Case, M., Mengert, E., and Bradbury, D. (1931). *Speech Sounds of Young Children.* Iowa City: University of Iowa Studies in Child Welfare, no. 5.

Wertz, R. T., LaPointe, L. L., and Rosenbek, J. C. (1984). *Apraxia of Speech in Adults: The Disorder and Its Management.* New York: Grune & Stratton.

West, J., Sands, E., and Ross-Swain, D. (1998). *Bedside Evaluation Screening Test—Second Edition (BEST-2).* Austin, TX: Pro-Ed.

Westby, C. (1980). "Assessment of Cognitive and Language Abilities through Play." *Language, Speech and Hearing Services in Schools* 11:154–168.

Weston, A., and Shriberg, L. (1992). "Contextual and Linguistic Correlates of Intelligibility in Children with Developmental Phonological Disorders." *Journal of Speech and Hearing Research* 35:1316–1332.

Wetherby, A., Cain, D., Yonclas, D., and Walker, V. (1988). "Analysis of Intentional Communication of Normal Children from the Prelinguistic to the Multiword Stage." *Journal of Speech and Hearing Research* 31:240–252.

Wetherby, A., and Prizant, B. (1992). "Profiling Young Children's Communicative Competence. In *Causes and Effects in Communication and Language Intervention,* eds. S. Warren and J. Reichle (Baltimore, MD: Brookes).

Wetherby, A., and Prizant, B. (1998). *CSBS Developmental Profile.* Chicago: Applied Symbolix.

Wetherby, A., and Prizant, B. (2002). *Communication and Symbolic Behavior Scales.* Baltimore, MD: Brookes.

Wetherby, A., and Prutting, C. (1984). "Profiles of Communicative and Cognitive-Social Abilities in Autistic Children." *Journal of Speech and Hearing Research* 27:364–377.

Wetherby, A., and Rodriguez, G. (1992). "Measurement of Communicative Intentions in Normally Developing Children During Structured and Unstructured Contexts." *Journal of Speech and Hearing Research* 35:130–138.

Wetherby, A., Yonclas, D., and Bryan, A. (1989). "Communicative Profiles of Preschool Children with Handicaps: Implications for Early Intervention." *Journal of Speech and Hearing Disorders* 54:148–158.

White, S. (2004). "HCPCS Level II Codes." *The ASHA Leader* 9(11):3, 17.

White, S. (2009). "New ICM-9 Codes Take Effect Oct. 1." *The ASHA Leader* 14(12):3–6.

Whitehill, T. L. (2002). "Assessing Intelligibility in Speakers with Cleft Palate: A Critical Review of the Literature." *The Cleft Palate-Craniofacial Journal* 39:50–62.

Whurr, R. (1996). *Whurr Aphasia Screening Test.* London: M. Phil.

Wilcox, M. (1984). "Developmental Language Disorders: Preschoolers." In *Language Disorders in Children: Recent Advances,* ed. A. Holland (San Diego, CA: College-Hill).

Williams, G., and McReynolds, L. (1975). "The Relationship between Discrimination and Articulation Training in Children with Misarticulations." *Journal of Speech and Hearing Research* 18:401–412.

Williams, R., and Wolfram, W. (1977). *Social Differences vs. Disorders.* Washington, DC: American Speech and Hearing Association.

Wilson, D. K. (1987). *Voice Problems in Children,* 3rd ed. Baltimore, MD: Williams and Wilkins.

Wilson, F., and Rice, M. (1977). *A Programmed Approach to Voice Therapy.* Austin, TX: Learning Concepts.

Wilson, K., Blackmon, R., Hall, R., and Elcholtz, G. (1991). "Methods of Language Assessment: A Survey of California Public School Clinicians." *Language, Speech and Hearing Services in Schools* 22:236–241.

Winitz, H. (1969). "Articulatory Acquisition and Behavior." Englewood Cliffs, NJ: Prentice Hall.

Winitz, H. (1975). *From Syllable to Conversation.* Baltimore, MD: University Park Press.

Wisconsin Division of Health (1966). *Communication Status Chart.* Madison: Division of Health.

Wise, J., Sevcik, R., Morris, R., Lovett, M., and Wolf, M. (2007). "The Relationship Among Receptive and Expressive Vocabulary, Listening Comprehension, Pre-Reading Skills, Word Identification Skills and Reading Comprehension by Children with Reading Disabilities." *Journal of Speech, Language and Hearing Research* 50:1093–1109.

Wolfram, W. (1989). "Structural Variability in Phonological Development: Final Nasals in Vernacular Black English." In *Current Issues in Linguistic Theory: Language Change and Variation,* eds. R. Fasold and D. Schiffren (Amsterdam: John Benjamins).

Wolfram, W. (1991). *Dialects and American English.* Englewood Cliffs, NJ: Prentice Hall.

Wolfram, W. (1994). "The Phonology of a Sociocultural Variety: The Case of African American Vernacular English." In *Child Phonology: Characteristics, Assessment and Intervention with Special Populations,* eds. J. Bernthal and N. Bankson (New York: Thieme).

Wolfus, B., Moscovitch, M., and Kinsbourne, M. (1980). "Subgroups of Developmental Language Impairment." *Brain and Language* 10:152–171.

Woods, J., and Wetherby, A. (2003). "Early Identification of and Intervention for Infants and Toddlers Who Are at Risk for Autism Spectrum Disorder." *Language, Speech and Hearing Services in Schools* 34:180–193.

Woolf, G. (1967). "The Assessment of Stuttering as Struggle, Avoidance, and Expectancy." *British Journal of Disorders of Communication* 2:158–171.

World Health Organization (WHO) (2002). "Toward a Common Language for Functioning, Disability and Health (ICF)." Accessed September 25, 2006 from the ICF homepage at http:www3.who.int/icf/

Wright, L., and Ayre, A. (2000). *WASSP: Wright and Ayre Stuttering Self-Rating Profile.* London: Winslow Press.

Wuyts, F. L., DeBodt, M. S., Molenberghs, G., Remacle, M., Heylen, L., Millet, B., Van Lierde, K., Raes, J., and Van de Heyning, P. H. (2000). "The Dysphonia Severity Index: An Objective Measure of Vocal Quality Based on a Multiparameter Approach." *Journal of Speech, Language, Hearing Research* 43(3):796–809.

Wyatt, T. (1996). "Acquisition of the African American English Copula." In *Communication Development and Disorders in African American Children,* eds. A. Kamhi, K. Pollock, and J. Harris (Baltimore, MD: Brookes).

Yairi, E. (1997). "Home Environments of Stuttering Children." In *Nature and Treatment of Stuttering: New Directions,* eds. R. Curlee and G. Siegel (Boston: Allyn & Bacon).

Yairi, E., and Ambrose, N. (2005). *Early Childhood Stuttering.* Austin, TX: Pro-Ed.

Yairi, E., and Ambrose, N. (2005). *Early Childhood Stuttering for Clinicians by Clinicians.* Austin, TX: Pro-Ed.

Yairi, E., Ambrose, N., and Niermann, R. (1993). "The Early Months of Stuttering: A Developmental Study." *Journal of Speech and Hearing Research* 36:521–528.

Yairi, E., Ambrose, N., Paden, E., and Throneburg, R. (1996). "Predictive Factors of Persistence and Recovery: Pathways of Childhood Stuttering." *Journal of Communication Disorders* 29:51–77.

Yairi, E., and Lewis, B. (1984). "Disfluencies at the Onset of Stuttering." *Journal of Speech and Hearing Research* 27:155–159.

Yairi, E., and Seery, C. (2011). *Stuttering Foundations and Clinical Approaches.* Boston, MA: Pearson.

Yaruss, J. S. (1998). "Real-Time Analysis of Speech Fluency Procedures and Reliability Training." *American Journal of Speech Language Pathology* 7:25–37.

Yaruss, J. S. (1999). "Current Status of Academic and Clinical Education in Fluency Disorders at ASHA—Accredited Training Programs." *Journal of Fluency Disorders* 24:169–184.

Yaruss, J. S. (2000). "Converting Between Word and Syllable Counts in Children's Conversational Speech Samples." *Journal of Fluency Disorders* 25:305–316.

Yaruss, S., Coleman, B., and Quesal, R. (2006). Online version of "Assessment of the Child's Experience of Stuttering (ACES)." Accessed October 12, 2006 from http://www.stutteringcenter.org

Yaruss, J. S., and Logan, K. J. (2002). "Evaluating Rate, Accuracy, and Fluency of Young Children's Diadochokinetic Productions: A Preliminary Investigation." *Journal of Fluency Disorders* 27:65–86.

Yaruss, J. S., and Quesal, R. W. (2002). "Academic and Clinical Education in Fluency Disorders: An Update." *Journal of Fluency Disorders* 27:43–63.

Yaruss, J. S., and Quesal, R. (2006). "Overall Assessment of the Speaker's Experience of Stuttering (OASES)." *Journal of Fluency Disorders* 31:90–115.

Yavas, M., and Goldstein, B. (1998). "Phonological Assessment and Treatment of Bilingual Speakers." *American Journal of Speech-Language Pathology* 7:49–60.

Yendle, K. (2010). "Influence of Syllable Train Length and Performance End Effects on Phonation Threshold Pressure in Females." Unpublished master's thesis, Auburn University.

Yiu, E. M. (2002). "Impact and Prevention of Voice Problems in the Teaching Profession: Embracing the Consumer's View." *Journal of Voice* 16:215–228.

Yoder, P., Warren, S., and McCathren, R. (1998). "Determining Spoken Language Prognosis in Children with Developmental Disabilities." *American Journal of Speech-Language Pathology* 7:77–87.

Yont, K., Hewitt, L., and Miccio, A. (2000). "A Coding System for Describing Conversational Breakdowns in Preschool Children." *American Journal of Speech-Language Pathology* 9:300–309.

Yorkston, K. M., Beukelman, D. R., and Bell, K. R. (1988). *Clinical Management of Dysarthric Speakers.* Boston, MA: College-Hill.

Yorkston, K., Beukelman, D., Stand, E., and Hakel, E. (2010). *Management of Motor Speech Disorders in Children and Adults.* Austin, TX: Pro-Ed.

Yorkston, K., Spencer, K. A., and Duffy, J. R. (2003). "Behavioral Management of Respiratory/Phonatory Dysfunction from Dysarthria: A Systematic Review of the Evidence." *Journal of Medical Speech-Language Pathology* 11(2):xiii–xxxviii.

Yoss, K., and Darley, F. L. (1974). "Developmental Apraxia of Speech in Children with Defective Articulation." *Journal of Speech and Hearing Research* 17:399–416.

Young, E., Diehl, J., Morris, D., Hyman, S., and Bennetto, L. (2005). "The Use of Two Language Tests to Identify Pragmatic Language Problems in Children with Autism Spectrum Disorders." *Language, Speech and Hearing Services in Schools* 36:62–72.

Zimmerman, I., Steiner, V., and Pond, R. (1992). *Preschool Language Scale.* Columbus, OH: Merrill.

Zur, K., Cotton, S., Kelchnor, L., Baker, S., Weinrich, B., and Lee, L. (2007). "Pediatric Voice Handicap Index (pVHI): A New Tool for Evaluating Pediatric Dysphonia." *International Journal of Pediatric Otorhinolaryngology* 71(1):77–82.

INDEX